Animal Nutrition & Reproductive Physiology

(Recent Concepts)

Animal Nutrition & Reproductive Physiology

(Recent Concepts)

Edited by

K.T. SAMPATH
JYOTIRMOY GHOSH
RAGHAVENDRA BHATTA

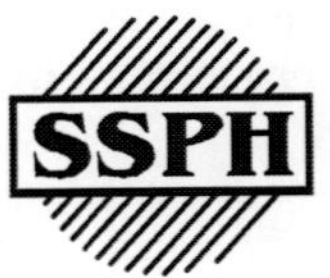

SATISH SERIAL PUBLISHING HOUSE
403, Express Tower, Commercial Complex, Azadpur, Delhi-110033 (India)
Phone : 011-27672852, Fax : 91-11-27672046
E-mail :info@satishserial.com, hkjain1975@yahoo.com
Website : www.satishserial.com

Published by :

SATISH SERIAL PUBLISHING HOUSE

403, Express Tower, Commercial Complex, Azadpur, Delhi-110033 (INDIA)
Phone : 011-27672852 Fax : 91-11-27672046
E-mail : info@satishserial.com, hkjain1975@yahoo.com

Reprint, 2019

ISBN 978-93-81226-23-0

Composed, Designed & Printed in India

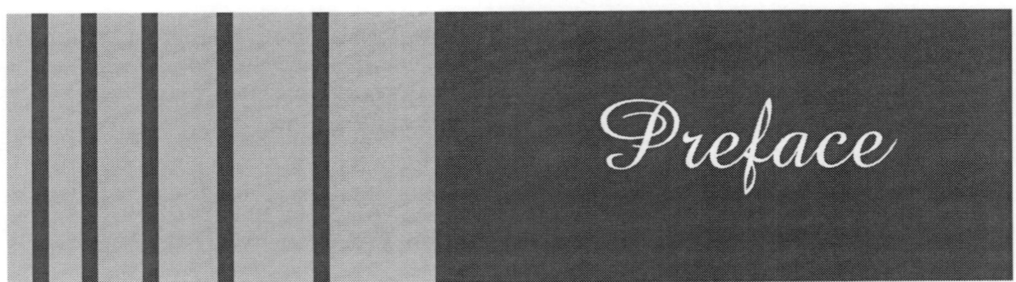

Preface

Animal nutrition and reproductive physiology are two independent but intertwined fields of study which cannot be looked separately. The general perspective of a nutritionist is to keep the livestock in good health during growth, physical work, production and reproduction without affecting other body functions. The goal of reproductive physiologists is to improve the efficiency of reproduction from the genetically superior animals for increasing the production of milk, meat or eggs for human consumptions. Thus, both nutrition and reproduction faces a tremendous pressure to perform in demanding situations and are considered critical for the researchers and policy makers. The idea of writing this book came from that urge and looking into the demand of research community who wants to understand the recent development in these areas. It is a daunting task to select few relevant topics from the vast areas of both the subjects. Attempts have been made to incorporate important topics that are useful and effective for postgraduate and doctorate students including the researchers. It may be that some aspects were left out not because those are unimportant but choices had to be made at certain stage and was purely based on the judgment of the editors.

Translation researches always emerges from the basic knowledge. Therefore, attempts have been made to describe each chapter in that light focusing on the development and applications. Thus the book is more appealing for those who are in forefront of applied research. The entire book elaborated the themes which have relevance on present day research considering 36 very important topics spreading over five sections *viz.*, the technologies for livestock production and nutrition, assisted reproduction, emerging technologies, interactions between environment and livestock, and lastly the feed safety and quality control.

The section-one provided up-to date knowledge necessary to understand the multiple aspects of nutritional principles such as improvement of fiber digestibility by exogenous treatments, genetic and non-genetic manipulation of rumen microbes, advances in mineral nutrition, probiotic and prebiotics, significance of poly unsaturated fatty acid supplementations in animals, and designer animal products. The reproduction is the luxury of the body system as it happens only when everything goes well so the section-two is dedicated to the topics of assisted reproduction. On female reproduction mechanism of ovarian follicular development and its *in vivo* modulation, the *in vitro* production of embryos, storage, and the *in vitro* preantral follicular technology are described. The uterus controls about forty percent success of conception therefore the organ microenvironment is important to understand. Topics are thus selected to describe conceptus signaling, use of conceptus proteins, the antioxidant mechanism in reproductive organs and the possible manipulation strategies. All of these would help trouble shooting the conception failure in animals. Males are considered half of the herd interms of contributing genetic merits to the offspring. Thus recent development in sperm evaluation techniques for good sire selection, paternal transcripts and their significance, and sex selection at gamete level are also elaborated.

The emerging technologies in stem cells, nanotechnology, application of next generation sequencing technology in ruminal microbial genome analysis, meta-analysis of research results, bioinformatics analysis of protein sequence are the theme of chapters in section-three. Interactions between environment and livestock are important to understand which is dealt in the section-four. It contains two important chapters on enteric methane emission, climate change, and abiotic stress in livestock production system.

Animals feed safety and quality issues are becoming important because of increasing human health concerns. The excess toxic principles in feed if consumed alter the animal's physiology and leave toxic levels of residues in the body. The section-five deals with these concerns with four dedicated chapters describing the recent development on mycotoxins, xenobiotics, antinutritional factors and its amelioration from feeds including a major concern fluorosis which contributes the sufferings of animal and human in many parts of the country. Lack of knowledge on feed safety and quality regulations sometimes results in rejection of our animal products and feed ingredients so a chapter is also included in this section which describes regulations in the countries.

This endeavor would not have been successful without the help of the contributing authors who had taken the pain of compiling the up to date information on the topics and responded well in time to incorporate suggested changes in their manuscripts. Care has been taken to make this book technically correct, but there might be a scope of improvement always. It would be appreciated if such inadvertent mistakes are noticed and pointed. We hope the comprehensive, compact and up-to-date information offered in this book would empower animal science by helping to design and improve research programs in different institutions of the country.

Editors

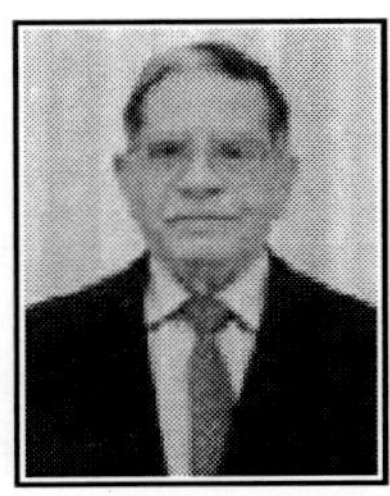

PROF. K PRADHAN, Ph D
FNAVS, FNAAS, FNABS
Former Vice Chancellor
OUAT Bhubaneswar and RAU Bikaner
Chancellor SOAU, Bhubaneswar

C-24/HIG
HB Colony, Baramunda
Bhubaneswar- 754 003
India

Foreword

The subjects of animal nutrition and physiology are the essential core text for all those engaged in research and teaching of nutritional physiology and biochemistry. The advances that have taken place in these two fields during the last four to five decades are spectacular. Understanding the fundamentals of metabolic processes including digestion, absorption, transportation and utilization of nutrients in animals for maintenance, growth, production and reproduction requires widely diverse research competencies in both basic and applied sciences. I am happy to know that a book on **'Animal Nutrition and Reproductive Physiology (Recent Concepts)'** is being published focusing on these aspects. I am particularly pleased that the authors have tried to address various issues associated with these aspects. I am confident that the book will be of use not only to scientists, but also to the students particularly, at master's and doctoral levels. The present publication is a welcoming attempt in this direction.

Compiling and editing a book requires lot of imagination, pragmatic judgment and immense energy in organizing the theme and chapters. This book provides extensive account of recent developments in the field of animal nutrition and reproductive physiology. Attempts have been made to design this book by incorporating important topics that are useful and effective for teachers, researchers and students. The readers will find in this book a variety of chapters and concepts that may help understand the subject much more comprehensively and far less arduously than was previously possible. Added to that, it does so with the information and inputs that one would expect of the scientists who have authored and edited it. Many recent subjects of scientific interest and exploration such as nanotechnology, stem cell technology, next generation sequencing, meta-analysis and their applications are incorporated in this book. The growing numbers at work in the field of animal nutrition and physiology have in their turn begun to ask fundamental questions about the practical uses of these technologies. Most of these questions are critically examined in this book. The scientific curiosity coupled with skepticism that led to conceptualize and then to develop a new way of presenting the recent developments is praiseworthy.

The editors and all contributors deserve thanks and appreciation for having been precise and update in their write-up and successfully produce this major piece of work. The task in preparing this Book incorporating almost all important aspects of animal nutrition and physiology and their orderly presentation is highly commendable. The topics have full relevance to the present day livestock scenario and would definitely contribute in updating the knowledge of students and researchers to understand the recent advances. This book will certainly garner the attention of all professionals involved in animal nutrition and physiology teaching and research.

I congratulate the authors lead by Dr. K.T. Sampath for bringing out this valuable publication.

K. PRADHAN

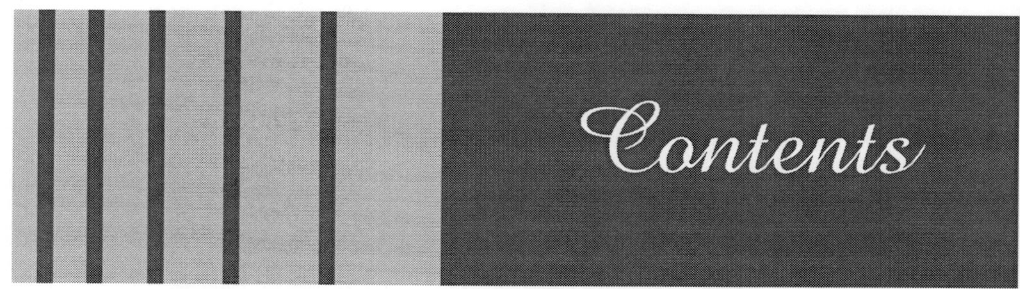

Contents

SECTION-5 : FEED SAFETY AND QUALITY CONTROL

Section - 1

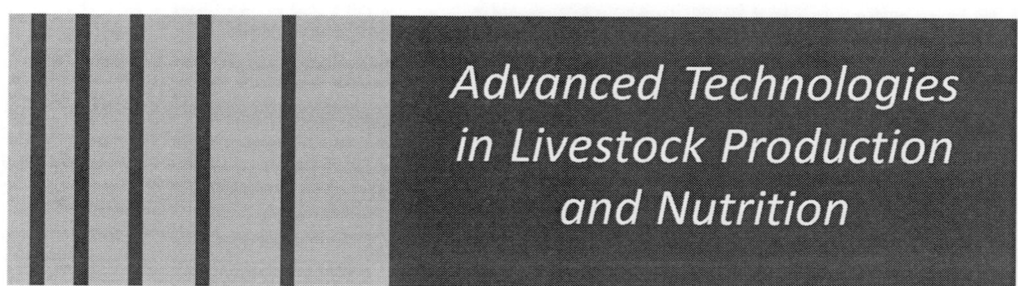
Advanced Technologies
in Livestock Production
and Nutrition

Chapter 1

Biotechnological Approaches for Enhancing Fiber Digestibility of Roughages in Ruminants

M. Sridhar, R. Bhatta, R.U. Suganthi, S.Senani, A.K. Samanta, A. Dhali, A.P. Kolte
National Institute of Animal Nutrition and Physiology, Adugodi, Bangalore-560030, Karnataka, India

Summary

Biotechnologies for enhancing fiber digestibility and productivity in ruminants utilize native micro-organisms including those produced through recombinant DNA technology. Several methods to manipulate rumen fermentation to enhance fiber digestibility have been employed including inoculants of native and recombinant rumen microorganisms. Fermentation technologies are used to improve the digestibility of animal feeds though solid state fermentation (SSF) of lignocellulosic materials to improve the quality of crop residues and forages. Fiber-degrading enzymes are used to increase animal productivity and decrease environment pollutants. Microorganisms that decompose lignocellulose are being studied as producers of enzymes to perform enzymatic hydrolysis of the lignocellulosic material present in the residues from the agro industries. Although the cellulose and hemi-cellulose present in these materials have their nutritive value for feeding ruminants, their bioavailability requires breakdown of bonds with indigestible lignin. Pre digestion of such materials with ligninases, xylanases and pectinases may transform the lignocellulosic substrate into a feed with higher digestibility and quality for ruminants. The development and use of genetically improved crops for animal feeds–including forages having low lignin would also help to mitigate the problem of low fiber digestibility. In this chapter, progress and problems related to solid-state fermentation have been addressed. An overview of variables to be considered in the utilization of fungal plant depolymerizing enzymes produced by solid-state fermentation from agricultural production along with the advancements in engineering of exogenous fibrolytic enzymes to improve digestibility of fibrous diets is dealt with special reference to the applications of ligninolytic enzymes of *Basidiomycetes* and expression and production of recombinant enzymes. The advances in approaches to modify lignin content employing genetic manipulation of lignin biosynthesis as well as genetic engineering of crops (transgenic) for genetically improved feed are also described.

The major feed resources for ruminants in many parts of the country are fibrous residues originating from cereal crops and pasture or cut grasses which are low in both nitrogen and digestibility. The presence of lignin in these crops has a detrimental effect on their digestibility by ruminants (Cherney *et al.*, 1991) owing to the resistance of lignin to degradation by gut microorganisms. Apart from maximizing the efficiency of breakdown and digestion of plant cell walls in the rumen by the native microorganisms which has a marked effect on animal productivity (McSweeney *et al.*, 1994) several biotechnological approaches are currently employed to enhance the digestibility of fibrous feeds for ruminants.

The use of solid state fermentation (SSF) for protein enrichment of lignocellulosic residues has been the focus of attention due its direct applicability of the fermented product for ruminant feed purposes as well as the production of recombinant exogenous microbial enzymes for increasing digestibility of fibrous diets. Improvements in fermentation technology and the biotechnological development of more defined enzyme preparations with techniques like immobilization have prompted a renewed interest in the use of enzymes in ruminant diets. Biotechnological techniques such as cloning, mutation and overproduction of lignocellulolytic enzymes would help to overcome the present limitations. Following the isolation and characterization of ligninase, several laboratories began to apply recombinant DNA technology to lignin degradation. The large scale production of recombinant ligninolytic enzyme(s) in genetically engineered organisms is on the horizon. For lignocellulose biotechnology to make a meaningful impact, suitable bioconversion processes need to be developed in a much bigger way with a cooperative and integrated approach. Efforts have to be directed towards modern, advanced genomics and proteomics technologies for identifying novel lignocellulolytic enzymes and engineered enzymes with improved activities suitable for industrial-scale applications.

Altering the content and/or composition of lignin by genetic manipulation of genes in the lignin biosynthetic pathway can result in changes to the digestibility of fibrous plant materials. Numerous studies have shown that by down-regulating expression of certain genes in the lignin pathway the ratio of syringyl/guaiacyl (S/G) monomers can be manipulated. Along with changes in lignin content, even small changes in the S/G ratio can have a significant impact on fiber digestibility. Recent advances in plant biotechnology may revolutionize the commercial enzyme industry by offering alternative, cost-effective methods of enzyme production and delivery. Large quantities of plant biomass can be produced inexpensively through the use of existing agricultural infrastructure. Expression of enzymes in plant species commonly used for animal feed will minimize downstream processing as the whole or parts of the producing plants are fed directly to livestock.

1. Fiber in ruminant nutrition

Structural carbohydrates (cellulose, hemicelluloses, pectin *etc.*) represent approximately 50 to 70% of total dry matter basal roughages of Indian livestock and are not generally digested by animal enzymes. The ability of animals to trap energy hidden in the structural carbohydrates depends on the presence of symbiotic microbial consortia comprising of all classes of life including bacteria, protozoa archea, yeasts and fungi. The absorption of nutrients is high in the small intestine but low in the large intestine and so post-gastric decay is generally of low nutritive importance. Moreover, the utilization of feeds with high fiber contents (structural carbohydrates) is generally higher in animals with a pre gastric digestion site such as ruminants.

The possibility of increasing fiber digestibility of high fiber content feeds by ruminants is of particular interest in developing countries to ensure higher productivity. Because these feedstuffs constitute the main or only dietary component for animals, where as, feeds of higher energy and protein value (cereals, legumes *etc.*) are reserved for human consumption.

2. Cell wall constituents

The primary component of fiber are cellulose, hemicellulose and lignin, which are organized into macrofibrils that mediate structural stability in the plant cell wall. Cellulose and hemicellulose represent the largest fraction of the plant cell wall and bond with the lignin in the cell wall matrix which needs to be broken in order to be accessible by enzymatic hydrolysis. For this reason, the direct feeding of fiber does not yield the expected favorable results considering the nutritional and energetic potential of these fibers (Colombatto *et al.,* 2003).

Lignin is composed of three major phenolic components, namely *p*-coumaryl alcohol (H), coniferyl alcohol (G) and sinapyl alcohol (S). It is synthesized by polymerization of these components and their ratio within the polymer varies between different plants, wood tissues and cell wall layers. Some organisms, particularly fungi, have developed the necessary enzymes to break lignin apart. The initial reactions are mediated by extracellular lignin and manganese peroxidases, primarily produced by white-rot fungi. Lignin degradation is primarily an aerobic process, and in an anaerobic environment lignin can persist for very long periods. Higher the proportion of lignin in the feed stuff lower is the bioavailability of the substrate. The effect of lignin on the bioavailability of other cell wall components is thought to be largely a physical restriction, with lignin molecules reducing the surface area available to enzymatic penetration and activity.

Chemically, cellulose consists of linear chains of glucose. Starch, the carbohydrate source in grains and nutritionally available to animals, also consists of glucose molecules. However, the glucose molecules in cellulose are linked by β-1, 4-glycosidic bonds whereas, starch has α-1, 4 and α-1,6 glucosidic bonds. The simplicity of the cellulosic structure, using repeated identical bonds, means that only a small number of enzymes are required to degrade this material. Only microbial enzymes are able to digest the β-1, 4 glucosidic bond of cellulose. Cows and other ruminant animals create a reducing and anaerobic environment in their rumen which encourages this microbial degradation, converting cellulose to volatile fatty acids and microbial biomass which the ruminant can then digest and use.

Unlike cellulose, hemicelluloses are heteropolysaccharides comprising of xylose, arabinose, galactose, mannose, and glucose. It binds with bundles of cellulose fibrils to form microfibrils, which enhance the stability of the cell wall. The digestion of hemicellulose also depends on microbial enzymes because of its complex structure, mainly xylose linked by β-1, 4 glucosidic bonds. They also cross-link with lignin, creating a complex web of bonds which provides structural strength, but not only exerts a strong negative influence on fiber digestion (Kung, 2006) but also challenges microbial degradation.

The breakdown of the bonds between lignin and cellulose, and particularly hemicelluloses, transforms the lignocellulosic substrate into a high-quality feed for ruminants (El-Nasser *et al.,* 1997). Enzymes such as xylanases, pectinases and endoglucanases have also been applied to release nutrients from cellulose fibers (Sørensen *et al.,* 2004; Eun *et al.,* 2006). Cellulose and hemi-cellulose are potentially digestible in the rumen by microbes, even though it is well known that these polymers are actually incompletely digested. The incomplete digestion of structural carbohydrates is partly due to the outflow rate of feeds from the rumen. It can thus be assumed that the time required for complete digestion of fiber is longer than the residence time in the rumen.

3. Degradation of lignin in the rumen

Initially, lignin was considered 'indigestible' in ruminants, and was used as an internal marker for evaluating the digestibility of feedstuffs. Subsequently it is proved that lignin is apparently digested to a variable extent with values ranging between 2 to 55% and there is evidence that lignin disappears from feeds incubated in bags suspended in the rumen. Under aerobic conditions, degradation has been shown to occur in the white rot fungi *Basidiomycetes,* a process which involves extracellular peroxidases, oxygenated compounds in the presence of readily available substrate. While, under anaerobic conditions, the degradative process is much more complicated. In microbial consortia, aromatic compounds serve as carbon sources and HCO^- as the electron acceptor. Degradation of lignin-derived monomers can occur in mixed cultures in the presence of methanogenic bacteria, which can use hydrogen as an electron donor in the CO_2 reduction process (Wuhrmann, 1982). The hydrogenation of polyunsaturated fatty acids, naturally present in vegetable oils, could be an additional sink for hydrogen. Anaerobic degradation of lignin fragments has also been reported, caused by bacteria and fungi, with the production of soluble compounds (Colberg, 1988).

4. Rumen microorganisms, their enzymes and biotechnological intervention for enhancing fiber digestibility

The rumen is a very diverse and complex microbial ecosystem and there is mounting evidence for genotypic and phenotypic diversity of the major functional groups of microorganisms in different ruminant species and geographical regions. *Butyrivibrio fibrisolvens, Ruminococcus albus, R. flavefaciens* and *Fibrobacter succinogenes* were identified as the primary fiber degrading bacteria in the rumen. DNA-DNA hybridization studies have shown that *Butyrivibrio* can be divided into at least five groups, suggestive of five different species (Mannarelli *et al.*, 1990). Biotechnological strategies for the manipulation of ruminal bacteria include expression of heterologous genes coding for fibrolytic enzymes into the rumen. Application of gene transfer technologies has been successfully employed for construction of recombinant anaerobic bacteria, designed for modification of the rumen environment. Rumen bacteria have also been selected as hosts for heterologous gene expression thereby executing the introduction of new genetic information to the ruminal environment. Research on construction of more effective expression systems and introduction of additional genes encoding fibrolytic enzymes into native ruminal species has been carried out.

With regard to fiber degradation in the rumen concerted effort has been expended in developing genetically modified bacteria that would have superior fiber-degrading abilities. The construction of genetically modified bacteria has proceeded under the assumption that the rumen micro biota does not produce the correct mixture of enzymes to maximize plant cell degradation. *Butyrivibrio fibrisolvens* and *Prevotella ruminicola* are present predominantly in ruminants and are the choice to introduce new or enhanced genetic material into the rumen. Six genera of anaerobic *Chytridomycetous* fungi have been isolated from the rumen: *Piromyces, Caecomyces, Neocallomastix, Anaeromyces, Orpinomyces* and *Cyllamyces* (Ho and Barr, 1995; Sridhar *et al.*, 2007) and are believed to play an important role in fiber degradation.

The rumen is also well known as a source of superior fibrolytic enzymes. Over 100 different genes encoding enzymes for fiber digestion have been identified and cloned from ruminal bacteria such as *Butyrivibrio fibrisolvens, Fibrobacter succinogenes, Prevotella ruminicola, Ruminococcus albus* and *Ruminococcus flavefaciens*. Cellulases and xylanases produced by ruminal fungi are among the most active fibrolytic enzymes and 50% of the fibrolytic genes cloned have been sequenced (Bowman and Sowell, 2003).

In order to elucidate the mechanisms of fiber digestion and to find efficient enzymes for industrial applications, technological developments now allow the genetic manipulation of rumen microorganisms and a number of genes from ruminal bacteria and fungi have also been cloned. Protein bioengineering has been used to increase the catalytic activity and substrate diversity of these fibrolytic enzymes from ruminant microbes (Sajjad *et al.*, 2008). This has resulted in enzymes which with up to 10 times higher specific activity, changed pH and temperature optima and increased substrate binding activity than the enzymes from which they originated (Selinger *et al.*, 1996).

New genetically modified organism (GMO) strains having superior fiber degrading capabilities are introduced into the rumen to increase fiber degradation which are found persistent in sufficiently high numbers and substantially increase the fiber digestion.

5. Solid-state fermentation in animal nutrition

The use of SSF to upgrade the nutritive value of agricultural byproducts represents a potential solution to feeding animals in developing countries (Robinson and Nigam, 2003; Graminha *et al.*, 2008). The SSF is a process that occurs in or near absence of any fluid in the space between particles (Lonsane *et al.*, 1985). In this system, water is present in the solid substrate whose capacity for liquid retention varies with the type of material. The liquid phase is represented by the aqueous film that surrounds the cells while the space between particles is occupied by the gas phase. Although replacement of the liquid phase with the gas phase increases the transfer of oxygen, this prevents the diffusion of solutes and substrates and markedly interferes with microbial growth (Gervais *et al.*, 1996). The three phases, *i.e.*, solid, liquid and gas phases are present in both liquid and solid medium but not in the same proportions; they differ in diffusion kinetics and rheological and thermodynamic (water activity, *a*w, osmotic pressure) characteristics.

In addition, in the solid process the proportion of each phase depends on the type of substrate being used. However, the main difference between solid and liquid fermentation is related to the fact that in the latter, the mixture between components of the process (microorganisms, nutrients and metabolites) is homogenous and uniformly distributed throughout the fermentor. Fungi have been considered to be the organisms most adapted to

SSF because their hyphae can grow on particle surfaces and penetrate into the inter particle spaces and thereby colonizing solid substrates (Santos *et al.*, 2004). In SSF, the solid material can serve as a physical support and as a source of carbon and nutrients to sustain microbial growth or only as an inert physical support to which nutrients and the carbon source are added. This solid material generally is a natural compound consisting of agricultural and agro industrial by-products and residues, urban residues, or a synthetic material (Pandey, 2003). Fungal spores produced by a SSF culture are more stable, more resistant to dehydration and have a higher germination rate after freezing than spores obtained by SmF (Holker *et al.*, 2004).

5.1 Enhancement of nutritional value of agricultural by-products through SSF

The SSF of lignocellulosic materials by white-rot fungi has received enormous attention, primarily because of the possibility of converting these materials into more digestible feedstuffs for ruminants as well as for the direct applicability of the fermented product for ruminant feeds purposes. The degradation of wheat and rice straws and other lignocellulosic materials using white rot fungi that degrade lignin has been extensively studied (Zadrazil and Puniya, 1995; Mishra *et al.*, 2007; Kinfemi *et al.*, 2009; Shrivastava *et al.*, 2011). The primary objective of lignocellulose treatment is to access the potential of the cellulose encrusted by lignin within the lignocellulose matrix. Thus, a combination of SSF technology with the ability of an appropriate fungus to selectively degrade lignin would make industrial scale implementation of lignocellulose-based biotechnologies feasible.

The white-rot basidiomycetes degrade lignin more rapidly and extensively than other studied microbial groups, and so this potential have been harnessed in SSF. They utilize cellulose and hemicelluloses at approximately the same rate relative to the original amounts present, whereas lignin is usually utilized at a faster relative rate. Fungal growth showed decrease in the neutral detergent fiber, acid detergent fiber and hemicellulosic contents of lignocellulosic fibers, increased the bioavailability of nutrients and there were also reports of a decrease in the anti nutritional factors such as phytic acid, polyphenols and tannins (Elyas *et al.*, 2002). Thus, two nutritionally important contributions can be obtained from fermentative process: first, depolymerizing enzyme and second, a protein-enriched and high degradability of feed material.

The use of SSF for protein enrichment of lignocellulosic residues has been a focus of attention due its direct applicability of the fermented product for ruminant feeds purposes. This material has low protein content and the fungal growth can improve it by around 10-15% (Shojaosadati *et al.*, 1999) further on increases its digestibility (Iluyemi *et al.*, 2006). Zadrazil and Puniya (1995) reported that culturing bagasse with *Pleurotus eryngii* raised organic matter digestibility (OMD) (3-16%). Similarly, Kinfemi *et al.* (2009) reported an increase in OMD (45.65-62.14%) and ME (6.97-9.41 MJ/kg DM), while degrading cowpea husk using *P. ostreatus* for ruminant feed production. Arora and Sharma (2009) reported an increase in dry matter intake (DMI) along with hemicellulose and cellulose degradation and *P. ostreatus* was found to dominantly degrade the lignin over hemicellulose and cellulose. Adamovic *et al.,* (1998) while studying the biodegradation of wheat straw by *P. ostreatus* for cattle feed production also reported a similar pattern of degradation. In our studies on SSF *P. chrysosporium* and *P. ostreatus* proved the most promising white rot fungi strains for improving digestibility of finger millet straw for ruminants (Sridhar *et al.,* 2011). Fungal fermentation of wheat straw effectively improved crude protein (CP) content, organic matter (OM) digestibility, single chain fatty acids (SCFAs) production, ME value and simultaneously lowered the carbon/nitrogen (C/N) ratio, thus showing potential for bioconversion of lignin rich wheat straw into high energy cattle feed (Shrivastava *et al.,* 2011).

5.2 Production of enzymes through SSF

With a ban on the use of growth promoters in animal diets since 2006, new agents are being investigated (Hruby and Cowieson, 2006). The potential use of enzymes such as cellulases, xylanases and other fiber-degrading enzymes in ruminant diets is likely to increase both in developed and developing countries provided a consistent and large response is achieved and their cost is low. The potential of fiber-depolymerizing enzymes for use in animal feeding has been recognized for partial degradation of agro industrial residues that serve as feed ingredients (Pandey *et al.,* 2000). Solid state fermentation is a promising biotechnology to produce fungal microbial enzymes using lignocellulosic materials from agricultural wastes due to low capital investment as well as operating costs. Lignocellulose-decomposing microorganisms can be selected as producers of enzymes under specific growth conditions using substrates of low commercial value including agricultural and agro industrial residues. The microorganisms grow under conditions closer to their natural habitats and are thus more capable of producing enzymes and metabolites which will not be produced or will be produced only in low yield under submerged conditions. Production of enzymes like cellulases and xylanases (Carmona *et al.,* 2005; Kang *et al.,* 2004; Kalogeris *et al.,* 2003), chitinases (Binod *et al.,* 2005) and ligninases (Couto and Sanrom´an, 2005; Sridhar *et al.,* 2011) have yielded very good results. The list of enzymes produced by fungi using by-products for animal nutrition use is given in Table 1.

Table 1 : Enzymes produced by fungi using by-products for animal nutrition use

Substrate	Microorganism(s)	Enzyme(s)	Author(s)/year
Ragi straw	*Phanerochaete chrysosporium* *Pleurotus ostreatus* *Pleurotus sajor caju* *Voriella volvoraceae*	Laccase Lignin peroxidase Manganese peroxidase	Sridhar *et al.* (2011)
Paddy straw	*Phlebia brevispora,* *Phlebia fascicularia,* *Phlebia floridensis* *Phlebia radiata.*	Laccase, Xylanase Carboxymethyl cellulase.	Sharma and Arora, (2011)
Rice straw	*Trichoderma reesei* *Bacillus licheniformis*	Cellulase Hemicellulase Protease	Eun *et al.* (2006)
Barley	*Talaromyces emersonii*	Endo-glucanase	McCarthy *et al.* (2005)
Corn silage	*Thermoascus aurantiacus*	Xylanase	Colombatto *et al.* (2004)
Corn stalk	*Fusarium oxysporum*	Endoglucanase Celobiohydrolase β-Glucosidase Xylanase β-Xylosidase	Panagiotou *et al.* (2003)
Corn straw	*Penicillium decumbens*	CMCase β-Glucosidase Xylanase	Yang *et al.* (2001)
Alfalfa	*Gliocladium* spp.	Cellulase, xylanase	Schimidt *et al.* (2001)
	Orpinomyces joyonii *Caecomyces communis*	Endoglucanase β-Glucosidase	Hodrov´a *et al.* (1998)
Forage silage	*Streptomyces*	Cellulase, hemicellulase	Hill *et al.* (2001)
Wheat straw	*Neurospora crassa*	Cellulase	Romero *et al.* (1999)
	Several fungi	Cellulase, hemicellulase Lignin peroxidase	Peiji *et al.* (1997)
	Trichoderma reesei	Cellulase	Kansoh *et al.* (1999)
	Phanerochaete chrysosporium	Ligninase	El-Gammal *et al.* (1998)
Sugarcane bagasse	*Coriolus versicolor* *Streptomyces* *Viridosporus* White rot fungi	Ligninase	Zadrazil and Puniya (1995)

contd....

Table 1 contd....

Substrate	Microorganism(s)	Enzyme(s)	Author(s)/year
Sugarcane bagasse, wheat straw, corn cobs, rice husks, peanut shells, *etc.*	*Phanerochaete chrysosporium* *Coriolus versicolor*	Cellulase, xylanase Glucanase	El-Nasser *et al.* (1997)
Soy hulls	*Chaetomium globosum* *Coriolus versicolor* *P. chrysosporium* *Trichoderma reesei* *Neurospora*	Cellulase	Jha *et al.* (1995)

The degradation of the lignocellulosic matrix is a complex phenomenon controlled by a large number of variables that limit the use of such fungi. Most of these studies used lignin degradation and improvement in the *in vitro* digestibility of dry matter as indicators for assessment of the efficacy of the biological treatment (Zadrazil *et al.*, 1991). However, few studies have tested direct addition of these enzymes to ruminant diets. Most commercially available enzymatic products that have been tested as food additives for ruminants were not designed specifically for this purpose. Instead enzymatic preparations containing cellulases and xylanases destined for use in the food, pulp, paper, textile, fuel and other chemical industries have been used (Beauchemin *et al.*, 2003). Martins *et al.* (2006) evaluated supplementation with fibrolytic enzymes (cellulase and xylanase, Fibrozyme ®) on the efficiency of microbial synthesis and enzymatic activity of β-1, 4-endoglucanase in animals fed on diets containing corn silage and Tifton 85 hay (*Cynodon* spp.). Addition of these engymes to the hay increased β-1, 4 endoglucanase activity but did not affect the other ruminal variable. According to Morgavi *et al.* (2000) commercial preparations of enzymatic complexes normally are standardized according to their capacity to degrade cellulose or xylan. However, multi-enzyme commercial products might present different fibrolytic activities which warrants greater quality control that may otherwise alter the performance of the enzyme complex. Another aspect regarding use of enzymes as diet additives is the production cost. The fermentation medium is one of the important components that determine the final price of the product. Normally low cost substrates are desired. Economic analysis of the production of lipase by *Penicillium restrictum* in SSF and SmF cultures showed that the investment capital for SmF was 78% higher than SSF; consequently, the price of the SSF product was 47% lower.

5.3 Advantages and disadvantages of SSF

Advantages of SSF as compared to the traditional submerged process are:

1. The production of higher cell mass within a short period of time;
2. Similarity to the natural habitat of the filamentous fungi that permits use of wild-type microorganisms which often show a better performance than genetically modified strains and may enhance biosafety;
3. Downstream steps are facilitated due to the higher concentration of the product. However, problems of scale-up production are:
   i. difficulties in control of pH, heating, nutrient supply and humidity;
   ii. impurity of the product because fiber degradation on microbial activity can generate complex and
   iii. colored compounds such as melanoidins that are difficult to separate and may block columns and degrade resins during downstream processes are some disadvantages;
   iv. also the high cost involved in transport and processing of the straw before inoculation with white rot fungi, considerable loss in energy from lignocellulosic material during fermentation and difficulty in up scaling the process have been reasons for the failure of SSF with regard to ruminant feeds. The quality of the feed obtained after fermentation is not commensurate with the efforts and money spent.

In short, the technology has not proved itself profitable. The greatest obstacle to the industrial use of SSF is the lack of knowledge about various aspects of the process and the lack of adequate fermentors. Probably for these reasons, this technology has never got off the ground but SSF for producing enzymes, especially fiber degrading enzymes and phytases for animal feeding is being employed commercially and appear to be the most promising nutrition related biotechnology to be used in future.

6. Lignocelluloytic enzymes

Lignocellulosic residues have been shown to stimulate enzyme production by basidiomycetes. These ligninolytic enzymes play a crucial role in the global carbon cycle. The demand for application of ligninolytic enzymes complexes of white-rot fungi in industry and biotechnology is ever increasing due to their use in a variety of processes (Vikineswary *et al.*, 2006). Basidiomycetes species are considered to be a very interesting group of fungi given their exceptional adjustment abilities to accommodate detrimental conditions of the environment where they continue to act as natural lignocellulose destroyers and include very different ecological groups such as white rot, brown rot, and leaf litter fungi (Cho *et al.*, 2009). The ligninolytic system is an extracellular enzymatic complex that includes peroxidases, laccases and oxidases responsible for the production of extracellular hydrogen peroxide (H_2O_2). The enzymes responsible for lignin degradation are mainly: lignin peroxidase (LiP), manganese peroxidase (MnP) and a copper containing phenoloxidase, known as laccase along with some others.

Laccases (benzenediol: oxygen oxidoreductase EC 1.10.3.2) belong to multicopper oxidase family. These copper-containing enzymes catalyze the oxidation of various substrates with the simultaneous reduction of molecular oxygen to water. All fungi that have been examined so far produce more than one isoform of laccase. The catalytic site of laccase is quite conserved among different species of fungi, but the rest of the enzyme structure shows high diversity. Fungal laccases are mostly inducible, extracellular, monomeric glycoproteins with carbohydrate contents of 10-20% which may contribute to the high stability of laccases. Laccases are usually the first ligninolytic enzymes secreted to the surrounding media by the fungus that normally oxidizes only those lignin compounds which have a free phenolic group. They form phenoxy radicals, a group of low molecular-weight organic compounds as the mediators required to degrade high redox-potential compounds.

Lignin peroxidases (EC 1.11.1.14) belong to the family of oxidoreductases, were first described in the basidiomycete *Phanerochaete chrysosporium* (Burdsall). These enzyme have been recorded for several species of white-rot basidiomycetes. The LiP is an extracellular hemeprotein, dependent of H_2O_2, with an unusually high redox potential and low optimum pH. It is capable of oxidizing a variety of reducing substrates including polymeric substrates. It has the distinction of being able to oxidize methoxylated aromatic rings without a free phenolic group, generating cation radicals that can react further by a variety of pathways, including ring opening, demethylation, and phenol dimerization. In contrast with laccases it does not require mediators to degrade high redox-potential compounds but it needs hydrogen peroxide to initiate the catalysis.

Manganese peroxidases (EC 1.11.1.13) belong to the family of oxidoreductases. The MnP secreted from *Phanerochaete chrysosporium* was found as another lignin degrading enzyme distributed in almost all white-rot fungi (Hofrichter, 2002). Manganese peroxidases (MnP) seem to be more widespread among white rot fungi than lignin peroxidase (Hammel and Cullen, 2008). Manganese peroxidase (MnP) oxidize Mn^{2+} to Mn^{3+}, which oxidize phenolic structures to phenoxyl radicals (Hofrichter, 2002). The Mn^{3+} product is highly reactive and complex with chelating organic acid, as oxalate or malate. The redox potential of the Mn peroxidase system is lower than lignin peroxidase and it has shown the preferential capacity to oxidize phenolic substrates *in vitro*.

Studies have been conducted to identify white-rot fungi that can degrade lignin bonds but preserve cellulose fibers and thereby improve the quality of lignocellulosic substrates for ruminant feeding. Limiting amounts of lignocelluloytic enzymes are produced by wood decay fungi, which impede their commercial use and also prevent true assessment studies of various potential applications. Biotechnology techniques such as cloning, mutation and overproduction of lignocellulolytic enzymes through techniques like immobilization on various matrices have helped to overcome these limitations. The technology involves isolation of fungal genomic DNA, restriction endonuclease treatment of the genomic DNA, ligation of the restriction fragments into a plasmid, and transformation of *E. coli* with the recombinant plasmid and should be applicable to the overproduction of more commercially important cellulases and ligninases.

7. Screening for organisms with novel enzymes

For more than fifty years one of the main areas of biotechnology research into lignocellulose has been driven by the need to isolate and identify organisms which are either hyper-producer and/or sufficiently robust to withstand conditions of the intended application and/or are producers of novel lignocellulolytic enzymes. In terms of enzyme novelty from an applications perspective, interest is focused on not only to find enzymes which could break down lignocellulose rapidly but also enzymes which could withstand pH, temperature and inhibitory agents more resiliently depending on the intended application. Screening of the environment for lignocellulolytic microorganisms is continuing using genomics and metagenomics which are more productive approaches in bio-mining for unique lignocellulolytic genes which could then be cloned and expressed in industrial strains. Although this technology holds out the best opportunity for discovering unique genes, issues such as representative cloning, quantitative analysis, and expression still require refining.

Enormous amount of data and information have been gathered over the years on the different organism's lignocellulolytic genes and controlling elements, their sequences and organization, protein sequence data, identification of catalytic amino acids and protein structural data including an increase in three-dimensional modular protein structures obtained from crystallographic studies.

8. Optimizing mixtures

Enzyme mixtures with properties of a possible increased specific activity could be created by combining purified individual proteins or individual domains either from the producing organisms or from recombinant organisms expressing a single cloned ligninase encoding gene. These combinations could either consist of pure enzymes from different organisms or the supplementation of crude enzymes with a pure enzyme or supplementing the pure enzyme with a purified cellulose-binding domain from another organism or with specific co-factors.

9. Production of recombinant enzymes

Two similar, simple methods for isolating high-quality DNA and/or RNA that appear general for filamentous fungi have been developed with basidiomycetes, including *P. chrysosporium*. Ligninase gene (s) encoding isoenzymes of *P. chrysosporium* have been cloned and sequenced. Besides ligninase, many other genes have also been cloned from *P.chrysoporium*. The major hosts used for expression of recombinant proteins are *Escherichia coli, Bacillus subtilis,* and *Saccharomyces cerevisiae*. Other bacterial host that are currently being studied and developed include *Pseudomonas* sp.; other yeasts host, *Aspergillus nidulans, Aspergillus niger;* mammalian systems; to a lesser extent plant and insect systems and finally *Trichoderma reesei*. The highest expression levels have been demonstrated in *E. coli,* which has the disadvantage of inability to glycosylate the protein enzyme. This fungus has the ability to recognize heterologous promoters and secretion signals, and a high capacity for accumulating protein in the extracellular medium. *Aspergillus* is an excellent choice as a host organism for expression of recombinant ligninolytic enzymes owing to physiological similarities to fungi such as *P. chrysosporium*. For recombinant ligninase production, heme incorporation is required *in vivo* and *in vitro*. Future molecular work will include the cloning of more ligninolytic genes and comparison of their expression and gene products in a variety of hosts.

Recombinant DNA technology and protein engineering used apart or in combination are powerful modern approaches holding potential for making significant improvements in several aspects of lignocellulolytic enzymes such as increased production, increased specific activity, pH and temperature stability and also creating 'synthetic' designer enzymes for specific applications. DNA technology also offers the possibility of fusing different lignocellulolytic genes or sections of genes from different organisms to give rise to novel chimeric gene-products with altered properties. Unique lignocellulolytic enzymes with multiple activities can be created by artificial gene-fusion.

10. Gene expression and delivery systems

The cost of livestock performance-enhancing enzymes can be reduced through the use of more effective expression and delivery systems. Recombinant bacterial and plant systems are being examined for their efficacy in producing and delivering enzymes on a continuous basis to livestock. Recent advances in plant biotechnology have revolutionized the commercial enzyme industry by offering cost-effective methods of enzyme production and delivery. Plant biomass can be produced inexpensively through the use of existing agricultural infrastructure. Expression of enzymes in plant species, commonly used for animal feed, minimizes downstream processing as, the whole or parts of the producing plants are fed directly to livestock. Transgenic plants also offer the added advantage of a safe and stable formulation system if product is obtained in the form of seeds. The recombinant enzymes would be stable in seeds if stored for up to one year at 4°C and room temperature.

Technological developments enabling introduction of genetic material into domestic animals have validated the concept of direct expression of glucanases and xylanases in the animal itself as an option to adding microbial enzymes to the feed. To be of benefit to the animal, the enzymes should be expressed in the appropriate tissue, secreted into the lumen of the gastrointestinal tract, resistant to proteases, and active in environmental conditions (*e.g.*, pH, temperature, osmolarity) prevailing in the lumen.

11. Genetic manipulation of plant lignin biosynthesis

Lignin is a major component of secondary cell wall of all crops, and is a heterogeneous three-dimensional phenolic polymer resulting from the oxidative polymerization of monolignols. During plant development, it is deposited primarily in the vascular tissues and provides additional strength and imperviousness to the cell wall. Deposition of lignin during defense responses is considered to function as a physical barrier against infection of pathogens.

Lignin is solely responsible for the lack of digestibility, of forage crops, with small increase in plant lignin content resulting in relatively high decrease in digestibility (Sridhar and Senani, 2009). Crops with reduced lignin content provide more efficient forage for cattle, with the yield of milk and meat being higher relative to the amount of forage crop consumed. Since lignin has a negative impact on digestibility, modifying the lignin content and composition can improve the digestibility of the forage crops to ruminants. In industries, lignin is removed from the cellulose by chemical treatment to enhance pulp quality and yield. These treatments are costly, energy-consuming and environmentally hazardous, making this approach unsuitable for enhancing digestibility to ruminants. Thus, approaches based on genetic modification of the trees/plants have gained importance.

11.1 Genes involved in lignin biosynthesis

All of the genes known to be involved in lignin biosynthesis have been targeted for manipulation or mutation in model plants such as *Arabidopsis,* tobacco, or poplar. There are currently ten genes known to be involved in monolignol production. The roles of each of these genes have been characterized following up or down-regulation of gene activity in transgenic plants, either in a single construct or in combination with other lignin genes. Mutants have also been isolated for some of the lignin genes.

12. Approaches to modify lignin content

12.1 Over-expression of white-rot fungi lignin-degrading enzymes

White-rot fungi produce extra cellular lignin-modifying enzymes, the best characterized of which are laccases, lignin peroxidases and manganese peroxidases. The genes encoding these lignin-degrading enzymes have been cloned and over-expressed in various forage crops. Transgenic alfalfa plants expressing *Bacillus licheniformis* alpha-amylase and manganese-dependent lignin peroxidase (Mn-P) from the wood-rot fungus *Phanerochaete chrysosporium* have been produced using the Agro bacterium-mediated transformation.

12.2 Down-regulation of genes involved in lignin biosynthesis

Various enzymes of the monolignol pathway have been targeted for down-regulation, primarily using the antisense strategy and RNA interference (RNA). Genes encoding seven enzymes of the monolignol pathway were independently down-regulated in alfalfa using antisense and/or RNA interference (Chen *et al.,* 2006). Similarly, down-regulation of genes involved in lignin biosynthesis has been attended in tobacco (Chabannes *et al.,* 2001; Pingon *et al.,* 2001; Abbott *et al.,* 2002), *Leucaena leucocephala* (Rastogi and Dwivedi, 2006) and tall fescue (Chen *et al.,* 2003) etc.

Numerous studies have shown that by down-regulating expression of certain genes in the lignin pathway the ratio of S/G monomers can be manipulated. Along with changes in lignin content, even small changes in the S/G ratio can have a significant impact on fiber digestibility as can changes to lignin structure. CAD- and COMT-deficient transgenic tobacco and alfalfa have also been shown to have slightly improved digestibility (Bernard-Vailhe *et al.,* 1996, 1998).

12.3 Gene discovery using reverse genetics

Mutant collections using T-DNA/transposon tagging (insertion as well as activation tagging) have been developed. Phenotypic evaluation of these mutants might identify lignin-deficient lines, which can be used for forward genetics to unravel gene(s) controlling the phenotype. Reverse genetics approach involving phenotypic evaluation for lignin is expected to reveal the role of tagged gene in lignin biosynthesis apart from any other associated adverse phenotypic changes.

12.4 Genetic engineering of crops for genetically improved feed

Lignin confers strength, rigidity, and impermeability to water in plants but higher proportions of lignin are of concern due to the reduced availability of crop cell wall polysaccharides brought about by it with respect to forage digestion in rumen. For these reasons it is desirable to alter lignin biosynthesis in order to develop improved plant varieties that can be more efficiently utilized for specific industrial or agricultural purposes. Attempts have been made to reduce lignin content in crops by down-regulating specific, rate limiting enzymes which control carbon flux into the lignin biosynthesis pathway. On the other hand, as the metabolic pathway leading to lignins is well known the characterization of several genes involved in the biosynthesis of lignins has been takeup for manipulation.

Antisense transgenic constructs are being developed, for all enzymes in the phenylpropanoid pathway and are utilized to determine their effect on plant lignin concentration and composition. Much of the genetic variation that has been generated in typical novel-lignin transgenic plants is parallel to that observed in natural populations of non-transgenic plants including variation in lignin concentration and composition. Phenotypic changes in transgenic plants, including changes in lignin concentration and composition and the reddish-brown coloration of some low-lignin plants, are both qualitatively and quantitatively similar to natural variation for these traits. The relative increases observed in *in vitro* digestibility are similar regardless of whether lignin is modified by conventional selection, mutagenesis, or transformation. Genetic modifications to lignin concentration and/or composition would thus be economically important in many woody or herbaceous perennials.

Soon it will be possible to manipulate lignin 'content' in plants in a way which is compatible with normal development. Plants genetically modified for reduced lignin must be evaluated for fitness in multiple environments that include an array of physiological stress factors. Selection among novel-lignin transgenic and their progenies may be required to ensure adequate agricultural fitness. Recurrent selection strategies for increased IVDMD or reduced lignin should include field testing of plants to ensure that fitness is retained throughout the selection process.

Lignocellulose biotechnology is based on the utilization of readily available residual plant biomass considered as 'waste' to produce numerous value-added products. It is an attractive technology for developing countries from a capital costs investment perspective since its biodegradation could follow solid-state fermentation comparable to silage or mushroom production, thus making such technology suitable for farms and small industrial plants without the need for large engineering infrastructure. By knowing to what extent it is possible to manipulate lignin content in plants it would be possible to reduce the plant cell wall for optimal utilization. Besides the immediate opportunities for exploitation, future work along these lines will undoubtedly result in a wide range of potential applications.

Conclusions

Lignocellulose biotechnology is an attractive technology for developing countries from a capital investment perspective since its biodegradation could follow solid-state fermentation comparable to silage or mushroom production. Such technology is considered suitable for farms and small industrial plants without the need for large engineering infrastructure. Besides the immediate opportunities for exploitation, future work along these lines will undoubtedly result in a wide range of potential applications. The degradation potential of lignocelluloses by ruminants has been under investigation by microbiogists and nutritionists, for utilization of these compounds and their subsequent transformation into animal products. This would be an alternative means to the oxidation achieved generally by aerobic degradation such as burning or other industrial processes. One most important step forward in that direction would be to isolate and identify the microorganisms which are able to convert lignin anaerobically and enzymatically into simpler compounds. The enzymatic degradative ability of such organism can be propagated to the rumen microbial species using engineering. Extensive efforts are made in that direction with some success which needs further improvement in terms of cost, efficacy and practical value.

Agricultural by-products vary widely in their chemical composition, nutritional value, and are sometimes too high in low-quality fibers, that a secific enzyme complex is required to break it down in order to use in the ruminant feed. Their nutritional value could be increased by biodegradation of fiber in the rumen, through efficient delignification. Agro-industrial residues can be utilized as substrate for the production of enzymes by solid-state fermentation that can be used as feed additives for ruminants. Solid-state fermentation of lignocellulosic materials is although categorized as low-tech, they have not been practically used at all. The reasons for failure is the high cost involved in transport and processing of straw before inoculation with white rot fungi, considerable loss in energy from lignocellulosic material during fermentation and difficulty in up-scaling the process. The quality of the feed obtained after fermentation do not commensurate with the efforts and money spent. In short, the technology has not proved itself profitable. The use of exogenous fibrolytic enzymes produced by SSF however, holds promise as a means of increasing forage utilization and improving the productive efficiency of ruminants. Biotechnology techniques such as cloning, mutation and over production of lignocellulolytic enzymes would help to overcome the present limitations. Following isolation and characterization of ligninase, several laboratories began to apply recombinant DNA technology for lignin degradation. The large scale production of recombinant ligninolytic enzymes(s) in genetically engineered organisms is on the horizon. The potential for improvement of the efficiency of non-ruminant and ruminant livestock feed utilization by enzyme supplementation is widely recognized. However, the cost of this technology has inhibited its widespread application in the industry. Reducing the cost of feed enzymes through improved enzymes and more efficient production systems is the focus of current research in this area. Microbial isolates from the rumen produce a wide array of enzymes and comprise an immense and under-utilized gene pool. The isolation of more potent enzymes is certain as exploration of this enzymological and genetic resource progresses from domestic ruminants to those animals adapted for survival in diverse habitats worldwide.

References

Abbott J.C., Barakate A., Pincon G., Legrand M., Lapierre C., Mila I., Schuch W., Halpin C. (2002). Simultaneous suppression of multiple genes by single transgenes. Down-regulation of three unrelated lignin biosynthetic genes in tobacco. *Plant Physiology* **128**: 844-853.

Adamovic M., Grubic G., Milenkovic I., Jovanovic R., Protic R., Sretenovic L., Stoicevic L. (1998). The biodegradation of wheat straw by Pleurotus ostreatus mushrooms and its use in cattle feeding. *Animal Feed Science and Technology* **71**: 357-362.

Arora D.S., Sharma R.K. (2009). Enhancement in *in vitro* digestibility of wheat straw obtained from different geographical regions during solid state fermentation by white rot fungi. *Bioresources* **4:** 909-920.

Austin S., Bingham E.T., Mathews D.E., Shahan M.N., Will J., Burgess R.R. (1955). Production and field performance of transgenic alfalfa (Medicago sativa L.) expressing alpha-amylase and manganese-dependent lignin peroxidase. *Euphytica* **85**: 381-393.

Beauchemin K.A., Colombatto D., Morgavi D.P., Yang W.Z. (2003). Use of exogenous fibrolytic to improve feed utilization by ruminants. *Journal of Animal Sciences* 81 (E.*Suppl.2*): E37-E47.

Bernard-Vailhe M.A., Besle J.M., Maillot M.P., Cornu A., Halpin C., Knight M. (1998). Effect of down-regulation of cinnamyl alcohol dehydrogenase on cell wall composition and on degradability of tobacco stems. *Journal of Food Science and Agriculture* **76:** 505-514.

Bernard-Vailhe M.A., Migne C., Cornu A., Maillot M.P., Grenet E., Besle J.M., Atanassova R., Martz F., Legrand M. (1996). Effect of modification of the O-methyltransferase activity on cell wall composition, ultrastructure and degradability of transgenic tobacco. *Journal of Food Science and Agriculture* **72:** 385-391.

Binod P., Pusztahelyi T., Nagy V., Sandhya C., Szak´acs G., P´ocsi I., Pandey A. (2005). Production and purification of extracellular chitinases from *Penicillium aculeatum* NRRL 2129 under solid-state fermentation. *Enzyme and Microbial Technology* **36:** 880-887.

Bowman J.G.P., Sowell B.F. (2003). Technology to complement forage-based beef production systems in the west. *Journal of Animal Sciences* **81:** E18-E26.

Carmona E.C., Fialho M.B., Buchgnani E.B., Coelho G.D., Brocheto-Braga M.R., Jorge J.A. (2005). Production,purification and characterization of a minor form of xylanase from *Aspergillus versicolor. Process Biochemistry* **40:** 359-364.

Chabannes M., Barakate A., Lapierre C., Marita J.M., Ralph J. Pean M., Danoun S., Halpin C., Grima-Pettenati J., Boudet A.M. (2001). Strong decrease in lignin content without significant alteration of plant development is induced by simultaneous down-regulation of cinnamoyl CoA reductase (CCR) and cinnamyl alcohol dehydrogenase (CAD) in tobacco plants. *Plant Journal* **28:** 257-270.

Chen F., Srinivasa Reddy M.S., Temple S., Jackson L., Shadle G., Dixon R.A. (2006) Multi-site genetic modulation of monolignol biosynthesis suggests new routes for formation of syringyl lignin and wall-bound ferulic acid in alfalfa (*Medicago sativa* L.). *Plant Journal* **48:** 113-124.

Chen L., Auh C.K., Dowling P., Bell J., Chen F., Hopkins A., Dixon R.A., Wang Z.Y. (2003). Improved forage digestibility of tall fescue (*Festuca arundinacea*) by transgenic down-regulatin of cinnamyl alcohol dehydrogenase. *Plant Biotechnology Journal* **1:** 437-449.

Cherney J.H., Cherney D.J.R., Akin D.E., Axtell J.D. (1991). Potential of brown-midrib, low lignin mutants for improving forage quality. *Advances in Agronomy* **46:** 157-198.

Cho N.S., Wilkolazka A.J., Staszczak M., Cho H.Y., Ohga S. (2009). The role of laccase from white rot fungi to stress conditions. *Journal of the Faculty of Agriculture, Kyushu University* **54:** 81-83.

Clough R.C., Pappu K., Thompson K., Beifuss K., Lane J., Delaney D.E., Harkey R., Drees C., Howard J.A., Hood E.E. (2006). Manganese peroxidase from the white-rot fungus phanerochaete chrysosporium is enzymatically active and accumulates to high levels in transgenic maize seed. *Plant Biotechnology Journal* **4:** 53-62.

Colberg P.J. (1988). Anaerobic microbial degradation of cellulose, lignin, oligolignols and mono aromatic lignin derivatives. In: *Biology of anaerobic microorganisms* (AJB Zehnder, ed), John Wiley & Sons, New York, pp 333-372.

Colombatto D., Mould F.L., Bhat M.K. (2003).Use of fibrolytic enzymes to improve the nutritive value of ruminant diets. A biochemical and in vitro rumen degradation assessment. *Animal Feed Science and Technology* **107:** 201-209.

Couto S.R., Sanrom´an M.A. (2006). Application of solid-state fermentation to food industry—a review. *Journal of Food Engineering* **76:** 291-302.

Eichlerova I., Homolka L., Nerud F., Zadrazil F., Baldrian P., Gabriel J. (2000). Screening of Pleurotus ostreatus isolates for their ligninolytic properties during cultivation on natural substrates. *Biodegradation* **11:** 279-287.

El-Gammal A.A., Kamel Z., Adeeb Z., Helmy S.M. (1998). Biodegradation of lignocellulosic substances and production of sugars and lignin degradation intermediates by four selected microbial strains. *Polymer Degradation and Stability* **61:** 535-542.

El-Nasser N.H.A., Helmy S.M., El-Gammal A.A. (1997). Formation of enzymes by biodegradation of agricultural wastes with rot fungi. *Polymer Degradation and Stability* **55:** 249-253.

Elyas S.H.A., El Tinay A.H., Yousif N.E., Elsheikh E.A.E. (2002). Effect of natural fermentation on nutritive value and *in vitro* protein digestibility of pearl millet. *Food Chemistry* **78:** 75-79.

Eun J.S., Beauchemin K.A., Hong S.H., Bauer M.W. (2006). Exogenous enzymes added to untreated or ammoniated rice straw: effects on in vitro fermentation characteristics and degradability. *Animal Feed Science and Technology* **131:** 87-102.

Gervais P., Marrchal P.A., Molin P. (1996).Water relations of solid state fermentation. *Journal of Scientific and Industrial Research* **55:** 343-357.

Graminha E.B.N., Goncalves A.Z.L., Pirota R.D.P.B., Balsalobre M.A.A., Da Silva R., Gomes E. (2008). Enzyme production by solid-state fermentation: Application to animal nutrition. *Animal Feed Science and Technology* **144:** 1-22.

Gupta R., Beg Q.K., Lorenz P. (2002). Bacterial alkaline protease: Molecular approaches and industrial applications. *Applied Microbiology and Biotechnology* **59:** 15-32.

Hall J., Ali S., Surani M.A., Hazlewood G.P., Clark A.J., Simons J.P., Hirst B.H., Gilbert HJ (1993). Manipulation of the repertoire of digestive enzymes secreted into the gastrointestinal tract of transgenic mice. *Nature Biotechnology* **11:** 376-379.

Hammel K.E., Cullen D. (2008). Role of fungal peroxidases in biological lignolysis. *Current Opinion in Plant Biology* **11:** 349-355.

Hill J., Xiao G.Q., Ball A.S. (2001.) Effect of inoculation of herbage prior to ensiling with *Streptomyces achromogenes* ISP 5028 on chemical composition of silage. *Animal Feed Science and Technology* **89:** 83-96.

Ho Y.W., Barr D.J.S. (1995).Classification of anaerobic gut fungi from herbivores with emphasis on rumen fungi from Malaysia. *Mycologia* **87:** 655-677.

Hodrov´a B., Kopecn´y J., K´as J.(1998). Cellulolytic enzymes of rumen anaerobic fungi *Orpinomyces joyonii* and *Caecomyces communis*. *Research in Microbio*logy **149**: 417-427.

Hofrichter M. (2002). Review: lignin conversion by manganese peroxidase (MnP). *Enzyme and Microbial Technology* **30:** 454-466.

Hofrichter M., Scheibner K., Bublitz F, Schneegaß I., Ziegenhagen D., Martens R., Fritsche W. (1999). Depolymerization of straw lignin by manganese peroxidase from*Nematoloma frowardii* is accompanied by release of carbon dioxide. *Holzforschung* **53:** 161-166.

Holker U., Hofer M., Lenz J. (2004). Biotechnological advantages of laboratory-scale solid-state fermentation with fungi. *Applied Microbiology and Biotechnology* **64:** 175-186.

Hruby M., Cowieson A.J. (2006). The role of enzymes and betaine in antibiotic growth promoter free nutrition. In: *Antimicrobial growth promoters: Where do we go from here?* (D. Barug, J. de Long, A. K. Kies, and M. W. A. Verstegen, ed.) Wageningen Acad. Publ., Wageningen, The Netherlands, pp 269-287.

Iluyemi F.B., Hanafi M.M., Radziah O., Kamarudin M.S. (2006). Fungal solid-state culture of plam kernel cake. *Bioresource Technology* **97:** 477-482.

Jha K., Khare S.K., Gandhi A.P. (1995). Solid-state fermentation of soy hull for the production of cellulase. *Bioresource Technology* **54:** 321-322.

Kalogeris E., Christakopoulos P., Katapodis P., Alexiou A., Vlachou S., Kekos D., Macris B.J. (2003). Production and characterization of cellulolytic enzymes from the thermophilic fungus *Thermoascus aurantiacus* under solid state cultivation of agricultural wastes. *Process Biochem*istry **38:** 1099-1104.

Kang S.W., Park Y.S., Lee J.S., Hong S.I., Kim S.W. (2004). Production of cellulose and hemicellulases by *Aspergillus niger* KK2 from lignocellulosic biomass. *Bioresource Technology* **91:** 153-156.

Kansoh A.L., Essam S.A., Zeinat A.N. (1999). Biodegradation and utilization of bagasse with *Trichoderma reesie. Polymer Degradation and Stability* **63:** 273-278.

Kinfemi A.A., Mohamed M.I., Ayoade J.A. (2009). Biodegradation of cowpea shells by Pleurotus species for its use as ruminant feed. *World Journal of Agricultural Sciences* **5:** 639-645.

Kung Jr., L. (2006). The role of fiber in ruminant ration formulation. http://ag. udel.edu/anfs/faculty/kung/articles/roleof fiber in ruminant ration.htm.

Lonsane B.K., Ghildyal N.P., Butiatman S., Ramakrishma S.V. (1985). Engineering aspects of solid state fermentation. *Enzyme and Microbial Technology* **7:** 258-265.

Manmdebvu P., West J.W., Froetschel M.A., Hatfield R.D., Gates R.N., Hill G.M. (1999). Effects of enzyme and microbial treatment of bermudagrass forages before ensiling on cell wall composition, end products of silage fermentation and in situ digestion kinetics. *Animal Feed Science and Technology* **77:** 317-329.

Mannarelli B.M., Evans S., Lee D. (1990). Cloning, sequencing and expression of a xylanase gene from the anaerobic ruminal bacterium *Butyrivibrio fibrisolvens. Journal of Bacteriology* **172:** 4247-4254.

Martins A.S., Vieira P.F., Berchielli T.T., Prado I.N., Garcia J.A.S. (2006). Efici^encia de s´ýntese microbiana eatividade enzim´atica em bovinos submetidos ʻa suplementac¸ ˜ao com enzimas fibrol´ýticas. *Revista Brasileira de Zootecnia* **35:** 1194-1200.

McCarthy T., Hanniffy O., Lalor E., Savage A.V., Tuohy M.G.(2005). Evaluation of three thermostable fungal endo-β-glucanases from *Talaromyces emersonii* for brewing and food applications. *Process Biochemistry* **40:** 1741-1748.

McSweeney C.S., Mackie R.I., White B.A. (1994). Transport and intracellular metabolism of major feed compounds by ruminal bacteria; the potential for metabolic manipulation. *Australian Journal of Agricultural Research* **45:** 731-756.

Misra A.K., Mishra A.S., Tripathi M.K., Prasad R., Vaithiyanathan S., Jakhmola R.C. (2007). Optimization of solid state fermentation of mustard (*Brassica campestris*) straw for production of animal feed by white rot fungi (*Ganoderma lucidum*). *Asian-Australasian Journal of Animal Sciences* **20:** 208-213.

Morgavi D.P., Newbold C.J., Beever D.E., Wallace R.J. (2000). Stability and stabilization of potential feed additive enzymes in rumen fluid. *Enzyme and Microbial Technology* **26:** 171-177.

Panagiotou G., Kekos D., Macris B.J., Christakopoulos P. (2003).Production of cellulolytic and xylanolytic enzymes by *Fusarium oxysporum* grown on corn stover in solid state fermentation. *Industrial Crops and Products* **18:** 37-45.

Pandey A. (2003). Solid-state fermentation. *Biochemical Engineering Journal* **13:** 81-84.

Pandey A., Soccol C.R., Nigam P., Soccol V.T. (2000). Biotechnological potential of agro-industrial residues. I. Sugarcane bagasse. *Bioresource Technology* **74:** 69-80.

Peiji G., Yinbo Q., Xin Z., Mingtian Z., Yongcheng D. (1997). Screening microbial strain for improving the nutritional value of wheat and corn straws as animal feed. *Enzyme and Microbial Technology* **20:** 581-584.

Pingon G., Chabannes M., Lapierre C., Pollet B., Ruel K., Joseleau J.P., Boudet A.M., Legarand M. (2001). Simulataneous down-regulation of caffeic/5-hydroxy ferulic acid-O-methyltransferase I and cinnamoyl-coenzyme A reductase in the progeny from a cross between tobacco lines homozygous for each transgene. Consequences for plant development and lignin synthesis. *Plant Physiology* **126:** 145-155.

Rastogi S., Dwivedi U.N. (2006). Down-regulation of lignin biosynthesis in transgenic leucaena leucocephala harboring O-methyltransferase gene. *Biotechnology Progress* **22:** 609-616.

Robinson T., Nigam P. (2003). Bioreactor design for protein enrichment of agricultural residues by solid state fermentation. *Biochemical Engineering Journal* **13:** 197-203.

Romero, M.D., Aguado, J., Gonz´alez, L., Ladero, M. (1999). Cellulase production by *Neurospora crassa* on wheat straw. *Enzyme and Microbial Technology* **25:** 244-250.

Sajjad, M., Andrabi S.M.H., Akhter S., Afzal M. (2008). Application of biotechnology to improve post-ingestion forage quality in the rumen. *Pakistan Journal of Nutrition* **7:** 70-74.

Santos M.M., Rosa A.S., Dal'boit S., Mitchell D.A., Kriger N. (2004). Thermal denaturation: is solid state fermentation really a good technology for the production of enzymes? *Bioresource Technology* **93:** 261-268.

Schimidt J., Szak´acs G., Cenkv´ari ´ E., Sipocz J., Urb´anszki K., Tengerdy R.P. (2001) Enzyme assisted ensiling of alfalfa with enzymes by solid substrate fermentation. *Bioresource Technology* **76:** 207-212.

Selinger L.B., Forsberg C.W., Cheng K.J. (1996). The rumen: a unique source of enzymes for enhancing livestock production. *Anaerobe* **2:** 263-284.

Sharma R.K., Arora D.S. (2011) Biodegradation of paddy straw obtained from different geographic locations by means of *Phlebia* spp.for animal feed. *Biodegradation* **22:** 143-152.

Shojaosadati S.A., Faraidouni R., Madadi-Nouei A., Mohamadpour I. (1999). Protein enrichment of lignocellulosic substrates by solid state fermentation using *Neurospora sitophila*. *Resources Conservation and Recy*cling **27:** 73-87.

Shrivastava B., Thakur S., Khasa Y.P., Gupte A., Puniya A.K., Kuhad R.C. (2011). White-rot fungal conversion of wheat straw to energy rich cattle feed. *Biodegradation* **22:** 823-831.

Sørensen J.F., Kragh K.M., Sibbesen O., Delcour J., Goesaert H., Svensson B., Tahir T.A., Brufau J., Perez-Vendrell A.M., Bellincampi D., D'ovidio O., Camardella L., Giovane A., Bonnin E., Juge N. (2004). Review: potential role of glycosidase inhibitors in industrial biotechnological applications. *Biochimica et Biophysica Acta* **1696:** 275-287.

Sridhar M., Kumar D., Anandan S., Prasad C.S., Sampath K.T. (2007). First report of occurrence and prevalence of *Cyllamyces* genus- a putative anaerobic gut fungus, in Indian cattle and buffaloes. *Current Science* **92:** 1356-1358.

Sridhar M., Senani S. (2009) Novel approaches for reducing lignin content in wheat and rice straw for enhancing their nutritional value for livestock feeding. *Indian dairyman* **61**(8): 50-54.

Sridhar M., Senani S., Bhatta R. (2011). Production of proteases and lignolytic enzymes during solid state fermentation (SSF) of finger millet straw (*Eleusine coracana*). *Indian Journal of Animal Sciences* **81:** 723-729.

Vikineswary S., Abdullah N., Renuvathani M., Sekaran M., Pandey A., Jones G.E.B. (2006). Productivity of laccase in solid substrate fermentation of selected agro-residues by *Pycnoporus sanguineus*. *Bioresource Technology* **97:** 171-177.

Wuhrmann K. (1982). Ecology of methanogenic systems in nature. *Experentia* **38:** 193-198.

Yang X., Chen H., Gao H., Li Z. (2001). Bioconversion of corn straw by coupling ensiling and solid-state fermentation. *Bioresource Technology* **78:** 277-280.

Zadrazil F., Galletti G.C., Piccaglia R., Chiavari G., Francioso O. (1991). Influence of oxygen and carbon dioxide on cell wall degradation by white-rot fungi. *Animal Feed Science and Technology* **32:** 137-142.

Zadrazil F., Puniya A.K. (1995). Studies on effect of particle size during solid state fermentation of sugarcane bagasse into animal feed using white-rot fungi. *Bioresource Technology* **54:** 85-87.

❑❑❑

Chapter 2

Advances in Mineral Nutrition Research

D.T. Pal, N.K.S. Gowda, K.S. Prasad, K.T. Sampath and C.S. Prasad
National Institute of Animal Nutrition and Physiology, Adugodi, Bangalore 560030, Karnataka, India

Summary

Minerals play a vital role in animal nutrition, being part of the structural materials, constituents of the soft tissues and cells and regulate many important biological processes. In order to determine efficient utilization of dietary minerals by animals, one must know the relative bioavailability of minerals from a specific feed ingredient, complete diet or minerals salts. Chelated minerals are more bioavailable, thus are more useful in improving the productive and reproductive efficiency in animals. It protects the minerals from unwanted reactions at the site of absorption. There has been positive impact in use of these organic minerals for environment also. Traditional biomarkers provide useful but frequently inadequate indices of minerals status. The expression of genes which changes on dietary trace minerals have recently been identified which has the potential to use as molecular markers of trace minerals status. Identification of transporters and chaperones at transcriptional and translation levels have the greater potential to use for this purpose in animals. When metals are present as minor or trace components in substrates as food, they are probably associated with macromolecular compounds such as proteins, lipids or carbohydrates. The chemical form or species of the element must be assessed which critically influences its bioavailability, essentiality, or toxicity. Speciation studies are therefore necessary to identify the distribution of trace elements in biological and environmental samples. The speciation study involves separation of biomolecules followed by on-line, real-time, sensitive element-specific detection. HPLC with inductively coupled plasma-mass spectrometry (ICP-MS) is a useful and most widely used technique for multi-element biomolecules analyses present at trace levels. Regarding supplementation of minerals to animals, recently area-specific mineral mixture has got much popularity because of cost-effectiveness and judicious use of minerals salts based on the minerals profile in soil-plant-animals in a particular zone.

Minerals are essential nutrients for all animals. They have a wide range of activities and functions within the body, individually or collectively *viz.*, in general metabolism, reproduction, immune system, growth, development and repair of various tissues and so on. It is important for the nutritionists to know the bioavailability of any element in the natural feed ingredients or mineral sources which are used as a dietary supplement. Recently organic mineral sources have begun to gain popularity because of a number of perceived benefits of their use in comparison to inorganic sources of mineral. Chelates and other complexes are useful in animal nutrition to protect trace minerals during digestion. Chelated and other complexed minerals are administered especially during high nutritional demand, such as pregnancy, weaning, or other reproductive stress, rapid growth, environmental or health stress. Mineral chelates have been studied mainly to evaluate their effect on improvement of immunity, reproductive performance and herd health.

The use of biomarkers to evaluate intake and nutritional status is a rapidly changing field. No sensitive indices are currently available to assess the trace elements status in animal populations. The indices of mineral status include growth rate, concentrations in tissue and physiological fluids physiological functions, chemical balances, mobilizable stores and immune competence. These are either not very sensitive enough or are very difficult to determine. The emergence of post-genomic technologies has led to the development of strategies aimed at identifying specific and sensitive biomarkers from thousands of molecules present in a tissue or biological fluid. Genes that change their expression in response to trace minerals availability constitute potential biomarkers of trace minerals status in animals. The total amount of an element present in food tells us very little about its possible absorption and fate inside the body. Therefore, speciation studies are focused to obtain more complete information about the form of trace elements in foods and are becoming mandatory to assess in the field of nutrition. To gain this information, the chemical form or species of the element must be assessed as this critically influences its bioavailability, essentiality, or toxicity. Thus elemental speciation has become a prominent topic of present research in food science.

1. Organic minerals

Minerals occur naturally in most feed ingredients but the amount and bioavailability varies considerably. Most of the green fodders, leguminous fodders and tree leaves contained more copper but will not necessarily have a higher supplementary value if its availability is lower (Gowda *et al.*, 2004). Mineral analysis of feed and forage samples determines concentration of specific elements present in it, however, availability of mineral to the animal is more difficult to measure.

For many years, nutritionists have been using the inorganic forms of minerals with the concept that the addition of these trace elements is sufficient to meet the animal's biological needs. Research conducted on the solubility and nutritional availability of these minerals has revealed that there is considerable variation in the availability of minerals to animal's body. Uncertain bioavailability of minerals in the source often led to the supplementation of higher than the minimum requirement for optimum performances. This ultimately results in over-supply with the risk of mineral toxicity, environmental pollution and affect the utilization of other nutrients or the levels may be too low to impart any impact on production. It is generally accepted that animal performance can be improved by judicious use of organic forms of essential elements which are more bioavailable than inorganic sources. However, the cost effectiveness of use of such organic minerals is a matter of debate. As the recent insight to the new assay procedures and its utility improves, the interest in chelated minerals is likely to increase.

1.1 Relative mineral bioavailability

In order to determine how efficiently an animal utilizes dietary minerals, one must know the relative bioavailability of that mineral from a feed ingredient or complete diet. Natural feedstuffs such as corn, wheat, soybean meal, grain and their by products contain essential trace elements that are required by animals. However, these trace elements are often in a form, which renders them unavailable to the animal. Also, even if the elements are totally available, they may not be in adequate concentrations to meet the animal's requirement. Further, some of the antinutritional factors like tannins, oxalates and silica present in feed can inhibit the utilization of minerals. It is advantageous for nutritionists to know the bioavailability of any element in the natural feed ingredient or mineral source used as a dietary supplement. With this knowledge the proper amount of the trace element can be supplied to the animal.

Relative Bioavailability

Inorganic Sources Organic Sources

Oxides < Carbonates < Sulfates < Proteinates < Amino Acid Complexes

1.2 Factors affecting bioavailability

There are many factors that influence the bioavailability of minerals, especially trace elements These include:- i) level of mineral intake, ii) chemical form, iii) overall diet digestibility, iv) particle size, v) interactions with other minerals and nutrients, vi) chelators, inhibitors, vii) physiological state of the animal, viii) water quality, ix) processing conditions to which the individual ingredients or complete diet have been exposed, and x) the age and species of the animal. Release of minerals form the forage and interactions with microbial cells, other minerals present, or other forage components in the rumen can influence availability for absorption by the animal (Pal *et al.*, 2011).

1.3 Chelates and organo-mineral complexes

A chelate is best described as a metal complex in which the metal atom is held in the complex through more than one point of attachment to a nonmetal entity referred to as ligand (chelating agent), with the metal atom occupying a central position in the complex. Ligand is a molecule containing an atom which has a lone pair of electrons. In the process of chelation, the ligand acts as chelating agent and encircles the metal atom to form a heterocyclic ring structure. So the metal atom is bonded to the ligand through donor atoms such as the oxygen of the carboxyl group, nitrogen or sulfur of the amino acid or peptide. When such ligands bond to a metal ion via two or more donor atoms, the complex formed contains one or more heterocyclic rings and they are called "chelates". Theoretically, the introduction of chelated minerals would increase absorption and utilization of the mineral because of more favourable binding or stability constant. The organic minerals utilize peptide and/or amino acid uptake mechanisms in the intestine. The mineral within the complex or chelate remains as chemically inert form due to coordinate, covalent and ionic bonding by the amino ligands hence, more stable and less prone to interactions. The mineral is protected from physiochemical factors or from negative interactions with dietary components such as phytate, which binds cations making them unavailable for absorption. In addition, the organic trace minerals remained to be electrically neutral at certain pH conditions. Thus, the mineral chelate/complex is absorbed intact through the intestinal mucosa, traversing the mucosal cell membrane into the plasma (Power and Horgan, 2000). Minerals using either amino acid or peptide uptake mechanism would therefore be expected to be absorbed and circulated to target tissues very efficiently (Power and Horgan, 2000) hence, highly bio-available (Fig. 1).

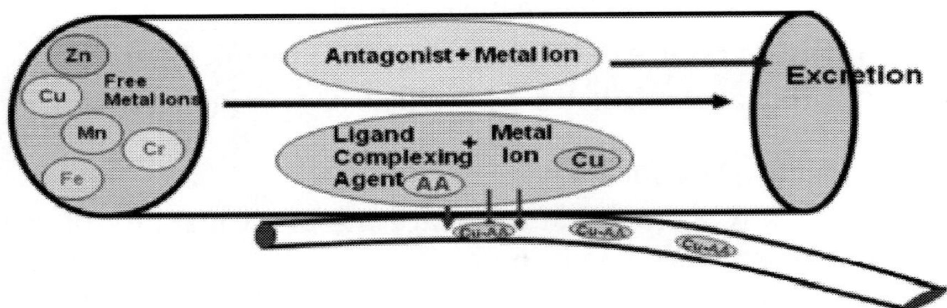

Fig. 1 : Intestinal absorption of trace minerals from inorganic and chelated sources

There are various categories of organic trace minerals as defined by Association of American Feed Control officials (AAFCO, 1998): metal (specific amino acid) complexes, metal amino acid complex, metal proteinates, metal amino acid chelates, metal polysaccharide complexes, metal propionates, and yeast derivative complexes.

1.4 Organic mineral complexes: their effect on livestock production and reproduction

More recently, the inclusion of organically complexed or chelated mineral supplements for livestock diets has been suggested on the basis that they supply more bioavailable mineral than the inorganic forms. However, limited research has been carried out to compare the biological availability of organic and inorganic mineral sources in ruminants (Ward *et al.*, 1996; Pal *et al.*, 2010). Use of mineral chelates in ruminant diets has increased growth and milk production and decreased somatic cell counts in milk compared with animals fed inorganic forms of the mineral (Prasad *et. al.*, 2003). Relative bioavailability of copper from copper-lysine, copper-methnionine (Pal *et al.*, 2010) or copper-proteinates is generally more than copper sulfate or copper oxide. Supplementation of Cu and Zn through organic sources (Cu-methionine, Zn-methionine) as compared to inorganic sources ($CuSO_4$, $ZnSO_4$) improved gut absorption, activity of Cu/Zn-SOD enzyme and tissue retention of Cu and Zn, suggesting better bioavailability through organic/chelated sources (Pal *et al.*, 2010; Table 1). Harmon *et al.* (1998) showed that the copper-proteinate supplement has advantage over copper sulfate at restoring Cu stores, particularly at the critical peri-parturient period. Liver Cu was two-fold higher in the Cu-proteinate than copper sulfate supplement at calving. They concluded that liver and plasma Cu contents and plasma ceruloplasmin activities tended to support the idea that organic Cu supplements had increased bioavailability over that of inorganic forms in peri-parturient heifers.

Table 1 : Relative bioavailability values (RBV) of Cu and Zn estimated based on multiple regressions slope ratios and from gut absorption (Pal *et al.*, 2010)

Attribute	Slope		RBV (%)*
	Cu-Sulf + Zn-Sulf	Cu-Meth + Zn-Meth	
Liver			
Cu	267.98	406.79	151.79
Zn	1057.5	1408.0	133.14
Plasma			
Cu	11.675	17.522	150.08
Zn	10.447	13.836	132.44
Gut absorption	Gut absorption %		
Cu	21.88	33.11	151.32
Zn	30.12	40.40	134.13

* Assumed that bioavailability of Cu and Zn from Cu- and Zn-sulfate was 100%.

Although the mode of action is unclear, research suggests that supplementing certain organic forms of zinc can improve animal production response (growth, milk production and/or reproduction) compared with those observed in ruminants that are supplemented with only inorganic Zn (Kessler *et al.*, 2003; Wright and Spears, 2004). The udder health can be improved through reduced somatic cell count in the herd by supplementing the organic mineral sources. Several studies have demonstrated a reduction in somatic cell count in dairy cattle which were supplemented with combinations of mineral proteinates (Boland *et al.*, 1996), suggesting better udder health.

More recently, the use of organic trace minerals has been evaluated for the impact on fertility. Boland *et al.* (1996) found that cows receiving organic trace minerals (Cu, Zn & Mn-proteinate and Se yeast) improved the first conception rate from 57.7% to 65.2%. Improving reproductive performance of beef and dairy cows by achieving better conception rates early in the breeding period ensure higher economic returns to the producer.

Prasad *et al.* (2006) showed that the Cu and Zn concentration in wool increases by 26-30% along with liver Cu and Zn content (41% Cu and 14% Zn) in sheep on supplementation of organic sources of these trace minerals as compared to in organic sources. Organic selenium in selenized yeast results in much larger increase in blood and milk selenium concentrations than selenite. Because of Se being a potential antioxidant agent in maintaining cellular integrity the role of organic selenium or selenized yeast has received greater significance.

It appears that organic trace minerals may have a place in dairy and beef diets when situations involving mineral antagonisms are encountered. In addition, organic mineral supplementation may be considered in the following situations: a) dry period b) peri-parturient dairy cattle c) during stress d) in advance of breeding (30-60d). A general recommendation is the inclusion of 25 to 30% of the supplemented mineral in an organic form, especially when proper supplementation with inorganic sources of trace mineral has not been effective (Harmon, 2000).

1.5 Economic considerations

Even if organic mineral sources are more bio-available than inorganic sources, cost of these sources will be a major factor in the decision on whether or not to use them. Dietary requirements for minerals may be greatly reduced by the addition of organic minerals to animal diets, but cost-to-benefit ratio need to be established (Jerry, 1996; Prasad *et. al.*, 2003). If inorganic elements are 40-50% bioavailable, chelated minerals are 2-2.5 times more bioavailable. So the cost calculation should be based on the level of bioavailability. Another approach to this problem would be to supply only a portion of the supplemental minerals in the organic form and see its effect with the same levels of inorganic salt supplementation. Uchida *et al.* (2001) and Ballantine *et al.* (2002) replaced a portion of an inorganic mineral supplement with organic sources (Zn, Mn, Cu and Co) in dairy cow and found higher first service conception rate, fewer services per conception and more milk production. Nocek and Patton (2002) also reported increased milk production and improved reproductive performance in cows fed mineral supplements containing a combination of inorganic and organic mineral sources. These studies suggest that replacing a portion of inorganic mineral supplements with organic sources may be a viable approach and would certainly help to address cost concerns.

1.6 Environmental applications

Another potential application for organic mineral sources, that is currently receiving a lot of attention, is the use of organic sources of minerals for challenging issues to sustainable agriculture. The rationale for this approach is that if organic sources are more bioavailable, then the beneficial effects of high levels of inorganic sources should be achieved with much lower concentrations of organic sources. Feeding lower levels will reduce the total amount of mineral excreted in the feces. Carlson *et al.* (2004) found that organic Zn either as a polysaccharide or proteinate had no effect on growth performance however, feeding the lower levels of organic Zn greatly decreased Zn excretion. Veum *et al.* (2004) reported that replacing 250mg Cu/kg as copper sulfate in nursery diets with 50 or 100mg Cu/kg as Cu-proteinate increased groth performance of pigs and Cu-proteinate reduced Cu excretion by 61-77% compared with higher concentration of inorganic copper sulfate source. Results of the studies suggest that there is the potential for using organic sources of Cu and Zn to reduce the negative environmental impact of inorganic Cu and Zn sources. As environmental issues impose restrictions it becomes necessary to lower supplemental trace mineral levels and adjust proportions of inorganic to organic in order to maintain optimum performance, profitability and environmental stability.

2. Biomarkers of trace minerals status

A nutritional biomarker can be any biological specimen that is an indicator of nutritional status with respect to intake or metabolism of dietary constituents. It can be a biochemical, functional or clinical index of status of an essential nutrient or other dietary constituent. The use of biomarkers to evaluate intake and nutritional status is a rapidly changing field. The discovery of new biomarkers of nutritional intake and status and the critical evaluation of them are essential to our continuing progress in nutritional epidemiology. The most commonly used indices for determining minerals deficiency in animals are reduced serum/plasma minerals concentration and decreased activity of plasma/serum enzymes (*e.g.*, ceruloplasmin for Cu and erythrocyte Cu/Zn superoxide dismutase for Cu and Zn). However, these indicators are influenced by many factors unrelated to minerals status, thus limiting their usefulness in many situations. Currently there is a need for more biomarkers that clearly relate to intake, which would be useful for validation of dietary instrumentation and in measurement-error research. If we are to gain a better understanding of the roles of feed components and nutrients in chronic disease and health, we must establish better markers of intake. Improved understanding of bioavailability and the metabolism of nutrients is important for the interpretation of most biomarkers of intake.

2.1 Assessing trace mineral status by gross changes and biochemical analysis

There are numerous measures of essential mineral element status, including growth rate, tissue and physiological fluids concentrations, enzyme concentrations and activities, chemical balance and mobilizable stores. Commonly used indices of mineral element adequacy are as follows:

Growth rate	Blood and plasma/serum concentrations
Hair, wool, hoof concentrations	Biopsy tissue concentrations
Enzyme concentrations and activities	Physiological functions
Chemical balance	Mobilizable stores/Turnover rates
Immune competence	Behaviour and appearance

Growth rate is an excellent measure of the adequacy of some mineral elements during the development phase of animals, but of course it is of no value in assessment of adult animals. For some elements appetite and growth rate are not significantly impaired by mild deficiency, even in young animals. Chemical balance and mobilizable stores provide valid measures but are difficult to determine.

2.1.1 Diet analyses

Diet analyses provide useful supporting data if representative samples of all feeds can be obtained. Actual chemical analyses need to be performed and should include those elements with important interactions (*e.g.*, Mo, S and Cu). Tabular values and feed tags should not be relied on for estimating trace element intakes (Kincaid, 1999).

2.1.2 Blood measures

Blood measures are frequently used for assessment because they are significantly correlated to nutritional status of some trace elements (Mills, 1987) and blood is less invasive to sample than liver. Despite the penchant for using plasma/serum samples in both clinical practice and epidemiologic research, of the trace minerals, only selenium assays in plasma/serum are a primary choice of biomarker. However, there are several limitations to blood analyses. Homeostatic control mechanisms can limit changes in concentrations of some trace minerals in plasma until endogenous reserves are substantially depleted. Cellular blood components are used quite rarely and then primarily for research purposes. The combination of the demanding sample preparation and, in general, their limited and/or inadequately defined potential has restricted enthusiasm for these sample materials. Whole blood selenium is sensitive to intake of this micromineral and provides a longer-term biomarker. Erythrocyte-membrane zinc has been found to be sensitive to dietary zinc restriction in some but not all studies.

2.1.3 Hair, wool and hoof concentrations

For several of the trace minerals, hair and wool analyses have provided a tantalizing potential biomarker. For assessing the zinc status, hoof concentration of this trace mineral sometimes provides a useful index. The values of minerals in hair, wool and hoofs lack reference standards and are too slowly responsive to intakes and can be easily contaminated.

2.1.4 Body stores

Liver is the organ that often represents the status of several trace elements in animals (McDowell, 1992). Liver concentrations of Cu had been found more effective in indicating the Cu status of sheep (Prasad *et al.,* 2006). Other tissues do not consistently reflect trace mineral status. Iron is the most notable example of a mineral that is stored by the body when intake of bioavailable iron is generous and released as required when intake is less adequate.

2.1.5 Analyses of milk and urine

Analyses of minerals in milk and urine are seldom useful in mineral assessment because most cations in milk are actively transported into the mammary gland and concentrations are regulated. Values of Se and I in milk and urine could have a role in indicating excess intakes if references values were established. Urine excretion rates of trace minerals for which the kidneys have a prominent role in homeostasis such as iodide provide useful biomarkers of dietary intake of these minerals. For those minerals for which the kidneys are not involved in maintaining homeostasis, measurement of urine excretion rates does not provide useful information on dietary intake and nor do these measurements provide biomarkers of mineral status.

2.1.6 Functional indices and mineral-dependent enzymes activity

Functional indices are of special putative practical value because they indicate when intake and status are sufficiently compromised to cause measurable disturbance of normal physiology and biochemistry. To be of value, these perturbations have to be more or less specific for deficiencies of a single micronutrient. Examples include a low haemoglobin, haematocrit and red cell morphology consistent with iron-deficiency anaemia, low circulating concentrations of thyroid hormones that result from iodide deficiency and low blood levels of glutathione in selenium deficiency. In vitamin B_{12} deficiency, methylmalonic acid accumulates, and the elevated concentrations of this metabolite in plasma and urine may be used for differential diagnosis of cobalt deficiency.

Blood and its specific nutrient concentrations provide a useful but frequently inadequate index. The first limiting biochemical system should provide the most valid index, but in many cases it is unknown or not easily measured. There have been expectations for many years that assays of the activity of selected metalloenzymes would provide invaluable functional indices of trace minerals status and possible surrogate biomarkers of dietary trace minerals. Most current approaches use cuproenzymes of one form or another for assessing Cu status. Many studies have used ceruloplasmin to predict the Cu status in animals (Milne, 1998; Pal *et al.*, 2011, unpublished) and its activity is reported to decrease in response to severe Cu deficiency, so that it has value for indicating moderate/severe Cu deficiency (Feillet-Coudray *et al.*, 2000). Other cuproenzymes that have been tested with greater or lesser success include Cu/Zn-superoxide dismutase (Cu/Zn-SOD), platelet cytochrome-c oxidase (CCO), lysyl oxidase and peptidylglycine α-amidating monooxygenase. Similarly alkaline phosphatase for Zn, glutathione peroxidase for Se. Recently, Pal *et al.* (2011, unpublished) observed that the combination of mineral-dependent enzymes with one common enzyme for two or three minerals and one specific enzymes for specific minerals could be more useful and better indicators of two or three trace minerals. They also validated their findings with liver storage as well as plasma levels of trace minerals which were regressed on mineral-dependent enzymes activities for assessing the trace minerals status in sheep.

2.2 Significance of different metal transporters

2.2.1 Metal transporters and metallochaperones

The emergence of post-genomic technologies has led to the development of strategies aimed at identifying specific and sensitive biomarkers from the thousands of molecules present in a tissue or biological fluid. Eukaryotic cells, genetically altered mice (such as knockout mice), and inborn errors of metabolism in humans have provided scientists with new opportunities for the application of molecular techniques. This has led researchers to conclude that there are multiple levels of protein regulation, and they hypothesize that metal-responsive transcription factors exist (Rutherford and Bird, 2004). Although many of these discoveries have yet to be made in mammals, even fewer have been made in non-rodent mammals such as livestock species. The recent identification of metal transporters and chaperones gives researchers the opportunity to understand the regulation of minerals trafficking where the proteins are modified by posttranslational mechanisms. It is essential that these new molecular findings be used to evaluate the bioavailability of and nutritional need for trace minerals in livestock.

The limits of homeostatic regulation of trace minerals in animals make it difficult to define the trace mineral status in deficient or adequate. In these regards, the expression analysis of biomarker genes could provide a robust assay to monitor trace minerals status. Genes that change their expression levels in response to trace minerals availability constitute potential biomarkers of trace minerals status in animals (Gonzalez *et al.*, 2008).

a) Copper transporters

Copper is a redox active metal that is essential for biological function. Copper is potentially toxic; thus, its homeostasis is carefully regulated through a system of protein transporters. In general proteins involved in copper homeostasis can be divided in two main and broad categories: *copper chaperones* and *membrane transporters* (O' Halloran and Culotta, 2000; Prohaska, 2008). Copper is taken up across the lumen surface of the small intestinal microvilli as cuprous ion by copper transporter protein-Ctr1. Cupric ion may also be taken up, but those processes are less well understood. Within the cell, intestinal as well as others, copper is escorted to specific compartments by metallochaperones. One, copper chaperone for superoxide dismutase (CCS), donates copper to superoxide dismutase. Another, COX17, delivers copper to additional chaperones within the mitochondria for synthesis of cytochrome c oxidase. A third chaperone, Atox1, delivers copper to the secretory pathway by docking with two P-type ATPases. One, ATP7A, is the protein required for cuproenzyme biosynthesis, and in the enterocyte it is required for copper efflux to portal blood. The second, ATP7B, predominantly expressed in liver, is required for copper metallation of ceruloplasmin and biliary copper excretion. Additional intracellular hepatic copper-binding proteins COMMD1 (copper metabolism MURR1 domain) and XIAP (X-linked inhibitor of apoptosis protein) may also be required for excretion. Other proteins involved in copper homeostasis may include metallothionein (MT) and amyloid precursor protein (APP). Plasma protein transport of copper from the intestine to liver and in systemic circulation probably includes both albumin and alpha2-macroglobulin. Changes in the expression of copper 'transporters' may be useful to monitor copper status of animals.

The last decade many proteins involved in copper homeostasis have been identified, and particular interest has been focused on the high affinity copper transporters belonging to the Ctr family, whose members share sequence homology and likely structural and functional features (Dumay *et al.*, 2006). In mammals only two different members of this family have been identified, a high-affinity Cu transport protein (Ctr1) and low-affinity Ctr2 (Bertinato *et al.*, 2008; Kim *et al.*, 2008; van den Berghe *et al.*, 2007) and the divalent metal transporter protein (DMT1) in the brush border, also called nramp (Cater and Mercer, 2005).

b) Copper chaperone for superoxide dismutase (CCS)

Most recently, the protein known as copper chaperone for SOD (CCS) has been studied for its potential possibility to become a good biomarker for copper. The CCS is a copper chaperone that shuttles copper to SOD for incorporation into its structure (Linder and Hazegh-Azam, 1996). A number of rodent studies have documented changes in CCS expression levels in response to various copper concentrations (Prohaska *et al.*, 2003; West and Prohaska, 2004). In contrast to ceruloplasmin and SOD, CCS levels vary inversely with copper status. In rats fed with diet containing either marginal or deficient copper amounts, liver and erythrocyte CCS protein expression was found to increase markedly (Prohaska *et al.*, 2003; West and Peohaska, 2004), indicating that CCS is highly responsive to low copper status. Mild copper deficiency induced by moderately high zinc intake in rats also resulted in increased CCS protein expression in the liver, erythrocytes and white blood cells (Iskander *et al.*, 2005). Cu deficiency increases CCS levels in liver and erythrocytes of cattle calves (Hepburn *et al.*, 2009), rat and mice (West and Prohaska, 2004). An increase in CCS level is observed in duodenal mucosal cells of Cu-deficient vs. Cu-adequate calves (Hansen *et al.*, 2009). These evidences suggest that CCS can be a sensitive indicator of copper deficiency in animals.

c) Copper chaperones for cytochrome c oxidase (CCO)

The cytochrome-c oxidase Cu chaperone (COX17) transports Cu to the mitochondria, where it transfers Cu to cytochrome c oxidase in the mitochondrial intermembrane space (Maxfield *et al.*, 2004). Whereas COX17 delivers Cu to the mitochondria and two other proteins SCO1 and SCO2 may be involved in the incorporation of Cu into the cytochrome c oxidase molecule (Bertinato and L'Abbe, 2004).

d) Atox1

Another Cu chaperone protein (Atox1) delivers Cu to ATP7A (Cu-transporting ATPase 1) and ATP7B (Cu-transporting ATPase 2) through direct interaction with these proteins. These two closely related P-type ATPases that deliver Cu to cuproenzymes normally are found in the trans-Golgi network, where Cu is incorporated into Cu enzymes such as lysyl oxidase, ceruloplasmin, and so forth (Cater and Mercer, 2005). If Cu concentrations in the cell are increased, ATP7A moves to the plasma membrane to expel Cu, and ATP7B takes Cu to the vesicular compartments for storage. Thus, besides the role of Cu delivery to essential cuproenzymes, these ATPases help the cell to eliminate excess Cu or sequester Cu as a means of detoxification.

The discovery of Cu chaperones that are involved in facilitating Cu absorption into proteins may provide an excellent status indicator.

e) Zn transporters

Like copper, zinc transporters are also having the potential as biomarkers of zinc status. At the cellular level, Zn concentrations are adjusted by uptake and secretion, by redistribution, and even by sequestration. Hence, the transportation of Zn is essential for life. Two families of Zn transporters - ZnT and ZiP have been investigated using quantitative PCR as potential indicators of Zn status (Gibson *et al.*, 2008).

i) ZnT

Cousins *et al.* (2006) reported that ZnT1 is located at the plasma membrane, ZnT2 is involved in vesicular localization of pancreatic acinar cells, and ZnT5 is present in the secretory vesicles of the pancreatic β cells and at the apical membranes of the enterocytes. The ZnT9 protein is found in the nucleus during mitosis. Using immunohistochemical analysis, Yu *et al.* (2007) reported that in the mouse, ZnT1 is expressed in the epithelium of several parts of the gastrointestinal tract (*i.e.*, the esophagus, duodenum, and caecum), whereas ZnT4 is primarily found in the large intestine. The ZnT6 protein was detected in the stomach, jejunum, cecum, colon, and rectum. The ZnT7 protein has been found in all parts of the gastrointestinal tract, with the greatest expression in the small intestine (Yu *et al.*, 2007). Given the importance of maintaining the appropriate amounts of Zn for the growing embryo and fetus, it is not surprising that the ZnT proteins are found in the placenta. Helston *et al.* (2007) reported that the expression of ZnT in the mouse placenta is responsive to dietary Zn. Metallothionein (Mt), ZnT1, and ZnT4 transcript concentrations are reduced when dietary Zn concentrations are below or 3-fold above the adequate amount (Helston *et al.*, 2007). The ZnT protein, ZnT1, is regulated differently among tissues by metal-responsive transcription factor 1 and the abundance of mRNA when Zn is supplied in the diet at different concentrations (Martinez, 2004 and Martinez *et al.*, 2005).

ii) Zip

The Zip proteins, which are involved in Zn transport activity, are Zip1 to Zip8 and Zip14. Although Zip proteins are specific for Zn, they can be inhibited by several other cations. Most Zip proteins are thought to be located at the plasma membrane, but Zip7 is located at the Golgi apparatus. To serve their role, Zip proteins are able to change, depending on Zn availability and the physiological condition. The transport protein Zip4 will increase in the plasma membrane of enterocytes when Zn is restricted and will decrease its expression to basal conditions if Zn is fed again (Cousins *et al.*, 2006). The Zip14 protein increases Zn uptake in the hepatocyte during an acute-phase response (Cousins *et al.*, 2006). Thus, the regulation of Zip genes by dietary Zn, and hence the presence of Zip proteins, may be important in managing Zn in livestock species, yet it appears that this family has not been investigated in farm species.

f) Metallothionein

PCR assays are being used increasingly to measure mRNA for some of the proteins involved in Zn regulation. For example, metallothionein mRNA in lymphocytes which decreases markedly in response to mild Zn depletion (Allan *et al.*, 2000). Metallothionein protein expression was more in pigs liver supplemented higher level of Zn in the diet (Hill and Link, 2009). Metallothionein synthesis is up-regulated in response to cellular copper exposure.

g) Nickel chaperones

Metallochaperones are also believed to deliver nickel ions to enzymes such as urease, hydrogenase, and CO dehydrogenase. Future studies of this system are likely to yield new paradigms of metallochaperone function.

h) Other metallochaperones

The recent advances in understanding copper and nickel chaperones underscore the possibility that additional metallochaperones exist for biologically relevant metal ions. Numerous gene products involved in assembly of other metal cofactors have been identified and may function as metallochaperones. As more biochemical, spectroscopic, and structural data become available, additional mechanisms of metallo chaperone-mediated metal cofactor assembly are likely to emerge.

2.3 -omics technologies for biomarker identification

Functional genomics approaches (*e.g.*, transcriptomics, proteomics and metabolomics) have enormous potential for advancement of nutritional research by providing new insights into diet-gene interactions and for the development of new robust biomarkers of nutritional status. In mammals, multiple proteins associated with copper metabolism are regulated by post-translational mechanisms (Petris *et al.*, 2003). However, regulation also occurs at the transcriptional level. The above mentioned metal transporters and metallochaperones proteins expression are regulated either transcriptional or translational levels at varying levels of dietary trace minerals and may have the potential to use as sensitive and valid biomarkers of trace elements status. In animal studies, CCS protein but not mRNA was shown to be consistently elevated in copper deficiency (Prohaska *et al.*, 2003). Recently, it was shown that the protein expression of the CCS is increased in erythrocytes of rodents with mild Cu deficiency. The genes associated with respiration are down-regulated in Cu deficiency (Van Bakel *et al.*, 2005). Sun *et al.* (2007) has found that there are 62 genes expression affected by Zn deficiency and excess in rats and Tom Dieck *et al.* (2005) reported the expression of 268 genes transcripts altered on Zn deficiency. On Fe deprivation, 20 genes increased and 4 genes decreased at rat duodenum (Collins *et al.*, 2005).

The proteomics also presents an emerging and promising tool for elucidation of mechanisms of action and development of relevant biomarkers of health and disease. Proteomics has the advantage over transcriptome profiling in that it measures the functional product of gene expression, and allows the identification of modifications that may relate to the activation or inactivation of proteins by dietary interventions. Current proteomics approaches include the use of protein separation, visualization and identification by 2D gel electrophoresis combined with mass spectrometry.

Metabolomics technologies determine broad-brush assessments of a very large spectrum of plasma metabolites. For example, comparison of plasma metabolites in individuals exposed to high and low Se intakes may reveal metabolite changes and may provide novel biomarkers of Se exposure.

The emerging science of '*metallomics*', involves the detection, mapping, and/or quantification of trace elements in biological systems at organ, cell, and sub-cell levels which may have the potential to identify metal-specific proteins for using as molecular markers of trace elements status. It requires the development of versatile measurement tools allowing for trace detection, identification, and quantification of metals associated with proteins. The association of LA-ICPMS (laser ablation -inductively coupled plasma mass spectrometry) with MALDI-TOF MS/MS (matrix-assisted laser desorption ionization time-of-flight tandem mass spectrometry) is a powerful tools in metallomics studies applied to determine differences in metal-containing proteins, being able to play an important role on the discovery of potential markers for trace elements.

Micronutrients are involved in specific biochemical pathways (*Network Biology*) and have dedicated functions in the body, but they are also interconnected in complex metabolic networks, such as oxidative-reductive and inflammatory pathways, defense mechanisms (Se, Zn, Cu, Fe) and hormonal regulation (I), in which the overarching function is to optimise health. The majority of trace element research to date has focused on the biological activity of single element or on the interactions between limited combinations of trace elements. A more global view of their metabolic effects is therefore needed to appraise their impact on health. And with the development of system biology (the study of multiple processes that together determine molecular/cellular and whole body physiology) it is needed to reconsider the function of trace elements in the context of an integrated perspective (van Ommen *et al.*, 2008).

3. Trace minerals speciation: Importance and tools for analysis

Total element determinations of trace and toxic metals, both in environmental and in biological materials or in living organisms, are increasingly demanded by society. The total concentration of trace elements does not always provide adequate information on bioavailability and toxicity. So speciation analysis is required to obtain a correct risk assessment regarding trace elements in feed. A trace element, and so a toxic metal can exist in a given sample (*viz.*, a sediment, urine, serum, *etc.*), in a most varied number of physico-chemical forms (*e.g.*, in the case of lead: $Pb^{+}2$, $Pb(OH)_2$, $Pb(OH)_4$, $(CH_3)_4Pb$, $(CH3\text{-}CH2)_4Pb$, *etc.*). More recently, the scientific community has concluded that toxicity, bioavailability, bioactivity, transport in the organism, bio-geological distribution/transportation and thus, the eventual impact of the toxic element in our body and environment, will be dictated by the particular species or form of mineral present in the sample. In this sense, total element determinations by atomic spectroscopy, of a toxic element as As, Hg or Sn are insufficient today, and sometimes misleading, to assess the toxicity of a food or sediment (*e.g.*, arsenobetaine is not toxic, methylmercury is much more toxic than $Hg^{+}2$; similarly tributyltin is a most potent biocide, while Sn (IV) is not). Therefore, additional "speciation" information to complement total toxic element determinations is demanding, both in environmental and in clinical/biological issues (Libonsky, 1997; Sanz-Medel, 1998a).There is an enormous interest in the last decades to develop analytical strategies and methods which is able to tackle this challenge of "speciating" trace element concentrations in the different forms or species actually present in the samples under scrutiny.

A definition of chemical species, speciation and speciation analysis was suggested by Templeton *et al.* (2000) which state that a *chemical species* is a specific form of an element defined as to isotopic composition, electronic or oxidative state, and/or complex or molecular structure. *Speciation* of an element is the distribution amongst defined chemical species in a system. The *speciation analysis* is the activities of identifying and/or measuring the quantities of one or more individual chemical species in a sample.

3.1 Analytical tools for trace elements speciation

The quest for molecular information on the chemical species has become a challenging task for analytical chemists. Elemental detection became more sensitive and hence more compounds were detected. Atomic absorption methods are by definition non-speciating methods as the atomiser destroys the molecules because measurement of atoms or ions is aimed at. Speciation analytical approaches are different to provide reliable molecular information of the sought particular species of the toxic metal. It must be ensured that species are preserved all along the steps of the analysis (sampling, storage, pretreatment, separation and measurement). The so-called "hybrid" techniques (that is, the coupling of a powerful separation with an element-specific atomic detector) are preferred method to solve real-life speciation problems (Sanz-Medel, 1998a). It appears much more convenient to couple online a powerful separation unit *viz.*, gas chromatography (GC), high performance liquid chromatography (HPLC), capillary electrophoresis (CE) with an adequate atomic detector operating in a continuous manner to provide on-line, real-time, sensitive element-specific detection (*e.g.*, analytical plasma). The selection of the separation technique depends on the nature and physical properties of the species of the trace element to be determined.

Various analytical methodologies have been applied for speciation analysis of heavy metals in both feed and food (Fig. 2). The analytical methods can be divided into a separation part and an element-selective detection part. Mainly liquid chromatography (LC), GC and CE has been used for the separation of the species prior to detection. Various kinds of separation approaches for LC have been applied: size exclusion, ion exchange, reversed phase and ion pairing. The detection of the element of interest is subsequently performed by element-selective detectors such as ICP-MS (inductively coupled plasma mass spectrometry) or AF (atomic fluorescence). Most commonly used is the coupling of HPLC to ICP-MS. Although this approach is used in many laboratories, there is still a need for development of new, fast and inexpensive methods for speciation of heavy metals to be used in routine laboratories for future monitoring and control in both food and feed.

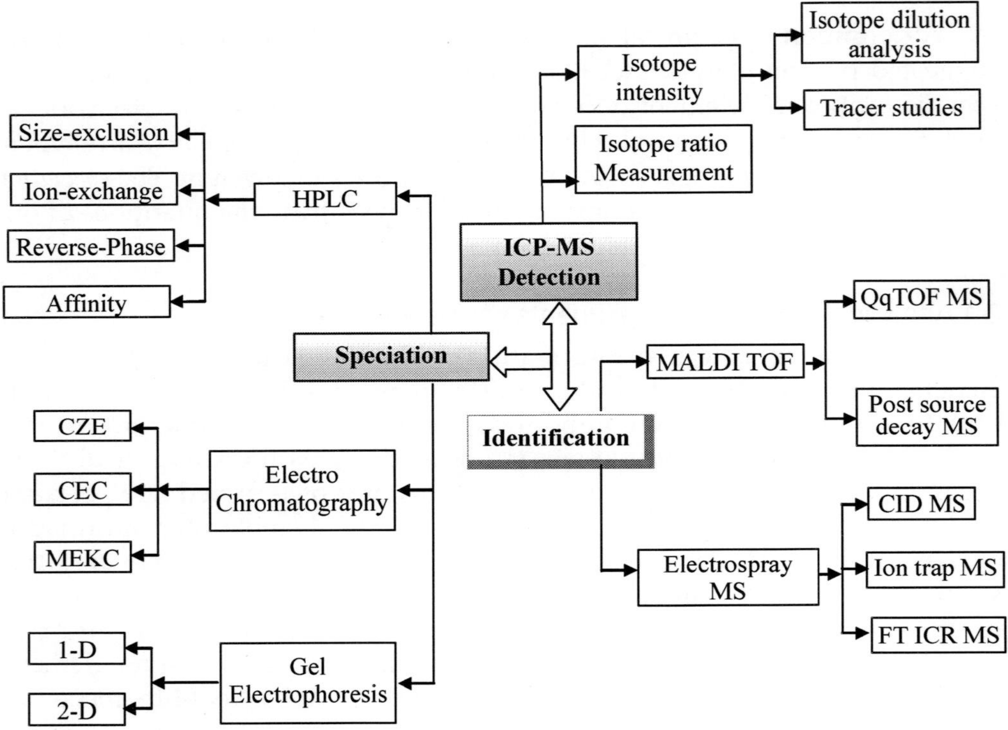

Fig. 2 : Schematic diagram for hyphenated techniques using ICP-MS detection

3.2 Arsenic and mercury speciation

More than fifty different naturally occurring arsenic (As) containing chemical species have been identified, mainly in samples from the marine environment (Francesconi *et al.*, 2004). Inorganic arsenic comprises the arsenite; As (III) and arsenate, As (V) which are readily interconverted and therefore often found together. Simple methylated arsenic species such as monomethylarsonic acid (MA), dimethylarsinic acid (DMA), trimethylarsine oxide (TMAO) and tetramethylarsonium ion (TETRA) are metabolites obtain from reduction and methylation of As(V) and are often found together (Challenger, 1945). Organo-arsenic compounds such as arsenobetaine is the predominant species in fish and crustaceans usually constituting more than 80% of the total arsenic content (Francesconi and Edmonds, 1997), whereas other species like arsenocholine (AC) and trimethylarsoniopropionate (TMAP) are usually only minor constituents in marine animals. Another group of arsenic species called arsenosugars (dimethylated and trimethylated arsenic-riboside compounds) have also been found at low concentrations in various marine animals.

A novel group of arsenic compounds have been recently discovered, namely the thioarsenicals, in which arsenic is bound to sulphur (Kahn *et al.*, 2005; Raml *et al.*, 2005). Arsenic may also be present in lipid-soluble compounds, so-called arsenolipids (Taleshi *et al.*, 2010). Analysis of fish oils for feed production showed total arsenic concentrations in the range of 9.1-13.5 mg per kg and it was estimated that approximately one third of the arsenic present in marine-based complete feedstuff can be lipid bound (Sloth *et al.*, 2005a). Inorganic As species, such as As (III) and As (V), have been classified as carcinogens and methylated forms, such as MMA and DMA have been labelled as cancer promoters. Arsenobetaine, the predominant As species in marine fish is believed to have negligible toxicity (Wrobel *et al.*, 2005; Borak and Dean Hosgood, 2007). Since seafood is the main dietary source of arsenic for humans (EFSA, 2009) as well as animals and poultry birds, speciation of this element is crucial in order to provide relevant input on both feed and food safety questions.

Mercury (Hg) is generally considered to be among the highest priority environmental pollutants on the global scale and it causes continuously concern as a contaminant in both feed and food. Mercury exists in the environment as elemental mercury (Hg^0), inorganic mercury and organic mercury (primarily methylmercury) (Horvat *et al.*, 2005). Elemental mercury is referred to as mercury vapour when present in the atmosphere or as metallic mercury when present in liquid form. It has a high vapor pressure and is slightly soluble in water. It has a high lipophilicity, which makes it dissolve easily in lipid compartments. The high affinity of Hg^{2+} to S-groups provides an explanation of the toxicity mode of action of Hg^{2+}. Interestingly the affinity for SeH groups is even higher, explaining the proposed antagonistic effect of selenium on mercury intoxication (Yoneda *et al.*, 1997). Organic mercury compounds comprise in practice alkyl-, aryl- and alkoxy-mercury compounds, where the two latter groups are labile and biodegrade relatively easy, whereas alkyl compounds are more resistant.

3.3. Selenium speciation

Selenium (Se) is an essential trace element required by both animals and humans. During last decade, the pharmaceutical market became overwhelmed with nutritional supplements or 'Nutraceuticals' based on Se. In recent years, increased research attention has focused on understanding the relationships between the Se-species content in foods and supplements and their nutritional benefits (Wrobel *et al.*, 2003) such as absorption, tissue distribution, bioavailability and disease preventive properties. It is of interest to understand which biochemical mechanisms and chemical forms of Se may give rise disease-preventive effect and so Se in feeds is currently a target for speciation studies. The identification and quantification of the elemental species, particularly Se, is crucial in understanding the metabolism of an element and its importance in biology, toxicology, clinical chemistry and nutrition. The list of identified Se compounds in foods, feeds and supplements is given below (Dumont *et al.*, 2006):

Dimethylselenide	Dimethyldiselenide
Selenate (Selenic acid)	Selenite (Selenous acid)
Trimethylselenonium ion	Se Protein
Se-containing Protein	Se-Cysteine
Se-Cystine	Se-Methionine
Se-Methyl-Se-Csyteine	Selenobetaine
Se-Homocysteine	Se-Methyl-Se-Methionine
Se-Cystamine	Se-Cystathione
Se-Cystathionine	Se-Lanthionine
γ-glutamyl-Se-Methyl-Se-Cysteine	Se-adenosyl-homocysteine

The continuous development of new and improvement of existing analytical techniques has provided different powerful tools to unravel the Se species and their function. The water soluble or insoluble and protein bound or polysaccharide bound Se compounds in yeast supplements and foods have been extracted and fractions have been analyzed by LC-ICP-MS or SEC-ICP-MS or MALDI-TOF-MS. Although it is mainly LC which has been used for the separation of Se species, some applications relied on the use of GC for the determination of volatile species. Se-Yeast is an attractive dietary supplement of Se in cows which can increase milk Se, improve antioxidant status and reproductive efficiency as well as improve health condition of calf and cow. As diverse Se compounds can be nutritional source and their chemical structures affect their absorption and distribution, Se in Se-Yeast is currently a target for speciation studies.Some of the Se species identified in yeast are Se-Methionine, Se-Cysteine, Se-Methyl-Se-Cysteine, Se-Cystine, Selenite, γ-glutamyl-Se-Methyl-Se-Cysteine, Se-Lanthionine, Se-Cystathionine (Wrobel *et al.*, 2002; Pal, 2011, Fig. 3).

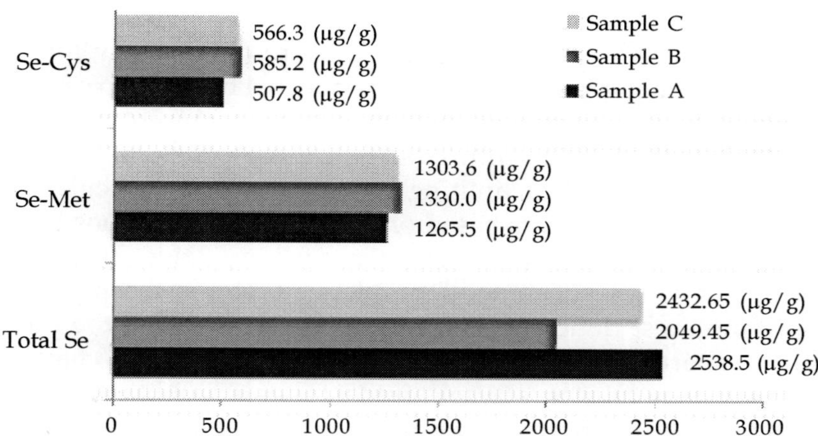

Fig. 3 : Mass balance of Se and Se species fractioned during the sample preparation and Ion Exchange Chromatography separation in yeast using detection as ^{78}Se by ICP-MS (Pal, 2011)

Speciation analysis of Se in blood comprises the determination of different proteins or amino acids which is achieved by separation of the proteins and subsequent detection of Se. In plasma Se is mainly present as selenoprotein P, glutathione peroxidise and associated to albumin. In urine Se is mainly excreted as $TMSe^+$, Se-Met, DMSe (Francesconi and Pannier, 2004) and Se-methylselenogalactosamine *etc.*, whereas in milk it is present as L-enantiomer of Se-Met (Gomez-Ariza, 2004). In the liver and kidney, cellular GPx has been detected as the carrier of endogenous Se (Chen and Berry, 2003). Selenoprotein P and Se-methyl-N-acetygalactosamine and Se-methyl-N-acetyl Se hexamine have been detected in liver tissues (Suzuki and Ogra, 2002; Suzuki, 2005).

The traditional feed control measures have only included measurement of total amounts of the above elements. However, the biological activity, mobility, bioavailability and also the toxicity of an element also depend on the chemical form in which the element is present. Thus in order to achieve correct information concerning these factors, analytical procedures that are able to distinguish between the different chemical forms are required, *i.e.* speciation analysis. Speciation studies for heavy metals and essential trace mineral elements are required to establish the links between health benefits and particular element species.

4. Mineral supplementation to animals: Recent advances

4.1 Relevance in use of area-specific mineral mixture

Traditionally, mineral mixture consisted of almost all the mineral salts were supplemented to animals irrespective of these minerals deficiency or sufficiency in the diets. This approach of mineral supplementation to animals had been found very costly and provide more opportunity for interaction and imbalances among the minerals. There may not be necessary to supplement all minerals as some of the minerals are adequately present in various feeds/fodders consumed by the animals. The most practical approach is to supplement the deficient or limiting minerals in that particular zone/area. Judicious use of mineral salts based on mineral concentrations in soil, plants and animals in different agro-climatic zones is imperative. The most practical and cost effective way of mineral supplementation is through strategically providing the most deficient minerals. In order to know the deficiency of minerals in a particular agro-climatic zone, there is a need to have a detailed survey on the mineral status in soil, feeds, fodders and blood of animals. On detailed survey throughout the whole country under All India Coordinated Research Project (AICRP), it has been found that some of the minerals are present in excess in soil, plant and animals which are not needed to supplement to animals. Hence, area-specific mineral mixture had been developed for different agro-eco zones of India which were found to be cost-effective and beneficial in terms of animal production and reproduction. Under the AICRP project, the minerals profile in soil, feeds and fodders and animals blood samples in different agro-eco zones of India has been analyzed. Also the most limiting micronutrients for animals feeding under various agro-climatic zones have been determined. Based on these mineral profiles, state-wise mineral mapping for whole country has been made (Fig. 4) and area-specific mineral mixtures are being prepared for supplementation to livestock of different agro-eco zones of the country.

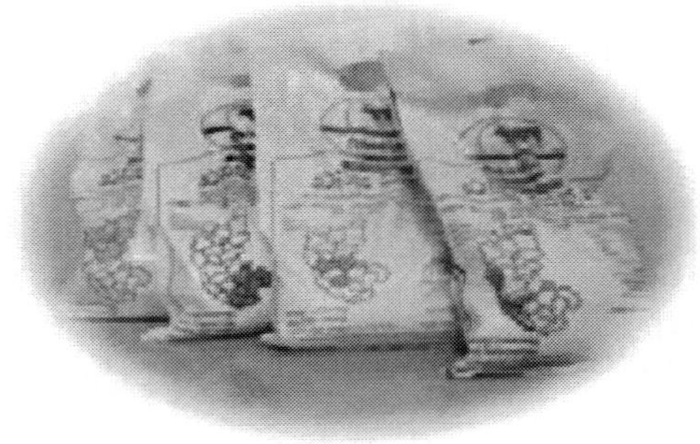

The detailed study conducted at NIANP, Bangalore at ten different agro-eco zones of Karnataka State in India has shown that the Ca, P, Cu and Zn are the most limiting minerals considering the minerals profile in soil, plant and animals in different agro-climatic zones of in state (Fig. 5). Based on these minerals profile, NIANP has developed area-specific mineral mixture, which are being used by the farmers for livestock production. Supplementary feeding with area-specific mineral mixture is able to correct the reproductive problems of animals like anestrous, repeat breeding, silent heat, conception in almost 80% of the cases (Prasad *et al.*, 2003; Prasad *et al.*, 2007). The developed technology is simple and easy to handle; it does not require huge investments and easy to adopt. The cost of feeding area-specific mineral mixture @ 40-45g per animal per day is Rs 0.65/- and works out to about Rs 230/- per animal per year and for productive life (10years) is Rs 2300/- (Prasad *et al.*, 2007). The value of saving on maintenance cost of animals by reduction in age at first calving through reduced postpartum breeding period, improvement in general health, better reproductive efficiency in terms of additional calves and the value of additional milk yield, all put together are to be at least 8 times higher than the cost of traditional mineral supplements. So, the concept of area-specific mineral mixture is cost-effective and farmer friendly approach. This technology needs popularization and commercialization.

The supplementation of area-specific mineral mixture based on minerals profile in soil, plant and animal in the region is the cost-effective way of mineral supplementation to animals. Animals can be supplemented with locally available mineral-rich feeds and fodders for providing required levels of minerals to their diets and this is the most economic and practical approach of mineral supplementation.

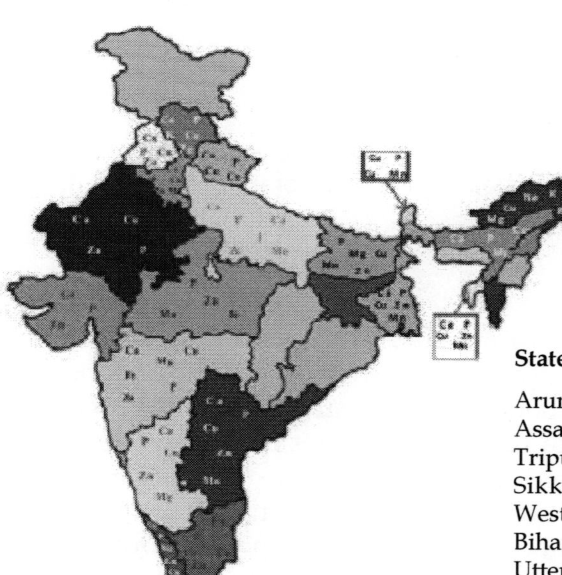

Fig. 4 : State-wise mineral mapping of India

State	Mineral deficiency
Arunachal Pradesh	Na, K, Mg, Cu, Mn
Assam	Ca, P, Mg, Cu
Tripura	Ca, P, Cu, Zn, Mn
Sikkim	Ca, P, Cu, Mn
West Bengal	Ca, P, Cu, Zn, Mn
Bihar	P, Mg, Cu, Z, Mn
Utter Pradesh	Ca, P, Cu, Zn, Mn, I
Uttaranchal	Ca, P, Cu, Co
Madhya Pradesh	P, Zn, Mn, Fe
Rajasthan	Ca, P, Cu, Zn
Gujarat	Ca, P, Zn
Punjab	Ca, P, Cu, Zn
Haryana	Ca, P, Cu, Zn, Mn
Himachal Pradesh	Ca, P, K, Cu, Zn
Maharashtra	Ca, P, Cu, Zn, Mn, Fe
Karnataka	Ca, P, Mg, Cu, Zn
Kerala	Ca, P, Mg, Cu, Zn, Mn
Tamil Nadu	Ca, P, Cu, Zn, Co
Andhra Pradesh	Ca, P, Cu, Zn, Mn

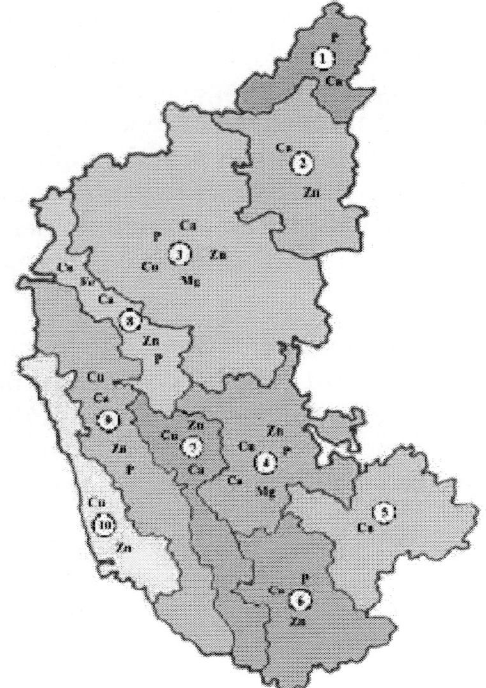

Agro-eco zones and limiting minerals in Karnataka

Agro-eco zone	Limiting minerals
1. North east transition zone	Ca, P
2. North east dry zone	Ca, Zn
3. Northern dry zone	Ca, P, Mg, Cu, Zn
4. Central dry zone	Ca, P, Mg, Cu, Zn
5. Eastern dry zone	Ca
6. Southern dry zone	Ca, P, Zn
7. Southern transition zone	Ca, Cu, Zn
8. Northern transition zone	Ca, P, Cu, Zn, Fe
9. Hilly zone	Ca, P, Cu, Zn
10. Coastal zone	Cu, Zn

Fig. 5 : Mineral mapping of Karnataka state showing mineral deficiency in different agro-climatic zones

Conclusions

Mineral elements have an important role in animal production, reproduction, health and immunity, as they are functional components of numerous metabolic events in the body. More recently, the inclusion of organic sources of mineral supplements to livestock diets has been suggested on the basis that they supply more bioavailable mineral than the inorganic forms. Adding organic mineral complexes significantly improved the animal production response (growth, milk production and reproduction). Another potential application, that is currently receiving a lot of attention, is the use of organic sources of minerals for challenging issues to sustainable agriculture by reducing the environmental pollution. Even if organic mineral sources are more bioavailable than inorganic sources, cost of the sources will be a major factor and so cost to benefit ratio is needed to be established before supplementing the minerals from organic sources. The emerging animal health importance of trace minerals and the continuing animal health challenges of trace mineral elements draw attention to the unmet need for improved biomarkers of trace element status. Currently available biomarkers of trace elements are critiqued including the outstanding lack of satisfactory biomarkers for the assessment of trace minerals intake and status. Emerging research into nutritional biomarkers will enhance our understanding, and hopefully it will also increase our precision in assessing nutritional status for a variety of dietary constituents. Ultimately having good biomarkers of nutritional intake and status is of considerable importance for animal health and clinical practice. The emergence of new molecular techniques is especially promising for the development of a new generation of biomarkers. Gene expression-based biomarker development still poses a major challenge. The understanding of the mechanisms of biological activities and biotransformation of trace elements such as arsenic and mercury has improved during recent years with the help of chemical speciation studies. However, the most important practical application of elemental speciation is in the area of toxicology. Toxicological knowledge on the individual trace element species can lead to more specific legislation of hazardous substances found in feed. Further, disease-preventive and nutritional health- benefits effects of elemental species has now the area of strong interest. Hence, speciation analysis is required to obtain a correct risk assessment regarding trace elements in feed. There is a need for methods for future monitoring and control of heavy metals in both food and feed. At last, proper mineral supplementation is essentially required for optimum production and reproduction in animals and in this regard most practical approach of mineral supplementation is through area-specific mineral mixture and through locally available mineral-rich feeds and fodders to animals.

References

AAFCO. (1998). Official publication of the association of American feed control officials incorporated (P. M. Bachman, ed). pp 237-238.

Allan A.K., Hawskworth G.M., Woodhouse L.R., Sutherland B., King J.C., Beattie, J.H. (2000). Lymphocute metallothionein mRNA responds to marginal zinc intake in human volunteers. *British Journal of Nutrition* **84:** 747-756.

Ashmead H.D. (1993). Comparative intestinal absorption and subsequent metabolism of metal amino acid chelates and inorganic metal salts. In: *The roles of amino acid chelates in animal nutrition*. Noyes Publishers, New Jersey, pp 306-319.

Ballantine H.T., Socha M.T., Tomlinson D.J., Johnson A.B., Fielding A.S., Shearer J.K., Van Amstel S. R. (2002). Effects of feeding complexed zinc, manganese, copper, and cobalt to late gestation and lactating dairy cows on claw integrity, reproduction, and lactation performance. *Professional Animal Scientist* **18:** 211.

Bertinato J., Iskandar M., L'Abbe M.R. (2003). Copper deficiency induces the upregulation of the copper chaperone for Cu/Zn superoxide dismutase in weanling male rats. *Journal of Nutrition* **133:** 28-31.

Bertinato J., Swist E., Plouffe L.J., Brooks S.P., L'abbé M.R. (2008). Ctr2 is partially localized to the plasma membrane and stimulates copper uptake in COS-7 cells. *Biochemical Journal* **409:** 731-740.

Blezinger S. (2000). Bioavailability of minerals in cattle is an important concern. In: *Cattle Today* online: *htpp//www. cattletoday.com*

Boland M.P., O'Donnell G., O'Callaghan D. (1996). The contribution of mineral proteinates to production and reproduction in dairy cattle. In: *Biotechnology in the feed industry*. (T.P. Lyons and K. Jacques, eds). Nottingham University Press, Nottingham, UK, p 95.

Borak J., Dean Hosgood H. (2007). Seafood arsenic: implications for human risk assessment. *Regulatory Toxicology and Pharmacology* **47:** 204-212.

Carlson M.S., Boren C.A., Wu C., Huntington C.E., Bollinger D.W., Veum T.L. (2004). Evaluation of various inclusion rates of organic zinc either as polysaccharide or proteinate complex on the growth performance, plasma, and excretion of nursery pigs. *Journal of Animal Science* **82:** 1359.

Cater M.A., Mercer J.F.B. (2005). Copper in mammals: Mechanisms of homeostasis and pathophysiology. In: *Molecular biology of metal homeostasis and detoxification: Topics in current genetics.* No. 14. (M. J. Tamás and E. Martinoia, eds). Springer Verlag, Berlin, Germany, pp 101-129.

Challenger F. (1945). Biological methylation. *Chemical Reviews* **36:** 315-361.

Chen C.Y., Berry M.J. (2003). Selenium and selenoproteins in the brain and brain diseases. *Journal of Neurochemistry* **86:** 1-12.

Collins J.F., Franck C.A., Kowdley K.V., Ghishan F. K. (2005). Identification of differentially expressed genes in response to dietary iron deprivation in rat duodenum. *American Journal of Physiology, Gastrointestinal and Liver Physiology* **288:** G964-G971.

Cousins R.J., Liuzzi J.P, Lichten L.A. (2006). Mammalian zinc transport, trafficking, and signals. *The Journal of Biological Chemistry* **281:** 24085-24089.

Dumay Q.C., Debut A.J., Mansour N.M., Saier Jr. M.H. (2006). The copper transporter (Ctr) family of Cu^{+} uptake systems. *Journal of Molecular Microbiology and Biotechnology* **11:** 10-19.

Dumont E., Vanhaecke F., Cornelis R. (2006). Selenium speciation from food source to metabolites: A critical review. *Analytical and Bioanalytical Chemistry* **385:** 1304-1323.

EFSA. (2009). Scientific opinion on arsenic in food. *EFSA Journal* **7:** 1351-1550.

Feillet-Coudray C., Coudray C., Bayle D., Rock E., Rayssiguier Y., Mazur A. (2000). Response of diamine oxidase and other plasma copper biomarkers to various dietary copper intakes in the rat and evaluation of copper absorption with a stable isotope. *British Journal of Nutrition* **83:** 561-568.

Francesconi K., Pannier F. (2004). Selenium metabolites in urine: a critical overview of past work and current status. *Clinical Chemistry* **50:** 2240-2253.

Francesconi K.A., Edmonds J.S. (1997). Arsenic and marine organisms. *Advances in Inorganic Chemistry* **44:** 147-189.

Francesconi K.A., Kuehnelt D. (2004). Determination of arsenic species: a critical review of methods and applications, 2000-2003. *Analyst* **129:** 373 – 395.

Gibson R.S., Hess S.Y., Hotz C., Brown K.H. (2008). Indicators of zinc status at the population level: a review of the evidence. *British Journal of Nutrition* **99:** S14-S23.

Gomez-Ariza J.L., Barnal-Daza V., Villegas-Portero M.J. (2004). Comparative study of the instrumental couplings of high performance liquid chromatography with microwave-assisted digestion hydride generation atomic fluorescence spectrometry and inductively coupled plasma mass spectrometry for chiral speciation of selenomethionine in breast and formula milk. *Analytica Chimica Acta* **520:** 229-235.

Gonz´alez-Guerrero M., Arguello J.M. (2008). Mechanism of Cu+-transporting ATPases: soluble Cu+ chaperones directly transfer Cu+ to transmembrane transport sites. *Proceedings of the National Academy of Sciences, USA* **105:** 5992-5997.

Gowda N.K.S., Ramana J.V., Prasad C.S., Singh K. (2004). Micronutrient content of certain tropical conventional and unconventional feed resources of Southern India. *Tropical Animal Health and Production* **36:** 77-94.

Hansen S.L., Ashwell M.S., Legleiter L.R., Fry R.S., Lloyd K.E., Spears J.W. (2009). The addition of high manganese to a copper-deficient diet further depresses copper status and growth of cattle. *British Journal of Nutrition* **101:** 1068-1078.

Harmon R.J. (2000). When are chelated minerals justified? *Kentucky Ruminant Nutrition.* 47-54.

Harmon R.J., Trammell D.S., Smith B.A., Scaletti R.W. (1998). Effects of dietary copper insufficiency and sources of dietary copper on copper status and intramammary infections at calving. *Journal of Dairy Science* **81** (Suppl.1): 43.

Hedegaard R.V., Sloth J.J. (2011). Speciation of arsenic and mercury in feed: why and how? *Biotechnology Agronomy Society and Environment* **15**(S1): 45-51.

Helston R.M., Phillips S.R., McKay J.A., Jackson K.A., Mathers J.C., Ford D. (2007). Zinc transporters in the mouse placenta show a coordinated regulatory response to changes in dietary zinc intake. *Placenta* **28:** 437-444.

Henry P.R., Ammerman C.B., Littell R.C. (1992). Relative bioavailability of manganese from a manganese-methionine complex and inorganic sources for ruminants. *Journal of Dairy Science* **75:** 3473-3478.

Hepburn J.J., Arthington J.D., Hansen S.L., Spears J.W., Knutson M.D. (2009). Technical note: copper chaperone for copper, zinc superoxide dismutase: a potential biomarker for copper status in cattle. *Journal of Animal Science* **87:** 4161-4166.

Hill G.M., Link J.E. (2009). Transporters in the absorption and utilization of zinc and copper. *Journal of Animal Science* **87:** E85-E89.

Horvat M., Gibièar D. (2005). Speciation of mercury: environment, food, clinical and occupational health. *In: Handbook of elemental speciation II* (R.Cornelis, ed), Wiley, Chichester, UK.

Iskandar M., Swist E., D. Trick K.D., Wang B., L'Abbé M.R., Bertinato J. (2005).Copper chaperone for Cu/Zn superoxide dismutase is a sensitive biomarker of mild copper deficiency induced by moderately high intakes of zinc. *Nutrition Journal* **4:** 35.

Jerry W.S. (1996). Organic trace minerals in ruminant nutrition. *Animal Feed Science and Technology* **58:** 151-163.

Kahn M. (2005). Two novel thio-arsenosugars in scallops identified with HPLC-ICPMS and HPLCESMS. *Environmental Chemistry* **2:** 171-176.

Kellog D.W. (1990). Zinc methionine affects performance of lactating cows. *Feedstuffs* **62:** 15-20.

Kessler J., Morel I., Dufey F.A., Gutzwiller A., Stern A., Geyes H. (2003). Effect of organic zinc sources on performance, zinc status, and carcass, meat, and claw quality in fattening bulls. *Livestock Production Science* **81:** 161-171.

Kim B.E., Nevitt T., Thiele D. J (2008). Mechanisms for copper acquisition, distribution and regulation. *Nature Chemical Biology* **4:** 176-185.

Kincaid R.L. (1999). Assessment of trace mineral status of ruminant: A review. In: *Proceedings of the American Society of Animal Science,* pp 1-10.

Linder M.C., Hazegh-Azam M. (1996).Copper biochemistry and molecular biology. *American Journal of Clinical Nutrition* **63:** 797S-811S.

Lobinsky R. (1997). Elemental speciation and coupled techniques. *Applied Spectroscopy* **51:** 260-278.

Martinez M.M. (2004). Effects of pharmacological zinc and phytase supplementation on metallothionein, hepatic differential gene expression, zinc transporter-1, mineral excretion, and apparent retention in newly weaned pigs. *PhD Dissertation,* Michigan State University, East Lansing, USA.

Martinez M.M., Link J.E., Hill G.M. (2005). Dietary pharmacological or excess zinc and phytase effects on tissue mineral concentrations, metallothionein, and apparent mineral retention in the newly weaned pig. *Biological Trace Element Research* **105:** 97-115.

Maxfield A.B., Heaton D.N., Winge D.R. (2004). Cox17 is functional when tethered to the mitochondrial inner membrane. *Journal of Biological Chemistry* **279:** 5072-5080.

McDowell L.R. (1992). Minerals in animal and human nutrition. Academic Press, New York.

Mills C.F. (1987). Biochemical and physiological indicators of mineral status in animals: copper, cobalt and zinc. *Journal of Animal Science* **65:** 1702-1711.

Milne D.B. (1998). Copper intake and assessment of copper status. *American Journal of Clinical Nutrition* **67:** 1041S-1045S.

Nocek J.E., Patton R.S. (2002). Effect of chelated trace mineral supplementation for inorganic sources on production and health of Holstein cows. *Journal of Dairy Science* **85** (*Suppl.1*): 107.

O'Halloran T.V., Culotta V.C. (2000). Metallochaperones, an intracellular shuttle service for metal ions. *The Journal of Biological Chemistry* **275:** 25057-25060.

Pal D.T. (2011). Identification of Selenium species in selenium-enriched yeast and their quantification by ion-exchange chromatography-inductively coupled plasma mass spectrometry. NAIP Report, pp 1-34.

Pal D.T., Gowda N.K.S., Prasad C.S., Amarnath R., Bellur S.R., Sampath K.T. (2010). Effect of copper- and zinc-methionine supplementation on bioavailability, mineral status, tissue concentrations of copper and zinc in ewe. *Journal of Trace Elements in Medicine and Biology* **24:** 89-94.

Pal D.T., Gowda N.K.S., Prasad C.S., Sampath K.T. (2011). Evaluation of copper- and zinc-dependent metalloenzymes as biomarkers of copper and zinc status in sheep (unpublished).

Pal D.T., Singh Pramod., Prasad C.S., Sampath K.T. (2011). Minerals release kinetics in the rumen from five commonly available dry fodders. *Indian Journal of Animal Sciences* **81:** 954-960.

Petris M.J., Smith K., Lee J., Thiele D.J. (2003). Copper-stimulated endocytosis and degradation of the human transporter, hCtr1. *Journal of Biological Chemistry* **278:** 9639-9646.

Power R., Horgan K. (2000). Biological chemistry and absorption of inorganic and organic trace metals. In: *Biotechnology in the Feed Industry.* (T.P. Lyons and K. A. Jacques, eds.), Nottingham University Press, Nottingham, UK, pp 277-291.

Prasad C.S., Pal D.T., Gowda N.K.S. (2007). Area-Specific mineral mixture for increased animal productivity. *Indian Farming* **8:** 53-54.

Prasad C.S., Gowda N.K.S., Pal D.T. (2003). Mineral: Importance with special reference to tropical animal husbandry practice. *Indian Journal of Dairy and Biosciences* **14:** 61-67.

Prasad C.S., Gowda N.K.S., Pal D.T. (2003). Supplementation of minerals in the ration of animals and significance of developing area specific mineral salts. In: Workshop on *"Feeding strategies for efficient utilization of existing resources to reduce cost of milk production"* organized by NDDB, Anand, Gujarat, India on 19-20 November 2003.

Prasad C.S., Pal D.T., Gowda N.K.S., Amarnath R. (2006). Inorganic and organic sources of copper and zinc supplementation on wool growth and tissue availability in sheep. In: *Prceedings of VI Biennial Conference of Animal Nutrition Association on 'Strengthening animal nutrition research for food security, environment protection and poverty alleviation'*, Jammu, J&K, India, p 125.

Prasad C.S., Pal D.T., Gowda N.K.S., Amarnath R. (2006). Inorganic and organic sources of Cu and Zn supplementation on wool and tissue availability in sheep. In: VI th Biennial Animal Nutrition Association Conference on *"Strengthening animal nutrition research for food safety, environment protection and poverty alleviation"* held at Sher-e-Kashmir University of Agricultural Science & Technology, Jammu, 15-17 September, 2006.

Prohaska J.R. (2008). Role of copper transporters in copper homeostasis. *The American Journal of Clinical Nutrition* **88:** 826S-829S.

Prohaska J.R., Broderius M., Brokate B. (2003). Metallochaperone for Cu,Zn-superoxide dismutase (CCS) protein but not mRNA is higher in organs from copper-deficient mice and rats. *Archives of Biochemistry and Biophysics* **417:** 227-234.

Raml R., Goessler W., Traar P., Ochi T., Francesconi K.A. (2005). Novel thioarsenic metabolites in human urine after ingestion of an arsenosugar,2′,3′-dihydroxypropyl 5-deoxy-5-dimethylarsinoylbeta-D-riboside. *Chemical Research in Toxicology* **18:** 1444-1450.

Rutherford J.C., Bird A.J. (2004). Metal-responsive transcription factors that regulate iron, zinc, and copper homeostasis in eukaryotic cells. *Eukaryotic Cell* **3:** 1-13.

Sanz-Medel A. (1998a). Trace element analytical speciation in biological systems: importance, challenges and trends. *Spectrochimica Acta, Part. B* **53:** 197.

Sanz-Medel A. (1998b). Toxic trace metal speciation: importance and tools for environmental and biological analysis. *Pure and Applied Chemistry* **70:** 2281-2285.

Sloth J.J., Julshamn K., Lundebye A.K. (2005a). Total and inorganic arsenic content in Norwegian fish feed products. *Aquaculture Nutrition* **11:** 61-66.

Spears J.W. (2003). Trace mineral bioavailability in ruminants. *Journal of Nutrition* **133:** 1506S.

Spears J.W. (1989). Zinc methionine for ruminants: Relative bioavailability of zinc in lambs and effects of growth and performance of growing heifers. *Journal of Animal Science* **67:** 835.

Spears J.W., Kegley E.B. (2002). Effect of zinc source (zinc oxide vs zinc proteinate) and level on performance, carcass characteristics, and immune response of growing and finishing steers. *Journal of Animal Science* **80:** 2747-2752.

Sun J.Y., Wang J.F., Zi N.T., Jing M.Y., Weng X.Y. (2007). Gene expression profiles analysis of the growing rat liver response to different zinc status by cdna microarray analysis. *Biological Trace Element Research* **115:** 169-185.

Suzuki K.T. (2005). Metabolomics of selenium: Se metabolites based on speciation studies. *Journal of Health Science* **51:** 107-114.

Suzuki K.T., Ogra Y. (2002). Metabolic pathway for selenium in the body: speciation by HPLC-ICP MS with enriched S., *Food Additives and Contaminants* **19:** 974-983.

Taleshi MS, Edmonds JS, Goessler W, Ruiz-Chancho MJ, Raber G, Jensen KB, Francesconi KA (2010). Arsenic-containing lipids are natural constituents of sashimi tuna. *Environmental Science and Technology* **44:** 1478-1483.

Templeton D.M. et al. {2000). Guidelines for terms related to chemical speciation and fractionation of elements. Definitions, structural aspects, and methodological approaches. *Pure Applied Chemistry* **72:** 1453-1470.

Tom Dieck H., Doring F., Fuchs D., Roth H.P., Daniel H. (2005). Transcriptome and proteome analysis identifies the pathways that increase hepatic lipid accumulation in zinc-deficient rats. *Journal of Nutrition* **134:** 1716-1723.

Uchida J., Mandebvu P., Ballard C.S., Sniffen C.J, Carter M.P. (2001). Effect of feeding a combination of zinc, manganese, and copper amino acid complexes, and cobalt glucoheptanate on performance of early lactation high producing dairy cows. *Animal Feed Science and Technology* **93:** 193.

Van Bakel H., Srengman E., Wijmenga C., Holstege F.C. (2005). Gene expression profiling and phenotype analyses of S. cerevisiae in response to changing copper reveals six genes with new roles in copper and iron metabolism. *Physiological Genomics* **22:** 356-367.

van den Berghe P.V., Folmer D.E., Malingre H.E. (2007). Human copper transporter 2 is localized in late endosomes and lysosomes and facilitates cellular copper uptake. *Biochemical Journal* **407:** 49-59.

van Ommen B., Fairweather-Tait S., Freidg A., Kardinaal A., Scalbert A., Wopereis S. (2008). A network biology model of micronutrient related health. *British Journal of Nutrition* **99:** S72-S80.

Veum T.L., Carlson M.S., Wu C.W., Bollinger D.W., Ellersieck M.R. (2004). Copper proteinate in weanling pig diets for enhancing growth performance and reducing fecal copper excretion compared with copper sulfate. *Journal of Animal Science* **82:** 1062.

Ward J.D., Spears J.W., Kegley E.B. (1996). Bioavailability of copper proteinate and copper carbonate relative to copper sulfate in cattle. *Journal of Dairy Science* **79:** 127.

West E.C., Prohaska J.R. (2004). Cu,Zn-superoxide dismutase is lower and copper chaperone CCS is higher in erythrocytes of copper-deficient rats and mice. *Experimental Biology and Medicine (Maywood)* **229:** 756-764.

Wright, C. L., Spears, J. W. (2004). Effect of zinc source and dietary level on zinc metabolism in Holstein calves. *Journal of Dairy Science* **87:** 1085-1091.

Wrobel K., Kannamkumarath S.S., Caruso J.A. (2003). Hydrolysis of proteins with methanesulfonic acid for improved HPLC-ICP-MS determination of seleno-methionine in yeast and nuts. *Analytical and Bioanalytical Chemistry* **375:** 133.

Wrobel K., Wrobel K., Caruso J.A. (2002). Selenium speciation in low molecular weight fraction of Se-enriched yeasts by HPLC-ICP-MS: detection of selenoadeno-sylmethionine. *Journal of Analytical and Atomic Spectrometry* **17:** 1048-1054.

Wrobel K., Wrobel K., Caruso J.A. (2005). Pretreatment procedures for characterization of arsenic and selenium species in complex samples utilizing coupled techniques with mass spectrometric detection. *Analytical and Bioanalytical Chemistry* **381:** 317-331.

Yoneda S., Suzuki K.T. (1997). Equimolar Hg-Se complex binds to selenoprotein P. *Biochemical and Biophysical Research Communications* **231:** 7-11.

Yu Y.Y., Kirschke C.P., Huang L. (2007). Immunohistochemical analysis of ZnT1, 4, 5, 6, and 7 in the mouse gastrointestinal tract. *Journal of Histochemistry and Cytochemistry* **55:** 223-234.

❑❑❑

Chapter **3**

Genetic Manipulation of Rumen Ecosystem for Improved Utilization of Crop Residues in Ruminants : Problems and Potentials

M. Chandrasekharaiah, A. Thulasi, K.T. Sampath
National Institute of Animal Nutrition and Physiology, Adugodi, Bangalore-560 030 Karnataka, India

Summary

Livestock production system in developing countries including India is mainly based on crop residues and agricultural by products. Despite their availability in huge quantities, these crop residues are poorly utilized by the ruminants because of unbalanced nutrient profile. Several methods tried to improve the utilization of these crop residues have met with varying degrees of success. One of the approaches is the genetic manipulation of rumen ecosystem through construction of genetically modified organisms (GMOs), which is gaining momentum in recent years. However, the practical application of these approaches through genetic manipulation of rumen ecosystem to increase utilization of crop residues go a long way and awaits development of suitable gene transfer systems and the major technical difficulties needs to be addressed before the results of these basic studies find their way to application aspect. Though there are speculations and doubts about the success of these technologies and their practical and economic significance, the efforts need to be continued in this direction, by integrating the knowledge of emerging molecular biology techniques with nutritional principles since our livestock production system is predominantly based on crop residues. Therefore, this chapter discusses mainly the potential of genetic manipulation of rumen microbial ecosystem utilising the recent molecular biology methods developed for manipulation of rumen microbes for improved utilization of crop residues.

The ruminants are fed mainly on crop residues, pastures, straws and stovers in developing countries including India. The utilization of these crop residues are very poor leading to low productivity of ruminants. Efforts are being made worldwide to make use of these low quality feeds more efficiently for improved livestock production. Several methods used to manipulate rumen ecosystem by altering feeding patterns, altering the site of digestion of nutrients by physical or chemical treatments, incorporation of feed addivitives, probiotocs, enzymes and plant extracts have met with varying degree of success. The biotechnological approach for improving the digestion of crop residues employs the genetic manipulation of the rumen microorganisms. Nutritionists and microbiologists have long been interested in manipulating the microbial ecosystem of the rumen to enhance feed utilization, improve production efficiency and alleviate problems associated with current feeding process. Ruminants have adapted to a variety of ecological niches because of diverse rumen microbial populations, which consist primarily of bacteria, fungi and protozoa. These animals have the ability to convert low quality feeds into high quality protein. This is due to the fact that rumen microbes synthesize β $(1 \rightarrow 4)$ cellulase enzyme complex that hydrolyses plant cell walls. If a greater percentage of the total dietary energy from forages is available to ruminants, low cost diets could be formulated and environmental resources would be used more efficiently.

1. Rumen microbial ecosystem

The Hungate roll tube technique was developed fifty years ago for the enumeration and cultivation of strict anaerobic rumen bacteria (Hungate, 1950). The success of this technique had a significant impact on microbiology in general and saw that a new area of microbiology was opened. Hungate's appreciation of the need to simulate the natural ecology of microbial ecosystems and his demonstration of strict anaerobiosis opened up the entire area of anaerobic microbiology. The rumen, whose gut community has been extensively studied, contains bacteria (up to 10^{11} viable cells/ml comprising approximately 200 species), ciliate protozoa (10^{4}-10^{6}/ml spread over 25 genera), anaerobic rumen fungi (Zoospore densities of 10^{3}-10^{5}/ml comprised of 5 genera) and bacteriophages (10^{8}-10^{9}/ml). Despite this information the enumeration and identification of community members have tremendous limitations, as there is no complete phylogenetic classification of the rumen microbes (Kamra, 2005). More information has been obtained these days by the application of the molecular biology techniques to the study of rumen ecology.

2. Rumen ecology, phylogenetics and taxonomy

It is necessary to understand the factors controlling rumen microbial activity to modify the rumen ecology and create conditions that will optimize the use of poor quality roughages by ruminant livestock. The simplest way to improve rumen function in an animal is to introduce digestion-enhancing bacterial species from other animals or to selectively increase populations of species that inhabit the rumen only at low levels.

Understanding the microbiological transformations that occur in the rumen has also explained much about the nature of ruminal fermentation and the way it affects ruminant nutrition. The physiological importance of volatile fatty acid (VFA) production by the ruminal microorganisms to the nutrition of the host was established early (Barcroft *et al.*, 1944); the mechanisms by which the fermentation acids are produced are for the most part similar to those established for non-ruminal bacteria (Russell and Wallace, 1988). A few species of bacteria, protozoa, and fungi carryout cellulolysis, and a more diverse population can hydrolyse starch and sugars (Stewart and Bryant, 1988). Protein is wasted by hydrolysis in the rumen because the rumen microorganisms use amino acids for energy production as well as for protein synthesis (Broderick *et al.*, 1991; Russell *et al.*, 1991). Ciliate protozoa are not essential for the fermentation, but their activity may be considered beneficial or detrimental to nutrition depending on the animal's nutritional status (Williams and Coleman, 1998). There are many other examples whereby an appreciation of microbiological events in the rumen has influenced nutritional practices.

Bacteria from one ruminant species have been shown to colonize others successfully. It has been demonstrated that the cross-inoculation of rumen fluid from wild to domestic ruminants alleviates tannin toxicity and enhances the productivity of livestock browsing tannin containing shrubs (MacMillan, 1996). Molecular methods are available to track individual organisms within complex mixtures when microbes are transferred between animal species. Without precise and quantitative tracking systems, the effectiveness of any particular organism within the microbial community in the rumen cannot be demonstrated. However, as the majority of the rumen microbes have not been isolated and characterized, it is essential to isolate them, characterize and study their taxonomy and *phylogenetics.*

2.1 Rumen bacteria

The rumen harbours various types of bacteria which are active in degradation of the components of the feed *viz.*, cellulose, hemicellulose, lignin, starch, protein and a very small quantity of oils. The interaction among themselves and with other microbial groups in the rumen is also responsible for synergistic effect on the production of VFA and microbial proteins in the rumen. Some of the common features of bacteria found in the rumen of animals fed on high roughage diet (Kamra, 2005) are as follows:

- Majority of the bacteria are gram-negative. The number of gram-positive bacteria tends to increase on increasing high energy diets in the ration.
- Most of the bacteria are obligate anaerobes. Some of them are so sensitive to oxygen that these are killed on exposure to oxygen. A few rumen

bacteria require a very low redox potential (indicating a high degree of anaerobiosis) and grow at a redox potential lower than -350 mV.

- The optimum pH for the growth of rumen bacteria lies between 6.0 and 6.9.
- The optimum temperature is 39°C.
- The bacteria can tolerate a considerably higher level of organic acids without affecting adversely their metabolism.

The bacteria such as *Ruminococcus albus, R.flavefaciens, Fibrobacter succinogenes, Butyrivibrio fibrisolvens, Clostridium lochheadii, C. Longisporu, Bacteroides amylophilus, Ruminococcus bromii* and *Selenomonas ruminantium* were isolated from the rumen of Indian cattle and buffaloes (Panjarathinum and Laxminarayana, 1977; Jalaludin *et al.*, 1992; Sinha and Ranganathan, 1983, Singh *et al.*, 2003) including a newly described bacterium, *Cellulosilyticum ruminicola* H1 isolated from yak (*Bos grunniens*) rumen and is characterized by its ability to grow on a variety of hemicelluloses and degrade cellulosic materials (Cai *et al.*, 2010). This bacterium appears to produce polymer hydrolases that act on both soluble and crystal celluloses.

The total viable bacterial count and the proportion of cellulytic, amylolytic, proteolytic and lipolytic bacteria were enumerated in the rumen fluid of steers fed maintenance rations on rations with different proportions of finger millet straw, para grass and concentrate mixtures. It was observed that the amylolytic bacteria were consistently predominant in all the feeding regimens irrespective of time of sampling. The peak values of cellulytic bacteria were obtained at 16 hours after feeding where as the peak values of amylolytic and proteolytic bacteria were obtained at 8 hours after feeding. *Streptococcus bovis* was the numerically predominant bacteria obtained followed by *Ruminococcus albus, R. flavefaciens, Fibrofactor succinogenes* and *Butyrivibrio fibrosolvens* which were cellulolytic bacteria isolated and *prevotella ruminicola* was the predominant proteolytic bacteria obtained in this study (Chandrasekharaiah *et al.*, 2003; 2009).

2.2 Rumen fungi

The gut fungi are an unusual group of zoosporic fungi occupying a unique ecological niche, the anaerobic environment of the rumen. They exhibit two basic forms, with nuclear migration throughout the hyphal mass for polycentric species and with concentration of nuclear material in a zoosporangium for monocentric species. (Brookman *et al.*, 2000). The presence of large fungal populations in animals consuming pasture or diets largely composed of hay or straw together with the production of highly active fibre degrading enzymes lead to the belief that anaerobic fungi may have a significant role to play in the assimilation of fibrous feeds by ruminants. The extent of the contribution of anaerobic fungi to the nutrition of ruminants has also been established through studies of fungal populations in the rumen and the dietary factors that influence them (Gordon and Philips, 1998).

Anaerobic fungi play an important role in the degradation of carbohydrates in the rumen. The process starts with the attachment of fungal zoospores to plant carbohydrates. Fungal xylanases and cellulases may be extra cellular or associated with the cell wall or cytosolic fractions of the organism. A range of hydrolytic activities are associated with a high molecular mass protein complex secreted by some fungal species, which may act synergistically with enzymes secreted by other species. Fungi interact with protozoa and bacteria in the rumen. Large protozoa and some bacteria inhibit fungal growth and metabolism. However, some bacteria may stimulate fungal activity. Fungi have important roles in hydrolyzing complex carbohydrates and phenolic polymers in fibrous feeds (Stewart *et al.,* 1995).

3. Development of gene transfer systems for rumen microbes

The development of a gene transfer system is of great importance to genetically modify the rumen bacteria. To develop a gene transfer systems, it is essential to isolate a native plasmids of the existing bacteria for gene analysis and manipulation. At present many plasmids have been isolated from rumen bacteria these plasmids could be used for the construction of shuttle vectors gene manipulation. These systems are now being developed and refined for prominent species of ruminal bacteria (Forsberg *et al.,* 1997; Forsberg *et al.,* 1999; Chandrasekharaiah *et al.,* 2000). Though bacteriophages have also been discovered and studied in the rumen, none have been used for gene transfer. Plasmids isolated from the rumen bacteria have a size of 1.4 – 8 kb which lacks an antibiotic marker. Since antibiotic markers are not present, these regions from other sources are used for the construction of chimeric shuttle vectors and can be used for introduction of genes of interest into a desired host (Forano and Flint, 2000). Novel genes have been introduced into rumen bacteria and genetically modified organisms have been obtained. The DNA of interest is ligated into the vector and introduced into the host by transformation or mating and antibiotic selection. The expression of the genes in the new host was depends on the functionality of the indigenous promoter or another sequence to substitute for the promoter (Forsberg *et al.,* 1999). It has been observed that *Ruminococcus flavefaciens* and *Ruminococcus albus* posses a multi enzyme system for fibre degradation. The enzyme system comprises a cellulosome like structure as observed in *Clostridium thermocellum* (Miron *et al.,* 2001). The cellulase and hemicellulase activity can be improved by amplifying the specific genes in the host organism and by recognizing the promoter region to this gene. It is possible to introduce novel genes into different bacteria with electroporation. Xylanase and endoglucanase genes have been introduced in *Prevotella ruminicola* (Whitehead and Hespell, 1990) and *Streptococcus bovis* (Whitehead and Flint, 1995). When xylanase gene was introduced in *Butyrivibrio fibrisolvens* as a host, the enzyme was expressed and secreted through manipulation of promoter and signal peptide. Most of the work on improvement of fibre digestion by biotechnological approach is still at the initial *in vitro* stage only. The success of improving the fibre digestibility in the rumen depends upon the development of suitable gene transfer, gene regulation and stability of genetically modified organisms (GMOs).

3.1 Gene transfer systems utilizing Butyrivibrio

Teather, (1982) isolated and identified a large extra chromosomal super coiled DNA (250 mega Daltons) from *B. fibrisolvens* ATIC 19177. Mann *et al.*, (1986) isolated a plasmid from *B. fibrisolvens,* designated it as pOM1 and used for the construction of shuttle vectors with various *E. coli* plasmids. Though the construction of shuttle vectors was successful, these constructs were not stable after transformation and sub-culturing in *E. coli.* The sequence analysis of pOM1 revealed that the plasmid replicates via the rolling mechanism (Hefford *et al.*, 1997).

A cryptic plasmid was also isolated from *B. fibrisolvens* strain AR10 (Ware *et al.*, 1992). This plasmid, pBF1 does not appear to encode for any antibiotic resistant gene and no sequence data is available to assist in the identification of replication origin. Hefford *et al.* (1993), have reported the isolation of a number of small cryptic plasmids from *Butyrivibrio* isolates from wild deer. Many of the isolates of *Butyrivibrio* contained one or more distinct plasmids. One of these plasmids, pRJFI has been sequenced and used in the construction of shuttle vectors (Beard *et al.*, 1995).

Hespell and Whitehead, (1991) reported the introduction of heterologus plasmid, pAMb1 and transposon Tn916 and Tn916 E into *B fibrisolvens* by conjugal transfer. This transfer was the first to demonstrate that genes conferring antibiotic resistance from non-ruminant bacteria could be expressed in ruminant bacteria and could be used as marker genes for selection of recombinants.

3.2 Stability of gene transfer system

Most of the bacteria are equipped with restriction enzymes. Restriction enzymes are sequence specific endonucleases that recognize foreign DNA molecules that invade bacterial cell cytoplasm (*e.g.*, phage DNA). In some bacteria cognate modification systems are responsible for methylating self-DNA with the same recognition sequence, protecting it from endonucleolytic cleavage (Forsberg *et al.*, 1999). Restriction enzymes have been characterized for *B. fibrisolvens, Fibrobacter succinogenes, Ruminococcus albus, R. flavefaciens, Selenomonas ruminantium and Streptococcus bovis.* In *F. succinogenes,* the restriction enzymes were found to be highly active non specific endonucleases which have a deleterious influence on the efficiency of gene transfer by transformation/electroporation. These facts partially explain the difficulty in developing a gene transfer system for *F. succinogenes.*

The stability and expression of transferred genes in the rumen is complicated by the following (Varga and Kolver, 1997) factors:

- Maintenance of the plasmid within the bacteria;
- Metabolic burden of the plasmid on the host bacterium;
- Integration of the inserted gene into the chromosome of the host organism;
- A possible requirement of post translational modification of the gene product;
- A requirement for DNA sequences to encode for the export of proteins synthesized by the new gene: and
- The most important hurdle is the successful establishment of these modified bacteria in the rumen, given the various interactions and cross feeding that occur among the rumen species.

4. Fiber digesting enzyme genes in rumen microbes

Different genes have been isolated from the rumen bacteria and fungi and have been characterized. Over 100 different genes encoding enzymes for fibre digestion have been identified and cloned from ruminal bacteria such as *B. fibrisolvens, F. succinogenes, P. ruminicola, R. albus* and *R. flavefaciens.* At least 30 genes from ruminal fungi have been isolated that encode cellulases, xylanases, mannanases and endoglunases. Almost 50% of the fibrolytic genes cloned have been sequenced (Bowman and Sowell, 2003).

4.1 Studies on cellulase and xylanase genes in rumen bacteria

A cellulase gene *(endA)* was isolated from a library of *R. flavefaciens strain* 27 DNA fragments inserted in pUC13 by Cunnigham *et al.*, (1991). The *endA* product showed activity against acid-swollen cellulose, carboxy-methylcellulose, lichenan, cellopentaose and cellotetraose, but showed no activity against cellotriose or binding to avicel. Malburg and Forsberg, (1993) constructed genomic libraries of *F. succinogenes S85 in λ-Dash, λ-DashII,* and *pUC19,* and screened the recombinant clones for carboxy methylcellulose hydrolysis. This study indicated that *F. succinogenes S85* possessed at least nine distinct endoglucanase genes. Vercoe *et al.*, (1995) determined the nucleotide sequence of the *celD* gene, which encodes endoglucanase and xylanase activity, from *R. flavefacicns* FD-1. The DNA sequence of *celD* had an open reading frame of 1215 nucleotides that encoded a polypeptide of 405 amino acids with a molecular mass of 44 631 Da. The endo-beta-1,4- glucanase gene *(celA)* present in clone TCI from *R. albus* strain AR67 contained an open reading frame (ORF) of 414 codons, encoding a protein of calculated molecular weight 46 kDa. The N-terminal 26 amino acids had features characteristic of bacterial signal peptides and a typical Shine-Dalgarno sequence was present 8 bp upstream from the translation start site. (Vercoe and Gregg, 1995).

A gene encoding a specific β-(1,3-1,4)-glucanase from *Streptococcus. bovis* was obtained by Ekinci *et al.* (1997). This gene was introduced into PRRW10 and the construct PTRWCIR was obtained. This construct was used to transform *Lactococcus lactis* IL2661 and *Enterococcus faecalis* JH2-SS. It was observed that the small extracellular activity was 8- to 50-fold lower than that in *S. bovis JBI. S. bovis* was found to be tolerant to oxygen and depressed rumen pH, unlike most cellulolytic bacterial species in the rumen. In addition, there are convenient gene transfer methods available for this species that make it a candidate as a host for the expression of genes from other organisms (Bowman and Sowell, 2003).

Gasparic, (1996) isolated clones expressing xylanase activity from a ë EMBL3 genomic DNA library of *P. ruminicola B14.* These clones were shown to represent 4 distinct chromosomal regions, based on restriction enzyme analysis and DNA hybridization. Three groups of clones encoded xylanolytic activity but no carboxy methylcellulolase activity.

Miyazaki *et al.* (2003) found that the xylanase gene cluster from *Prevotella bryantii B14* included a gene (*xynR)* that encodes a multidomain regulatory protein. It was found to be downstream from the xylanase and beta-xylosidase genes *xynA* and *xynB*. The other genes identified upstream of *xynA* and *xynB* include *xynO,* (which encodes an integral membrane protein that has homology with Natsolute snnporters), *xynE,* (related to the genes encoding acyl hydrolases and arylesterases) and *xynF* (which has homology with the genes encoding alpha-glucuronidases). The xynR acts as a positive regulator that activates expression of *xynABD* in *P. bryantii B14.* This is the first regulatory protein with significant homology with the two-component regulatory protein super family and is involved in the regulation of polysaccharidase gene expression. Thulasi *et al.*, (2003, 2008), isolated the cellulase genes from *R. albus* and *R. flavifaciens* and cloned *in E. Coli* and the activity of cellulase enzyme in periplasmic protein fraction was also studied.

4.2 Studies on cellulase and xylanase genes in rumen fungi

Liu-JinHao *et al.*, (1999) isolated and characterised a xylanase gene (*xynC*) from Neocallimastix *patriciarum*. The gene was found to contain an N-terminal catalytic domain that exhibited homology to family 11 of glycosyl hydrolases, a C-terminal cellulose binding domain (CBD) and a putative dockerin domain in between.

The cellulosome produced by *Piromyces sp. strain E2* during growth on filter paper was purified by Steenbakkers *et al.*, (2002) using an optimized cellulose-affinity method. Three dominant proteins were identified in the cellulosome preparation, with molecular masses of 55, 80 and 90 kDa. To investigate the major 90 kDa cellulosome protein further, the corresponding gene, *ccl9A*, was isolated, using immunoscreening and N-terminal sequencing. The *cel9A* genomic organization revealed the presence of four introns, allowing the construction of a consensus for introns in anaerobic fungi. Cel9A includes a 445-residue glycoside hydrolase family 9 catalytic domain, and so was the first fungal representative of this large family.

Two cellulase cDNAs, *celB29* and *celB2*, were isolated from a cDNA library derived from mRNA extracted from the anaerobic fungus, *Opinomyces joyonii strain SG* by Qiu- Xiao *et al.*, (2000). The nucleotide sequences of *celB2* and *celB29* and the primary structures of the proteins encoded by these cDNAs were determined. The larger *celB29* cDNA was 1966 bp long and encoded a 477 amino acid polypeptide with a molecular weight of 54 kDa. Analysis of the 1451 bp *celB2* cDNA revealed an 1164 bp open reading frame coding for a 44 kDa protein consisting of 388 amino acids. Homology analysis showed that both enzymes belong to glycosyl hydrolase family 5 and was most closely related to endoglucanases from the *N. patriciarum, N. frontalis* and *Orpinomyces sp.* The classification of CelB29 and CelB2 as endoglucanases was supported by enzyme assays. Ekinci *et al.*, (2002) were able to use a β (1, 3-1,4)- glucanase promoter found in *S. bovis* to express a cellulase gene from the anaerobic rumen fungus *N.patriciarum.* These fungi are found in very low levels in the rumen and are important for the degradation of crystalline cellulose. The resulting enzyme product was active against a wide variety of cellulosic substrates. The advantages of using fungal enzymes are their stability at low pH and their high activity level.

A metagenomic (6000-clone) library with the average size of its inserts amounting to 15 bp has been constructed on the basis of total DNA isolated from cow rumen microorganisms (Shedova *et al.*, 2009). As the result of the screening of the library on plates with different substrates, a clone was selected that efficiently hydrolyzed lichenan and carboxy methyl cellulose. The clone contained the recombinant plasmid pBlue-13 bearing a 12071 bp long metagenomic fragment carrying ten open reading frames, two of them being identified as glycosyl hydrolase genes. No homology of the metagenomic DNA with any known microorganism genomes was revealed. The amino acid sequence, deduced on the basis of frame 4 and denoted by Xyl3A, bears resemblance with beta-xylosidases of glycosyl hydrolase Family 3. Frame 6 encodes polypeptide Cel5A homologous to cellulases of glycosyl hydrolase Family 5. The amino acid sequences deduced on the basis of seven out of ten open reading frames were homologous to proteins of microorganisms belonging to the *Bacteroides sp.* family, the bacteria inhabiting mammalian intestines.

4.3 Studies on the genome of *Fibrobacter succinogenes*

Ogata *et al.*, (1997) constructed a genomic cleavage map of the type strain *F. succinogenes S85.* The restriction enzymes AscI, AvrII, FseI, NotI and SfiI generated DNA fragments of suitable size distribution that could be resolved by pulsed-field gel electrophoresis (PFGE). An average genome size of 3.6 Mb was obtained by summing the total fragment sizes. The genome of *F. succinogenes* was represented by the single circular DNA molecule. Southern hybridization with specific probes allowed the 8 genetic markers to be located on the restriction map. The genome of this bacterium contains at least 3 rRNA operons. The PFGE of the other 3 strains of *F. succinogenes* gave estimated genome sizes close to that of the type strain. However, RFLP patterns of these strains generated by AscI digestion are completely different. Pair wise comparison of the genomic fragment distribution between the type strain and the 3 isolates showed a similarity level in the region of 14.3 to 31.3%. No fragment common to all of these F. *succinogenes* strains could be detected by PFGE. There was a marked degree of genomic heterogeneity among members of this species makes genomic RFLP a highly discriminatory and useful molecular typing tool for population studies.

5. Activity of various fiber digesting enzymes in bacteria

5.1 Activity of cellulase

Kirby *et al.* (1997) analysed the *endA cellulase gene* from *R. flavefaciens 17* and found that it encodes a product of 759 amino acids, and an example of a multi-domain cellulase from a *Ruminococcus sp*. The C-terminal sequences of EndA contain a 34-amino acid threonine-rich linker connected to an 81-amino acid region, both of which show strong similarities to sequences present in 2 xylanases from R. *flavefaciens* 17. A distant relationship is evident between regions of the 80-amino acid sequences of endA, xynD and xynB and the duplicated 23-amino acid dockerin sequences found in cellulolytic *Clostridium sp.* The properties of the recombinant proteins derived from *Fibrobacter succinogenes* endoglucanase F (EGF) [cellulase], AD2 and AD4, were characterized by Mitsumori *et al.* (2002).

Ohara *et al.* (2000b) isolated the cellulosome complex from the culture supernatant of *Ruminococcus albus strain F-40*. The cellulolytic complex produced by *R. albus* resembles the cellulosome specified for the cellulolytic complex of several *Clostridia i.e.*, the cellulosome is formed by the interaction between a dockerin domain of catalytic components and a cohesin domain of a scaffolding protein. Ohara *et al.*, (2000a) also found that the *Ruminococcus albus F-40 egV* gene, encoding endoglucanase V (EGV), consisted of an open reading frame of 1833 nucleotides and encodes 611 amino acids with a deduced molecular weight of 67103. The deduced EGV is a modular enzyme composed of a catalytic domain of family 5 of glycosyl hydrolases, a domain of unknown function, and a dockerin domain responsible for cellulosome assembly, suggesting that *R. albus F-40* produces a cellulosome, and EGV is a component of the cellulosome.

Effects of urea infusion on the endoglucanase (CMCase) and xylanase activities in solid and liquid fractions of rumen contents in steers were investigated by Pan *et al.* (2003). The solid fraction consistently exhibited much greater activities of CMCase and xylanase than liquid fraction, but the response to urea infusion was somewhat different between these two fractions. Activities of fibrolytic enzyme (CMCase and xylanase) in the rumen digesta were increased by urea infusion, and then the extent of the increase was higher for liquid than for solid fractions. Regardless of urea infusion, activities of fibrolytic enzyme from solid fractions were higher in ventral sac than dorsal sac, while opposite results were obtained in liquid fractions. These results indicate that increased ruminal ammonia-N by urea infusion could enhance fibrolytic enzyme activity of liquid-associated microbes at an early stage after feeding, and those of particle-associated microbes at a later stage, through stimulating growth of cellulolytic microbes

Ko *et al.* (2011) isolated a novel anaerobic microorganism termed AN-C16-KBRB from the bovine rumen and demonstrated cellulolytic activity on a NB agar plate containing azo-carboxymethyl cellulose. The 16S rRNA gene of the strain was 98% similar to that of *Clostridiaceae bacterium* SK082 (AB298754). A novel celEdx16 gene encoding a bifunctional endo-/ exocellulase (CelEdx16) was cloned by the shotgun method from AN-C16-KBRB, and the enzyme was characterized. CelEdx16 was overexpressed in *E.coli* and purified using Ni-NTA affinity chromatography. The specific endocellulase and exocellulase activities of CelEdx16 were 15.9 and 3.6×10^{-2} U/mg, respectively. CelEdx16 was optimally active at pH 5.0 and 40°C.

5.2 Activity of xylanase

In the rumen, the major xylanolytic species are *B. fibrisolvens* and *Bacteroides ruminicola*. A xylosidase gene has been cloned from *B. fibrisolvens*

113. Data from DNA hybridizations using a xylanase gene cloned from *B. fibrisolvens* 49 indicate that this gene may be present in other *B. fibrisolvens* strains. A cloned xylanase from *B. ruminicola* was highly expressed in *Bacteroides fragilis* and *Bacteroides uniformis.* Arabinosidase and xylosidase genes from *Bacteroides ovatus* have been cloned (Hespell and Whitehead, 1990).

An *Eubactereium ruminantium* xylanase gene (xynA) was inserted into pYK4, a shuttle vector replicable in both *E.coli* and *B. fibrisolvens,* and the resultant chimeric plasmid (pYK4XT) was electroporated into *B. fibrisolvens OB156C* by Kobayashi *et al.,* (1998), in an attempt to obtain a more xylanolytic *B. fibrisolvens.* The plasmid pYK4XT was maintained stably in the transformant for more than 100 generations. Logar *et al. (*1998) isolated four regions encoding xylanase activity from *P. bryantii B14.*

Ekinci *et al.* (2001) examined the polysaccharide-degrading enzymes of *R. flavefaciens strain 17* and demonstrated that it produces a complex array of enzymes active against cellulose, hemicellulose (xylan) and lignin. These enzymes are xylanase, avicellase, acid-swollen cellulase, carboxymethyl cellulase (CMCase), pNP-cellobiosidase (pNPC), pNP- glucopyranosidase (pNPG), pNP-xylopyranosidase (pNPX) and pNP-arabinofuranosidase (pNPA).

5.3 Activity of fiber digesting enzymes in fungi

Seven fractions rich in endoglucanase activity were separated from the extracellular cellulase system of *Neocallimastix frontalis* by Wood *et al.* (1995). The mode of action of the cellulase system of *N. frontalis* in degrading crystalline cellulose may be similar to that of other aerobic fungi.

Aylward *et al.* (1999) determined the complete nucleotide sequence of a cDNA encoding three catalytic domains of the *Neocallimastix patriciarum* cellulase CelD. The three domains have a very high degree of amino acid identity and are separated by two linker sequences rich in proline, threonine and glutamic acid. A third linker is followed by a probable protein-docking domain for the proposed cellulosome-like structure of *N. patriciarum.* Domain 2 of CelD was representative of the activity of the larger CelD enzyme and this domain would be suitable for the enrichment of the genome of rumen bacteria by genetic manipulation.

Cybinski *et al.* (1999) found that the extent of digestion of acetylated xylans by XynA appears to be limited by the acetylation. A *N. patriciarum* acetyl xylan esterase (BnaA) was expressed from the cloned gene in *E.coli.* Purified recombinant BnaA efficiently released acetate from soluble acetylated birch wood xylan (ABX), with a specific activity of 76 U/mg. In contrast, release of acetate was very inefficient from the insoluble substrates, spear grass and de-lignified spear grass. Addition of a recombinant xylanase, XynA, also expressed from a cloned *N. patriciarum* gene, had no effect on the release of acetate from ABX.

Five anaerobic fungi *(N. frontalis Nl-1, Pyromyces communis Pl-2, Orpinomyces sp. O2-2, Caecomyces communis Cl-5, Anaeromyces sp. Al-3)* isolated from the rumen by Kang *et al.* (2000) were compared in terms of fermentation characteristics and enzyme activities in order to select a proper fungal species with a high fibre-degrading capacity. All 5 fungal species produced CMCase, xylanase and amylase, and *N. frontalis* showed the highest fibre digesting ability among 5 fungal species.

Ye *et al.* (2001) purified a cellulase from the rumen fungus *Orpinomyces joyonii* cloned in *E. coli.* The cellulase represented the product of the cellulase gene cel B2. The purified enzyme was highly active against barley beta-glucan, lichenan, carboxymethyl cellulose (CMC), xylan, but not towards laminarin and pachyman. In addition, the cloned enzyme was able to hydrolyse p-nitrophenyl (PNP)-cellobioside, PNP-cellotrioside, PNP- cellotetraoside, PNP-cellopentaoside, but not PNP-glucopyranoside.

Samanta *et al.* (1999) identified various isoenzymes of endoglucanase and xylanase in an isolate of *Piromyces sp.* from the rumen of a riverine buffalo, following chromatographic and electrophoretic analyses. On SDS-PAGE, endoglucanase gave 4 activity bands having molecular weights of 100, 66, 40 and 33 kDa. Xylanase also gave 4 activity bands with molecular weights of 168, 80, 61 and 50 kDa.

Malik *et al.* (1998) demonstraed the production, purification and characterization of an endo-1,4-beta-glucanase (EG) from *R. albus* A-23, isolated from the rumen of buffaloes. The molecular weight of EG as determined by SDS-PAGE and EG activity staining in gel was around 45000 daltons. The EG exhibited temperature and pH optima of 40°C and 6.0, respectively.

A gene encoding a xylanase, named xynS20, was cloned from the ruminal fungus *N. patriciarum*. The DNA sequence of xynS20 revealed that the gene was 1,008 bp in size and encoded amino acid sequences with a predicted molecular weight of 36 kDa. The specific activity of purified XynS20 toward oat spelt xylan was 1,982.8 U mg(-1). The recombinant XynS20 was stable in the mild acid pH range from 5.0 to 6.0, and the pH optimum was 6.0. The optimal reaction temperature of XynS20 was 45°C; at temperatures below 30 and above 55°C, enzyme activity was less than 50% of that at the optimal temperature (Liu *et al.*, 2008). Qi *et al.* (2011) isolated a novel ferulic acid esterase gene (fae1A) from rumen fungus *Anaeromyces mucronatus*, cloned, heteroexpressed in *E.coli* and characterized. Gene product Fae1A was found to exhibit activity against a number of substrates including naphthyl fatty acid esters, p-nitrophenyl fatty acid esters and hydroxylcinnamic acid esters. It releases ferulic acid and p-coumaric acid from barley straw.

5.4 Fibrolytic activity from metagenomic library

A ruminal metagenomic library was constructed and functionally screened for cellulase activities and 61 independent clones expressing cellulase activities were isolated (Duan *et al.*, 2009). One novel cellulase gene, C67-1, was overexpressed in *E. coli*, and the purified recombinant enzyme showed optimal activity at pH 4.5 and stability in a broad pH range from 3.5 to 10.5. Its enzyme activity was stimulated by dl-dithiothreitol. The cellulases cloned in this work may play important roles in the degradation of celluloses in the variable and low pH environment in buffalo rumen. A xylanase-coding gene, XynGR40, was cloned directly from the environmental DNA of goat rumen contents and expressed in *E. coli* BL21 (DE3). Purified recombinant XynGR40 exhibited high activity at low temperatures, and remained active (~10% of the activity) even at 0°C. The optimal temperature of XynGR40 was 30°C, much lower than other xylanases from rumen. These properties suggest that XynGR40 is a novel cold active xylanase and has great potential for basic research and industrial applications (Wang *et al.*, 2011). The gene encoding feruloyl esterase enzyme (FAE) amplified from the metagenomic DNA of *Coptotermes formosanus* gut was cloned in the TA cloning vector and subcloned into a pET32a expression vector. The Ft3-7 gene has 84% sequence identity with *Clostridium saccharolyticum* and shows amino acid sequence identity with predicted xylanase/chitin deacetylase and endo-1,4-beta-xylanase. The sequence analysis reveals that probably Ft3-7 could be a new gene and that its molecular mass was 18.5 kDa. The activity of the recombinant enzyme (Ft3-7) produced in *Escherichia coli (E.coli)* was 21.4 U with substrate ethyl ferulate and its specific activity was 24.6 U/mg proteins. The optimum pH and temperature for enzyme activity were 7.0 and 37°C, respectively. The substrate utilization preferences and sequence similarity of the Ft3-7 place it in the type-D sub-class of FAE (Chandrasekharaiah *et al.*, 2011).

6. Improvement in the cellulose digestion through genetic manipulation

Potential strategies proposed for genetic manipulation (Forsberg *et al.*, 1986; Teather 1985; Varga and Kolver, 1997) of rumen microbes to develop new strains have included the following:

1. Increasing the competitiveness of cellulolytic organisms (F. *succinogenes, Ruminococcus)* by conferring the ability to utilize xylose and pectins, thereby allowing earlier colonization of particulate matter.
2. Inserting the cellulase gene into numerically pre dominant species (*Prevotella ruminicola*).

3. Increasing the competitiveness of cellulolytic species present in the rumen in low numbers (*Clostridium polysaccharolyticum*) by according them the ability to adhere to feed particles.
4. Inserting an acid-tolerant cellulase gene into acid-tolerant bacteria (Lactobacillus) to allow fiber fermentation at a ruminal pH less than 6.
5. Developing a cutinase activity in predominant bacteria; and
6. Allowing predominant species to degrade arabinose side chains, thereby overcoming the rate-limiting effect of lignin.

Genetic engineering of rumen bacteria for improved cellulose digestion has been proposed as one route to improve the animal productivity (Russel and Wilson, 1988). Two strategies were envisaged, where the first one involved improving the existing predominant primary rumen cellulolytic bacteria – *R. albus, R. flavefaciens* and *F. succinogenes*. These bacteria have evolved to digest cellulose relatively rapidly. The first order rate constant for the digestion of highly ordered cellulose by the three ruminal species under optimal growth conditions to be fixed. Therefore, any genetic modification in these strains to enhance the cellulolytic proprieties would be very complicated and hypercellulolytic strains may not be obtained. Rumen cellulolytic bacteria are sensitive to low pH and are non-motile and the digestion of thick walled cells is limited by the slow diffusion of rumen cellulolytic bacteria into the lumina of the secondary wall (Willson and Mertens, 1995). Hence the other alternative would be to remove the characteristic defects existing in this organism for example to improve the acid tolerance of the cellulolyitic bacteria or the introduction of motility. All theses complex functions cannot be genetically transferred and expressed into the rumen cellulolytic bacteria at this stage of research.

The second strategy is to introduce the cellulolytic function into a robust rumen bacterium or even into the dominant rumen bacteria. Many bacteria have been proposed as suitable candidates for this purpose. Russel and Willson, (1988) suggested *Prevotella ruminicla B14* strain was an attractive candidates for genetic modification to produce a cellulolytic rumen bacterium that was acid resistance. It can utilize the products of cellulose digestion, resist low pH and produces an acid stable beta 1, 4, endoglucanase. Crystalline cellulases studied from non rumen bacteria have shown that they have separated catalytic and cellulose binding sites. (Ghangas and Wilson, 1987; Gikes *et al.*, 1988; Hall *et al.*, 1988; Kraulis *et al.*, 1989; Matsushita *et al.*, 1990). This organism produces a carboxymethyl cellulase with a catalytic domain but without a cellulase binding domain. Hence this species does not have a strong adherence to cellulases (Minato and Suto, 1978). Even when the binding sites on these cellulases are lost, they retain the activity against carboxy methyl cellulose (CMC) but lose activity against crystalline cellulose (Gikes *et al.*, 1988 ; McGavin and Forsberg, 1989). Based on these observations, the addition of cellulase binding domain to the *Prevotella ruminicola* B 14, beta 1, 4 endoglucanase appears to be a means of creating an acid resistant cellulolytic bacterium. However, the Carboxy methylcellulase was produced as a single enzyme and therefore it may not have all the characteristics of the enzymes that are produced by the predominant cellulolytic bacteria. It was also felt that the cellulolytic capability of an engineered strain of this species may be modest, though it could be useful in the rumen of animal having a pH less than 6. *Thermonospora fusca* produces several cellulases and the DNA of each of these enzymes have been cloned and sequenced. When DNA, which encoded the cellulose binding domain *of T. fusca* E2 was ligated to the beta 1,4 endoglucanase gene of *P. ruminicola* B14 strain and expressed in *E.coli* the reconstructed chimeric gene caused an increase in cellulose digestion by 10 fold. Gene reconstruction appears to offer a means of turning *Prevotella* into an acid resistant bacterium and experiments are still underway to move the reconstructed gene to *P. ruminicola* B 14.

B. fibrisolvens, a secondary rumen cellulolytic bacterium was also proposed as a candidate for genetic manipulation. This species also has acid tolerance and some strains are moderately celluolytic. Limited success has been obtained in gene transfer by the use of electroporation (Whitehead, 1992) but the practical utility of this organism can be gauged only after the release of the organism into the rumen environment and the survival under the *in vivo* conditions.

While evidence from some sources have suggested that the likelihood of successfully introducing a bacterium of non-rumen origin into the rumen is low, as reported by Cotta *et al.* (1997). Strain BTX contains the xylanase gene from *P. ruminicola* 23, which was integrated into the chromosome of *B. thetaiotomicron,* using a suicide vector. The xylanase activity of the strain containing the chromosomally integrated xylanase was 30% lower than that observed when the xylanase gene was present on a plasmid vector. In addition, the xylanase was more stable when integrated into the chromosome than when present on the plasmid vector (White head *et al.,* 1991). Using a consecutive batch culture system, which mimics the rumen ecosystem, the researchers were unable to maintain strain BTX for more than 48 h. Hence, it is possible to clone and efficiently express genes isolated from rumen bacteria in other bacterial species and vice versa. These reports provide encouragement for the possibility of modifying other microorganisms, using genes which may be unique to rumen bacteria, as well as imparting to rumen bacteria unique features of other microorganisms.

7. Establishment of natural or genetically modified new micro-organisms in the rumen

Introduction of a defined genotype into a complex microbial ecosystem is probably more difficult than originally expected (Stewart *et al.*, 1988). The success of establishment of genetically modified organism or natural micro organisms of having desired characters may ultimately depend on a better understanding of the factors that determine establishment in a complex microbial ecosystem, survival and population density in the rumen (McSweeney *et al.*, 1999).

The ruminants in Australia were unable to utilize *Leucaena leucocephala*, due to the presence of a non protein amino acid, mimosine. This amino acid was converted to hydroxyl 4 (1H) pyridine (DHP) but was not metabolized further. The DHP had goitrogenic effect on the host. These sensitive animals were then inoculated with rumen fluid from goats adapted to consume *Leucaena leucocephala.* The DHP was further metabolized and the toxicity was avoided (Dawson and Allion, 1988). Certain species of rumen bacterium can be used to inoculate the rumen to enhance the rumen function. When *Megasphaera elsdenii* was added intraruminally, a large inoculum decreased the severity of acute acidosis in cattle and smaller doses enhanced the recovery of rumen pH (Robinson *et al.*, 1993). The other reports include protection of cattle from leucaena toxicity by inoculants of *Synergistes jonesii* (Jones and Megarrity, 1986), ruminal transfers that prevented toxicity from *A. angustissima* (Odenyo *et al.*, 1997a,b) and decreased susceptibility to rumen acidosis in feedlot cattle by additions of acid tolerant strains of the lactate utilizing organism Megasphaera *elsdenii* strain 407A (Hibbard *et al.*, 1993).

Gregg *et al.*, (1994) have reported the cloning of a dehalogenase gene from *Moraxella sp.* in to the *E.coli/ B. fibrisolvense* shuttle vector pBHerm and its introduction into the *B. fibrisolvens.* The dehalogenase gene detoxifies fluoraacetate, a potent plant toxin which is known to kill domestic livestock in Australia and Africa. This is the first report of a gene with practical, industrial and economic significance being expressed by a rumen bacterium, thus alleviating the need for speculation regarding the viability of using rDNA approach to modify ruminal bacterial. The promoter, signal sequence and plasmid were designed to function within the host. The clone was stable for over 500 generations without antibiotic selection. It is evedient, that the fluoroacetate was transported into the *B. fibrisolvense* cell, since no dehalogenase activity was detected extracellularly. Monitoring experiments have indicated that single strains of *B. fibrisolvens* can represent 0.1 to 1.0% of the rumen population (Gregg *et al.*, 1994 ; Gregg, 1995), suggesting that defluorination activity levels in *B. fibrisolvense* OB156 may be high enough to protect against the poisoning.

A number of non-rumen bacteria added to the rumen declined rapidly *in vivo*. Attwood *et al.* (1988), developed a probe to track *P. ruminicola B14* in the rumen fluid under *in vitro* and *in vivo* conditions. It was found that the strain had a half life of 9 hours under *in vitro* conditions and less than 30 minutes under *in vivo* conditions. However a report by Cotta *et al.* (1997) regarding the survival *B. thetaiotaomicron BTX* under rumen simulating conditions, provides some optimism that genetically modified strains can be maintained in the rumen.

Different *Ruminococcus* strains isolated from cattle and sheep were assessed for their ability to digest plant cell walls (Krause *et al.*, 1999a). Out of 26 strains studied, only three strains had the same genotype and the digestibility of fibre of a medium quality grass varied from 0-61%. Increasing the number of highly fibrolytic *Ruminococci* strains could potentially improve the fibre digestibility in the rumen, if this phenotypic diversity is represented within an individual rumen. Further, the highly fibrolytic *Ruminococcus* strains were evaluated for their ability to colonize the rumen and enhance fibre digestion (Krause *et al.*, 1999b). The inoculated *Ruminococcus* strains did not persist for more than 3 weeks before reaching undetectable levels. Ziemer *et al.* (2002) also reported increased fibre digestibility, when a natural bacterium *Butyrivivibrio thetaiotaomicron* was added to a rumen model.

The xylanase gene was isolated from the ruminal fungus *N.patriciarum,* cloned and expressed in *Butyrivibrio fibrisolvens* (Krause *et al.*, 2001). The recombinant *Butyrivibrio fibrisolvens* did not persist in the rumen for more than 22 days, though they showed an increased ability to digest fibre, indicating the difficulties in maintenance of newly introduced strains in the anaerobic environment and need to understand the mechanisms involved in survival of newly introduced strains in the rumen (Wallace, 1994).

The depression in survivability of the recombinants was mainly due to heat sensitive antibacterial factors associating with microbial cells in the rumen (Kobayshi and Yamamoto, 2002). Reestablishment of either natural or recombinant ruminal bacteria in the rumen is both variable and unpredictable and the disappearance of the newly introduced inoculants from the rumen after very short period of time also reported (Wallace and Walker, 1993; Miyagi *et al.*, 1995; Krause *et al.*, 2003). The probability of colonizing the rumen with a bacterium of non rumen origin is low (Wallace, 1994; Cotta *et al.*, 1997). The factors that affect the survivability of reintroduced bacterium in the rumen (McSweeney *et al.*, 1999) include:

1. Competition with indigenous microbes for substrates that are used for growth.
2. Growth at a rate faster than the dilution rate of the rumen.

3. Adaptation to and tolerance of the chemical and physical environment in the rumen.
4. Capability of withstanding engulfment by protozoa, and
5. Resistance to inhibition by bacteriocins and infection by bacteriophage.

Therefore, several methods are currently employed to manipulate rumen fermentation to enhance post ingestion nutritive value of fibrous forages through use of biotechnology including inoculants of native and recombinant rumen microorganisms, natural adaptation and microbial feed enzymes (Sajjad *et al.,* 2008). However, more research needs to be conducted in this area and the practical application of biotechnological approaches to increase utilization of crop residues go a long way and awaits development of suitable gene transfer systems and the major technical difficulties needs to be addressed before the results of these basic studies find their way to application aspect.

8. Newer molecular biology tools to study rumen microbes

The major technical problems encountered during studies in rumen microbial ecology and biotechnology are the bias introduced by a culture based enumeration and characterization techniques and the lack of a phylogenetically based classification scheme. The morphology, biochemical characteristics, fermentation characteristics, the ecological niche and any information pertaining to the rumen microbes was obtained from culture collections which were isolated by the conventional classic culture techniques. However, these traditional culture techniques used to classify bacteria based on phenotypic characteristics is not the perfect method of obtaining this information (Amann *et al.,* 1992, Lin and Stahl, (1995). Conventional culture-based methods for enumerating rumen microorganisms (bacteria, archaea, protozoa, and fungi) have been superseded and are now used mainly to obtain pure isolates of novel organisms and reference strains that are required for the development and validation of the nucleic acid approaches. These reference strains are also essential for physiological studies of the lifestyle of the organisms as well as sources of genomic DNA and RNA that can be analysed for functional gene activity. The focus of nucleic acid research is now shifting to the functional analysis of the ecosystem which involves the measurement of functional genes and their expression in the predominant or specific members of the rumen microbial community (McSweeney *et al.,* 2009).

McSweeney *et al.,* (2006) reviewed several molecular techniques *viz.,* qPCR and DGGE to monitor the abundance and diversity of different genera and species of rumen protozoa. The qPCR technique has been improved by the design of new primers to quantify the abundance of anaerobic rumen fungi

(ARF) (Denman *et al.*, 2008; Edwards *et al.*, 2008). Further, to address the issue of ARF community analysis, an automated ribosomal intergenic spacer region (ARISA) method has been developed for the detection and monitoring of ARF.

Metagenomic technologies are used to capture and study the entire microbiome from a complex microbial community in the rumen. The rumen-DNA metagenomic libraries were screened for several novel enzymes involved in depolymerisation of lignocellulose and starch including laccases (Beloqui *et al.*, 2006; Ferrer *et al.*, 2005; Ferrer *et al.*, 2007). Zhu *et al.* (2007) constructed a bacterial artificial chromosome library from the rumen of a dairy cow for screening the activities of novel enzymes.

Rapid high-throughput technologies such as microarray analysis were developed where in abundance of particular mRNA can be quantified by using DNA microarrays or by real-time RT-PCR. Limited studies have been carried out till today with regards to gene expression array profiling of rumen microorganisms (Krause *et al.*, 2003; Qi *et al.*, 2005).

The next generation sequencing technologies developed for mapping the human genome are now being used for studying microbial ecosystems. This technology delivers more information by metagenomic analysis of complex microbiomes. Recently, the metagenomic analysis of the specific glycoside hydrolases (fibre-degrading enzymes) that are associated with the fiber-adherent bovine rumen microbiome has been carried out by using the next generation sequencing technology (Brulc *et al.*, 2009).

Conclusions

Poor quality roughages, including agricultural by products continued to be the major source of feeding for ruminants in developing countries including India. The major objective would be to increase the digestibility of these feeds through treatments or genetic or non genetic manipulation of rumen ecosystem to degrade fiber. The basic approaches for be the manipulation of rumen eco system should be followed in such a way that the feeds given to ruminants must supply an appropriate array of nutrients needed for particular type of productive function. Construction of genetically modified organisms to improve the productivity of the ruminants is one of the important areas of research which is rapidly gaining importance. However, the practical application of biotechnological approaches through genetic manipulation of rumen ecosystem to increase utilization of crop residues go a long way and awaits development of suitable gene transfer systems and the major technical difficulties needs to be addressed before the results of these basic studies find their way to application aspect. The major problem encountered in using indigenous rumen microbes for manipulating rumen fermentation is their obligatory anaerobic physiology. Finally, whatever the technology that is used for ruminant production improvement would be determined by economic considerations. Though at present there are speculations and doubts about the success of these technologies and their practical and economic significance, the efforts need to be continued in this direction also, by integrating the knowledge of emerging molecular biology techniques with nutrition principles since our livestock production system is predominantly based on crop residues.

References

Amann R.I., Lin C., Key R., Montgomery L., Stahl D.A. (1992). Diversity among *Fibrobacter* isolates: towards a phylogenetic classification. *Systematic and Applied Microbiology* **15:** 23-31.

Attwood G.T., Lockington R.A., Xue G.P. Brooker J.D. (1988). Use of a unique gene sequence as a probe to enumerate a strain of *Bacteroides ruminicola* introduced into the rumen. *Applied and Environmental Microbiology* **54:** 534-539.

Aylward J.H., Gobius K.S., Xue-GangPing, Simpson G.D., Dalrymple B.P., Xue G.P. (1999). The Neocallimastix patriciarum cellulase, CelD, contains three almost identical catalytic domains with high specific activities on Avicel. *Enzyme and Microbial Technology* **24:** 609-614.

Barcroft H., Edholm O.G., McMichael J., Sharpey-Schafer E.P. (1944). Post-haemorrhagic fainting. Study by cardiac output and forearm flow. *Lancet* **1:** 489-491.

Beard C.E., Hefford M.A., Forster R.J., Sontakke S., Teather R.M., Gregg K. (1995). A stable and efficient transfermation system for Butyrivibrio fibrisolvens OB156. *Current Microbiology* **30:** 105-109.

Beloqui A., Pita M., Polaina J., Martínez-Arias A., Golyshina O.V., Zumárraga M., Yakimov M.M., García-Arellano H., Alcalde M., Fernández V.M., Elborough K., Andreu J.M., Ballesteros A., Plou F.J., Timmis K.N., Ferrer M., Golyshin P.N. (2006). Novel polyphenol oxidase mined from a metagenome expression library of bovine rumen: biochemical properties, structural analysis, and phylogenetic relationships. *Journal of Biological Chemistry* **281:** 22933-22942.

Bowman J.G.P., Sowell B.F. (2003) Technology to complement forage beef production systems in the west. *Journal of Animal Science* **81:** E18-E26.

Broaderick G.A., Wallace R.J., Orskov E.R. (1991). Control of rate and extent of protein degradation. In: *Physiological aspect of digestion and metabolism in ruminants.* (T. Tsuda, Y. Sasaki, and R. Kawashima, eds) Academic Press, Orlando,FI, pp. 541-592.

Brookman J. L., Ozkose E., Rogers S., Trinci A.P.J., Theodorou M.K. (2000). Identification of spores in the polycentric anaerobic gut fungi which enhance their ability to survive. *FEM Microbiology Ecology* **31:** 261-267.

Brulc J.M., Antonopoulos D.A., Miller M.E., Wilson M.K., Yannarell A.C., Dinsdale E.A., Edwards R.E., Frank E.D., Emerson J.B., Wacklin P., Coutinho P.M., Henrissat B.,

Nelson K.E., White B.A. (2009). Gene-centric metagenomics of the fiber-adherent bovine rumen microbiome reveals forage specific glycoside hydrolases. *Proceedings of the National Academy of Science, USA* **106:** 1948-1953.

Cai S., Li J., Hu F.Z., Zhang K., Luo Y., Janto B., Boissy R., Ehrlich G., Dong X. (2010). *Cellulosilyticum ruminicola,* a newly described rumen bacterium that possesses redundant fibrolytic-protein-encoding genes and degrades lignocellulose with multiple carbohydrate- borne fibrolytic enzymes. *Applied and Environmental Microbiology* **76:** 3818-3824.

Chandrasekharaiah M., Thulasi A., Bagath M., Kumar D.P., Santosh S.S., Palanivel C., Jose V.L., Sampath K.T. (2011). Molecular cloning, expression and characterization of a novel feruloyl esterase enzyme from the symbionts of termite (*Coptotermes formosanus*) gut. *Biochemistry and Molecular Biology Reports* **44:** 52-57.

Chandrasekharaiah M., Thulasi A., Sampath K.T. (2003). Diurnal variations in bacterial numbers and profile in crossbred steers fed different dietary regimes. *Indian Journal of Dairy and Biosciences* **14:** 8-12.

Chandrasekharaiah M., Thulasi A., Sampath K.T. (2009). Culturable rumen microbial population in steers fed with different dietary requires. *Indian Veterinary Journal* **86:** 819-822.

Chandrasekhariah M., Thulasi A., Sampath K.T. (2000). Development of gene transfer system in Rumen bacteria - a review. *Indian Journal of Dairy and Biosciences* **11:** 128-135.

Cotta M.A., Whitehead T.R., Rasmuseen M.A. (1997). Survival of the recombinant *Bacteroides thetaiotaomicron* strain BTX in in vitro rumen incubations. *Journal of Applied Microbiology* **82:** 743-750.

Cunningham C., McPherson C.A., Martin J., Harris W.J., Flint H.J. (1991). Sequence of a cellulase gene from the rumen anaerobe *Ruminococcus flavefaciens 17. Molecular and General-Genetics* **228:** 320-323.

Cybinski D.H., Layton I., Lowry J.B., Dalrymple B.P. (1999). An acetylxylan esterase and a xylanase expressed from genes cloned from the ruminal fungus *Neocallimastix patriciarum* act synergistically to degrade acetylated xylans. *Applied Microbiology and Biotechnology* **52:** 221-225.

Dawson K.A. Allison M.J. (1988). Digestive disorders and Nutritional Toxicity In rumen microbial ecosystem. (P.N.Hobson, ed), p. 449.

Denman S.E., Nicholson M.J., Brookman J.L., Theodorou M.K., McSweeney C.S. (2008). Detection and monitoring of anaerobic rumen fungi using an ARISA method. *Letters in Applied Microbiology* **47:** 492-499.

Duan C.J., Xian L., Zhao G.C., Feng Y., Pang H., Bai X.L., Tang J.L., Ma Q.S., Feng J.X. (2009). Isolation and partial characterization of novel genes encoding acidic cellulases from metagenomes of buffalo rumens. *Journal of Applied Microbiology* **107:** 245-256.

Edwards J.E., Kingston-Smith A.H., Jimenez H.R. Huws S.A., Skøt K.P., Griffith G.W., McEwan N.R., Theodorou M.K. (2008). Dynamics of initial colonization of nonconserved perennial ryegrass by anaerobic fungi in the bovine rumen. *FEMS Microbial Ecology* **63:** 141-142.

Ekinci M.S., Martin J.C., Flint H.J. (2002). Expression of a cellulase gene cel1A, from the rumen fungus *Neocallimastix patriciarum* in *Streptococcus bovis* by means of promoter fusions. *Biotechnology Letters* **24:** 735-741.

Ekinci, M.S., McCrae, S.I. and Flint, H.J. (1997). Isolation and overexpression of a gene encoding an extracellular beta-(l,3-1,4)-glucanase from *Streptococcus bovis JB1. Applied and Environmental Microbiology* **63:** 3752-3756.

Ekinci M.S., Ozcan N., Ozkose E. Hint H.J. (2001). A study on cellulolytic and hemicellulolytic enzymes of anaerobic nimen bacterium *Ruminococcus flavefaciens* strain 17. *Turk Veterinerlik ve Hayvancilik Dergisi.* **25:** 703-709.

Ferrer M., Beloqui A., Golyyshina O.V., Plou F.J., Neef A., Chernikova T.N., Fernández-Arrojo L., Ghazi I., Ballesteros A., Elborough K., Timmis K.N., Golyshin P.N. (2007). Biochemical and structural features of a novel cyclodextrinase from cow rumen metagenome. *Biotechnology Journal* **2:** 207-213.

Ferrer M., Golyyshina O.V., Chernikova T.N., Khachane A.N., Reyes-Duarte D., Santos V.A., Strompl C., Elborough K., Jarvis G., Neef A., Yakimov M.M., Timmis K.N., Golyshin P.N., (2005). Novel hydrolase diversity retrieved from a metagenome library of bovine rumen microflora. *Environmental Microbiology* **7:** 1996-2010.

Forano, E., Flint H.J. (2000). Genetically modified organisms: consequences for ruminant health and nutrition. *Annales De Zootechnie* **49:** 255-271.

Forsberg C.W., Crosby B., Thomas Y.D. (1986). Potential for manipulation of the rumen fermentation through the use of recombinant DNA techniques. *Journal of Animal Science* **63:** 310-325.

Forsberg C.W., Cheng, K.J., White, B.A. (1997). Polysaccaride degradationin the rumen and large intestine. In: *Gastrointestinal Microbiology*, (R.I. Mackie and B.A. White, eds.) Chapman and Hall. New York, pp 319-379.

Forsberg C.W., Egbosimba E.E., McLellan S. (1999). Recent advances in biotechnology of rumen bacteria (A review). *Asian-Australasian Journal of Animal Sciences* **12:** 93-103.

Gasparic A. (1996). Izolacija Stirih genov ksilanoliznega kompleksa vampne bakterije Prevotella ruminicola B14. *Zbornik Biotehniske Fakultete Univerze v Ljubljani, Kmetijstvo* **68:** 7-17.

Ghangas G.S., Wilson D.B. (1987). Cloning of the *Thermonospora fusca* endoglucanase E2 gene into *streptomyces lividans*: affinity purification and functional domains of the cloned geneproducts. *Applied and Environmental Microbiology* **54:** 1470.

Gikes N.R., Warren R.A.J., Miller R.C., Kilburgn D.J. (1988). Precise excision of the cellulose binding domains from two *Cellulomonas fime* cellulases by homologous protease and the effect on catalysis. *Journal of Biological Chemistry* **263:** 10401-10407.

Gordon G.L.R., Philips M.W. (1998). The role of anaerobic gut fungi in ruminants. *Nutrition research reviews* **11:** 133-168.

Gregg K. (1995). Engineering gut flora of ruminant livestock to reduce forage toxicity: progress and problems. *Trends in Biotechnology* **13:** 418-421.

Gregg K., Cooper C.L., Schafer D.J., Sharpe H., Beard C.E., Allen G., Xu J.W. (1994) Detoxification of the fluroacetate by a genetically modified ruminal bacterium. *Journal of Biotechnology* **12:** 1361-1365.

Hall J., Hazelwood G.P., Barker P.J., Gilbert H.J. (1988). Conserved restricted domains in *Clostrdium thermocellum* endoglucanases are not essential for catalytic activity. *Gene* **69:** 29-38.

Hefford M.A., Kobayashi Y., Allard S.E., Forster R.J., Teather R.M. (1997). Sequence analysis and characterization of pOM1, a small cryptic plasmid from *Butyrivibrio fibrisolvens*, and its use in construction of a new family of cloning vectors for Butyrivibrios. *Applied and Environmental Microbiology* **63:** 1701-1711.

Hefford M.A., Teather R.M., Forster R.J. (1993). The complete nucleotide sequence of a small cryptic plasmid from a rumen bacterium of the Genus *Butyrivibio*. *Plasmid* **29:** 63-69.

Hespell R.B.,Whitehead T.R. (1990). Physiology and genetics of xylan degradation by gastrointestinal tract bacteria, *Journal of Dairy Science*. **73:** 3013-3022.

Hespell R.B., Whitehead T.R. (1991). Conjugal transfer of Tn916, Tn916 delta E, and pAM beta 1 from Enterococcus faecalis to Butyrivibrio fibrisolvens strains. *Applied and Environmental Microbiology* **57:** 2703-2709.

Hibbard, B., Robinson, J.A., Greening, R.C., Smolenski, W.J., Bell, R.L., Peters, J.P. (1993). The effect of route of administration of isolate 407A (UC-12497) on feed intake and selected ruminal variables of beef steers in an acute acidosis in appetence model. In: *22nd Biennial Conference on "Rumen Function"*, Chicago, IL, USA, p 19.

Hungate R.E. (1950). The anaerobic mesophilic cellulolytic bacteria. *Bacteriological Reviews* **14:** 1-49.

Jalaludin S., Ho Y.W., Abdullah N., Kudo H., (1992). Rumen microorganisms of the water buffalo. *Buffalo Journal* **8:** 211-220.

Jones R.J., Megarrity R.G. (1986). Successful transfer of DHP degrading bacteria from Hawaiian goats to Australian ruminants to overcome the toxicity of Leucaena. *Australian Veterinary Journal* **63:** 259-262.

Kamra D. N. (2005). Rumen microbial ecosystem. *Current Science* **89:** 124-135.

Kang M.W., Lee S.S., Ha J.K. (2000). Estimation of cellulose-degrading enzyme activity by anaerobic rumen fungi. *Korean Journal of Animal Science*. **42:** 521-530.

Kirby J., Martin J.C., Daniel A.S. Flint H.J. (1997). Dockerin-like sequences in cellulases and xylanases from the rumen cellulolytic bacterium *Ruminococcus flavefaciens*. *FEMS Microbiology Letters* **149:** 213-219.

Ko K.C., Han Y., Choi J.H., Kim G.J., Lee S.G., Song J.J. (2011). A novel bifunctional endo-/exo-type cellulase from an anaerobic ruminal bacterium. *Applied Microbiology Biotechnology* **89:** 1453-1462.

Kobayashi Y., Okuda N., Mastsumoto M., Inoue K., Wakita M., Hoshino S. (1998). Constitutive Expression of a Heterologous Eubacterium ruminantium Xylanase Gene (xynA) in Butyrivibrio fibrisolvens. *FEMS Microbiology Letters* **163:** 388-396.

Kobayshi Y., Yamamoto M. (2002). Factors that limit maintenance of recombinant rumen bacterium in the sheep rumen. *Journal of Animal Science* **73:** 131-136.

Kraulis P.J., Clore G.M., Nilges M., Jones J.A., Peterson G., Knowles J., Gronenborn A.M. (1989). Determination of the three dimensional solution structure of C terminal domain of cellobiohydrolase I from *Trichoderma reesei. Biochemistry* **28:** 7241-7257.

Krause D.O., Denman S.E., Mackie R.I., Morrison M., Rae A.L., Attwood G.T. McSweeney C.S. (2003). Opportunities to improve fiber digestion in the rumen: microbiology, ecology and genomics. *FEMS Microbiology Review* **27:** 663-693.

Krause, D.O., Bunch, B.D., Dalrymple, K.S., Gobius, K.S., Smith, W.J.M., Xue, G.P. McSweeney C.S. (2001). Expression of a modified *Neocallimastix patriciarum* xylanase in *Butyrivibrio fibrisolvens* digests more cellulose but cannot effectively compete with highly fibrolytic bacteria in the rumen. *Journal of Applied Microbiology* **90:** 388-396.

Krause D.O., Bunch R.J., Smith J.M., McSweeney C.S. (1999a). Diversity of *Ruminococcus* strains: a survey of genetic polymorphisms and plant digesting ability. *Journal of Applied Bacteriology* **86:** 487-495.

Krause D.O., Dalrymple B.P., Smith J.M., Mackie W.J., McSweeney C.S., (1999b). 16S rDNA sequencing of Ruminococcus albus and Ruminococcus flavefaciens: design of a signature probe and its application in adult sheep. *Microbiology* **145:** 1797-1807.

Lin C., Stahl D.A. (1995). Taxon-specific probes for cellulytic the genus *Fabrobacter* reveal abundant and novel equine-associated populations. *Applied and Environmental Microbiology* **61:** 1348-1351.

Liu JinHao, Selinger B.L., Tsai Cheng Fang., Cheng Kuojaon., Liu J.H., Tsai C.F., Cheng K.J. (1999). Characterization of a *Neocallimastix patriciarum* xylanase gene and its product. *Canadian journal of Microbiology* **45:** 970-974.

Liu, J.R., Duan, C.H., Zhao, X., Tzen, J.T., Cheng, K.J., Pai, C.K. (2008). Cloning of a rumen fungal xylanase gene and purification of the recombinant enzyme via artificial oilbodies. *Applied Microbiology and Biotechnology* **79:** 225-233.

Logar R.M., Gasparic A., Nekrep F.V. (1998). Xylanolytic enzyme system of rumen bacterium *Prevotella bryantii B14. Zbornik Biotehniske Fakultete Univerze v Ljubljani. Kmetijstvo. Zootehnika.* **72:** 63-67.

MacMillan, S. (1996). Improving the Nutritional Status of Tropical Ruminants. *Biotechnology and Development Monitor* **27:** 8-9.

Malburg L.M. Jr., Forsberg C.W. (1993). *Fibrobacter succinogenes* possesses at least nine distinct glucanase genes. *Canadian Journal of Microbiology* **39:** 882-891.

Malik S., Rajput Y. S., Sunita-Grover., Mohanty A. K., Batish V. K., Malik S., Grover S. (1998). Purification and characterization of an endo-l, 4-beta-glucanase from *Ruminococcus albus* A-23. *Microbiologic, Aliments, Nutrition* **16:** 221-229.

Mann S.P., Hazelwood G.P., Orpin C.G. (1986). Characterization of a cryptic plasmid (pOM1) in *Butyrivibrio fibrisolvens* by restriction endonuclease analysis and its cloning in *Escherichia coli. Current Microbiology* **13:** 17-22.

Matsushita O., Russel J.B., Wilson D.B. (1990). Cloning and sequencing of a *B. rumincola* beta 1,4 endoglucanase gene. *Journal of Bacteriology* **172:** 3620-3630 .

McGavin M., Forsberg C.W. (1989). Catalytic and substrate binding domains of endoglucanase 2 from *B. succinogenes. Journal of Bacteriology* **171:** 3310-3315.

McSweeney C.S., Kang S., Gagen E., Davis C., Morrison M., Denman S. (2009). Recent developments in nucleic acid based techniques for use in rumen manipulation. *Revista Brasileira de Zootecnia* **38:** 341-345.

McSweeney C.S., Dalrymple B.P., Gobius K.S., Kennedy P.M., Krause D.O., Mackie R.I., Xue G.P. (1999). The application of rumen biotechnology to improve the nutritive value of fibrous feedstuffs: pre- and post-ingestion. *Livestock Production Science* **59:** 265-283.

McSweeney C.S., Denman S.E., Wright A.D.G., Yu Z. (2006). Application of recent DNA/ RNA-based techniques in rumen ecology. AAAP Conference, Korea. *Asian-Australasian Journal of Animal Science* **20:** 283-294.

Minato H., Suto T. (1978). Techniquefor fractionation of bacteria in rumen microbial ecosystem II. Attachment of bacteria isolated from bovine rumen to cellulose powder in vitro and elution of bacteria attached therefrom. *The Journal of General and Applied Microbiology* **24:** 1-16.

Miron J., Ben_Ghedalla D., Morrison M. (2001). Adhesion mechanisms of rumen cellulolytic bacteria. *Journal of Dairy Science* **84:** 1294-1309.

Mitsumori, M., Xu-LiMing, Kajikawa, H., Kurihara, M., and Xu, L. M., (2002). Properties of cellulose-binding modules in endoglucanase F from Fibrobacter succinogenes S85 by means of surface plasmon resonance. *FEMS Microbiology Letters.* **214:** 277-281.

Miyagi T., Kaneichi K., Aminov R.I., Kobayashi Y., Sakka K., Hoshino S., Ohmiya K. (1995). Enumeration of transconjugated *Ruminococcus albus* and its survival in the goat rumen ecosystem. *Applied and Environmental Microbiology* **61:** 2030-2032.

Miyazaki K., Miyamoto H., Mercer D.K., Hirase T., Martin J.C., Kojima Y., Flint H.J. (2003). Involvement of the multidomain regulatory protein XynR in positive control of xylanase gene expression in the ruminal anaerobe *Prevotella bryantii B14. Journal of Bacteriology* **185:** 2219-2226.

Odenyo A.A., Osuji P.O., Karanfil O., Adinew K., (1997a). Effect of multipurpose tree (MPT) supplements on ruminal ciliate protozoa. *Animal Feed Science and Technology* **67:** 169-180.

Odenyo A.A., Osuji P.O., Karanfil O., Adinew K. (1997b). Microbiological evaluation of *Acacia angustissima* as a protein supplement for sheep. *Animal Feed Science and Technology* **65:** 99-112.

Ogata K., Aminov R.I., Nagamine T., Sugiura M., Tajima K., Mitsumori M., Sekizaki T., Kudo H., Minato H., Benno Y. (1997). Construction of a *Fibrobacter succinogenes* genomic map and demonstration of diversity at the genomic level. *Current Microbiology* **35:** 22-27.

Ohara H., Noguchi J., Karita S., Kimura T., Sakka K., Ohmiya K. (2000a). Sequence of egV and properties of EgV, a *Ruminococcus albus* endoglucanase containing a dockerin domain. *Bioscience, Biotechnology and Biochemistry* **64:** 80-88.

Ohara H., Karita S., Kimura T., Sakka K., Ohmiya K. (2000b). Characterization of the cellulolytic complex (cellulosome) from *Ruminococcus albus. Bioscience, Biotechnology and Biochemistry* **64:** 254-260.

Pan J., Suzuki T., Koike S., Ueda K., Kobayashi Y., Tanaka K., Okubo M. (2003). Effects of urea infused into the rumen on liquid- and particle-associated fibrolytic enzyme activities in steers fed low quality grass hay. *Animal Feed Science and Technology* **104:** 13-27.

Panjarathinum R., Laxminarayana H. (1977). Studies on rumen microflora in cows and buffaloes under different feeding regimes. 4. Distribution of bacteria and in vitro studies. *Indian Journal of Animal Sciences* **45:** 173-182.

Qi M., Nelson K.E., Daugherty S.C., Nelson W.C., Hance I.R., Morrison M., Forsberg C.W. (2005). Novel molecular features of the fibrolytic intestinal bacterium Fibrobacter intestinalis not shared with *Fibrobacter succinogenes* as determined by suppressive subtractive hybridization. *Journal of Bacteriology* **187:** 3739-3751.

Qi M., Wang P., Selinger L.B., Yanke L.J., Forster R.J., McAllister T.A. (2011). Isolation and characterization of a ferulic acid esterase (Fae1A) from the rumen fungus *Anaeromyces mucronatus. Journal of Applied Microbiology* **110:** 1341-1350.

Qiu-Xiao, Selinger B., Yanke LJ., Cheng K.J., Qiu X. (2000). Isolation and analysis of two cellulase cDNAs from *Orpinomyces joyonii. Gene.* **245:** 119-126.

Robinson J.A., Greening R.C., Smolenski W.J., Bell R.L., Ogilve M.L., Barsuhn K. (1993). Effect of inoculums of *Meghasphaera elsdenii* 407A on rumen pH, Lactate and VFA in bovine model of acute acidosis. *Journal of Animal Science* **71**(*Suppl*): 269.

Russel J.B., Wilson D.B. (1988). Potential oppurtunites and problems for genetically engeeiered rumen microorganisms. *Journal of Nutrition* **118:** 271-279.

Russell J.B., Onodera R., Hino T. (1991). Ruminal protein fermentation: New perspectives on previous contradictions. In: *Physiological Aspects of Digestion and Metabolism in Ruminants.* (T. Tsuda, Y. Sasaki, R. Kawashima, eds.) Academic Press, London, p 681.

Russell, J. B., Wallace. R. J., (1988). Energy yielding and consuming reactions. In : *The Rumen Microbial Ecosystem*. (P. N. Hobson, ed), Elsevier, Barking, Essex, UK p185.

Sajjad., M., Andrabi, S.M.H., Akhter, S., Afzal M. (2008). Application of Biotechnology to Improve Post-Ingestion Forage Quality in the Rumen. *Pakistan Journal of Nutrition* **7:** 70-74.

Samanta A.K., Walli T.K., Rajput Y.S., Batish V.K, Grover S., Mohanty A.K. (1999). Fractionation and partial purification of endoglucanase and xylanase from *Piromyces* sp. isolated from rumen of buffalo. *Microbiologic, Aliments, Nutrition* **17:** 81-91.

Shedova E.N., Berezina O.V., Lunina N.A., Zverlov V.V., Schwartz W.H., Velikodvorskaia G.A. (2009). Cloning and characterization of a large metagenomic DNA fragment containing glycosyl-hydrolase genes. *Molecular Geneneral Mikrobiology Virusol* **1:** 11-15.

Singh S., Bhatia S.K., Pradhan K., Singh S. (2003). Relative ruminal ciliates distribution and physiology of bacteria isolated in buffalo and cattle fed wheat straw- preformed protein diets. *Indian journal of Animal-Sciences* **73:** 663-667.

Sinha R.N., Ranganathan B. (1983). Cellulolytic bacteria in buffalo rumen. *Journal of Applied Bacteriology* **54:** 1-6.

Steenbakkers P.J.M., Ubhayasekera W., Goossen H.J.A.M., Lierop E.M.H.M.V., Drift C.V.D.R., Vogels G.D., Mowbray S.L., Camp H.J.M.O.D. (2002). An intron-containing glycoside hydrolase family 9 cellulase gene encodes the dominant 90 kDa component of the cellulosome of the anaerobic fungus *Piromyces sp.* strain E2. *Biochemical Journal* **365:** 193-204.

Stewart C.S., Bryant M.P. (1988). The rumen bacteria. In: *The rumen microbial ecosystem*. (P.N. Hobson, ed.), Elsevier Applied Science Publication Ltd., England, pp. 21-75.

Stewart C.S., Fevre M., Prins R.A. (1995). Factors affecting fermentation and polymer degradation by anaerobic fungi and the potential for manipulation of rumen function. In: *Ruminant Physiology, Digestion, Metabolism, Growth and Reproduction. Proceedings of the 8th International Symposium on Ruminant Nutrition*. (W. von Engelhardt, S. Leonhard-Marek, G. Breves, D. Gieseke, eds.), Ferdinand Enke Verlag, Stuttgart, Germany pp 249-268.

Stewart C.S., Fonty G., Gouet P.H., (1988). The establishment of rumen microbial communities. *Animal Feed Science and Technology* **21:** 69-97.

Teather A.M. (1982). Isolation of plasmid DNA from *Butyrivibrio fibrisolvens*. *Applied and Environmental Microbiology* **43:** 298-302.

Teather R.M. (1985). Application of gene manipulation to rumen micro?ora. *Canadian Journal of Animal Science* **65:** 563-574.

Thulasi A., Chandrasekharaiah M., Sampath K.T. (2003). Cloning of endobeta 1,4 gluconase gene from *Ruminococcus albus* gene and its expression in *Escherchia coli* JM109. *Indian Journal of Dairy and Biosciences* **15:** 14-18.

Thulasi A., Chandrasekharaiah M., Sampath K.T. (2008). Cloning of cellulase gene from *Ruminococcus albus* in *Escherichia coli* and the activity of cellulase in the periplasmic protein fraction, *Indian Veterinary Journal* **85:** 361-362.

Varga, G.A., Kolver, E.S. (1997). Microbial and Animal Limitations to Fiber Digestion and Utilization. *Journal of Nutrition* **127**(Suppl5): 819S-823S.

Vercoe, P. E., Gregg, K. (1995). Sequence and transcriptional analysis of an endoglucanase gene from *Ruminococcus albus AR67. Animal Biotechnology* **6:** 59-71.

Veroe, P.E., Spight, D.H., White, B.A. (1995). Nucleotide sequence and transcriptional analysis of the celD beta-glucanase gene from Ruminococcus flavefaciens FD-1. *Canadian Journal of Microbiology* **41:** 27-34.

Wallace R.J. (1994). Ruminal microbiology, biotechnology, and ruminant nutrition. *Journal of Animal Science* **72:** 2992-3003.

Wallace R.J., Walker N.D. (1993). Isolation and attempted introduction of sugar-utilizing bacteria in sheep rumen. *Journal of Applied Bacteriology* **74:** 353-359.

Wang G., Luo H., Wang Y., Huang H., Shi P., Yang P., Meng K., Bai Y., Yao B. (2011). A novel cold-active xylanase gene from the environmental DNA of goat rumen contents: directcloning, expression and enzyme characterization. *Bioresource Technology* **102:** 3330-3336.

Ware C.E., Bauchop T., Hudman J.F., Gregg K. (1992). Cryptic plasmid pBfl from *Butyrivibrio fibrisolvens* AR10. *Current Microbiology* **24:** 193-197.

Whitehead T.R. (1992). Genetic transformation of the ruminal bacteria *B. Fibrosolvens* and *S. Bovis* by electroporation. *Letters in Applied Microbiology* **15:** 186-189.

Whitehead T.R., Cotta M.A., Hespell R.B. (1991). Introduction of the *Bactereoides ruminicola* xylanase gene into the *Bacteroides thetaiataomicron* chromosome for production of xylanase activity. *Applied and Environmental Microbiology* **57:** 277-282.

Whitehead T.R., Flint H.J. (1995). Heterologus Expression of an Endoglucanase Gene (end A) from the Ruminal Anaerobe *Ruminococcous flavefaciens* 17 in *Streptococcus bovis* and *Streptococcus Sangius*. *FEMS Microbiology Letters* **126:** 165-169.

Whitehead T.R., Hespell R.B. (1990). Heterologous expression of the Bacteroides ruminicola xylanase gene in Bacteroides fragilis and Bacteroides uniformis. *FEMS Microbiology Letters* **66:** 61-65.

Williams A.G., Coleman G.S. (1998). The rumen protozoa, In: *The rumen microbial ecosystem*. (P.N. Hobson, C.S. Stewart, eds.) Blackie Academy Professional, New York, USA, pp73-139.

Willson J.R., Mertens D.R. (1995). Cell wall accessibility and cell structure limitations to microbial digestion of forage. *Crop Science* **35:** 251-259.

Wood T.M., Wilson C.A. McCrae S.I. (1995). The cellulase system of the anaerobic rumen fungus *Neocallimastix frontalis:* studies on the properties of fractions rich in endo-(1—>4)-beta-D-glucanase activity. *Applied Microbiology and Biotechnology* **44:** 177-184.

Ye, X.Y., Ng,T.B., Cheng, K.J. (2001). Purification and characterization of a cellulase from the ruminal fungus *Orpinomyces joyonii* cloned in *Escherichia coli*. *International Journal of Biochemistry and Cell-Biology*. **33:** 87-94.

Zhu Y.X., Wang J.Q., Ma R.L., Huang L., Dong Z.Y. (2007). Construction and analysis of rumen bacterial artificial chromosome library from a dairy cow rumen microflora. *Acta Microbiologica Sinica* **47:** 213-217.

Ziemer C.J., Sharp R., Stern M.D., Cotta M.A., Whitehead T.R., Stahl D.A. (2002). Persistence and functional impact of a microbial inoculant on native microbial community structure, nutrient digestion and fermentation characteristics in a rumen model. *Systematic and Applied Microbiology* **25:** 416-422.

❑❑❑

Chapter 4

Bypass Nutrient Technology for Meeting the Requirement of High Yielding Dairy Animals

M. Chandrasekharaiah, K.T. Sampath, A. Thulasi
National Institute of Animal Nutrition and Physiology, Adugodi, Bangalore-560 030 Karnataka, India

Summary

Feed cost accounts for more than half of the recurring cost of milk production. For maintaining profitable dairy production/operations, the dairy animals should be fed with proper rations with minimum cost. In this context the concept of bypass nutrients technology assumes special significance and this technology is useful not only for better utilization of nutrients but also to minimize the ruminal fermentation losses there by reducing the wastage of nutrients in to the environment. Feeding of bypass nutrients such as bypass protein and bypass fat has the potential to increase productive as well as reproductive performance of dairy animals under Indian conditions. The responses are likely to be more favourable in high yielding animals in the early part of lactation or fast growing animals. These are typical situations where the demand for nutrients is high and where the animals may be in negative protein and energy balance with lower body condition score. The importance of bypass nutrients technology with particular reference to proteins and fats are discussed here in this chapter.

In dairy animals, most of the feed nutrients ingested are degraded by microorganisms present in the rumen at varying degrees / proportions. Bypass nutrients are the nutrient fractions, which gets fermented at a lower degree in the rumen, which becomes available at the lower part of the gastrointestinal tract for the subsequent digestion and absorption. In addition to this the bypass nutrients provide a steady supply of nutrients instead of providing all the nutrients immediately with sudden bursts from easily soluble nutrients (Walli *et al.*, 1995). Initially the concept of bypass nutrients was used for proteins, to describe the protein quality in ruminants, but subsequently this term has been extended to other nutrients like carbohydrates and fats that could also escape rumen fermentation partially and digested and absorbed in the small intestine. These concepts are useful not only for better utilization of nutrients but also minimize the ruminal fermentation losses thereby reducing the wastage of nutrients into the environment.

Bypass nutrients –natural or manipulated?

Some nutrients have bypass characteristics in their natural forms. In some feedstuffs, nutrients are bound to other feed components, thus reducing their rumen degradability. The bonds with which nutrients are linked remain intact in the natural environment (pH: 6.7) of the rumen, but they are broken in the acidic environment of the abomasum (pH: 2-3). These are referred to as naturally occurring bypass nutrients. However, others are required to be manipulated to reduce their degradability for optimization of ratios between degradable and undegradable nutrients in diet.

1. Bypass protein technology

In ruminants protein digestion is dominated by microbial transformation in the fore- stomach. A varying portion of feed protein is degraded into peptides, amino acids and ammonia, all of which can be used for synthesis of microbial protein. Microbial proteins and non-degraded feed proteins are digested in the lower tract. Dietary proteins that resist degradation in the rumen and pass to lower tract are called bypass proteins.

1.1 Microbial protein synthesis in ruminants

Approximately more than 50% of the amino acids are absorbed by the ruminants are derived from microbial protein synthesized in the rumen, thus, the microbial protein forms a major source of protein to the ruminants under normal feeding conditions. In order to establish the amounts and ratios of nutrients necessary for optimal microbial and animal response, one must first adequately predict the degree to which nutrients are made available in the rumen from a variety of ingredient sources (Nocek, 1988). The quality of intestinally degraded protein is largely determined by the extent and efficiency of microbial protein synthesis in the rumen (Oosting *et al.,* 1995).

To effectively understand the process of ruminal demand and supply of nutrient to host animal, there is a need to quantify the microbial protein production. The purine nitrogen index (PNI) and nitrogen capture efficiency (NCE) are new potential parameters, which can be used for determining the overall efficiency of utilization of ruminant diets. The PNI, which refers to the ratio of PD nitrogen to total nitrogen in urine (Chen *et al.,* 1999), could indicate the NCE. These parameters have been proposed as an index of utilization of nitrogen in the rumen compared to the amount wasted in the urine. The diet with higher PNI and NCE values will produce more microbial protein and proportionally less nitrogen will be excreted in urine. Endogenous nitrogen excretion, protein intake, degradability, digestibility and efficiency of observed amino acid all can affect the value of PNI. However, these parameters are not sensitive for detecting small differences and have certain limitations, which could be overcome by using in a "grouping system". The recent studies conducted by Chandrasekharaiah *et al.* (2010) in sheep fed on straw based diets with different rumen degradable nitrogen levels indicated that PNI and NCE could be effectively used in the evaluation of protein efficiency of ruminant diets in India. Further, the work carried out by Chandrasekharaiah *et al.* (2011) revealed that the optimum microbial protein synthesis occurred at 12 -18 g rumen degradable nitrogen (RDN) per Kg of digestible organic matter (DOM) in sheep fed on straw based diet. However, more studies needed to be conducted in this direction to evaluate straw based diets for ruminant under Indian conditions.

1.2 Bypass protein requirement in dairy animals

The microbial protein synthesis is energy dependent process. Deficiency of dietary energy especially during early part of the lactation, which is not uncommon, result in correspondingly lower synthesis of bacterial protein in the rumen leading to reduced availability of protein for milk production. Therefore, for sustaining higher level of milk yield and faster growth rate, ruminants need more dietary protein than the flora in the rumen can utilize. However, higher dietary protein intake especially rumen degradable protein (RDP) often results in increasing loss of ammonia from the rumen. Excess ammonia is converted in to urea in the liver, the major part of which is excreted through urine resulting in the loss of part of dietary protein. Increased ammonia levels also leads to reduced fertility besides causing stress on the liver. Adequate protein supply to high yielding cows without stress from excess ammonia can be ensured by decreasing the degradability of dietary proteins. This has lead to the development of techniques to protect greater proportion of dietary proteins from the degradation in the rumen.

1.3 Evaluation and expression of protein requirements in dairy animals

Over the last two decades, more and more quantitative knowledge on the protein requirement of ruminants has been acquired and on this basis new systems for protein evaluation of feeds and for expression of protein requirement of ruminants have been proposed (NRC, 1989). These systems require that the protein needs of the ruminants must be supplied in terms of:

a) *Rumen degradable protein (RDP)* to meet the nitrogen requirement of the rumen microorganisms and

b) *Undegradable dietary protein (UDP) or bypass protein, i.e.,* the fraction which escapes degradation in the rumen and passes to the lower tract, which should be made available to the animal whenever the microbial protein formed in the rumen is not sufficient to meet the protein requirement of the animal.

An important pre-requisite for the implementation of the new protein evaluation system mentioned above is the expression of protein requirement of ruminants on RDP and UDP basis and also the description of the protein content of ruminant feeds on RDP and UDP basis. Ruminants consume a wide variety of proteins and non protein nitrogen sources. From the work carried out in different laboratories during last few years, the protein degradability values of a large number of feeds are available now. Various methods (*in vivo, in vitro, in situ*) have been employed for the estimation of degradability of proteins in the rumen with their own limitations. Of the different methods, *in situ* nylon bag technique which involves the suspension of feed materials in the rumen of fistulated animals is generally accepted method (Mehrez and Orskov, 1977; Orskov and McDonald, 1979). The RDP and UDP requirement of different categories of dairy cattle based on publications of NRC, (1989) is given in Table1. The RDP and UDP content of some of the commonly used feed stuffs (Sampath *et al.*, 1999; Chandrasekharaiah *et al.*, 2001, 2002,) based on the result of the studies conducted in different parts of the world are given Table 2.

Table 1 : Daily nutrient requirement of lactating cows (NRC, 1989)

Live weight (kg)	Fat (%)	Milk (kg)	TDN (kg)	Protein	
				UDP	RDP
400	4.5	8.0	6.44	511	753
400	4.5	14.0	8.48	710	1052
400	4.5	20.0	10.51	880	1355
400	4.5	26.0	12.54	1026	1662
400	4.5	32.0	14.58	1220	1962

It can be observed from table 2 that some of the feedstuffs have ruminal degradability value of more than 60% and are poor sources of UDP/bypass protein. It is difficult to obtain absolute protein degradability values for a wide variety of feedstuffs. Several factors introduce considerable variations into what is supposed to be standard for comparison. It is more realistic therefore to determine the relative RDP and UDP values. These values rank the protein sources and diets relative to one another. The commonly used feedstuffs can be divided into three categories depending up on their degradability (Table 3) in the rumen.

Table 2 : Crude protein (CP), rumen degradable protein (RDP) and undegradable protein (UDP) / bypass protein content of feeds and fodders

Feedstuffs	CP	RDP	UDP (bypass protein)	Feedstuffs	CP	RDP	UDP (bypass protein)
	gram per kg dry matter				gram per kg dry matter		
Concentrates				**Concentrates**			
Bajra	120	38	82	Neem seed kernel cake	386	217	169
Barley	100	79	21	Niger cake	330	244	86
Brewers grains	260	122	138	Oats	100	84	16
Coconut cake (solvent extracted)	270	62	208	Rice bran	140	91	49
Coconut cake (expeller)	240	173	67	Rice bran extraction	160	64	96
Corn gluten meal (60% CP)	600	126	474	Rice broken	110	35	75
Corn gluten meal (40% CP)	400	148	252	Rice polish	120	61	59
Cotton seed	170	78	92	Rubber seed cake	280	202	78
Cotton seed cake	350	179	171	Safflower cake	220	141	79
Cotton seed cake (solvent extracted)	360	137	223	Salseed meal	90	27	63
Distillers dried grain	290	133	157	Silk cotton seed cake	370	289	81
Gingelly / sesame/ til cake	350	266	84	Soyabean meal extractions	460	276	184
Groundnut cake (GNC), expeller	450	315	135	Sunflower meal	300	165	135
GNC (formaldehyde treated 1g/100g CP)	450	194	256	**Roughages**			
GNC (heat treated 130°C 3h)	450	194	256	Alfalfa, dehydrated	200	80	120
GNC (heat treated 130°C 2h)	450	234	216	Alfalfa fresh (*Medicago sativa*)	200	152	48
GNC (deoiled/ solvent extracted)	480	408	72	Berseem (*Trifolium alexndrium*)	259	127	132
Horse gram	240	137	103	Grass hay	29	13	16
Jowar	100	20	80	Guninea grass	82	33	49
Karanja cake	320	173	147	Maize early cut	165	96	69
Kokam cake	140	17	123	Oats (*Avena Sativa*)	126	65	61
Linseed cake	280	162	118	Para grass	71	34	37
Mahua seed cake	185	105	80	Rice straw	40	15	25
Maize bran	160	59	101	Subabul (*Leucaena leucocephola*)	250	80	170
Maize grain	90	27	67	Sugar cane tops, chaffed, ensiled	68	10	58
Mustard cake	350	263	87	Wheat straw	33	18	15

1. High ruminal degradability (values ranging from 61 to 100 percent).
2. Medium ruminal degradability (values ranging from 31 to 60 percent).
3. Low ruminal degradability (values ranging from 0 to 30 percent).

Table 3 : Feedstuffs of low, medium and high degradability.

Low degradability (<30 %)	Medium degradability (30-60%)	High degradability (>60 %)
Concentrates		
Kokam cake	Bajra	Safflower cake
Jowar Corn gluten meal (60% CP) Coconut cake (solvent extracted)	Rice broken Corn gluten meal (40% CP) Maize bran	Rice bran Groundnut cake (expeller) Coconut cake (expeller)
Maize grain	Cotton seed cake (Solvent extracted)	Rubber seed cake
Salseed meal	Rice bran extraction Cotton seed	Niger cake Mustard cake
	Distillers dried grain	Gingelly / sesame / til cake
	Brewers grains Cotton seed cake Rice polish Karanja cake	Silk cotton seed cake Barley Oats Groundnut cake (Deoiled / solvent extracted)
	Sunflower meal Neem seed kernel cake Horse gram Mahua seed cake Linseed cake Soyabean meal extractions	
Roughages		
Sugar cane tops, chaffed, ensiled	Subabul (*Leucaena leucocephala*)	Alfalfa fresh (*Medicago sativa*)
	Rice straw Alfalfa, dehydrated Guniea grass Grass hay Para grass Berseem (*Trifolium alexandrium*) Oats (*Avena Sativa*) Wheat straw Maize early cut	

1.4 Methods to increase bypass protein content of feedstuffs

Although considerable proportions of dietary proteins are resistant to fermentative digestion in the rumen, the quantities which bypass the rumen do not appear to be sufficient to supplement the microbial protein completely in some feeding situations. Methods which can be adopted for increasing the bypass protein content are

1. Selection of feed ingredients on the basis of their degradability
2. Protection of proteins from degradation in the rumen

1.4.1 Selection of ingredients

Relatively good proportion of bypass protein can be provided by selecting the ingredients of high bypass protein value while formulating the rations. Some of the feed ingredients which are known to have high bypass protein value are dried byproducts of fermentation industry (Barley, Corn and Potato), Corn milling byproducts (e.g., corn gluten meal), dehydrated alfalfa, heat treated protein sources etc.

In selecting the ingredients attention must be given to the amino acid profile of the undegraded protein fraction in combination with microbial protein. This must then be related to the tissue needs of the animal in question.

1.4.2 Protection of proteins from degradation in the rumen

Several approaches have been tried to protect the dietary protein from ruminal degradation. They include closure of esophageal groove, post ruminal infusion, physical processing, heat treatment, chemical treatments *viz.*, formaldehyde treatment and tannic acid treatment, non enzymatic browning technique and using of acids, alkalies, alcohol and metal ions. There are also reports indicating the effectiveness of calcium soaps of long chain fatty acids in protecting the proteins from ruminal degradation.

i) Physical processing

Alterations in the physical form influence the behaviour of the feed particles in the rumen environment. The most often applied way of changing the physical form of the diet is grinding. Increasing the surface of degradability, but the reduced particle size may reduce the retention time in the rumen resulting in increased bypass.

ii) Heat treatment

Subjecting certain feeds to controlled higher heat decreases the solubility of proteins by creating cross linkages within and among peptide chains to carbohydrates, thus lowering their susceptibility to ruminant degradation.

However, high temperature and extended heating times render protein less digestible through Millard reaction between sugar aldehyde groups and free amino groups thus lowering the digestibility of constituent amino acids. In general, the beneficial effects of reduced rate of degradation in rumen appear to be greater than the reduced whole tract protein digestibility caused by limited heat damage. Walli *et al.,* (2000) observed 150°C for 2 h as the optimum temperature-time combination. Sampath *et al.,* (1997) reported that the ruminal protein degradability of groundnut cake was reduced by 35% and 45% due to heat treatment for 2 hours and 3 hours at 130°C, respectively. Further, they observed that heat treatment at that temperature and time duration did not have any negative effect on *in vivo* apparent CP digestibility.

iii) Chemical treatment

Certain chemical agents form reversible cross linkages with amino and amide groups which decreases solubility of proteins at the pH of the rumen. Chemically treated proteins are subsequently made available to the host animal by destruction of these linkages in acidic abomasum. Agents investigated include aldehydes and tanning materials.

Formaldehyde treatment

Formaldehyde (1 to 1.5 g per 100g crude protein) treatment was used to reduce the protein degradability of highly degradable cakes and also to study the impact of its feed on the productive response of dairy animals (Gupta and Walli, 1987; Bhagwat and Srivastava, 1993; Kumar and Walli, 1994; Tiwari and Yadav, 1994; Ramachandra and Sampath, 1995; Chatterjee and Walli, 2003a). Chatterjee and Walli, (2003b) also optimized the formaldehyde as 1.0 to 1.2g/100g CP for the treatment of mustard and groundnut-cake at which level protein degradability is substantially reduced without having adverse effect on post ruminal degradability.

Tannic acid treatment

The presence of tannins in food sources for monogastric animals is generally viewed adversely. However, in ruminants, tannins can induce beneficial effects. For example, in sheep higher retention of nitrogen has been observed with low to moderate levels of tannins in forages (Egan and Ulyatt, 1980). In these cases, the lower apparent and true digestibility of nitrogen was compensated for by reduced urinary loss of nitrogen. Tanins can have beneficial responses in ruminants, resulting in higher growth rates and milk yield. (Marten and Ehle, 1984; Larsen *et al.,* 1974).

Several mechanisms have been suggested to explain how tannins influence protein utilization by ruminants (Reed, 1995). Tannins may complex protein at the pH of the rumen and protect protein from microbial enzymes. These complexes are unstable at the acid pH of the abomasum and the proteins become available for digestion (Jones and Mangan, 1977; Barry and Manley, 1984). Another hypothesis is that tannins may increase efficiency in nitrogen recycling to the rumen. Tannins lower the rate of protein degradation and deamination in the rumen resulting in lower rumen ammonia concentration. This results in lower plasma urea nitrogen (PUN). Lower PUN means lower urinary nitrogen excretion with less wastage of nitrogen (Robbins *et al.*, 1987). Larger amounts of nitrogen are recycled because tannins stimulate increased saliva production. In diets based on tanniferous forages, rumen nitrogen outflow is often larger than nitrogen intake. Several studies have reported an increase in protein flow when moderate doses of tannins were used. This has been attributed to increased rumen escape of dietary proteins, increase in microbial protein flow (up to 28% in sheep) (Reed *et al.*, 1990). The larger microbial flow could be the result of increased saliva production, increased rumen turnover rate, and hence, increased microbial outflow, increased nitrogen recycling to the rumen.

iv) Other methods

- *Non enzymatic browning technique*: Involves the mixing of a protein source with xylose sugar or sucrose and heating it. (Chalupa, 1975; Stern, 1984; Cleale *et al.*, 1986).
- *Using metal ions*: Involves using of zinc salts (Britton and Klopfenstein, 1986; Gaynor *et al.*, 1988)
- *Using corn protein zein*: Involves the protein supplement or the amino acid coated with zein by mixing it with zein along with binding agent and extrusion.
- *Using acids and alkalis*: such as acetic acid, propionic acid and hydrochloric acid (Waltz and Loerch, 1986; Khorasani *et al.*, 1989) and sodium hydroxide (Bowman *et al.*, 1988; Mir *et al.*, 1984; Gould *et al.*, 1976; Friedman1982).
- *Using alcohols (ethanol, propanol, iso propanol)*: with or without addition of heat (Lynch *et al.*, 1987; Lynch *et al.*, 1988).

v) Genetic engineering approach

Alfalfa and other forage legumes are high in protein but deficient in S-amino acids cysteine and methionine. The protein content of forage legumes can be improved for ruminants by introducing into them functional genes encoding for proteins rich in sulfur amino acids that are ruminally stable. The delta and beta-zein proteins contain proportionately high levels of S-amino acids. Bagga *et al.* (2004) in their preliminary studies, transformed alfalfa with CaMV 35S- beta -zein and CaMV 35S- delta -zein gene constructs individually and in combination. The results indicate that as in tobacco both the beta - and the delta -zeins accumulate in the leaves of alfalfa and that the co-expression of the two zein genes has a stabilizing effect on the delta-zein. However, the level of accumulation of the zeins in alfalfa leaves is not high enough to make a significant change in the methionine levels. The data on rumen incubation experiments have demonstrated that the zeins are completely stable in the rumen of cows and thus qualify as the suitable rumen bypass protein that is rich in methionine.

1.5 Effect of bypass protein supplementation on growth, milk production and reproduction

1.5.1 Growth

Sampath *et al.* (1996) did not observe any effect on growth rate in crossbred calves fed formaldehyde treated groundnut cake. Pachauri *et al.*, (1999) also reported that inclusion of formaldehyde treated groundnut cake replacing untreated groundnut cake did not have any additional positive effect on body weight gain and UDP was not important for calves growing at a rate of 450-485g per day. A significant increase in growth rate was observed in goat kids, on feeding formaldehyde treated groundnut cake (Mudgal and Sengar, 1980). Feeding of formaldehyde treated GN cake resulted in increase in the growth rate of crossbred claves (Kumar and Walli, 1994). Similarly, the feeding of formaldehyde treated mustard cake gave significant increase in growth performance of buffalo calves (Chatterjee and Walli, 1998). The feeding of bypass protein in the form of formaldehyde treated mustard cake can be proven economically beneficial for raising of buffalo calves (Chatterjee and Walli, 2003b) on wheat straw based rations.

1.5.2 Milk production

In India several studies have been conducted to study the effect of feeding higher bypass protein on milk production and the results of few studies are presented below.

Dahiya *et al.* (1991) reported a significant increase in milk yield (2-3 kg per day) in buffaloes in early lactation fed on urea treated straw supplemented with 1.5 and 3.0 kg cottonseed cake (bypass protein source). Sampath *et al.*, (1997) studied the effect of two levels of UDP in the diet on milk production. Fourteen cows whose previous lactation yield was 8 to 10 kg/d were divided into two groups of seven cows each and fed Ragi straw and isocaloric concentrate mixtures with RDP: UDP in the ratio of 65:35 (Group I) and 50:50 (group II) from 15th day after calving up to 36 weeks. The average yield of fat corrected milk per day per cow was significantly higher in group II (9.40 kg) than in group I (7.80 kg) and also the decline in milk yield with progress of lactation was much slower in group II. An experiment of short duration (four months) on paddy straw based diet also yielded similar results (Ramachandra and Sampath, 1995). Kalbande and Thomas, (1999) reported an average milk yield of 10.11, 7.18 and 6.32 kg in lactating Jersey crossbred cows fed on iso nitrogenous concentrate mixtures containing RDP/UDP in the ratio of 37:63, 52:48 and 70:30, respectively. Further, they observed that higher levels of UDP in the concentrate mixture stimulated the feed consumption resulting in better availability of nutrients for higher milk production. Bharadwaj and Sengupta, (1999) studied the effect of protected and unprotected protein on lactation performance of Murrah buffaloes and observed increased average daily milk yield, FCM yield, fat, protein and total solid content in animals fed with bypass protein. The effect of feeding rumen bypass protein in the form of formaldehyde treated mustard cake protein on milk yield and milk composition in Murrah buffaloes was determined by Chatterjee and Walli, (2003a). The average daily yield of protein, fat, SNF and total solid were also significantly higher, the feed cost was lower, indicating that the diet containing formaldehyde treated mustard cake was more economical than the control diet containing untreated mustard cake. Supplementation of 1.0 kg protected protein in the form of formaldehyde treated sunflower and rapeseed meals in the ration of cows was found to be economical, compared to feeding a similar quantity of untreated protein meal straw based rations (Garg *et al.*, 2002, 2005). Reported 15% increase in milk yield on feeding of formaldehyde-protected mustard-cake to crossbred cows.

Several on–farm trials (Sampath *et al.*, 2004; Chandrasekharaiah *et al.*, 2008) conducted to study the effect of bypass protein on milk production performance in medium yielding cows revealed that the feeding of bypass protein is beneficial even in medium yielding cows. The feeding practice followed by the farmers was refined by partly replacing the groundnut cake with cottonseed cake which provided more bypass protein than groundnut cake. By this refinement, milk production increased by 1 to 1.5 litre /cow/ day and the cost of feed was reduced and the overall income of the farmers was increased by about Rs. 12-17/cow/day.

1.5.3 Reproduction

Protein nutrition can affect reproduction through toxic effects of ammonia and it's metabolites on gametes and early embryos, through deficiencies of amino acids and by exacerbations of negative balances of energy. Excess degradable protein acts through some unidentified mechanism to decrease uterine pH during luteal phase which may play a role to reduce fertility. Energy cost of detoxifying large amounts of ammonia to urea may aggravate an existing post partum energy shortage. Higher UDP in late dry period improves post partum performance and also reduces metabolic disorders.

Limited studies were carried out in India on the effect of bypass protein supplement on male and female reproductive performance. Bulls with bypass protein feeding along with exercise showed highest improvement in erection, protrusion, intensity of thrust reaction time, total time taken to successful mount and required less added stimulus and had a lower flehmen response which was slightly better than bypass protein feeding group alone. A combination of exercise and bypass protein feeding had a highest beneficial effect on semen quality (sperm abnormality, live / dead sperm and acrosomal integrity) and quantity in Mehasana bull (Prajapati *et al.,* 1996, 1998 a,b). Reduced service period was also observed in buffaloes by feeding a commercial bypass protein feed (Bharadwaj *et al.,* 2000). Supplementation of formaldehyde treated GNC in place of untreated GNC in the concentrate mixture of crossbred cows on paddy straw based ration improved the production and reproductive performance economically (Mishra *et al.,* 2006).

1.6 Beneficial aspects of feeding protein of low degradability to ruminants

In ruminants, the microbial protein synthesized in the rumen is the major protein source utilized for body functions. However, higher growth rates and milk production levels require higher protein than usually provided from microbial protein alone. Supplementation with UDP may enhance growth rate and milk production, especially under such conditions. Egan, (1988) explained that the enhanced growth or milk production is mediated by :

- Dietary protein intact or as peptide delivered to the lower tract can improve the amino acid availability for lean tissue,
- Slow degradation of proteins can result in more constant N supply to the rumen which may improve the supply of NH_3 and possibly peptides for the growth and fermentative activity of rumen micro-organisms, thus improving the supply of microbial protein to the lower tract,
- The extra amino acids absorbed as a result of feeding more ruminal escapes protein may be used with high efficiency as an amino acid source for the body protein synthesis, but they may also alter the hormonal balance e.g. between growth hormone and insulin and improve growth through lean tissue growth. Similarly, beneficial effects of UDP supplementation to cows in early lactation could also be due to alteration in the hormonal concentration of insulin and the growth hormone apart from providing more amino acids to the mammary gland. Lower insulin and higher growth hormone levels are likely to favour tissue mobilization of fat and increase milk production.

1.7 Reasons for lack of response to bypass protein feeding

1. Increased amount of bypass protein feeding some times results decreased microbial protein synthesis in the rumen. Even though high amount of bypass protein is there in the ration, but there will be no change in amount of total amino acids supplied to the rumen.

2. Bypass protein supplements in some cases, though having high bypass value, they may be poorly digested in the intestine and contains a deficient amino acids profile *e.g.*, over protected (heat/formaldehyde) proteins supplements, feather meal etc.,

3. Essential amino acid profile in the bypass protein fraction may be poor. For *e.g.*, corn gluten meal is good source of methionine in bypass protein fraction but deficient in lysine (Sampath *et al.*, 2002, 2003). Fishmeal is good source of lysine and methionine. Protected soybean meal is a good source of lysine and methionine. Hence, correct matching of these bypass supplements is necessary to achieve maximum production.

1.8 How to balance bypass protein

1.8.1 Optimization /maximization of microbial protein production

Ruminal microbial protein synthesis depends upon the supply of ammonia, digestible energy and carbon skeleton for amino acid synthesis. Nearly 50 to 75% of the amino acids absorbed by the ruminants are derived from the microbial protein synthesized in the rumen, thus making it an important protein source for the animals. Though the ammonia, supplies nitrogen requirement of rumen microbial population, preformed amino acids and peptides increase the efficiency of microbial growth compared to ammonia alone. The work carried out by Chandrasekharaiah *et al.* (2011) revealed that the optimum microbial protein synthesis occurred at 12-18 g rumen degradable nitrogen (RDN) per kg of digestible organic matter (DOM) in sheep fed on straw based diet. Hence, in order to ensure the beneficial effect of bypass protein feeding in high yielders, a minimum 50-60% of the dietary crude protein should be supplied with or in the form of rumen degradable protein (RDP).

i) Combination of supplements (protein/bypass protein) should be used in order to meet the amino acid profile in high yielding animals.

ii) *Essential /limiting amino acids*:

Lysine and methionine are considered to be first or co-limiting amino acids for milk production in dairy animals. The other limiting amino acids are assumed to be one or more of the following-phenylalanine, histidine and threonine. These can be included in the ration of high producing cows.

Inclusion of higher level of bypass protein in the ration of lactating crossbred animals improves the milk production performance under the Indian conditions of feeding and management. It is observed that the feeding of bypass protein is even beneficial for medium production animals, although the benefits could be more pronounced on high producing animals. Therefore it is desirable to include feed materials of medium or high bypass protein content in the ration of high yielding animals especially in the early stages of lactation. However, it is essential to ensure that sufficient amount of rumen degradable protein (50 to 60% of total crude protein) is supplied in the ration of these animals to maintain optimum rumen fermentation for better utilization of fiber. The practice of feeding protected proteins will only be successful in affecting the animal performance if the proteins/amino acids are not over protected and the animal has the metabolic capacity to respond to increased amino acid supply. A key to efficient feed utilization is to formulate rations that optimize microbial protein synthesis and also supply amounts of rumen undegradable or bypass protein needed for growth, production and reproduction in ruminants.

2. Bypass fat technology

The majority of diets based on crop residues, agricultural by products and local mixed grasses/pastures used in countries like India are extremely low in fat compared with diets used in temperature countries. Green fodders and concentrates that are the major feeds that contribute to the fat/EE (ether extract) content of the rations in dairy animals. As per specifications of Bureau of Indian Standards (BIS), concentrate mixture should contain at least 2.5-3.0% EE. The dietary fats are metabolized by rumen micro-organisms for synthesis of microbial lipids, which involves two important steps i.e. lipolysis and biohydrogenation (Jenkins, 1993). Dietary fats ingested by the animals are hydrolyzed in rumen to glycerol and fatty acids. While the glycerol is fermented to propionic acid, the unsaturated fatty acids are either partially or completely bio-hydrogenated to increase the quantity of saturated fatty acids leaving rumen. Inclusion of fat in the diet can increase its energy density, because the energy value fat is 2.25 times higher than carbohydrate or protein.

2.1 The need for addition of bypass fats

During the early part of lactation in cows, the feed intake is reduced due to stress of calving and milk production. The energy available from the diet during this period may not be sufficient to meet the energy needs for body maintenance and milk production. Hence, body fat reserves will be mobilized during this period which ultimately lead to metabolic disorders like ketosis and reduced immune status and other reproductive related problems.

(Bell, 1995; Drackley, 1999). The cereal grains/concentrates or fats can be added to the rations to meet the energy requirement during the periods. But the addition of concentrates at higher level decreases fibre intake and leads to acidosis (Palmquist and Jenkins, 1980).

During heat stress animals undergo metabolic changes (Okab *et al.*, 2008; Olexiková *et al.*, 2007), leading to low productive performance (Brouèek *et al.*, 2009). This effect can be minimized by supplementation of fats in the ratios of dairy animals (Gaugha *et al.*, 2008; Warntjes *et al.*, 2008; Wang *et al.*, 2009). Supplementation of dietary fat on early-lactating cows during hot weather can alter milk components and blood parameters, which may be beneficial for enhancement of energy balance and alleviation of heat stress (Zhang *et al.*, 2011).

It may be beneficial to add fat to a diet to increase its energy density. However, addition of fats have certain disadvantages that include, inhibitory effects on ruminal fermentation leading to decrease in fiber digestibility, lower intestinal absorption at higher intake, low contribution to total oxidation of nutrients and sensitivity to nutrient imbalance causing reduced energy intake (Palmquist, 1994). The reduction in fiber digestibility is mainly due to (i) coating of fibrous portion of diet with lipids thereby preventing attack by rumen microorganisms (ii) modification in rumen population concerned with cellulose digestion (iii) inhibition of the activity of rumen microorganisms due to an effect on cell permeability brought about by absorption of FA on cell wall or due to an antimetabolite effect (iv) reduction in availability of minerals (Ca and Mg), essential for microbial activity due to formation of mineral complexes with FA (Devendra and Lewis, 1974; Naik, 2012). So in order to use fats supplements for ruminants, they must be either protected from rumen fermentation or converted to soaps. Under these circumstances, bypass fats assume special significance in feeding of dairy animals. Bypass fat is defined as the fat source specially designed to resist bio-hydrogenation by rumen microbes and modify fatty acid profile of body tissues and milk.

The fats can be protected by physical or chemical agents to bypass the rumen and to get digested in the lower tract (Kundu *et al.*, 2008). Feeding of protected lipids to dairy animals increase the energy density of the diet without compromising fibre digestion in rumen (Scott *et al.*, 1995). Apart from increasing the energy intake of the animals, there is an added advantage of feeding protected unsaturated fat to cows, as the milk produced by such cows shall have higher unsaturated fatty acids in milk fat, which makes a softer butter, and is also safer for humans, especially the heart patients. Bypass fat can be supplemented to get designer milk with higher content of long chain unsaturated fatty acids for human beings (Gulati *et al.*, 2001).

Oil seeds provide natural partial protection from lipolysis and biohydrogenation in rumen due to their hard outer seed coat (Ekeren *et al.*, 1992). However, ruminal protection is very inconsistent as processing (ground, extruded, pelleted) of oilseeds reduces their resistance to biohydrogenation. Cottonseed and full fat soya are good sources of both rumen protected protein and fat (Naik, 2012). Feeding of these source increases the supply of protein and energy to the animal for higher productivity.

2.2 Preparation of rumen protected fat

Several methods have been used to make fats protected from ruminal lipolysis and biohydrogenation that include,

1. Encapsulation of protein-fat complex in crushed oil-seeds with formaldehyde. Major limitation of this technology is the inconsistency in the level of rumen protection due to physical breakdown of the treated oil seeds during mastication by animal (Bines *et al.*, 1978).
2. Conversion of fatty acids into calcium salt of fatty acids. In rumen, calcium salts of long chain fatty acids (Ca-LCFA) are inert, if pH remains more than 5.5. At normal rumen pH, dissociation of Ca salts of unsaturated fatty acids (USFA) are relatively higher than Ca salts of saturated fatty acids (SFA) (Sukhija and Palmquist, 1990)
3. Crystalline/ prilled fatty acids are made up of SFA or from hydrogenated fat by liquefying and spraying under pressure into a cooled atmosphere, resulting in dried Prilled fatty acids, which are inert in rumen (Chalupa *et al.*, 1986).
4. Fatty acyl amides fatty acyl amides are amides of USFA and are known to be resistant to ruminal biohydrogenation, Generally; fatty acyl amide is supplemented in diet of lactating cows to increase the desired FA (especially USFA) content of milk fat (Naik, 2012). Butylsoyamide is a fatty acyl amide consisting of an amide bond between soy FA and a butylamine, which increases linoleic acid content of milk fat (Jenkins, 1998). Conversion of oleic acid to fatty acyl amide (oleamide) increases MUFA concentration in milk, when fed to dairy cows (Jenkins, 1999), while amide of soybean FA is effective in enhancing post-ruminal flow of oleic acid (Lundy *et al.*, 2004).

Out of all these methods, the calcium salt of fatty acids is the most commonly used method, as the method may be cheaper and more effective (Kundu *et al.*, 2008). Generally, two methods are used for the production of calcium salt of fatty acids, viz. Fusion method and double decomposition method.

2.2.1 Fusion method

In this method, oils and fatty acids are heated with calcium oxide or calcium hydroxide in the presence of catalyst, in a closed vessel at a required temperature and pressure. Water is produced in the reaction and the added water is driven off as steam and the resulting product of calcium saponified salts or bypass fat. Naik *et al.*,(2007a,b, 2009a) developed a simple, indigenous technology for preparation of Ca-LCFA (PF) by treating vegetable FA oil with calcium hydroxide under specific conditions. This technology of preparation of Ca-LCFA (PF) is user- friendly and pro-small farmer (Naik, 2012).

2.2.2 Double decomposition method

In this method, Ca-LCFA is prepared in two steps (Jenkins and Palmquist, 1984; Sampelayo *et al.*, 2004). This method requires heating of the known quantity of fat supplement in metal container, followed by addition of an alkali (aqueous sodium hydroxide solution). Then the heating is stopped. While the contents are still warm, calcium chloride solution is added slowly to the water soluble sodium soap with constant stirring, which ultimately causes precipitation of calcium soaps. Excess water is then removed by filtration. The calcium-soap is dried at low temperature and the lumps are broken and ground, to be used bypass fat.

During the refining of edible oils, free fatty acids are removed by treating with sodium hydroxide and then acid. The free fatty acids thus removed by centrifugation are termed as 'acid oil' which has roughly one-third the price of edible oils and can be converted in to calcium salts. Hence, in developing countries, where cost of fats is very high, acid oils can be converted in to calcium salts and fed. At present, India is importing protected fat or may be some industries have hooked up with some foreign firms for the manufacture of this product. However, the indigenous methodologies for the production of fat and the development and scaling of the technologies are being tried at many research centers in the country (Kundu *et al.*, 2008). Different byproducts from edible/non-edible oil industries and other unconventional oil supplements have been tried, for the protection of their fat and for the preparation of bypass fat by the above two methods. The purpose of trying to make use of non-conventional and non edible fat sources is to make the technology of bypass fat commercially viable and cost effective.

2.3 Supplementation of fats in rations

As per NRC, (2001), dairy ration (mixture of cereals and forages) contains about 3% fat, and total dietary fat in ration should not exceed 6 -7% of DM (Naik, 2012). Addition of 3-5% fat of total ration DM has beneficial effect on milk production (Palmquist and Jenkins, 1980); and decrease in production occurs, when fat level exceeds 6% of ration DM (Jenkins and Palmquist, 1984), which probably results from the effects of fats, especially unesterified FA on rumen cellulolytic microbial activity. Although, protected fats can be incorporated up to 9% of dietary DM due to its inertness in rumen (Sharma, 2004), feeding of Ca-LCFA at 9% of dietary DM is not beneficial in lactating dairy cows (Schauff and Clark, 1992), However, it is always better to supplement different types of fat in dairy ration. First 3% fat of the DM intake of animal should be provided by oilseed sources and that in excess of 3% should be as protected fats (Palmquist, 1990) or rations of high yielders should have 4-6% fat, containing 1/3rd fat from each source of natural feed, oil seed and bypass fat (Sharma, 2004).

2.4 Considerations prior to using supplemented fat

- In high yielding animals especially during the first 120 days of lactation.
- Quantity of grains and natural high fat feeds in the ration to be taken into consideration before adding the fats.
- Source and quality of fats and cost economics.

2.5 Effect of bypass fat supplementation on growth, milk production and reproduction

2.5.1 Growth

Inconsistent results were reported by feeding fats in animals. The loss of body weight is more in primiparous cows than multiparous cows (Sklan *et al.*, 1994). The studies conducted by Fallon *et al.*, (1986) and Ngidi *et al.*, (1990) showed decrease in average daily gain (ADG), and the other studies (Van Houtert *et al.*, 1990; Alexander *et al.*, 2003; Kumar *et al.*, 2004) revealed significant influence of supplemental protected fat up to 10% level on ADG and feed efficacy in ruminants.

2.5.2 Milk production

Increased milk yield as well as milk fat was observed by feeding of bypass fat supplements to dairy animals (Hermanson, 1989; Eastridge and Firkins, 1991). The milk yield and composition is affected by breed, parity, stage of lactation of animal; level of supplementation and FA composition of bypass fats (Naik, 2012). Effect of supplementation of Ca-LCFA in dairy cows on milk yield and FCM yield is more in primiparous cows than multiparous cows (Sklan *et al.*, 1994) and more in early and peak lactation (Schneider *et al.*, 1988) than mid or late lactation due to decreased transfer efficiency of plasma FA to mammary tissue as lactation progresses (Grummer, 1988). Studies carried out by Garg and Mehta, (1998) on lactating dairy animals showed that milk yield and milk fat content significantly increased by feeding protected fat supplements. Milk yield increased 3.2 kg/d (19.6%) and FCM yield increased

2.8 kg/d (22.3%) on supplementation of Ca-LCFA in crossbred lactating cows during early lactation, (Naik *et al.*, 2009b). Supplemental Ca-LCFA increases FCM yield of lactating cows up to 6% of dietary DM, but yield is decreased at 9% of dietary DM (Schauff and Clark, 1992). Wu *et al.*, (1993) supplemented tallow, Ca salts of palm oil fatty acids and prilled fat at 2.5% to mid-lactation cows. Added fat increased milk yield over control but source of fat did not affect milk yield. Similarly, Schroeder *et al.*, (2002) demonstrated an increase in FCM yield from 23.4 to 26.3 kg/ d on supplementing partially hydrogenated oil to lactating Holstein cows under grazing conditions.

Milk fat percentage is either increased (Sklan *et al.*, 1991) or decreased (Chouinard *et al.*, 1998) or not affected (Naik *et al.*, 2009b) due to bypass fat supplementation in lactating animals. Thakur and Shelke, (2009) reported an improvement of 12.4 % in milk yield of buffaloes fed 4% Ca salts of fatty acids. Tyagi *et al.*, (2009) reported that bypass fat supplementation @ 2.5 per cent of DMI for 90 days postpartum increased the milk production and its persistency up to 120 days after cessation of bypass feeding.

Effect of bypass fat supplementation on milk protein content is influenced by parity and stage of lactation of animal. Decline in milk protein content is reported in primiparous cows (Sklan *et al.*, 1992); but decline is apparent only in late lactation, not in early lactation (Sklan *et al.*, 1992). Dietary protein should be increased, when fat supplemented diets are fed to animals (Palmquist and Moser, 1981). The lactose content is altered in quadratic pattern, due to supplementation of bypass fat in the ration (Chouinard *et al.*, 1997). Tyagi *et al.*, (2009) reported that supplementation of protected fat @ 2.5 % DM significantly increased the proportion of unsaturated FA and LCFA in milk fat of cross bred cows.

2.5.3 Reproduction

The higher milk yield is associated phenotypically and genetically with reduced reproductive performance in lactating cows (Nebel and McGilliard, 1993). Several hypotheses are suggested regarding role of FA on improvement of reproductive performance of dairy animals (Sklan *et al.*, 1994). These include (i) improved energy balance, resulting in an earlier return to post-partum ovarian cycling; (ii) increase linoleic acid may provide increase PGF2a and stimulate return to ovarian cycling and improve follicular recruitment; and (iii) increase in progesterone secretion either from improvement energy balance or altered lipoprotein composition of dietary fat. Dietary supplementation of Ca-LCFA reduces number of artificial inseminations required per conception (Naik *et al.*, 2009b), which indicates better reproductive performance of dairy animals (Naik, 2012).

Improved energy balance could result in an earlier return to postpartum ovarian cyclicity (Palmquist and Jenkins, 1980). Since the feeding of bypass fat invariably results in increased blood cholesterol concentration, it in turn, increase the plasma progesterone concentration, which can improve the fertility of the cows (Staples *et al.*, 1998). Supplemental fat also improved the fertility through the reduction in PGF2α and/or by modifying circulating concentration of insulin, GH and enhance the synthesis of insulin-like growth factor-1 (IGF-1) in ovarian cell (Williams and Stanko, 1999).

Hence, feeding of protected fats, mostly as calcium salts of fatty acids can increase milk yields and also the efficiency of energy utilisation in high yielding animals that receive diets of too low energy content (Walli *et al.*, 1995). Although in many parts of India, the supply of energy feeds for ruminants is limited, normally it may not pose an acute problem because many cows are low yielders. The minimum dietary fat level should be 3 percent in high yielding cows. However, in countries where animals are fed primarily on crop residues, feeding of bypass fat could help increasing milk production and growth. In developing countries, where cost of fatty acids (fat) is very high, acid oils can be converted into calcium salts and fed. However, efforts need to do to commercialize the technology with cheaper sources of fat.

Conclusions

Inclusion of higher level of bypass protein in the ration of dairy animals improves the milk production performance under the Indian conditions of feeding and management. It is observed that the feeding of bypass protein is even beneficial for medium and low yielders, although the benefits could be more pronounced on high producing animals. Therefore it is desirable to include feed materials of medium or high bypass protein content in the ration of animals yielding large quantities of milk especially in the early stages of lactation, under such feeding regimes. However, it is essential to ensure that sufficient amount of rumen degradable protein (50 to 60% of total crude protein) is supplied in the ration of these animals to maintain optimum rumen fermentation for better utilization of fibre. Therefore, feeding of bypass nutrients such as bypass protein and bypass fat has the potential to increase productive as well as reproductive performance of dairy animals under Indian conditions. The responses are more likely to be more favourable in high yielding animals in the early part of lactation or fast growing animals. These are typical situations where the demand for nutrients is high and where the animals may be in negative protein and energy balance with lower body condition score.

References

Alexander G., Rao Z.P., Rama Prasad J. (2003). Effect of sunflower acid oil or its calcium soap supplementation to rations of growing lambs. *Indian Journal of Animal Nutrition* **20:** 36-41.

Bagga S., Armendaris A., Klypina N., Ray I., Ghoshroy Endress M., Sutton D., Kemp J.D., Sengupta Gopalan C. (2004). Genetic engineering ruminal stable high methionine protein in the foliage of alfalfa. *Plant Science* **166:** 273-283.

Barry T.N., Manley T.R. (1984). The role of condensed tannins in the nutritional value of Lotus pedunculatus for sheep 2. Quantitative digestion of carbohydrates and protein. *British Journal of Nutrition* **51:** 493-504.

Bell A.W. (1995). Regulation of organic nutrient metabolism during transition from late pregnancy to early lactation. *Journal of Animal Science* **73:** 2804-2819.

Bhagwat S.R., Srivastava A. (1993). Effect of feeding unprotected and protected soybean cake on growth, feed conversion and certain blood constituents of calves. *Indian Journal of Dairy Science* **46:** 237-242.

Bharadwaj A., Sengupta B.P., Sethi R.K. (2000). Effect of feeding rumen protected and unprotected protein on nutrients intake and reproductive performance of lactating buffaloes. *Indian Journal of Animal Sciences* **70:** 428-430.

Bharadwaj A., Sengupta B.P. (1999). Effect of sources of dietary unprotected and protected protein on lactational performance of Murrah buffaloes. *Buffalo Journal* **15:** 269-278.

Bines J.A., Brumby P.E., Storry J.E., Fulford R.J., Braithwaite G.D. (1978). The effect of protected lipids on nutrient intakes, blood and rumen metabolites and milk secretion in dairy cows during early lactation. *Journal of Agricultural Science* **91:** 135-150.

Bowman J.M., Grieve P.G., Buchnan Smith J.G., Macleod G.K. (1988). Response of dairy cows in early lactation to sodium hydroxide-treated soybean meal. *Journal of Dairy Science* **71:** 982-989.

Britton R.A., Klopfenstein T.J. (1986). Zinc treated soybean meal; A method to increase bypass. *Nebraska Beef Cattle Report, MP 50.* University of Nebraska, Lincoln, USA, pp 45-57.

Brouèek J., Novák P., Vokøálová J., Šoch M., Kišac P., Uhrinèa M. (2009). Effect of high temperature on milk production of cows from free-stall housing with natural ventilation. *Slovak Journal of Animal Science* **42:** 167-173.

Chalupa W. (1975). Rumen bypass and protection of protein and amino acids. *Journal of Dairy Science* **58:** 1198-1218.

Chalupa W., Vecchiarelli B., Elser A.E., Kronfeld D.S., Sklan D., Palmquist D.L. (1986). Ruminal fermentation in vivo as influenced by long-chain fatty acids. *Journal of Dairy Science* **69:** 1293-1301.

Chandrasekharaiah M., Sampath K.T., Praveen U.S. (2008). Effect of feeding bypass protein on milk production performance in crossbred cows. *Indian Journal of Animal Sciences* **78:** 527-530.

Chandrasekharaiah M., Thulasi A., Sampath K.T. (2010). Effect of variable rumen degradable nitrogen levels on microbial protein synthesis estimated with purine derivatives in sheep urine and PDC index. *Indian Journal of Animal Sciences* **80:** 674-678.

Chandrasekharaiah M., Thulasi A., Suresh K.P., Sampath K.T. (2011). Rumen degradable nitrogen requirements for optimum microbial protein synthesis and nutrient utilization in sheep fed on Finger Millet straw (*Eleucine coracana*) based diet. *Animal Feed Science and Technology* **163:** 130-135.

Chandrasekharaiah M., Sampath K.T., Thulasi A. (2002). Rumen protein degradability of certain feedstuffs in cattle determined by nylon bag technique. *Indian Journal of Dairy and Biosciences* **13:** 18-21.

Chandrasekharaiah M., Sampath K.T., Thulasi A., Anandan S. (2001). *In situ* protein degradability of certain feedstuffs in the rumen of cattle. *Indian Journal of Animal Sciences* **71:** 261-264.

Chatterjee A., Walli T.K. (1998). Effect of feeding formaldehyde treated mustard cake on growth performance of Murrah buffalo calves. *Indian Journal of Animal Production* **30:** 163.

Chatterjee A., Walli T.K. (2003[a]). Effect of formaldehyde treatment on effective protein degradability and in vitro post rumen digestibility of mustard cake. *Indian Journal of Animal Nutrition* **20:** 143-148.

Chatterjee A., Walli T.K. (2003[b]). Economics of feeding formaldehyde treated mustard cake as bypass protein to growing buffalo calves. *Indian Journal of Dairy Science* **56:** 241-244.

Chen X.B., Subba D.B., Orskov E.R., Jayasuriya M.C.N. (1999). Purine Nitrogen Index, potentially a new parameter for rapid feed evaluation in ruminants. *IAEA-IECDO* **109:** 97-110.

Chouinard P.Y., Girard V. Brisson G.J. (1997). Lactational response of cows to different concentrations of calcium salts of canola oil fatty acids with or without bicarbonates. *Journal of Dairy Science* **80:** 1185-1193.

Chouinard P.Y., Girard V. Brisson G.J. (1998). Fatty acid profile and physical properties of milk fat from cows fed calcium salts of fatty acids with varying un-saturation. *Journal of Dairy Science* **81:** 471-481.

Cleale R.M., Klopfenstein T.J., Britton R.A., Satterlee L.D. (1986). Induced non-enzymatic browning of soybean meal for enhancing efficiency of protein utilization by ruminants. *Journal of Animal Science* **63** (Suppl. 1): 139 (Abstr.).

Dahiya S.S., Sengar S.S., Mugal V.D. (1991). Effect of feeding urea (ammonia) treated wheat straw with cotton seed cake on nutrient utilization and milk production in buffaloes. *International Journal of Animal Science* **61:** 133-137.

Devendra C., Lewis D. (1974). The interaction between dietary lipids and fibre in the sheep. *Journal of Animal Production* **19:** 67-76.

Drackley J.K. (1999). ADSA Foundation Scholar Award. Biology of dairy cows during the transition period: the final frontier? *Journal of Dairy Science* **82:** 2259-2273.

Eastridge M.L., Firkens J.L. (1991). Feeding hydrogenated fatty acids and triglycerides to lactating dairy cows. *Journal of Dairy Science* **74:** 2610-2616.

Egan A.R. (1988). Ration formulation and evaluation of protein provisions from diets of mixed components with particular reference to milk production systems in India. In: *Fibrous crop residues in animal feed* (Kiran Singh and J.B. Schiere, eds) ICAR. New Delhi/India, pp168-179.

Egan A.R., Ulyatt M.J. (1980). Quantitative digestion of fresh herbage by sheep: VI. Utilization of nitrogen in five herbages. *Journal of Agricultural Science* **94:** 47-56.

Ekeren P.A., Smith D.R., Lunt D.K. Smith S.B. (1992). Ruminal bio hydrogenation of fatty acids from high-oleate sunflower seeds. *Journal of Animal Science* **70:** 2574-2580.

Fallon R.J., Williams P.E.V., Innes G.M. (1986). The effects on feed intake, growth and digestibility of nutrients of including calcium soaps of fat in diets for young calves. *Animal Feed Science and Technology* **14:** 103-105.

Friedman M. (1982). Relationship of Composition to Protein Functionality. In: *Food protein denaturation*, (J.P. Cherry, ed). *ACS symposium series* **206:** 231.

Garg M.R., Sherasia P.L., Bhanderi B.M., Gulati S.K., Scott T.W. (2002). Effect of feeding rumen protected nutrients on milk production in crossbred cows. *Indian Journal of Animal Nutrition* **19:** 191-198.

Garg M.R., Sherasia P.L., Bhanderi B.M., Gulati S.K., Scott T.W. (2005). Effect of feeding rumen protected protein on milk production in low yielding crossbred cows. *Animal Nutrition and Feed Technology* **5:** 1-8.

Garg M.R., Mehta A.K. (1998). Effect of feeding bypass fat on feed intake, milk production and body condition of Holstein Friesian cows. *Indian Journal of Animal Nutrition*. **15:** 242-245.

Gaugha J.B., Mader T.L., Holt S.M. (2008). Cooling and feeding strategies to reduce heat load of grain-fed beef cattle in intensive housing. *Livestock Science* **113:** 226-233.

Gaynor P.J., Montgomery M.J. Holmes C.R. (1988). Effect of zinc chloride or zinc sulfate treatment of protein supplement on milk production. *Journal of Dairy Science* **71:** 2175-2180.

Gould D.H., Macgregor J.J. (1976). Symposium on cross linking: 31, (M. Friedman, ed.) Plenum publications, New York.

Grummer R.R. (1988). Influence of prilled fat and calcium salt of palm oil fatty acids on ruminal fermentation and nutrient digestibility. *Journal of Dairy Science* **71:** 117-123.

Gulati S.K., Ryde I, Kaur R., Scott T.W., Garg M.L., Sherasia P.L., Singh D.K. (2001). Role of protected nutrients in sustainable milk production. In: *Proc. of Xth Animal Nutrition Conference on "Emerging nutritional technologies for sustainable animal production and environmental protection" held during 9th to 11th November, at Karnal, Haryana,* pp 1-9.

Gupta H.K., Walli T.K. (1987). Growth rate feed conversion efficiency and feed utilization in crossbred kids fed HCHO treated cake as such and partly replaced by urea. *Indian Journal of Animal Nutrition* **4:** 94-99.

Hermansen J.E. (1989). Feed intake, milk yield and milk composition by replacing unprotected fat by Ca-soaps for dairy cows. *Animal Feed Science and Technology* **22:** 193-203.

Jenkins T.C. (1993). Lipid metabolism in the rumen. *Journal of Dairy Science* **76:** 3851-3863.

Jenkins T.C. (1999). Lactation performance and fatty acid composition of milk from Holstein cows fed 0 to 5% oleamide. *Journal of Dairy Science* **82:** 1525-1531.

Jenkins T.C. 1998. Fatty acid composition of milk from Holstein cows fed oleamide or canola oil. *Journal of Dairy Science* **81:** 794-800.

Jenkins T.C., Palmquist D.L. (1984). Effect of fatty acids or calcium soaps on rumen and total nutrient digestibility of dairy rations. *Journal of Dairy Science* **67:** 978-986.

Jones W.T., Mangan J.L. (1977). Complexes of the condensed tannins of sainfoin (*Onobrychis uiciifolia*) with fraction 1 leaf protein and with submaxillary mucoprotein, and their reversal by polyethylene glycol and pH. *Journal of the Science of Food and Agriculture* **28:** 126-136.

Kalbande V.H., Thomas CT. (1999). Effect of bypass protein on yield and composition of milk in crossbred cows. *Indian Journal of Animal Sciences* **69:** 614-616.

Khorasani G.R., Robinson P.H., Kennelly J.J. (1989). Effect of chemical treatment on *in vitro* and *in situ* degradation of canola meal crude protein. *Journal of Dairy Science* **72:** 2074-2080.

Kumar V. Walli T.K. (1994). Effect of urea treated wheat straw supplemented with HCHO treated GN cakes on growth performance of cross bred calves. *Indian Journal of Animal Nutrition* **4:** 29-33.

Kumar R., Sivaiah K., Ekambaram B., Reddy Ramana Y., Reddy T. J., Reddy G.V.N. (2004). Influence of dietary rumen inert lipids on growth and carcass characteristics in Deccani sheep. *Indian Journal of Animal Nutrition* **21:** 217-220.

Kundu S.S., Sirohi S.K., Singh S. (2008). Significance of bypass fat feeding to dairy animals. *Indian Dairyman* **60:** 55-59.

Larsen H. J., Tenpas G. H. Jensen E. L. (1974). Birds foot trefoil-grass vs. alfalfa-grass haylage in the dairy cow diet. *Journal of Dairy Science* **57:** 169-174.

Lundy F.P., Block E., Bridges W.C.Jr., Bertrand J.A. Jenkins T.C. (2004). Ruminal biohydrogenation in Holstein cows fed soybean fatty acids as amides or calcium salts. *Journal of Dairy Science* **87:** 1038-1046.

Lynch G.L., Vander-Aar P.J. Berger L.L., Fahey G.C., Merchens N.R. (1988). Proteolysis of alcohol-treated soybean meal proteins by *Bacteroides ruminicola, Bacteroides amylophilus*, pepsin, trypsin, and in the rumen of steers. *Jounal of Dairy Science* **71:** 2416.

Lynch G.L., Berger L.L., Merchens N.R., Fahey G.C., Baker E.C. (1987). Effects of ethanol and heat treatments of soybean meal and infusion of sodium chloride into the rumen on ruminal degradation and escape of soluble and total soybean meal protein in steers. *Journal of Animal Science* **65:** 1617.

Marten G. C., Ehle F. R. (1984). Influence of quality variation in four legume species on weight gains of grazing heifers. Agronomy Abstract, American Society of Agronomy, Madison, WI, USA, p 159.

Mehrez A.Z., Orskov E.R. (1977). A study of artificial fibre bag technique for determining the degradability of feeds in rumen. *Journal of Agricultural Science, Cambridge* **88:** 645-650.

Mir A., Macleod G.K., Buchnan Smith J.G. Grovum W.L. (1984). Effect of feeding soybean meal protected with sodium hydroxide, fresh blood, or fish hydrolysate to growing calves and lactating dairy cows. *Canadian Journal of Animal Science* **64:** 853-865.

Mishra B.B., Swain R.K., Sahu B.K., Samantaray D.P. (2006). Effect of Bypass Protein Supplementation on Nutrient Utilization, Milk Production and Its Composition in Crossbred Cows on Paddy Straw Based Ration. *Animal Nutrition and Feed Technology* **6:** 123-133.

Mudgal V.D., Sengar S.S. (1980). Effect of feeding protecting and non protected protein on the growth rate and body composition of goats. *Journal of Nuclear Agriculture and Biology* **9:** 19.

Naik P.K., Saijpaul S. Rani N. (2007a). Evaluation of rumen protected fat prepared by fusion method. *Animal Nutrition and Feed Technology* **7:** 95-101.

Naik P.K, Saijpaul S., Rani N. (2007b). Preparation of rumen protected fat and its effect on nutrient utilization in adult buffaloes. *Indian Journal of Animal Nutrition* **24:** 212-215.

Naik P.K., Saijpaul S. Rani N. (2009a). Effect of ruminally protected fat on in vitro fermentation and apparent nutrient digestibility in buffaloes (*Bubalus bubalis*). *Animal Feed Science Technology* **153:** 68-76.

Naik P.K., Saijpaul S., Sirohi A.S. Raquib M. (2009b). Lactation response of crossbred dairy cows fed on indigenously prepared rumen protected fat – a field trial. *Indian Journal of Animal Science* **79:** 1045-1049.

Naik P.K. (2012). Feeding rumen protected fat to high yielding dairy cows. In: Animal nutrition advances and developments. (U.R. Mehra, Putan Singh, A.K.Verma, Eds.) SSPH publishers, Delhi, India, pp. 529-548.

Nebel R.L., McGilliard M.L. (1993). Interactions of high milk yield and reproductive performance in dairy cow. *Journal of Dairy Science* **76:** 3257-3268.

Ngidi M.E., Loerch S.C., Fluharty F.L. Palmquist D.L. (1990). Effect of calcium soaps of long chain fatty acids on feedlot performance, carcass characteristics and ruminal metabolism of steers. *Journal of Animal Science* **68:** 2555-2565.

Nocek J.E. (1988). In vitro and other methods to estimate ruminal protein and energy digestibility – review. *Journal of Dairy Science* **71:** 2051-2069.

NRC (1989). Nutrient requirements of dairy cattle. 6th revised edition, National Acadamy of Science. Washington DC.

NRC (2001). Nutrient requirements for dairy cattle. 7th revised edition, National Acadamy of Science . Washington, DC.

Okab A.B., EL-Banna S.G., Koriem A.A. (2008). Influence of environmental temperatures on some physiological and biochemical parameters of New-Zealand rabbit males. *Slovak Journal of Animal Science* **41:** 12-19.

Olexiková L. Makarevič A.V. Chrenek P., Kubovièová E., Pivko J. (2007). Development of rabbit preimplantation embryos under thermal stress *in vitro*. *Slovak Journal of Animal Science* **40:** 63-65.

Oosting S.J., Van Bruchem J., Chen X.B. (1995). Intake, digestion and small intestinal protein availability in sheep in relation to ammoniation of wheat straw with or without protein supplementation. *British Journal of Nutrition* **74:** 347-368.

Orskov E.R., MeDonald I. (1979). The estimation of protein degradability in the rumen from incubation measurements weighted according to rate of passage. *Journal of Agricultural Science* **92:** 499-503.

Pachauri V.C., Majumdar A.B, Mahanta S.K. (1999). Effect of feeding formaldehyde treated groundnut cake incorporated diets on nutrient utilization and growth in crossbred female calves. *Indian Journal of Animal Science* **69:** 197-198.

Palmquist D.L. (1990). Using fat strategically in dairy cattle rations. *In: Proc. International Animal Nutrition Symposium*. National Renderer's Association, Brussels, Belgium, p 35.

Palmquist D.L., Jenkins T.C. (1980). Fat in lactation rations: Review. *Journal of Dairy Science* **63:** 1-14.

Palmquist D.L., Moser E.A. (1981). Dietary fat effects on blood insulin, glucose utilization, and milk protein content of lactating cows. *Journal of Dairy Science* **64:** 1664-1670.

Palmquist D.L. (1994). The role of dietary fats in efficiency of ruminants. *Journal of Nutrition* **124:** 1377S-1382S.

Prajapati K.B., Nagpaul P.K., Singh D.V., Walli T.K. Dave A.S. (1996). Influence of exercise and by-pass protein feeding on sexual behavior in Mehsana buffalo bulls. *Indian Journal of Animal Production and Management* **12:** 164-169.

Prajapati K.B., Nagpaul P.K., Raina V.S. (1998a). The effect of exercise and feeding bypass protein on semen quality measures in Mehsana buffalo bulls. *Indian Journal of Animal Reproduction* **19:** 143-145.

Prajapati K.B., Nagpaul P.K., Chauhan M.K., Singh D.V., Walli T.K., Raina V.S. (1998b). Influence of exercise and by-pass protein feeding on seminal attributes of Mehsana buffalo bulls. *Indian Journal of Animal Production and Management* **14:** 10-15.

Ramachandra K.S., Sampath K.T. (1995). Influence of two levels of rumen degradable protein on milk production and performance of lactating cows maintained on paddy straw based rations. *Indian Journal of Animal Nutrition* **12:** 1-6.

Reed J.D., Soller H., Woodward A. (1990). Fodder tree and straw diets for sheep: Intake, growth, digestibility and the effects of phenolics on nitrogen utilisation. *Animal Feed Science and Technology* **30:** 39-50.

Reed J. D. (1995). Nutritional toxicology of tannins and related polyphenols in forage legumes. *Journal of Animal Science* **73:** 1516-1528.

Robbins C. T., Hanley T. A., Hagerman A. E., Hjeljord, O., Baker, D. L., Schwartz, C. C., Mautz. W. W. (1987). Role of tannins in defending plants against ruminants: reduction in protein availability. *Ecology* **68:** 98-107.

Sampath K.T., Prasad C.S., Ramachandra K.S., Sundareshan K., Subba Rao A. (1996). Effect feeding two levels of undegradable dietary protein (UDP) on growth and nutrient utilization in crossbred female cows. *Indian Journal of Animal Science* **13:** 1-6.

Sampath K.T., Chandrasekharaiah M., Praveen U.S. (2004). Effect of bypass protein on milk production of crossbred cows – a field study. *Indian Journal Animal Nutrition* **22:** 41-43.

Sampath K.T., Prasad C.S., Ramachandra K.S, Sunderashan K, Subbarao A. (1997). Effect of feeding undegraded dietary protein on milk production of crossbred cows. *Indian Journal of Animal Science* **67:** 706-708.

Sampath K.T., Chandrasekharaiah M., Thulasi A., Anandan S. (1999). Bypass protein for ruminants. *Technical bulletin II* National Institute of Animal Nutrition and Physiology, Bangalore, pp 1-19.

Sampelayo M.R., Sanz Alonso J.J., Martin Perez L., Extremera F., Gil Boza J. (2004). Dietary supplements for lactating goats by polyunsaturated fatty acid-rich protected fat. Effects after supplement withdrawal. *Journal of Dairy Science* **87:** 1796-1802.

Schauff D.J., Clark J.H. (1992). Effects of feeding diets containing calcium salts of long-chain fatty acids to lactating dairy cows. *Journal of Dairy Science* **75:** 2990-3002.

Schneider P., Sklan D., Chalupa W., Kronfeld D.S. (1988). Feeding calcium salts of fatty acids to lactating cows. *Journal of Dairy Science* **71:** 2143-2150.

Schroeder G.F., Gagliostro G.A., Villalobos D.B., Mengido I.L. (2002). Supplementation with partially hvdrogenated oil in grazing dairy cows in early lactation. *Journal of Dairy Science* **85:** 580-594.

Scott T.A., Shaver R.D., Zepeda L., Yandell B. Smith T.R. (1995). Effects of rumen-inert fat on lactation, reproduction, and health of high producing Holstein herds. *Journal of Dairy Science* **78:** 2435-2451.

Sharma D.D. (2004). All India dairy husbandry officers' workshop. Dairy Extension Division, National Dairy Research Institute, Karnal, India, pp 28-33.

Sklan D., Moallem U., Folman Y. (1991). Effect of feeding calcium soaps of fatty acids on production and reproductive responses in high producing lactating cows. *Journal of Dairy Science* **74:** 510-517.

Sklan D., Ashkenazi R., Braun A., Devorin A., Tabori K. (1992). Fatty acids, calcium soaps of fatty acids, and cottonseeds fed to high yielding cows. *Journal of Dairy Science* **75:** 2463-2472.

Sklan D., Kaim M., Moallam U., Folman Y. (1994). Effect of dietary calcium soaps on milk yield, body weight, reproductive hormones, and fertility in first parity and older cows. *Journal of Dairy Science* **77:** 1652-1660.

Staples C.R., Burke J.M., Thatcher W.W. (1998). Influence of supplemental fats on reproductive tissues and performance of lactating cows. *Journal of Animal Science* **81:** 856-871.

Stern M.D. (1984). Effect of lignosulfonate on rumen microbial degradation of soybean meal protein in continuous culture. *Canadian Journal of Animal Science* **64:** 26 (Abstr.)

Sukhija P.S., Palmquist D.L. (1990). Dissociation of calcium soaps of long-chain fatty acids in rumen fluid. *Journal of Dairy Science* **73:** 1784-1787.

Thakur S.S., Shelke S.K. (2009). Milk production and nutrient utilization of Murrah buffaloes fed ration supplemented with bypass fat prepared from soybean acid oil. *Indian Journal of Animal Sciences* **79:** 1238-1241.

Tiwari D.P., Yadav L.S. (1994). Effect of growth, nutrient utilization and blood metabolites in buffaloe calves fed ration containing HCHO treated mustard cake. *Indian Journal of Animal Sciences* **64:** 625-630.

Tyagi N., Thakur S.S., Shelke S.K. (2009). Effect of bypass fat supplementation on productive and reproductive performance in crossbred cows. *Tropical Animal Health and Production*. **42:** 1749-1755.

Van Houtert M.F., Perdok H.B., Leng R.A. (1990). Factors affecting food efficiency and body composition of growing ruminants offered straw-based diets. Supplementation with lipids with and without protein meal. *Animal Production* **51:** 321-331.

Walli T.K., Das M.M., Rai S.N., Garg M.R. (2000). Effect of heat treatment on protein degradability, N solubility and Ammonia release of groundnut cake and soybean meal. *Indian Journal of Dairy Science* **57:** 361-368.

Walli T.K., Garg M.R., Sampath K.T., Srivastava A., Singh G.P., Gill M., Ibrahim M.N.M. (1995). Feeding of bypass nutrients to ruminants. Handbook for straw feeding systems (Kiran Singh and J B Schire, eds.), ICAR, New Delhi, pp 163-173.

Waltz D.M., Loerch S.C. (1986). Effect of acid and alkali treatment of soybean meal on nitrogen utilization by ruminants. *Journal of Animal Science* **63:** 879-887.

Wang Jian-ping., Wang Jia-qi., Bu Deng-pan., Huo Xiao-kai., Guo Tong-jun., Wei Hong-yang., Zhou Ling-yun., LI Fa-di., Liang Jian-guang., Wang Guang-wen., Yuan Yao-ming. (2009). Effects of supplementation of saturated fatty acid on milk production and milk fatty acid profile of mid-lactating cows during hot weather. *Chinese Journal of Animal Nutrition* **21:** 301-311.

Warntjes J.L., Robinson P.H., Galo E., Depeters E.G., Howes D. (2008). Effects of feeding supplemental palmitic acid (C16:0) on performance and milk fatty acid profile of lactating dairy cows under summer heat. *Animal Feed Science and Technology* **140:** 241-257.

Williams G.L., Stanko R.L. (1999). Dietary fat as reproductive nutraceuticals in beef cattle. In: *Proceedings of the American Society of Animal Science,* pp 1-12.

Wu, Z. Huber, J.T., Sleiman, F.T., Simas, J.M., Chen, K.H., Chan, S.C., Fontes, C. (1993). Effect of three supplemental fat sources on lactation and digestion in dairy cows. *Journal of Dairy Science* **76:** 3562-3570.

Zhang H., Wang Z., Liu G., He J., Su C. (2011). Effect of dietary fat supplementation on milk components and blood parameters of early-lactating cows under heat stress. *Slovak Journal of Animal Science* **44:** 52-58.

❑❑❑

Chapter 5

Nutritional Significance of Poly Unsaturated Fatty Acid Enriched Feed Supplementation in Animals

A. Mech, S.C. Roy, J. Ghosh, A. Dhali, K.S. Roy, R.U. Suganthi
National Institute of Animal Nutrition and Physiology, Adugodi, Bangalore-560 030, Karnataka, India

Summary

The polyunsaturated fatty acids (PUFA) are essential for normal growth, production and reproduction in human and all domestic animals. The role of PUFA supplementation in animals has been a topic of interest for the animal nutritionists. The main emphasis of PUFA enriched feed supplementation to animals is production of PUFA enriched animal products which may ultimately have potential health benefit in human. In addition, conjugated linoleic acid is a group of geometric and positional isomers of linoleic acid which has also been known to have nutraceutical value. There is considerable interest for including conjugated linoleic acid (CLA) in animal feed to improve lean meat production and provide value-added meat products for human consumption. In this chapter, some of the key aspects of nutrition, metabolism, benefits and limitations of dietary PUFA supplementation in animals are discussed from a comparative perspective. One of the most interesting aspects of PUFA biology is its interaction with nuclear receptor proteins like eicosanoids, their metabolism and effect on various physiological functions. Further dietary PUFA supplementation has also a role to play on reproduction and fertility in animals. Nevertheless there are some major limitations with respect to oxidative stability and sensory characteristics of PUFA enriched animal products. Currently, this is one of key challenges in the production of PUFA enriched functional animal products. Further, present knowledge and approaches to increase beneficial PUFA content in animal products of economic importance are discussed in nutshell.

Polyunsaturated fatty acids (PUFA) are integral structural component of biomembranes. They are actively involved in maintenance and functioning of essential cell components and act as precursors of signaling molecules and eicosanoids. The PUFAs also control gene transcription of enzymes involved in differentiation, growth and metabolism in animals. Besides providing a balanced nutrition to animals, researches on animal nutrition emphasize enriching animal diet with specific nutrients like PUFA, CLA (conjugated linoleic acid), vitamins, antioxidants *etc.* for production of functional animal products. However, PUFA deficiencies are extremely rare in animals (Muller *et al.,* 2001). Dietary supplementation of PUFA enriched feed to animals has been in practice with an aim to produce omega-3 PUFA or CLA enriched meat, milk or eggs, which may finally have a potential health benefit in human. The dietary PUFA supplementation to animals for improving nutritional quality of animal products are still an issue as PUFAs are chemically unstable due to presence of unsaturated double bonds in their carbon chain.

1. Classification of PUFA

The fatty acid molecules of 18 carbons or more with two or more double bonds are called as polyunsaturated or polyenoic fatty acids (PUFA). Further PUFAs are classified based on the positions of the double bonds from the terminal methyl group (denoted as Omega/ω/n):

1. Omega-3/ω-3/n-3 : first double bond is on the third carbon from the terminal methyl end;
2. Omega-6/ω-6/n-6 : first double bond is on the sixth carbon from the terminal methyl end;
3. Omega-9/ω-9/n-9 : first double bond is on the ninth carbon from the terminal methyl end.

These fatty acids have 2 or more *cis* double bonds that are usually non-conjugated and separated from each other by a single methylene group (Table1). This concept of grouping the PUFAs according to the position of terminal double bond was introduced by Holman in 1964. The PUFAs under different families cannot be interconverted. Conjugated linoleic acid refers to a group of isomers of linoleic acid (cis-9, cis-12 octadecadienoic acid) where the constituent double bonds are separated by a single carbon-carbon bond instead of a methylene group. The most biologically important CLA is *cis-9, trans-11* (rumenic acid).

Table 1 : List of nutritionally important PUFAs

Common name	Chemical name
Omega-3 fatty acid	
α-Linolenic acid	*all-cis*-9,12,15-octadecatrienoic acid, 18:3
Eicosapentaenoic acid	*all-cis*-5,8,11,14,17-eicosapentaenoic acid, 20:5
Docosapentaenoic acid	*all-cis*-7,10,13,16,19-docosapentaenoic acid, 22:5
Docosahexaenoic acid	*all-cis*-4,7,10,13,16,19-docosahexaenoic acid, 22:6
Omega-6 fatty acid	
Linoleic acid	*all-cis*-9,12-octadecadienoic acid, 18:2
Arachidonic acid	*all-cis*-5,8,11,14-eicosatetraenoic acid, 20:4
Docosapentaenoic acid	*all-cis*-4,7,10,13,16-docosapentaenoic acid, 22:5
Conjugated linoleic acid	
Rumenic acid	9Z,11E-octadeca-9,11-dienoic acid, 18:2 10E,12Z-octadeca-9,11-dienoic acid, 18:2

2. Nutritional significance and source of PUFA in animals

Dairy and beef cattle diets without additional fat supplementation contain approximately 2 to 3% long-chain fatty acids (LCFA) from vegetable origin that are predominantly polyunsaturated (Santos, 2001). The changes in length, degree of unsaturation and position of the double bonds in the *acyl* chain of fatty acids decides the effect of a particular fatty acid on animals' performance. Animals cannot incorporate double bonds into fatty acids beyond 9th carbon from the carboxyl end of a fatty acid. Hence, both linoleic acid (18:2, n-6) and α-linolenic acid (18:3, n-3) are considered to be essential PUFAs for animals that must be obtained from the diet (Squires, 2003). These fatty acids are converted through desaturation and elongation reactions to longer chain n-3 (Docosahexaenoic acid, DHA) and n-6 (Docosapentaenoic acid, DPA) fatty acids (Fig 1). In humans it has been observed that the conversion of linolenic acid to eicosapentaenoic acid (EPA) is more limited than rodent models and conversion to DHA is even more limited. It is because of the fact that stearidonic acid (18:4 Octadecatetraenoic Acid) biosynthesized from alpha-linolenic acid by the enzyme Δ-6-desaturase bypasses the limiting step in synthesis of EPA, but not DHA. Quantitative data on the synthesis of EPA and DHA from linoleic acid in domestic animals has not been reported so far, but conversion is limited in animals as well (Palmquist, 2009). Dietary fatty acids can be derived both from the plant as well as animal products. Animal fats are rich in saturated fatty acids whereas vegetable oils are rich in unsaturated fatty acids. Linolenic acid is found mainly in plant oils, while EPA and DHA are abundant in fish oil and marine algae products.

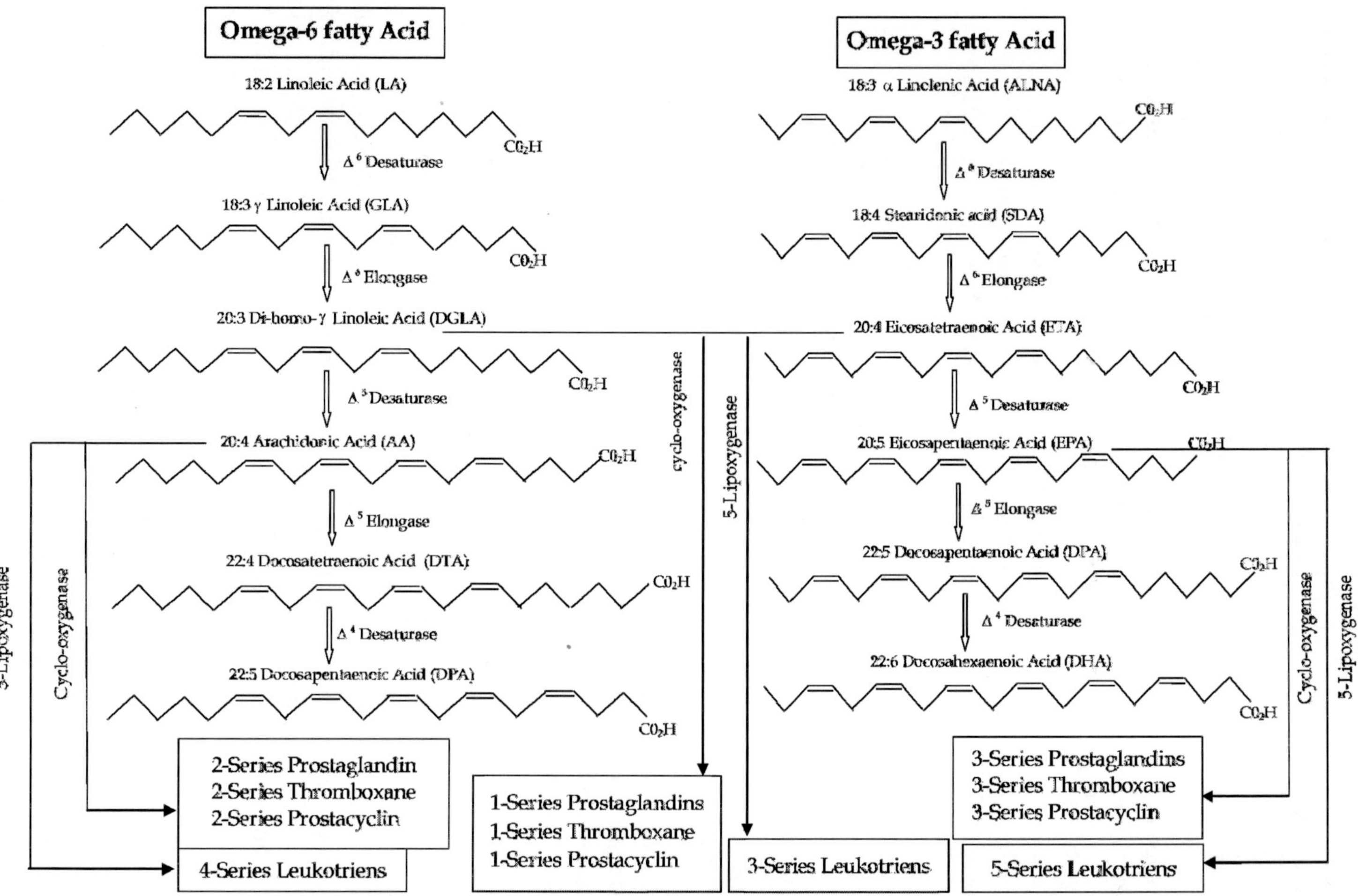

Fig. 1 : The mechanism of desaturation and elongation of linolenic acid (n-6) and linoleic acid (n-3)

3. Metabolism

3.1 Metabolism of omega-3 and omega-6 fatty acids: Cyclooxygenase pathway

Metabolism of C20 PUFAs by cyclooxygenase and 5-lipoxygenase yields a range of important signaling molecules known as the eicosanoids. The eicosanoids or the 'local hormones' have less than five minutes of half life. These molecules have specific effects on their target cells proximal to their site of production and are actively involved in autocrine or paracrine signaling pathways. These eicosanoids, more specifically named as prostaglandins, leukotrienes and thromboxanes are involved in modulation of several biological processes including vasodilatation, platelet aggregation and blood pressure. Arachidonic acid is the immediate precursor for the 2-series prostaglandins, prostacyclins, thromboxanes and 4-series leukotrienes, while the 3-series prostanoids and thromboxanes and 5-series-leukotrienes are derived from eicosapentaenoic acid. The 1-series prostaglandins, thromboxanes and 3-series leukotrienes originate from dihomo-γ-linolenic acid as well as eisosatetraenoic acid (Fig. 1).

3.2 Lipogenesis and carbohydrate metabolism

The PUFAs and their metabolites act as the regulators of enzymes involved in lipid and carbohydrate metabolism (Fig. 2). PUFAs are negative regulators of hepatic and adipose tissue lipogenesis. The mechanism of action for this negative effect is via decline in mRNA levels of hepatic enzymes like acetyl-CoA carboxylase, fatty-acid synthase and stearoyl-CoA desaturase which finally reduce hepatic lipogenesis. Dietary PUFAs act as the repartitioning agent increasing the oxidation of fatty acids rather than storage as triacylglycerols and increase glucose storage as glycogen (Squires, 2003). The PUFAs also effect gene expression by regulating the activity or abundance of different nuclear transcription factors like peroxisome proliferator activated receptors, retinoid X receptors, liver X receptors, hepatic nuclear factors-4a and sterol regulatory binding proteins 1 and 2 (SREBP).

The PUFAs selectively suppress hepatic SREBP-1, a key transcription factor for the regulation of lipogenic enzyme genes in the liver. The SREBPs are transcription factors that belong to the basic helix-loop-helix leucine zipper (bHLH-Zip) family and are profoundly involved in the transcriptional regulation of cholesterogenic and lipogenic enzymes. The three SREBP isoforms, SREBP-1a, SREBP-1c and SREBP-2 have different roles in lipid synthesis. SREBP-1c is responsible for regulating the genes required for *de novo* lipogenesis and SREBP-2 regulates the genes of cholesterol metabolism.

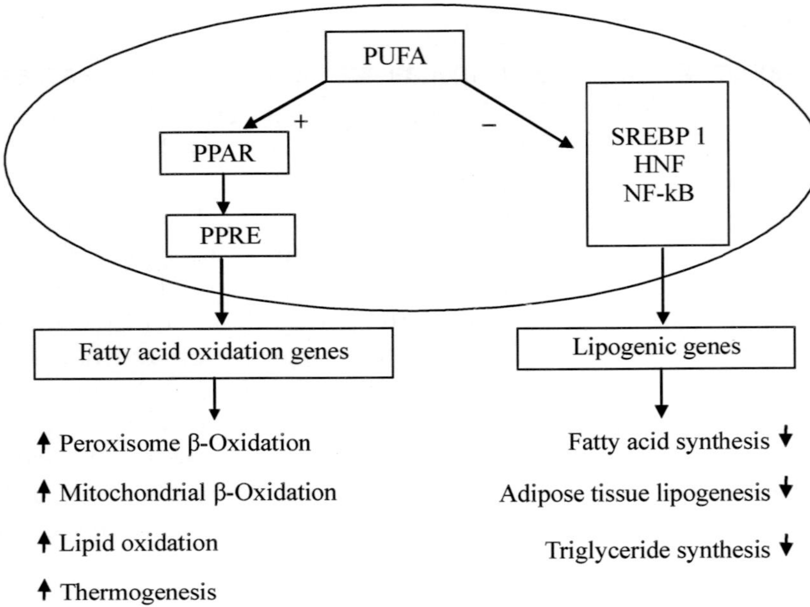

Fig. 2 : Effects of dietary PUFA metabolism. PPAR: peroxisome proliferator activated receptor; PPRE: peroxisome proliferator response element; SREBP: sterol regulatory element binding protein; HNF: hepatic nuclear factor; NFkB: nuclear factor kB. Down and up arrow indicates decrease or increase of the respective activities (Source: Palmquist, 2009).

In vivo study in male mice showed that there are two mechanisms involved in PUFA regulation of SREBP-1c (Takeuchi *et al.,* 2010).The primary mechanism for PUFA suppression of SREBP-1 expression is at the proteolytic processing level and this suppression in turn decreases the transcription of sterol regulatory element binding factor 1c (*Srebf1c*) through lowering SREBP-1 binding to sterol regulatory element (SRE) on the promoter *i.e.,* an autoloop regulatory circuit (Fig. 3).

Although the transcription factor SREBP-1c is described as a major mediator of the negative effects of PUFAs on lipogenic genes in liver, recently, carbohydrate-responsive element-binding protein (ChREBP) is implicated in the regulation of glucose metabolism by glycolytic and lipogenic genes. The ChREBP has been found to act in synergy with SREBP-1c to induce glycolytic and lipogenic gene expression. It has been found that fatty acids can suppress ChREBP gene expression in adipocyte cell line (Dentin *et al.,* 2005). The PUFAs (essential n-6 and n-3 fatty acids) down regulate ChREBP gene expression both *in vivo* and *in vitro* by increase decay of ChREBP mRNA. In addition, another PUFA regulatory mechanism acts via alteration of ChREBP translocation from the cytosol to the nucleus, independently of an activation of the AMP-activated protein kinase that was previously shown to regulate ChREBP activity (Dentin *et al.,* 2005). This ability of PUFAs in regulating cellular and organismal homeostasis gives us an opportunity to explore its use as potential nutraceuticals.

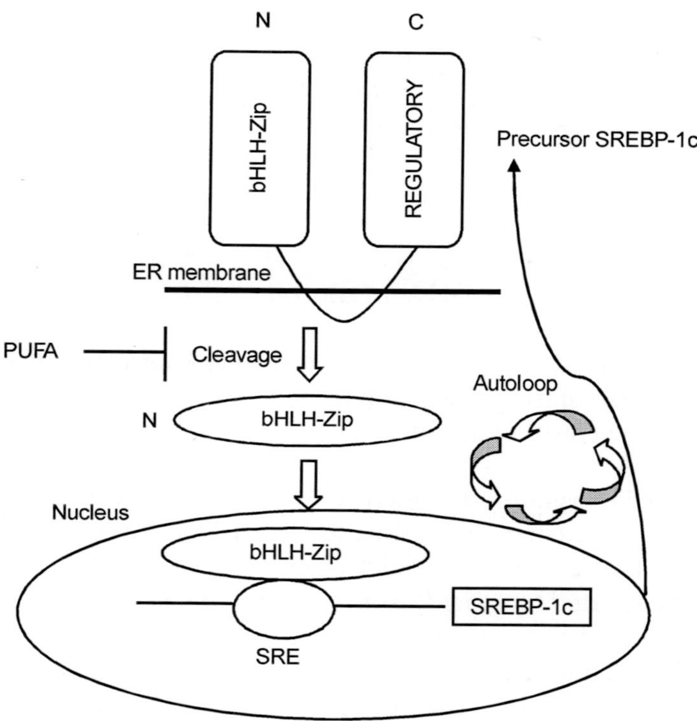

Fig. 3 : Molecular mechanisms for inhibitory effects of polyunsaturated fatty acid (PUFA) on SREBP-1c. bHLH-zip: basic helix loop helix zipper; ER membrane: endoplasmic reticulum membrane; SRE: sterol regulatory element SREBP1-c : sterol regulatory element binding factor1c (Source: Takeuchi *et al.*, 2010).

3.3 Metabolism in the rumen

In monogastric animals (pigs, poultry and rabbits), the fatty acid content of animal products is indicator of tissue fatty acid biosynthesis and fatty acid composition of ingested lipids. In contrast, the phenomenon is not similar in ruminants as dietary fatty acids are hydrogenated in the rumen by microbes. The amount of PUFAs absorbed from the small intestine is limited in ruminants due to extensive ruminal hydrogenation of dietary PUFA to saturated fatty acids. One of the major pathways of biohydrogenation of PUFA in the rumen is conversion of free C18 and PUFA to conjugated dienes or trienes, then to 18:1 and finally undergoing reduction to form stearic acid (Fig. 4). Respectively more than 70% linoleic acid and more than 85% α-linolenic acid fed as unprotected oils or as Ca salts of long chain fatty acid were reported to be biohydrogenated in the rumen of lactating cows (Juchem, 2007). However, *in vitro* studies suggest that the effect of rumen hydrogenation on PUFAs of more than C18 chain length *i.e.*, C20≥ PUFAs is negligible (Ashes *et al.*, 1992). A higher rate of biohydrogenation of C18:3, n-3 (80 to 93%) compared to C20:5, n-3 and C22:6, n-3 (72 to 79%) was observed in sheep supplemented with diets consisting of fish oil or linseed oil (Wachira *et al.*, 2000). Insignificant biohydrogenation of EPA (20:5) and DHA (22:5) was observed in the rumen followed by increase in their concentration in tissues after dietary supplementation (Bilby *et al.*, 2006). In contradiction to this concept, in few *in vivo* investigations extensive hydrogenation of EPA and DHA has been reported in cattle (Castaneda-Gutierrez *et al.*, 2007). Despite ruminal biohydrogenation, continual feeding of Ca salts of fish oil increase concentrations of EPA and DHA in uterine caruncles, endometrium, liver, mammary, muscle, subcutaneous and internal adipose tissues of dairy cows (Bilby *et al.*, 2006). Daily feeding of Ca salts of selective fatty acids is a practical approach for manipulating the tissue fatty acid composition according to the stage of the life cycle in cattle. In order to alter tissue concentrations of the long chain PUFA appreciably, the unsaturated fatty acid sources should be rumen protected or rendered rumen inert. Nevertheless the quantity should be optimum as excessive PUFA in the rumen can have negative effect on ruminal fermentation and total tract fiber digestion (Chilliard and Doreau, 1997). Polyunsaturated fatty acid supplementation has been reported to disturb the ruminal anaerobic ecosystem by altering the ruminal pH, volatile fatty acids (VFA) profile and micro-organisms (Liu *et al.*, 2012). Dietary fish oil supplementation in dairy cows caused significant decline in feed intake (Chilliard and Doreau, 1997). However, feeding PUFA in the form of oilseeds might be less detrimental than feeding free oils (Zhang *et al.*, 2007).

4. Biosynthesis of conjugated linoleic acid (CLA) in the rumen

Biohydrogenation is the process of conversion of unsaturated fatty acids to saturated fatty acids via isomerization and hydrogenation by rumen bacteria. This process is a defense mechanism by the rumen bacteria against potentially toxic unsaturated fatty acids. During this process of biohydrogenation, fatty acids and CLA intermediates are released from the rumen, get absorbed across the small intestine and finally get incorporated into milk fat. In cattle about 3 to 6% of fatty acids are provided through standard dietary means (Muller and Delahoy, 2008). The forages are higher in linoleic and linolenic acid contents, whereas, the grains have higher contents of linoleic acids. The PUFA supplements may also be given to cattle in the form of vegetable oils (18:2 and 18:3) and calcium salts of fat (18:2 and 18:3). There are several CLA isomers present in ruminant fat. The two isomers that are important from physiological point of view are cis-9, *trans* -11 and *trans-10, cis-12*. The *cis*-9, *trans -11* is the most prevalent one comprising 80 to 90% of total CLA in food products from ruminants, whereas *trans*-10, *cis*-12 is present only 3-5% of total CLA (Khanal and Dhiman, 2004). Biohydrogenation of linoleic and linolenic acid result in the formation of *trans-11* (18:1) in the rumen. The products and intermediates of biohydrogenation escape the rumen and get absorbed in the small intestine. Further these fatty acids are taken up by the mammary gland into milk. The ruminal trans-*11* (18:1) gets adsorbed into the small intestine and then incorporated into milk fat. Another major source of CLA is other intermediates of biohydrogenation and CLA synthesis in the mammary gland. Biohydrogenation of linoleic and linolenic acid result in formation of trans-11 (18:1); which is again converted to *cis-9, trans-11* CLA by the Δ9 desaturase enzyme in the mammary gland (Fig. 4). In addition, there is a minor pathway for the formation of *trans-l0, cis-12* CLA from linoleic acid in the rumen and mammary gland. It is suggested that a shift in biohydrogenation pathway of linoleic acid in the mammary gland to *trans-10, cis-12* CLA isomer is an indicative of milk fat depression in dairy cows (Muller and Delahoy, 2008). However, *the cis-9, trans-11 CLA* that is formed by the insertion of a double bond at the 9th carbon of *trans- 11, 18:1* in the mammary gland is the major pathway accounting up to 80% of CLA in ruminant milk. Nevertheless, the rate and extent of biohydrogenation by rumen bacteria are influenced by several factors like the rumen pH, available soluble carbohydrates and fatty acids.

5. Incorporation of CLA and essential PUFA in animal products

5.1 Incorporation of CLA in animal products

The mammary synthesis may account for up to 70 to 80% of the total CLA found in milk. Some literatures suggest that biohydrogenation converts linolenic acid to stearic acid without the formation of CLA (Lee and Jenkins, 2011). Nevertheless, a study was conducted by using a stable isotope tracer to investigate the biohydrogenation intermediates of ^{13}C-linolenic acid. A continuous culture fermenter was used to maintain a mixed microbial population obtained from the cattle rumen at pH 6.5 for 6 days in batch culture. The results of the study confirmed that mixed ruminal microbes are capable of forming several CLA and 18:3 isomers from linolenic acid indicating that linolenic acid biohydrogenation pathways are more complex than reported (Lee and Jenkins, 2011).

In recent years CLA has been established as a component with numerous health promoting benefits including potent cancer-fighting properties. As CLA is formed in the rumen as an intermediate product in the digestion of dietary PUFA, milk and meat from ruminants contains more CLA than non-

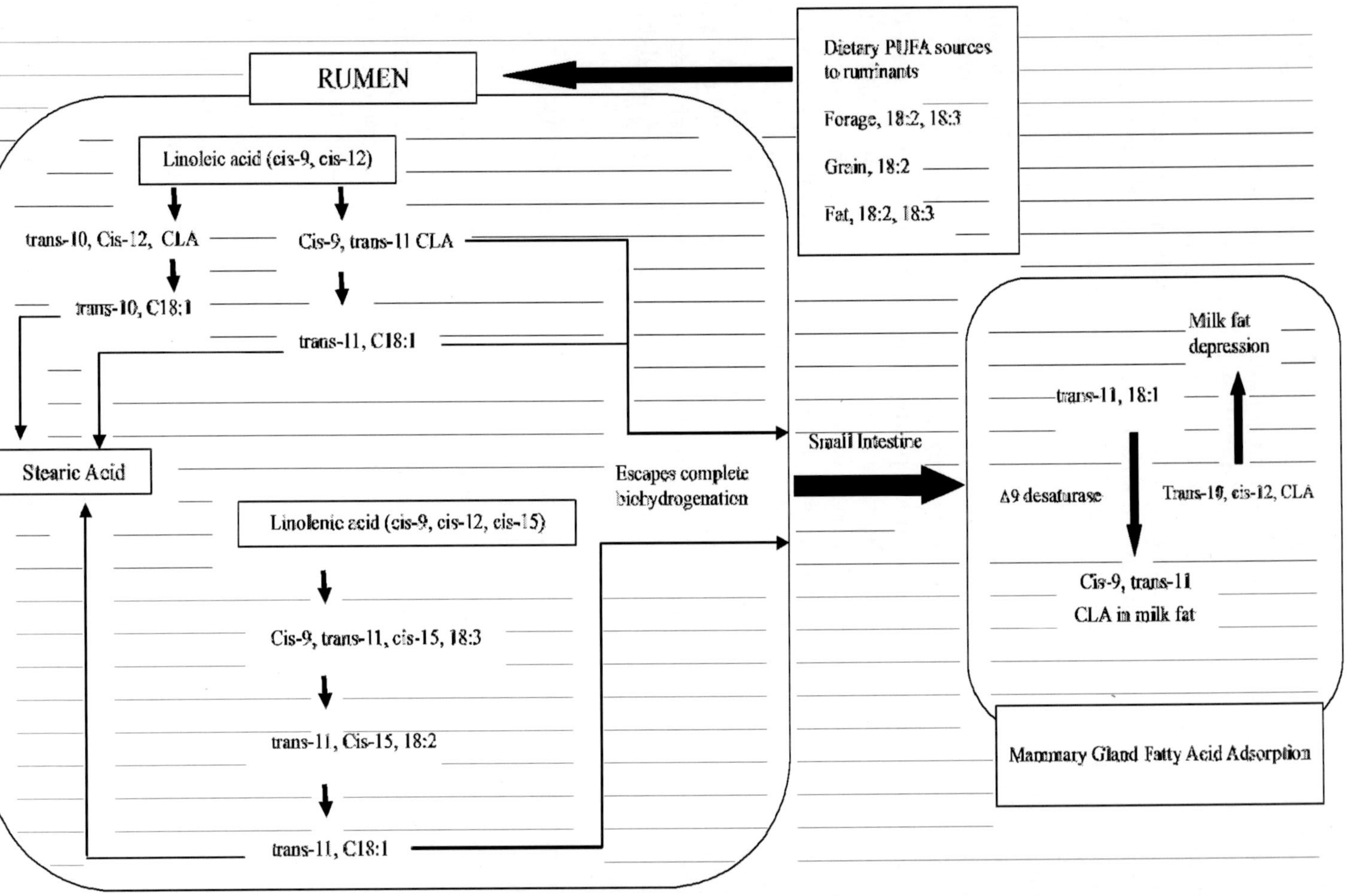

Fig. 4 : Rumen fatty acid metabolism and conjugated linoleic acid (CLA) biosynthesis (Source: Muller and Delahoy, 2008).

ruminants. However CLA content in meat is comparatively less than dairy products (Table 2). It has been reported that CLA acts as an effective repartitioning agent in pigs resulting in increase feed efficiency, decrease back fat and increase lean muscle in the carcass (Dugan *et al.,* 1997). Substantial variation in the concentration of CLA in bovine milk fat has been observed depending on the feeding strategy adopted. Pasture feeding has been found to result in a much higher milk fat CLA concentration compared to total mixed ration (22.1 mg/g fat vs. 3.8 mg/g fat) (Dhiman *et al.,* 1999). Similar enrichment of CLA in milk fat could be achieved through supplementation of unsaturated fat from oil seeds. Supplementation of 53 g/kg dry matter of peanut oil (high oleic acid), sunflower oil (high linoleic acid) or linseed oil (high linolenic acid) has resulted in CLA concentrations of 13.3, 24.4, and 16.7 mg/g milk fat, respectively (Kelly *et al.,* 1998).

Table 2 : CLA content of animal products (Source: Song and Kenelly, 2003).

Products	CLA content (mg/g of fat)
Dairy products	
Homogenized milk	5.5
Butter fat	4.7
Meat	
Ground beef	4.3
Lamb	5.6
Pork	0.6
Chicken	0.9

In cattle, diets supplemented with 4% DM of calcium salts of fatty acids from canola oil, soybean oil, or linseed oil resulted in respective milk CLA concentration of 13.0, 22.0 and 19.0 mg/g fat compared to control that yielded only 3.5 mg CLA/g of fat (Chouinard *et al.,* 1998). In lactating buffaloes, milk fat CLA concentrations of 7.12 mg and 6.74 mg/g fat could be achieved by respective feeding of mustard oil cake and ground nut cake (Tyagi *et al.,* 2006). Further, supplementation of 2% mustard oil along with mustard oil cake resulted in 185% increase in total milk fat CLA content (19.5 mg/g fat) compared to ground nut cake supplementation (6.84 mg/g fat) in buffaloes (Kathirvelan *et al.,* 2007). While in goats raised on berseeem feeding higher milk fat CLA content (13.3 mg/g fat) could be achieved as compared to goats reared on berseem plus concentrate feeding (8.5 mg/g fat) (Tyagi *et al.,* 2007). Such possibility for enhancing milk CLA concentration through dietary manipulation gives us an opportunity to produce CLA enriched dairy products.

5.2 Incorporation of omega-3 and omega-6 fatty acids in animal products

The health benefits of polyunsaturated fatty acids (PUFA) are well established. The recommended ratios for polyunsaturated: saturated fatty acid and n-6:n-3 in diet and meat products are 2:1 and ≤5:1, respectively. Several investigations have undertaken on the health benefits of PUFA in various animal models. These studies have mainly used diets supplemented with linseed as a source of n-3 fatty acids. The use of linseed based diets generally leads to an increase in n-3 fatty acid content in animal products (egg, meat, milk) in ruminants and monogastric animals. Feeding linseed or linseed oil increases linolenic acid content of products 2- to 3-folds and in some products EPA also increases. Fish oil and marine algae products are the rich source of biologically active long chain omega-3 fatty acids (EPA, C20:5 and DHA, C 22:6) therefore these products are fed to animals to increase EPA and DHA contents in animal products (Palmquist, 2009). However, for achieving 2- to 3-fold increase in total PUFA in ruminant tissues and milk, the supplementation of rumen protected linseed or a marine oil product is necessary.

Species specific differences have been observed in relation to fatty acid deposition in adipose and muscle tissues in animals. In pig, higher levels of linoleic acid and linolenic acid have been found in adipose tissue than muscle tissue (Teye *et al.*, 2006). In contrast, similar proportion of PUFAs in the adipose and muscle tissues has been observed by Wood and coworker (2008). In sheep, the full ranges of PUFAs are present in adipose tissue and muscle (Wood *et al.*, 2008), whereas cattle conserve long chain PUFA in muscle phospholipids. The α- linolenic acid is a major dietary fatty acid for ruminants since it constitutes over 50% of total fatty acids in grass and grass products. However, 85 to 100% α-linolenic acid and 70 to 95% linoleic acid undergoes biohydrogenation in rumen. Therefore, in ruminants, around 10% of the dietary linoleic acid is available for incorporation into tissue lipids and the availability of α-linolenic acid for incorporation into tissues is less compared to linoleic acid (Doreau and Ferlay, 1994). In contrast, in pig, dietary linoleic acid and linolenic acid passes through stomach without any change and get absorbed into blood through small intestine and finally incorporated into tissues. Although high n-3 content in meat is considered nutritionally beneficial for human, but rather than the n-3 contents alone it is the ratio of n-3 and n-6 which is more important. In pig, feeding of 15% full fat soyabean for 6 weeks prior to slaughter resulted in approximately 17% (18:2, n-6) and 20% total PUFA in back fat and 11% (18:2, n-6) and 15% total PUFA in the longissimus muscle (Warnants *et al.*, 1999). High PUFA may lead to soft muscle and its oxidative deterioration, which may eventually result in rejection of meat by consumers. Nevertheless, cured pork products do not cause off-flavors as long as there is less than 23% PUFA in back fat and if 18:2 (n-6) is the predominant PUFA in it (Warnants *et al.,* 1998). It is suggested that to avoid undesirable processing problems, back fat should contain less than 20% PUFA (Warnants *et al.,* 1998). A standard test for lipid oxidative stability in foods is the thiobarbituric acid reacting substances (TBARS) test that measures the oxidation product malondialdehyde. A TBARS value above ~0.5 is considered critical since it indicates a level of lipid oxidation that produces a rancid odor, which is detectible by the consumers. Dietary supplementation of antioxidants like α-tocopheryl-acetate/vitamin E has been found to play an important role in maintaining meat quality through stabilizing PUFA and preventing such lipid peroxidation.

Omega-3 fortified poultry eggs are considered as a good source of n-3 PUFA. The enrichment of laying-hen rations with vegetable oils such as linseed or canola oil that are rich in linolenic acid can readily promote the deposition of n-3 PUFA into egg yolk (Van Elswyk, 1997).

6. PUFA as methane inhibitor

The supplementation of fatty acid as one of the nutritional approaches to reduce methane emission and optimize energy metabolism in ruminants has been under investigation for some time. In the rumen, unsaturated fatty acids get saturated using available hydrogen and thereby inhibit methane production (Rasmussen and Harrison, 2011). It has been reported that PUFA supplementation in cattle significantly reduced methane emissions (Eugene *et al.,* 2008). However, PUFA supplementation also has a toxic effect on fiber digesting bacteria, protozoa and methanogens. In lactating dairy cows, 18% methane reduction was reported with the inclusion of 3.3% linseed oil. Although there was no change in VFA concentration, rumen pH, rumen protozoa population, milk yield and composition, digestibility was affected negatively (Beauchemin *et al.,* 2009). In lambs, 6.6% linseed oil supplementation reduced only 10% methane production with adverse effect on digestibility, total VFA concentration and rumen protozoa numbers (Machmüller *et al.,* 2000). There was a reduction in butyrate and acetate concentrations while propionate remained unchanged. Moreover, there was no significant effect on daily live weight gain. Supplementation with a PUFA source with roughage based diet, reduces the digestibility of cell wall carbohydrates, the production of hydrogen and finally reduces methane production in the rumen.

7. Role of PUFA on reproduction and fertility

7.1 Role in prostaglandin synthesis and metabolism

The PUFAs have specific roles in hormone production, tissue repair and function, immune function and embryonic development. They act as mediators in a series of processes in several reproductive tissues including fluidity of cell membrane, intracellular signaling and susceptibility to oxidative damage. It is suggested that supply of extra dietary rumen protected fat is a possible approach to improve fertility in dairy cows (Tamminga, 2006).

Strategic dietary supplementation of PUFAs can alter their respective concentrations in blood and key reproductive tissues. Several hypotheses have been proposed regarding the mechanisms by which dietary PUFA supplementation improves reproductive performance (Staples *et al.*, 1998), which are mentioned below.

- Amelioration of negative energy balance leading to an earlier resumption of postpartum estrus and thereby improving fertility
- Increasing steroidogenesis favorable to fertility
- Manipulating insulin and thereby stimulating ovarian follicular development
- Stimulating or inhibiting the production and release of PGF2α and thereby influencing the persistence of the corpus luteum

There are reports on the positive effect of dietary supplementation of n-3 and n-6 fatty acid on reproductive events like ovulation number, cyclicity, ovarian follicle dynamics, corpus luteum function, progesterone secretion and uterine health in dairy cattle (Robinson *et al.*, 2002; (Ambrose *et al.*, 2006; Bowen and Roy, 2008). In cattle, significantly longer duration of behavioural estrus and estradiol (E2) surge with greater area under the E2 curve have been observed as a result of dietary n-3 fatty acid feeding during pre and postpartum period. Simultaneously, lower concentration of prostaglandin-E2 in the E2 active follicles and alternations in the membrane fatty acid composition has been observed (Zachut *et al.*, 2011). The mechanism behind the effect of n-3 and n-6 fatty acid supplementation on the timings and characteristics of events in and around estrus has been linked to the alternation in prostaglandin metabolism.

7.2 Effect on innate immunity

The PUFAs of n-6 and n-3 families also act as nutraceuticals, altering the innate immune responses and subsequent gene expression within the uterus to complement the sequential processes of follicle and embryo development and survival of embryo and fetus. The threshold for triggering an immune response (pro-inflammatory state) can be altered due to feeding of linoleic acid which is a source of proinflammatory eicosanoids. This accelerates postpartum immunity, specifically innate immunity and causes secretion of acute phase proteins in milk of lactating dairy cows (Thatcher *et al.*, 2010).

It is suggested that feeding supplements enriched with linoleic acid can improve uterine health by increasing uterine production of dienoic prostaglandins, including PGF2α and other immuno-stimulatory eicosanoids (Robinson *et al.*, 2002). This promotes uterine involution and consequently resumption of estrous cycle.

7.3 Role in maternal recognition of pregnancy

For establishment of pregnancy in cows, suppression of luteolytic PGF2α secretion and maintenance of the CL are the obligatory steps. It has been hypothesized that the inclusion of n-3 fats in diet through fish oil or Ca-LCFA (long chain fatty acids) increases the length of conceptus, which is directly related to the production capacity of IFN-τ (Bilby *et al.*, 2006). Feeding calcium salts enriched with n-3 PUFA during the breeding period followed by C18:2 (n-6) supplementation in the transition period improved pregnancy rates (Silvestre *et al.*, 2009). Supplementation of n-3 PUFA increases systemic cholesterol and IGF-1 and CL size and any or all of these may mediate positive effect on maintenance of pregnancy (Childs *et al.*, 2008). In sheep, progesterone concentration in the follicular fluid has been found greater in animals consuming *n-3* fatty acids enriched ration compared to animals fed *n*-6 fatty acid enriched ration (Wonnacott *et al.*, 2010).

7.4 Role on oocyte and embryo development

The PUFAs of n-6 and n-3 families contribute to the development of oocytes and embryos. Incorporation of n-6 fatty acid to the oocyte maturation medium has been found to increase cumulus cell expansion and development of oocytes to metaphase II stage (Marei *et al.*, 2010). Subsequently, these stimulatory effects increased cleavage rates, enhanced blastocyst development and increased number of cells in both the inner cell mass and trophectoderm. In contrast, n-3 supplementation has been found to inhibit early embryonic development (Marei *et al.*, 2010). In Holstein Friesian cows, supplementation of n-3 PUFA had no effect on the number of good quality embryos recovered, but the number of degenerated embryos recovered was significantly less (Childs *et al.*, 2008). This was in concurrence to an increase in uterine EPA and decrease in arachidonic acid which might subsequently led to increased production of the 3-series prostaglandin resulting a more luteotrophic environment. Consequently, there was no effect on superovulation response, embryo recovery rate, embryo quality or on the expression of genes (BAX, LIF, Cx43 and E-CAD) related to early embryo development. Moreover, no effect was evident on peroxisome proliferator-activated receptors (PPARs)-α and δ. It has been suggested that the potential effects of dietary n-3 PUFA on the reproductive processes are not mediated through the effects on the embryo *per se* in cattle (Childs *et al.*, 2008).

7.5 Effect on spermatozoa

Sperm plasma membranes have high levels of long-chain PUFAs, especially DPA and DHA compared to somatic cells. Relatively a higher proportion of DPA is present in stallion and boar spermatozoa (Grady *et al.*, 2009) than other domestic animals. Enhanced fertility has been seen when the DHA: DPA ratio is increased in boars and humans (Grady *et al.*, 2009). In stallion, the poorest sperm membrane integrity along with a high level of lipid peroxidation was recorded in the ejaculate with lower concentration of DPA in the sperm plasma membranes and the PUFAs provided a higher fluidity of the plasma membrane. Similarly, the higher levels of DPA and DHA content in the boar sperm membrane make it more cryoprotectant due to initial higher membrane fluidity (Waterhouse *et al.*, 2006). Similarly, variations in sperm plasma membrane DPA and DHA levels have also been reported to be associated with the differences in cryotolerance in sperm isolated from Asian and African elephants, common wombats, grey kangaroos, koalas, blue foxes and silver foxes (Waterhouse *et al.*, 2006). Furthermore, a high PUFA:saturated fatty acid ratio in cold-resistant bee sperm and lower ratios in cold-sensitive ram and fowl sperm have been observed (Arav *et al.* 2000). Nevertheless, the high degree of polyunsaturation of n-3 fatty acids may result in a higher susceptibility of sperm to lipid peroxidation with the consequent risk of damage to the cellular structures (Grady *et al.*, 2009).

8. PUFA supplementation on poultry

8.1 Nutritional significance

Linoleic acid is considered to be the only essential fatty acid for poultry. Even though growth and performance studies have not revealed a need for α-linolenic acid in poultry, essential fatty acid deficiency symptoms have been recorded in poultry. Furthermore the long-chain (n-3) PUFAs are necessary for normal development of brain and retina. The linoleic acid requirement for growth in chickens, turkeys and quail is suggested to be 0.8-1% of the diet. It is also suggested that laying hens may have two requirements for linoleic acid, 0.9% for physiological purposes and an additional 2 to 4% for maximum egg size (Watkins, 1991).

8.2 Effect on immune response

Several studies have shown an enhanced immune response following the replacement of dietary linoleic acid with dietary linolenic acid in chickens. Such immunoregulatory effects of PUFA may be applied for enhancing immune response to vaccination in poultry (Puthpongsiriporn and Scheideler, 2005). It is suggested that linolenic acid supplementation stimulates the production of transforming growth factor 1 (TGF 1) which leads to an increase in lgA production (Fisher and Harbige, 1997). Dietary supplementation of omega-3 fatty acids are considered to be effective in treating metabolic diseases like ascites and sudden death syndrome in poultry. A dietary supplementation of 5% flaxseed has been reported to be effective in prevention of ascites. In layer, such dietary supplementation reduces fat accumulation in the liver of poultry and also provides a good dietary source of omega-3 fatty acid in poultry products for human consumption.

Conclusions

In recent years, a greater awareness of consumers about the nutritional implications on health has opened new market opportunities for essential fatty acid enriched animal products. The essential fatty acids, although key to normal growth, production and reproduction, have not traditionally been a priority in animal nutrition. It is because of the increasing interest in essential fatty acid for human nutrition and health and the potential to increase their content in human diets through animal products; the PUFAs have become a subject of interest in animal nutrition. Greater scopes are ahead for production of animal products enriched with essential PUFAs and CLA without expensive processes. However, the major limitation in inclusion of more amount of PUFA to animal diet is the increase possibility of lipid peroxidation in PUFA enriched animal products. This further decline the sensory characteristics leading to reduction in quality as well as shelf life of PUFA enriched animal products. Research is on progress to find out the effective means for protecting PUFA enriched animal products from lipid peroxidation. Another interesting aspect of PUFA biology is related to their interactions with nuclear receptor proteins like eicosanoids and their metabolism. Hence there is a scope of PUFAs to be used as nutraceutical or pharmaceutical agents. Moreover, PUFAs exert a broad range of beneficial effects on the reproductive tissues. Further research efforts in different animal models related to the effect of dietary PUFAs and antioxidant supplementations on molecular and enzymatic mechanisms influencing the synthesis and deposition of long-chain n-3 PUFA are required.

References

Ambrose D.K., Kastelic J.P., Corbett R., Pitney P.A., Petit H.V., Small J.A., Zalkovic P. (2006). Lower pregnancy losses in lactating dairy cows fed a diet enriched in α-linolenic acid. *Journal of Dairy Science* **89:** 3066-3074.

Arav A., Pearl M., Zeron Y. (2000). Does membrane lipid profile explain chilling sensitivity and membrane lipid phase transition of spermatozoa and oocytes? *Cryo Letters* **21:** 179-186.

Ashes J.R., Siebert B.D., Gulati S.K., Cuthbertson A.Z., Scott T.W. (1992). Incorporation of n-3 fatty acids of fish oil into tissue and serum lipids of ruminants. *Lipids* **27:** 629-631.

Beauchemin K.A., McGinn S.M., Benchaar C., Holtshausen L. (2009). Crushed sunflower, flax or canola seeds in lactating dairy cow diets: effects on methane production, rumen fermentation and milk production. *Journal of Dairy Science* **92:** 2118–2127.

Bilby T.R., Jenkins T., Staples C.R., Thatcher W.W. (2006). Pregnancy, bovine somatotropin and dietary n-3 fatty acids in lactating dairy cows: III. Fatty acid distribution. *Journal of Dairy Science* **89:** 3386-3399.

Bowen A., Roy Ax M.S. (2008). Cows fed MEGALAC®-R saw improved ovarian activity, reduced incidence of clinical and subclinical endometritis, and increased cumulative Research Bulletin: Arm and Hammer Animal Nutrition. Available at: http://www.ahdairy.com/uploads/articles/MEGALAC-R_Research_Bulletin-Repro_&_Uterine_Health.pdf.

Castaneda-Gutierrez E., de. Veth M.J., Lock A.L., Dwyer D.A., Murphy K.D., Bauman D.E. (2007). Effect of supplementation with calcium salts of fish oil on n-3 fatty acids in milk fat. *Journal of Dairy Science* **90:** 4149-4156.

Childs S., Hennessy A.A., Sreenan J.M., Wathes D.C., Cheng Z., Stanton C., Diskin M.G., Kenny D.A. (2008). Effect of level of dietary n-3 polyunsaturated fatty acid supplementation on systemic and tissue fatty acid concentrations and on selected reproductive variables in cattle. *Theriogenology* **70:** 595-611.

Chilliard Y., Doreau M. (1997). Influence of supplementary fish oil and rumen-protected methionine on milk yield and composition in dairy cows. *Journal of Dairy Research* **64:** 173-179.

Chouinard P.Y., Corneau L., Bauman D.E., Butler W.R., Chilliard Y., Drackley J.K. (1998). Conjugated linoleic acid content of milk from cows fed different sources of dietary fat. *Journal of Dairy Science* **81:** 223 (Abstr.).

Dentin R., Benhamed F., Pégorier J.P., Foufelle F., Viollet B., Vaulont S., Girard J., Postic C. (2005). Polyunsaturated fatty acids suppress glycolytic and lipogenic genes through the inhibition of ChREBP nuclear protein translocation. *The Journal of Clinical Investigation* **115:** 2843-2854.

Dhiman T.R., Anand G.R., Satter L.D., Pariza M.W. (1999).Conjugated linoleic acid content of milk from cows fed different diets. *Journal of Dairy Science* **82:** 2146-2156.

Doreau M., Ferlay A. (1994). Digestion and utilization of fatty acids by ruminants. *Animal Feed Science and Technology* **45:** 379-396.

Dugan M.E.R., Aalhus J.L., Schaefer A.L., Kramer J.K.G. (1997). The effect of conjugated linoleic acid on fat to lean repartitioning and feed conversion in pigs. *Canadian Journal of Animal Science* **77:** 723-725.

Eugene M., Mass´e D., Chiquette J., Benchaa C. (2008). Metaanalysis on the effects of lipid supplementation on methane production in lactating dairy cows. *Canadian Journal of Animal Science* **88:** 331-334.

Fisher B.A.C., Harbige L.S. (1997). Effect of omeaga-6 lipid rich borage oil feeding on immune function in healthy volunteers. *Biochemical Society Transactions* **25**: 343S.

Gardener N.H., Reynolds C.K., Phipps R.H., Jones A.K., Beever D.E. (1999). Effects of different diet supplements in the pre and postpartum period on reproductive performance in the dairy cow. In: *Fertility in the high producing dairy cow.* (M.G. Diskin, ed.), BSAS Occasional Symposium No. **26:** 313-322.

Grady S.T., Cavinder C.A., Brinsko S.P., Forrest D.W., Sawyer J.E., Scott B.D. (2009). Dietary supplementation of two varying sources of n-3 fatty acids and subsequent effects on fresh, cooled and frozen seminal characteristics of stallions. *The Professional Animal Scientist* **25:** 768-773.

Juchem S.O. (2007). Lipid digestion and metabolism in dairy cows: Effects on production, reproduction and health. *Doctorate Dissertation.* University of California, Davis, USA.

Kathirvelan C. (2007). Influence of mustard cake feeding on conjugated linoleic acid content of buffalo milk and its anticarcinogeneic potency. *Ph.D thesis,* NDRI (Deemed University), Karnal, India.

Kelly M.L., Berry J.R., Dwyer D.A., Griinari J.M., Chouinard P.Y., Amburgh M.E.V., Bauman D.E. (1998). Dietary fatty acid sources affect conjugated linoleic acid concentrations in milk from lactating dairy cows. *Journal of Nutrition* **128:** 881-885.

Khanal R.C., Dhiman T.R. (2004). Biosynthesis of conjugated linoleic acid (CLA): A Review. *Pakistan Journal of Nutrition* **3:** 72-81.

Lee Y.J., Jenkins T.C. (2011). Biohydrogenation of linolenic acid to stearic acid by the rumen microbial population yields multiple intermediate conjugated diene isomers. *Journal of Nutrition* **141:** 1445-1450.

Liu S.J., Bu D.P., Wang J.Q., Liu L., Liang S., Wei H.Y., Zhou L. Y., Li D., Loor J.J. (2012). Effect of incremental levels of fish oil supplementation on specific bacterial populations in bovine ruminal fluid. *Journal of Animal Physiology and Animal Nutrition* **96:** 9-16.

Machmüller A., Ossowski D.A., Kreuzer M. (2000). Comparative evaluation of the effects of coconut oil, oilseeds and crystalline fat on methane release, digestion and energy balance in lambs. *Animal Feed Science and Technology* **85:** 41-60.

Marei F.W., Wathes D.C., Fouladi-Nashta A.A. (2010). Impact of linoleic acid on bovine oocyte maturation and embryo development. *Reproduction* **139:** 979-988.

Muller G.H., Kirk, R.W., Scott D.W., Griffin C.E. (2001). Nutritional skin diseases. In: *Muller and Kirk's Small Animal Dermatology* (6th). Elsevier, Philadelphia, Pennsylvania.

Muller L.D., Delahoy J.E. (2008). Conjugated Linoleic Acid (CLA): Implications for animal production and human health. Available at: http://www.das.psu.edu/dairy-alliance/research-extension/dairy/nutrition/pdf/das0488cla.pdf.

Palmquist D.L. (2009). Omega-3 fatty acids in metabolism, health, and nutrition and for modified animal product foods. *The Professional Animal Scientist* **25:** 207-249.

Puthpongsiriporn U., Scheideler S.E. (2005). Effects of dietary ratio of linoleic acid to linolenic acid on performance, antibody production and *in vitro* lymphocytes proliferation in two strains of leghorn pullet chicks. *Poultry Science* **84:** 846-857.

Rasmussen J., Harrison A. (2011). The benefits of supplementary fat in feed rations for ruminants, with particular focus on reducing levels of methane production. *ISRN Veterinary Science*, Article ID 613172, doi:10.5402/2011/613172.

Robinson R.S., Pushpakumara P.G., Cheng Z., Peters A.R., Abayasekara D.R., Wathes D.C. (2002). Effects of dietary polyunsaturated fatty acids on ovarian and uterine function in lactating dairy cows. *Reproduction* **124:** 119-131.

Santos J.E.P. (2001). Dietary ingredients and nutritional management impact fertility in dairy cattle. In: *Proc. 36th Pacific Northwest Animal Nutrition Conference*. Boise, ID, pp 189-219.

Silvestre F. T., Carvalho T.S.M., Crowford C., Francisco N., Santos J.E.P., Kim S.C., Jenkins T., Staples C.R., Thatcher W.W. (2009). Feeding n-6 and n-3 fatty acids to dairy cows: Effects on immunity, fertility and lactation: In: *Proc. Florida Ruminant Nutritional Symposium*. **20:** 75-90.

Song M.K., Kennelly J.J. (2003). Biosynthesis of conjugated linoleic acid and its incorporation into ruminant's products. *Asian Australian Journal of Animal Science* **16:** 306-314.

Squires E.J. (2003). Manipulation of growth and carcass Composition. In: *Applied Animal Endocrinology* (1st ed). CABI Publishing, UK, pp 66-123.

Staples C.R., Burke J.M.,Thatcher W.W. (1998). Influence of supplemental fats on reproductive tissues and performance of lactating cows. *Journal of Dairy Science*. **81:** 856-871.

Takeuchi Y., Yahagi N., Izumida Y., Nishi M., Kubota M., Teraoka Y., Yamamoto T., Matsuzaka T., Nakagawa Y., Sekiya M., Iizuka Y., Ohashi K., Osuga J., Gotoda T., Ishibashi S., Itaka, K., Kataoka K., Nagai R., Yamada N., Kadowaki T., Shiman H. (2010). Polyunsaturated fatty acids selectively suppress sterol regulatory element-binding protein-1 through proteolytic processing and autoloop regulatory circuit. *The Journal of Biological Chemistry* **285:** 11681-11691.

Tamminga S. (2006). The effect of the supply of rumen degradable protein and metabolisable protein on negative energy balance and fertility in dairy cows. *Animal Reproduction Science* **96:** 227-239.

Teye G.A., Sheard P.R., Whittington F.M., Nute G.R., Stewart A., Wood J.D. (2006). Influence of dietary oils and protein level on pork quality. 1. Effects on muscle fatty acid composition, carcass, meat and eating quality. *Meat Science* **73:** 157-165.

Thatcher W.W., Silvestre F.T., Santos J.E.P., Staples C.R. (2010). Nutritional modulation of immune-function and compatibility with pregnancy. Available at: http://ag.arizona.edu/ans/swnmc/Proceedings/2010/03_Thatcher_2010.pdf

Tyagi A.K., Kewalramani N., Dhiman T.R., Kaur H., Singhal K.K., Kanawjia S.K. (2007). Enhancement of CLA content in buffalo milk through green berseem feeding. *Animal Feed Science Technology* **132:** 15-19.

Tyagi A.K., Saluja M., Singhal K.K. (2006). Effect of *berseem* feeding on nutrient utilization and milk yield in Goats. *Indian Journal of Dairy Science* **59:** 29-32.

Van Elswyk M. E. (1997). Comparison of n-3 fatty acid sources in laying hen rations for improvement of whole egg nutritional quality: a review. *British Journal of Nutrition* **78:** 61-69 (Suppl. 1).

Wachira A.M.,Sinclair L.A., Wilkinson R.G., Hallett K., Enser M.,Wood J. D. (2000). Rumen biohydrogenation of *n*-3 polyunsaturated fatty acids and their effects on microbial efficiency and nutrient digestibility in sheep. *The Journal of Agricultural Science* **135:** 419-428.

Warnants N., Van Oeckel M.J., Boucque C.V. (1998). Effect of incorporation of dietary polyunsaturated fatty acids in pork back fat on the quality of salami. *Meat Science* **49:** 435-445.

Warnants N., Van Oeckel M.J., Boucque C.V. (1999). Incorporation of dietary polyunsaturated fatty acids into pork fatty tissues. *Journal of Animal Science* **77:** 2478–2490.

Waterhouse K.E., Hofmo P.O., Tverdal A., Miller Jr.R.R. (2006). Within and between breed differences in freezing tolerance and plasma membrane fatty acid composition of boar sperm. *Reproduction* **131:** 887–894.

Watkins B.A. (1991).Importance of essential fatty acids and their derivatives in poultry. *Journal of Nutrition* **121:** 1475-1485.

Wonnacott K.E., Kwong W.Y., Hughes J., Salter A.M., Lea R.G., Garnsworthy P.C., Sinclair K.D. (2010). Dietary omega-3 and -6 polyunsaturated fatty acids affect the composition and development of sheep granulosa cells, oocytes and embryos. *Reproduction* **139:** 57-69.

Wood J.D., Enser M., Fisher A.V., Nute G.R., Sheard P.R., Richardson R.I., Hughes S.I., Whittington F.M. (2008). Fat deposition, fatty acid composition and meat quality. *Meat Science* **78:** 343–358.

Zachut M., Arieli A., Moallem U. (2011). Incorporation of dietary n-3 fatty acids into ovarian compartments in dairy cows and the effects on hormonal and behavioral patterns around estrus. *Reproduction*. Manuscript no. REP-10-0518, pp 1-32.

Zhang R.H., Mustafa A.F., Zhao X. (2007). Effects of feeding oilseeds on nutrient utilization by lactating ewes. *Small Ruminant Research* **67:** 307–311.

❑❑❑

Chapter 6

Future Trends in Poultry Nutrition

A.V. Elangovan
National Institute of Animal Nutrition and Physiology, Adugodi, Banglaore-560 030 Karnataka, India

Summary

Poultry is one of the fastest growing components of global meat production. Expansion in India is being driven by rising incomes and a shift in industry structure toward integrated ownership in poultry production. The concept of feeding has changed dramatically with the change in the genetic potential of broiler and layer stock. In the past, poultry nutrition focused on the nutrient requirements, feed ingredients, feed efficiency, feed additives and juvenile nutrition. However, over the next decade, it will be closely integrated with biotechnology, microbiology and computational technology to produce the quality poultry products at the most economical cost.

Poultry production is projected to increase the most among the livestock sector over the next decade according to the latest United States Department of Agriculture (USDA) agricultural projections report. Currently we have major poultry production in Americas, Europe and Asia. The Americas and Asia will continue to meet world demand, whereas Europe, to supply its own local market. Within the Americas, the United States and Brazil will continue to be the major producers and exporters, whereas in Asia, China will likely represent the major region for growth, both for domestic production and also for exports. In future, Brazil is expected to continue as the largest exporter of poultry products, as a result of low production costs and competitive export prices. Indian poultry sector has been growing annually at around 8-10%. As per the recent reports of International Credit Rating Agency, June 2011, overall domestic poultry market size is estimated at rupees forty seven thousand crore with broiler meat and table eggs contributing more than 95% of the market. Globally India ranks fourth in broiler meat production with annual production of 2.9 million metric tons (MMT) of broiler meat. India is ranked third in table egg production with annual production of 57 billion eggs.

The poultry sector has been able to withstand the escalating feed costs, mainly due to the efficient feed conversion rates of the commercial stock and shorter production process. The production capacity has responded with increased integration and penetration of contract poultry farming. The major hurdles in poultry expansion include high feed costs combined with short supply of conventional feed ingredients, inadequate cold chain and transportation facility and high vulnerability to disease outbreaks. In future, poultry industry has to face challenges not only on disease aspect; but also for the shortage of cereals and oilseed byproducts, as the production of crops may not be able to keep pace with the expanding growth rate of poultry industry.

Over the years, there has been a tremendous genetic improvement of both broiler and layer chicken stock. Geneticists have continued to make improvements to the performance of broilers but there has to be a limit to the rate at which these birds can grow. Today, we can achieve 2.5 kg broilers at 35 d of age with a feed conversion ratio close to 1.6 and egg layers capable of producing in excess of 330 eggs in 52 weeks of lay. Further, with the change in the performance of birds, the nature of feeding practices also has changed. Earlier, there was only two phases of broiler ration, starter and finisher, the chicks for the first two or three days were fed on only maize, now the concept of pre starter diet for first seven to ten days have changed the whole concept as well the importance of initial feeding. The feeding strategies are directed towards achieving the best-feed efficiency in a most cost effective manner. May be at times, we may have to sacrifice the best feed efficiency while utilizing alternate feed ingredients in broiler/layer chicken in most economical way.

1. Alternate feed ingredients

The nutrient requirement standard, National Research Council (NRC) has not been updated since 1994 but is still relevant for unit gain or egg production of broiler/layer stock. The diet formulation, feeding programs and production goals are continually changing, and it is these factors that affect diet specifications. Feed costs forms more than 60-70% of raw material costs for a poultry farm. Energy costs are high because of demand for maize and the fact that there are no viable alternative. Limitation to alternate feed ingredient use is often its inadequate supply and consistency. Distiller's grain is a relatively new alternate ingredient but has a considerable variation in composition and nutrient availability. The feed industry is faced with a number of challenges, not only the availability of feed ingredients but also to produce high quality products in a cost effective manner. The increase in ingredient price surely increases the cost of production of eggs and poultry meat and thus reduces the profitability of the farmers. In the coming times, poultry has definitely to look beyond maize and soybean meal because of its availability; cost and also maize-soybean production cannot keep pace with the ever-increasing poultry production. There is a scope for alternate feed ingredients in future with the expanding poultry production and stagnant conventional feed ingredients. There has been a lot of work done in the area of alternate feed ingredients (Raju *et al.*, 2003; Rao *et al.*, 2004; Elangovan *et al.*, 2004b; Mandal *et al.*, 2005a b; Mandal *et al.*, 2006; Kumar *et al.*, 2005; Chauynarong *et al.*, 2009) and we have to start employing these ingredients in diet formulations whenever economical. The incorporation of alterative feed ingredients in feed formulation call for use of digestible amino acid values. The use of digestible amino acid values ensures that the correct or appropriate price is paid for alternative feed ingredients and helps to ensure that predictable performance will be obtained when alternative feed ingredients are used in the formulation.

2. Feed amino acid content

The early development of digestive organs in chicken is associated with better growth and feed utilization through intake of nutrients, digestion and absorption of nutrients. Proportionately higher growth rate of gastrointestinal tract in younger birds signified the prioritization of nutrient partitioning towards development of digestive systems, *i.e.*, the organ of supply, which had been facilitated by higher level of amino acids in diets (Iji, 1999; Jin *et al.*, 1998; Noy *et al.*, 2001). In the recent years, the level of incorporation of amino acids has increased dramatically in the initial phase of broiler production. This has also been possible due to lower cost of synthetic amino acids. As the potential growth rate of broilers is increased by genetic selection, the amino acid and energy requirements of the bird also increase, but these do not increase in the same proportion. The amino acid requirements increase proportionately faster than does the energy requirement, thus a higher amino acid to energy ratio is required for meeting the genetic potential of broiler stock (Morris and Njuru, 1990). The amino acid and energy contents in the diet may not be capable of being increased indefinitely; to meet the ever increasing nutrient requirements of broilers as growth rate continues to be increased by selection is a great challenge. The amino acid digestibility values of cereal grains and protein meals determined using caecectomized cockerels might be appropriate for poultry diet formulations (Vasan *et al.*, 2008). Also, a large volume of published data on the amino acid digestibility for poultry feeds is available (Green *et al.*, 1987; Ravindran *et al.*, 1996a; 1996b). The knowledge on the digestibilities of amino acids in feed ingredients helps in improving the utilization of dietary protein and to minimize nitrogen in excreta thereby enhancing the performance of birds, reducing stress to birds and environmental pollution (Lemme *et al.*, 2004).

3. *In ovo* feeding

The early access to feed is critical, feeding the embryo external feed components (*i.e.*, carbohydrates, protein, *etc.*) before hatch by *in ovo* administration significantly enhances the enteric development for greater digestive and nutrient absorptive capacity. The intestines of hatchlings fed *in ovo* have been found to be functionally similar to conventionally fed two-day old chicks as a result of accelerated enteric development through increased absorptive surface area of the gut, increased brush border enzyme activity. Experiments have demonstrated that *in ovo* administration of nutrients influenced the gut physiology of broiler embryos prior to and after hatch. The *in ovo* feeding not only improves hatchability, but also provides superior nutritional status of the hatchling, greater vigour, and post-hatch growth (Bhanja *et al.*, 2004; Bhanja and Mandal, 2005). The avian embryo develops in a carbohydrate-free environment with a finite amount of *in ovo* energy and nutrients to support embryonic growth and hatching. The maintenance of glucose homeostasis during late-term embryonic development depends on the amount of glucose present as glycogen in the liver and also the glucose produced by gluconeogenesis from protein mobilized from amnion albumen and then from muscle. In case of insufficient glycogen and albumen, the embryo mobilizes more muscle protein toward gluconeogenesis, thus restricting growth potential and hatchability.

As the embryo grows, the yolk reserves and albumen decline transiently and are almost depleted prior to hatching. The yolk lipids and albumen protein provide the gluconeogenic substrates for endogenous production of glucose, which is stored as glycogen in the liver and muscles. Therefore, glycogen reserves provide the energy needed for growth, development and hatching and plays a crucial role for the survival of the avian embryo and neonate.

At hatch, glycogen reserves can be replenished with the immediate access and consumption of external feed. In commercial practice, the immediate access to feed is often not possible after hatch and the chicks have to mobilize critical body resources (primarily muscle) to provide the energy needed for maintenance, thermoregulation and activity. Thus, *in ovo* feeding serves as a way to overcome early growth constraints during embryonic and post-hatch development in broilers to reach their maximum genetic potential.

4. Juvenile nutrition

The first few days after hatch are the most crucial period for the development and survival of commercial chicken. During this period, chicks make the transition from nutrients stored in yolk to exogenous feed. The sooner the young bird achieves this functional capacity, the sooner it can utilize dietary nutrients, grow efficiently to its genetic potential and resist disease. Chicks are precocial and will start eating feed almost immediately after hatch. The degree of enteric development in the hatchling is dependent upon when they begin to consume external feed components. Under practical conditions, many chicks gain access to feed only 2-3 days of hatching because of variable hatching time, hatchling servicing, and delivery to the farm. This delay in feed consumption causes the mobilization of body reserves. Consequently, body weight gain, meat yield and overall growth performance is impaired. It has been seen that early access to feed had 3 to 5% higher body weights at market age along with 4 to 10% greater breast meat yield. Therefore, the onset of feeding is critical from the time of hatching of chicks and is definitely related to the future productive performance of commercial chicks. While the residual yolk fulfills hatchling nutrition for the first couple days of life, but this is not fully sufficient for optimum performance. The yolk lipids, oleic acid, are highly absorbed close to hatch, whereas, dietary carbohydrates and amino acids are not well utilized because of limitation in digestive and absorptive capacity. At the onset of feeding, the small intestine, liver and pancreas grow 2-5 times faster than the rest of the body. They also play a key role in supplying nutrients for growth of muscle and other tissues. The immune system requires adequate nutrient intake for full and rapid development.

Any delay in onset of feeding, the chicks may become more susceptible to disease, lower weight gain, and the development of critical tissues is restricted in an effort to conserve nutrient resources for enteric development. During this adjustment period, the hatchling draws on its limited body reserves to fuel the rapid physical and functional development of the gastrointestinal tract in order to attain the capacity to digest feed and assimilate nutrients necessary for growth and development. The sooner the chick achieves this functional capacity, the sooner it can utilize dietary nutrients, grow efficiently to its genetic potential and resist disease. Consumption of feed physically stimulates the motility of hatchling's gastro-intestinal tract and yolk sac, thereby delivering the critical nutrients from both yolk and feed necessary to accelerate enteric development.

The concept of using prestarter diets is to hasten the early growth with more of easily digestible nutrients. The idea in formulating prestarter diets is to provide critical nutrient needs and to increase early growth rate. During the initial phase of broilers, digestive capacity is not fully developed, measured enzymatic activities in the intestine are relatively low and the physiological development of the gastro-intestinal tract is not complete. Indeed, the digestibility of energy estimated by the MEn values of cereals and soybean meals were significantly lower at one and two weeks of age, compared with values obtained at three weeks of age (Mahagna *et al.*, 1995).

The selection pressures for high-growth and egg laying traits has increased the susceptibility to infectious diseases and compromised health status. The focus should be on determining the most appropriate nutrient feeding strategies to optimize the immune response and to study the influence of immune response on the growth and nutrient requirements of the bird (Klasing, 1998). A number of studies indicate nutrient levels adequate for growth, feed efficiency, egg production and reproduction may not be adequate for normal immunity and for optimizing the birds resistance to disease. Broiler nutrient needs for immunity does not parallel those for growth or breast meat accretion. Nutrients are required to provide the building blocks for immune cells and tissues, such as T and B lymphocytes, macrophages, and natural killer cells. Several nutrients are especially important in early development of the immune system. Studies indicate that the immune enhancement of dietary vitamin E is best between 25 and 50 IU/kg of diet of broilers (Leshchinsky and Klasing, 2001).

5. Nutrigenomics

The future of nutrition research will increasingly focus on the ways in which our bird's genes are affected by feed. The genome mapping of the birds together with the progress within information technology and molecular biology techniques will accelerate the future for in-depth research in nutrition. Epigenetics is the latest priority of nutrigenomic research, which includes any heritable influence on gene activity without involving a change in the DNA sequence. Common epigenetic mechanisms occurring during the pre-pubertal or peri-natal development include DNA methylation, histone modification, and regulatory non-coding RNAs. The feeding and management of breeders, incubation of eggs, or feed and management of chicks influences the physiological response, productive performance and health of the bird. Epigenetic programming plays a role to increase caloric efficiency, enhance nutrient utilization, improve disease resistance and stress tolerance, and modify behaviour of commercial poultry. The nutrients available to the embryo in the chemical form are transferred as an epigenetic message to its offspring. The digestive capacity begins to develop at the embryo stage, but most of the development occurs post-hatch when the neonatal chick begins consuming feed. The delay in feed intake initiation suppresses gastro-intestinal development and cause early malnutrition (Uni *et al.*, 2003), and inhibit satellite cell proliferation and muscle growth potential (Mozdiak *et al.*, 2002; Halevy *et al.*, 2003; and Moore *et al.*, 2005). Our future research in nutrigenomics should focus on the effect of specific nutrients on gene expression in poultry. This approach allows us to gain an understanding of the molecular and cellular processes that result from changes in poultry diet composition. Nutrigenomics is especially important in studying the antioxidant effect of organic micro-nutrients such as selenium, chromium.

6. Feed enzymes

The ban on antibiotics as growth promoters in the European Union and elsewhere has encouraged to search for potential alternatives and the feed additives particularly enzymes, probiotics and prebiotics have been receiving a lot of attention (Panda *et al.*, 2006; 2008; Vidanarachchi *et al.*, 2010; Elangovan *et al.*, 2011). Gut health is a complex relationship between the diet, the intestinal mucosal, and the intestinal microflora. The research and development attention in the coming years will definitely focus more on plant extracts, microbial fermentation products, and direct fed microbial. Since the introduction of exogenous enzymes in the past decades, their use has been more beneficial with viscous grains (wheat, barley, rye) rather than maize and sorghum. Although, the application of enzymes has proved to be highly beneficial, the use of enzymes in poultry rations has not yet reached to its full potential except for wheat/barley based diets (Choct, 2000; 2006) and for phytate phosphorus utilization (Rao, 1999).

The main anti-nutritional properties of non starch polysaccharide (NSP) include ß-D-glucans (barley, oat) with linear polymers of glucose (ß-(1-3), (1-4) glycosidic linkage), the arabinoxylans (wheat, rye, triticale), more complex being composed of two sugars, arabinose and xylose, in a branched structure. Even more complex polysaccharides are present in legumes. Most of the anti-nutritive activities of NSP in broiler performance have been attributed directly to solubility which increases the digesta viscosity and reduces the nutrient digestibility in poultry (Choct and Annison, 1992; Bedford and Classen, 1992; Choct, 2000; Bedford and Partridge, 2010). The improvement in the AME of cereal diets following enzyme addition is due to improvements in nutrient (starch, protein, fat) digestibility and not due to the availability of NSP itself since NSP is not completely broken down to monomers in the gastro intestinal tract. In our country, the alternate cereals viz., sorghum, pearl millet, broken rice and finger millet used in poultry diet do not contain soluble NSP. The evolution of digestive capability with age is expected to influence the response of birds to soluble NSP in the diet and also the response to enzyme supplementation targeted at NSP. Under current commercial conditions, the majority of the enzyme activity takes place in the small intestine wherein the pH is closely regulated. The exogenous enzyme has to survive the pH, the gastric enzymes and able to act in the short transit time of broiler chicken. Most of the exogenous enzymes have an optimum pH between 4.0 to 5.0.

The optimum pH for xylanases is 4.0-6.0 for maximum activity (de Vries and Visser, 2001) while for ß glucanases is 5.5 (Thacker and Baas, 1996). The beneficial effects of enzyme supplementations has not been very apparent in maize based diets (Elangovan *et al.*, 2004a,b) or in low soluble NSP wheat or triticale based diets (Elangovan *et al.* 2011).

The benefits of enzyme use are likely related to an increase in the rate of diet digestibility and production of short chain sugars (from fiber degradation). As a result of such improvements in diet digestibility, there is a significant change in the substrate quality and quantity available to the intestinal microflora in both the upper and lower gut. The effects of enzymes on gut microflora were classified by Bedford (2000) into two phases: an ileal phase and a caecal phase. In the ileum, enzymes simply reduce the number of bacteria by increasing the rate of digestion and limiting the amounts of substrates available to the microflora. In the caecal phase, enzymes produce soluble, poorly absorbed sugars which feed beneficial bacteria. The volatile fatty acids produced by such bacteria may be of benefit not only in controlling populations of pathogenic species, but also in providing an energy source for the bird (Snel *et al.*, 2002). The development of enzymes should be specially designed to use NSP as energy sources and to deactivate anti-nutrients in feed (Choct, 2006).

7. Enrichment and quality of egg and meat

In recent times with the increase in purchasing power and also as the consumers are becoming more health conscious, there is increased demand for designer and enriched food. The designer egg was developed with the concept of egg containing low cholesterol, rich in polyunsaturated fatty acids with antioxidants. Feeding strategies has been modified to produce foods that are enriched with an array of nutrients. The fatty acid profile of eggs and meat mirror that present in the diet and so it is a relatively easier to formulate diets for direct incorporation of diet fatty acids into poultry products. Flaxseed and fish oils have been the major ingredients incorporated into designer poultry feeds. Egg protein and carbohydrate content are not easily influenced by dietary manipulation, whereas, vitamins can be enriched in the eggs. As per the several reports, the efficiency transfer of vitamin E from diet to egg is quite variable; reports range from 10 to 50% while the average is about 20%. The efficiency of vitamin transfer into eggs as a function of intake ranges from 60% (riboflavin) to 5% (thiamine and folacin).

The manipulation of dietary nutrients affects meat composition at various stages of maturity. As energy level of the diet increases relative to dietary protein, fat deposition also increases, resulting in an undesirable carcass with proportionately more fat than protein. Studies have shown that increasing the levels of lysine or methionine or threonine above the levels required for optimal growth and feed efficiency has a positive impact on breast meat yield. Currently, the synthetic forms of essential amino acids - lysine, methionine, threonine, and tryptophan – are commercially available and can be used with different feedstuffs to formulate diets, which closely match the requirements of the bird. The availability of a growing number of synthetic amino acids has made the feed formulation more economical and precise.

A major concern in the food industry is safety. There is a direct link between animal-feed quality, hygiene and safety of foods of animal origin. In near future, there may be ban on the sale of live birds and only processed broiler meat will be available at retail outlets as frozen products, hence there has to be a change in nutritional aspect. Poultry meat is highly susceptible to oxidative rancidity or lipid oxidation during frozen storage. Naturally occurring antioxidant - vitamin E or alpha-tocopherol have been reported to be effective in improving self-life of poultry meat and meat products through delaying lipid oxidation. The supplementation of 225 IU vitamin E and 0.5 mg inorganic selenium per kg in diet of broiler chicken fed during 4-7 weeks of age before slaughter was sufficient for optimum meat stability (Tyagi *et al.* 2005b) and 300 mg/kg vitamin E 10 days prior to sacrifice improved the keeping quality of meat (Mandal *et al.*, 2005c).

8. Bio-informatics and meta-Analysis

The computational knowledge includes data mining and data analysis using bioinformatics, meta-analysis, and holo-analysis. Bioinformatics will be mainly used in poultry nutrition through applications, such as gene sequence analysis, analysis of gene expression (genomics), analysis of protein expression (proteomics), and analysis of metabolism (metabolomics). Meta-analysis comprises of very diverse methods of data collection analysis, ranging from simple averages to more complex statistical methods. Holo-analysis is a fully comprehensive statistical analysis of all available data and all available variables in a specified topic. The major applications of holo-analysis in poultry nutrition will be translation of work done under research conditions to commercial / field conditions, and definition of topics and priorities for future research (Rosan, 2006).

Conclusions

Poultry is one of the fastest growing components of global meat production. Expansion in India is being driven by rising incomes and a shift in industry structure toward integrated ownership in poultry production. The poultry nutrition over the next decade will be closely integrated with biotechnology, microbiology and computational technology to produce the quality poultry products at the most economical cost.

References

Bakyaraj S., Bhanja S.K., Majumdar S., Dash, B.B. (2012). Modulation of post-hatch growth and immunity through *in ovo* supplemented nutrients in broiler chickens. *Journal of the Science of Food and Agriculture* **92:** 313-320.

Bedford M.R. (2000). Exogenous enzymes in monogastric nutrition - their current value and future benefits. *Animal Feed Science and Technology* **86:** 1-13.

Bedford M.R., Partridge, G.G. (2010). Enzymes in farm animal nutrition. 2nd Edn. CAB Publishing, UK.

Bedford M.R., Classen, H.L. (1992). Reduction of intestinal viscosity through manipulation of dietary rye and pentosanase concentration is effected through changes in the carbohydrate composition of the intestinal aqueous phase and results in improved growth rate and food conversion efficiency of broiler chicks. *Journal of Nutrition* **122:** 560-569.

Bhanja S.K., Mandal A.B. (2007). Validating the current amino acid and energy requirements of coloured broiler chickens. *Journal of the Science of Food and Agriculture* **87:** 2131-2140.

Bhanja S.K., Mandal A.B. (2005). Effect of *in ovo* injection of critical amino acids on pre- and post-hatch growth, immunocompetence and development of digestive organs in broiler chickens. *Asian Australasian Journal of Animal Sciences* **18:** 524-531.

Bhanja S.K., Mandal A.B., Goswami T.K. (2004). Effect of *in ovo* injection of amino acid on growth immune response, development of digestive organs and carcass yield of broiler. *Indian Journal of Poultry Science* **39:** 212-218.

Chauynarong N., Elangovan A.V., Iji, P.A. (2009). The potential of cassava products in diets for poultry. *World's Poultry Science Journal* **65:** 23-35.

Choct M. (2000). Enzyme supplementation of poultry diets based on viscous cereals. In: Enzymes in Farm Animal Nutrition. (M.R. Bedford and G.G. Partridge, eds.). CABI Publishing, pp 145-160.

Choct M. (2006). Enzymes for the feed industry: past, present and future. *World's Poultry Science Journal* **62:** 2-6.

Choct M., Annison G. (1992). Antinutritive effect of wheat pentosans in broiler chicken: Role of viscosity and gut microflora. *British Poultry Science* **33:** 821-834.

Choct M., Sinlae M. Al-Jassim R.A.M., Pettersson D. (2006). Effects of xylanase supplementation on between-bird variation in energy metabolism and the number of Clostridium perfringens in broilers fed a wheat-based diet. *Australian Journal of Agricultural Research* **57:** 1017-1021.

de Vries R.P., Visser J. (2001). Aspergillus enzymes involved in degradation of plant cell wall polysaccharides. *Microbiology and Molecular Biology Reviews* **65:** 497-522.

Elangovan A.V., Bhuiyan M., Jessop R., Iji P.A. (2011). The potential of high-yielding triticale varieties in the diet of broiler chickens. *Asian Journal of Poultry Science* **5:** 68-76.

Elangovan A.V., Mandal A.B., Praveen K. Tyagi, Pramod K.Tyagi, Toppo, S. and Johri, T.S. (2004a). Use of enzymes in diets with varying energy levels on growth and egg production performance of Japanese quail. *Journal of the Science of Food and Agriculture* **84:** 2028-2034.

Elangovan, A.V., Mandal, A.B., Tyagi, K.Pramod, Tyagi, K. Praveen, Toppo, S. and Johri, T.S. (2004b). Utilization of sorghum and finger millet with or without feed enzyme in broiler chickens. *Journal of Applied Animal Research* **26:** 33-38.

Elangovan A.V., Mandal A.B., Shrivastav A.K., Yadav A.S. (2011). Supplementing probiotics (*gallipro*) to broiler chicken on growth performance, immunity and gut microbial population. *Animal Nutrition and Feed Technology* **11:** 169-176.

Green S., Bertrand S.L., Duron M.J.C., Maillard R. (1987). Digestibilities of amino acids in maize, wheat and barley meals, determined with intact and caecectomized cockerels. *British Poultry Science* **28:** 631-641.

Halevy O., Nadel Y., Barak M., Rozenboim I., Sklan, D. (2003). Early posthatch feeding stimulates satellite cell proliferation and skeletal muscle growth in turkey poults. *Journal of Nutrition* **133:** 1376-1382.

Iji P.A. (1999). The impact of cereal non-starch polysaccharides on intestinal development and function in broiler chickens. *World's Poultry Science Journal* **55:** 374-387.

Jin S., Corless A., Sell, J.L. (1998). Digestive system development in post-hatch poultry. *World's Poultry Science Journal* **54:** 335-345.

Klasing K.C. (1998). Nutritional modulation of resistance to infectious diseases. *Poultry Science* **77:** 1119-1125.

Kumar V., Elangovan A.V., Mandal A.B. (2005). Utilization of reconstituted high-tannin sorghum in the diets of broiler chickens. *Asian Australasian Journal of Animal Sciences* **18:** 538-544.

Lemme A., Ravindran V., Bryden W.L. (2004). Ileal digestibility of amino acids in feed ingredients for broilers. *World's Poultry Science Journal* **60:** 423-437.

Leshchinsky T.V., Klasing K.C. (2001). Divergence of the inflammatory response in two types of chickens. *Developmental and Comparative Immunology* **25:** 629-638.

Mahagna M., Nir I., Larbier M., Nitsan Z. (1995). Effect of age and exogenous amylase and protease on development of the digestive tract, pancreatic enzyme activities and digestibility of nutrients in young meat-type chicks. *Reproduction Nutrition Development* **35:** 201-212.

Mandal A.B., Elangovan A.V., Tyagi Praveen K. (2005a). Poultry nutrition for economic egg and meat production: A review. *Indian Journal of Animal Science* **75:** 1215-1226.

Mandal A.B., Elangovan A.V., Tyagi Praveen K., Tyagi Pramod K., Kaur S., Johri, A.K. (2005b). Effect of enzyme supplementation on metabolizable energy content of solvent-extracted rapeseed and sunflower seed meal for chicken, guinea fowl and quails. *British Poultry Science* **46:** 1-5.

Mandal A.B., Yadav A.S., Elangovan A.V., Tyagi Praveen K., Tyagi Pramod K., Toppo S. (2005c). Effect of pre-slaughter feed withdrawal and dietary supplementation of vitamin E and ascorbic acid on microbiological and keeping quality of broiler chicken meat. *Indian Journal of Poultry Science* **40:** 285-287.

Mandal A.B., Tyagi Praveen K., Elangovan, A.V., Tyagi Pramod K., Kaur, S., Johri, A.K. (2006). Comparative apparent metabolisable energy values of high, medium and low tannin varieties of sorghum in cockerel, guinea fowl and quail. *British Poultry Science* **47:** 336-341.

Moore D.T., Ferket P.R., Mozdziak P.E. (2005). Early post-hatch fasting induces satellite cell self renewal. *Comparative Biochemistry and Physiology-Part A: Molecular and Integrative Physiology* **142:** 331-339.

Morris T.R., Njuru, D.M. (1990). Protein requirement of fast- and slow-growing chicks. *British Poultry Science* **31:** 803-809.

Mozdiak P.E., Walsh T.J., McCoy D.W. (2002). The effect of early posthatch nutrition on satellite cell mitotic activity. *Poultry Science* **81:** 1703-1708.

Noy Y., Geyra A., Sklan D. 2001. The effect of early feeding on the growth and small intestine development in the posthatch poult. *Poultry Science* **80:** 912-919.

Panda A.K., Rama S.V.R., Raju M.V.L., Sharma S.R. (2006). Dietary supplementation of *Lactobacillus sporogenes* on performance and serum biochemico-lipid profile of broiler chickens. *Poultry Science* **43:** 235-240.

Panda A.K., Rama S.V.R., Reddy M.R. (2008). Growth promoters in poultry: Novel concepts. International Book Distributor, viii, p.134.

Raju M.V.L.N., Shyamsunder G., Elangovan A.V., Reddy M. R., Sadagopan V.R., Rao, S.V.R. (2003). Sorghum, bajra and ragi vis-à-vis maize as energy sources in broiler chicken diets. *Indian Journal of Animal Nutrition* **20:** 185-192.

Rao S.V.R., Reddy V.R., Reddy V.R. (1999). Enhancement of phytate phosphorus availability in the diets of commercial broilers and layers. *Animal Feed Science and Technology* **79:** 211-222.

Rao S.V.R., Raju M.V.L.N., Reddy, M.R., Panda A.K. (2004). Replacement of yellow maize with pearl millet (Pennisetum typhoides), foxtail millet (Setaria italica) or finger millet (Eleusine coracana) in broiler chicken diets containing supplemental enzymes. *Asian Australasian Journal of Animal Sciences* **17:** 836-842.

Ravindran V., Hew L.I., Ravindran G., Bryden W. L. (1996a). A comparison of ileal digesta and excreta analysis to determine the digestibility of amino acids for poultry. In: *Proceedings XX World's Poultry Congress,* of World's Poultry Science Association: New Delhi, volume IV p 150.

Ravindran V., Hew L.I., Ravindran G., Bryden W.L. (1996b). Ideal digestibilities of amino acids for broilers. In: *Proceedings, 10th Australian poultry and feed convention, Melbourne,* pp 209-215.

Rosen, G. D. (2006). Holo-analysis. *Poultry Science* **85:** 957-959.

Snel J., Harmssen H.J.M., van der Wielen P.W.J.J., Williams B.A. (2002). Dietary strategies to influence the gastrointestinal microflora of young animals, and its potential to improve intestinal health. In: *Nutrition and Health of the Gastrointestinal Tract.* (M. C. Blok, H. A. Vahl, L. de Lange, A. E. van de Braak, G. Hemke, and M. Hessing, eds). Wageningen Academic Publishers, Wageningen, The Netherlands, pp 37–69.

Thacker P.A., Bass T.C. (1996). Effects of gastric pH on the activity of exogenous pentosanase supplementation of the diet on the performance of growing-finishing pigs. *Animal Feed Science and Technology* **63:** 187-200.

Tyagi, Praveen K., Mandal A.B., Elangovan, A.V., Tyagi, Pramod K., Kaur, S., Johri, A. K. (2005a). Feeding value of coarse cereals in the diet of broiler chicken. *Indian Journal of Animal Nutrition* **22:** 27-31.

Tyagi, Praveen K., Tyagi, Pramod K., Singh R.P., Elangovan A.V., Mandal A.B. (2005b). Performance and meat quality of broilers as influenced by dietary Vitamin E and selenium during different phases of life. *Animal Nutrition and Feed Technology* **5:** 53-60.

Uni Z., Smirnov A., Sklan D. (2003). Pre-and post-hatch development of goblet cells in the broiler small intestine: effect of delayed access to feed. *Poultry Science* **82:** 320-327.

Vasan P., Mandal A.B., Dutta N., Maiti S.K., Sharma K. (2008). Digestibility of amino acids of maize, low tannin sorghum, pearl millet and finger millet in caecectomized roosters. *Asian Australasian Journal of Animal Sciences* **21:** 701-706.

Vidanarachchi J.K., Elangovan A.V., Mikkelsen L.L., Choct M., Iji, P.A. (2010). The effect of some plant extracts on growth performance, intestinal morphology and growth of intestinal microflora in broiler chickens. *Animal Production Science* **50:** 880-889.

❑❑❑

Chapter 7

New Innovations to Enhance Egg Production in Domestic Hen

I.J. Reddy, C.G. David
National Institute of Animal Nutrition and Physiology, Adugodi, Bangalore-560 030, Karnataka, India

Summary

Food security to all humans by 2020 is the cry of the hour since the demand for animal products especially eggs has increased tremendously due to varying lifestyle. The global market for eggs is projected to reach 1,154 billion by the year 2015. First with growing base of the middle class population and their increasing purchasing power, the per capita consumption of eggs is increasing constantly across major Asian nations such as China and India. Secondly, the sudden upward swing of consumer's preference towards functional foods in the western countries has increased the per capita consumption of eggs in the last 15 years especially in the US. These increasing demands ensure an increase in animal productivity paving way to horizontal growth in the poultry industry. Newer paradigms have been put to practice to increase egg production each day. In this chapter some of these newer methodologies that have the potential to increase egg production have been discussed.

Reproduction, health and nutrition are three key inter-dependant pillars of successful poultry production. Reproductive technologies such as the control of photoperiod and artificial insemination have significantly contributed to improve the efficiency and profitability of poultry production. To date, genetic selection has allowed the development of specific breeds with high producing performances. However, as observed in turkey and broiler breeders, birds with high genetic merit for growth do not have the best reproductive performances. Significant improvements in optimizing the existing management procedures will reduce the cost and increase profitability in such birds. In addition, lack of basic knowledge on the underlying mechanisms remained a major impediment to develop the next generation management procedures and genetic selection tools. Like most seasonal breeders, avian species rely upon the control of the hypothalamo-pituitary-gonadal axis. Understanding how external and internal stimuli control this axis will provide clues to optimize existing technologies and design future strategies. Furthermore, as 'super layers' have recently been introduced to the producers, it is becoming apparent that these birds may also display several reproductive abnormalities such as multiple ovulations resulting in double yolk and soft shell eggs.

The per capita consumption of egg has increased by about 3 folds in India despite an overall decline in the per capita consumption of egg in the western countries in the 90's (Surai and Sparks, 2001). The global market for eggs is projected to reach 1,154 billion by the year 2015 (Source: http://www.StrategyR.com). The exponential growth rate of population and the export of eggs to the Middle East have put the pressure to increase the egg production in our country. However, the increasing demand for eggs for human consumption is not met by merely increasing the vertical growth of poultry sector but also warrants horizontal growth of the poultry sector by increasing the egg producing rate of the layer and the desi- breeds in our country. At present poultry entrepreneurs are not much interested on horizontal expansion due to availability of feed resources and farm management constraints. Yet, it is ideal time to concentrate upon increasing the production beyond the one year production period of white leghorn strain of birds by adopting molting or other physiological interventions. At this juncture several methods are not made available to the farmers for horizontal expansion due to the lack of necessity.

Egg production is under the direct control of the hypothalamo-pituitary-gonadal axis as in other mammals (Etches, 1996), which is influenced by the environmental long days (Sharp *et al.,* 1992; Kobayashi *et al.,* 2004). The difference from the mammalian counterpart is that prolactin released from the anterior pituitary gland has a negative effect on egg production by triggering broodiness in birds and maternal instinct. Since, development of broodiness feeds back on the hypothalamic release of GnRH and thereby release of LH thus abolishing the egg laying cycle in birds temporarily. Albeit the fact that white leghorn birds were developed against broodiness and their annual egg production is about 300 eggs, all these hens do not have the same laying persistency. Layer hens continue to lay eggs in clutches taking a pause of one or two days in between. These inter sequence pause days generally vary with the genetic makeup of individual birds and also depending on the environmental and managemental conditions. Some birds have more than

5-6 days of inter sequence pause days. Research has thrown light on the inter-sequence pause days and related its occurrence to the circulating levels of prolactin (Reddy *et al.,* 2001). Following this relationship between prolactin and inter sequence pause days attempts were made to combat the increasing levels of prolactin by employing pharmacological or immunological interventions to maintain prolactin levels within physiological limits. The results obtained were encouraging (Reddy *et al.,* 2002). Secondly, several works are on the anvil to regulate the levels of prolactin in turkey hens where broodiness is a major problem hampering egg production thus affecting turkey breeding. Regulating the production of prolactin at the gene level by silencing PRL gene using RNA interference has shown remarkable results in turkey embryonic pituitary gland (Gen Hayama *et al.,* 2009). Applying gene silencing technology to commercial layer hens as well as desi birds will certainly improve egg production. This article will focus on these techniques adopted in other countries on species other than layer chicken, as well as certain protocols carried out at experimental level and the probable impact it would have, if adopted for use in layer hens.

1. Egg production: prolactin – gonadotropin connection

In birds, the secretion of luteinizing hormone (LH) and prolactin is controlled by the releasing hormones, gonadotrophin releasing hormone-I (GnRH-I) and vasoactive intestinal polypeptide (VIP), respectively. The secretion of LH is depressed and the secretion of prolactin is at its highest, during the time of incubation: brooding young and during the development of reproductive photo refractoriness. In incubating domestic chickens, decreased LH and increased prolactin secretion are correlated with decreased hypothalamic GnRH-I mRNA and increased hypothalamic VIP mRNA (El Halawani *et al.,* 1995). Increased plasma prolactin contributes to the suppression of LH secretion in incubating poultry, possibly acting at the levels of hypothalamus and anterior pituitary gland. During the development of photo refractoriness, decreased plasma LH and increased plasma prolactin are correlated with decreased hypothalamic GnRH-I and increased hypothalamic VIP (Saldanha *et al.,* 2001). High concentrations of plasma prolactin play a role in ensuring the rapid regression of the gonads but are not essential for the maintenance of the condition (Sharp *et al.,* 1989).

2. Egg production: dopamine – prolactin connection

Prolactin has been associated with broodiness in avian species (Scanes *et al.,* 1977). Increasing circulating concentration of prolactin is directly related to broodiness in bantam hens (Sharp *et al.,* 1989) and turkeys (Gumene and Etches, 1990). Under such conditions, disruption of nests or removal of eggs from the bird's sight has brought back the birds to laying by abolishing the negative impact of prolactin on hypothalamic GnRH (Yasuo and Yoshimura, 2009). This is possible in domesticated species alone since egg laying is dependent on environmental cues and is influenced by additional lighting over and above the natural 12h photoperiod and clutch size is not fixed in these birds unlike the wild birds.

In birds, the natural endogenous prolactin releasing factor is vasoactive intestinal peptide (VIP). Evidence that VIP is a physiologically relevant avian prolactin releasing hormone came from the finding that passive immunization against VIP blocks prolactin release in incubating chickens and active immunization prevents photo induced prolactin secretion (El halawani *et al.*, 1995). It has been shown that the neurotransmitter dopamine plays a significant role on the release of prolactin depending on the location of the dopamine receptors D1 and D2 on the mediobasal hypothamic neurons and anterior pituitary. Stimulation of the D2 receptors causes the release of prolactin from the anterior pituitary gland (Yongren *et al.*, 1998).

3. Innovating technologies to modulate prolactin levels

Upon developing the relationship between the increasing circulatory levels of prolactin and decreasing reproductive performance in terms of termination of clutch and occurrence of longer inter sequence pause days, it is felt to augment egg production by combating the increase in prolactin levels beyond physiological limits. Some of the methods employed to bring back prolactin levels within physiological limits includes:

1. Pharmacological intervention
2. Immunological intervention and
3. Gene silencing using RNA interference.

3.1 Pharmacological intervention by D2 receptor agonist bromocriptine

Albeit, the relationship between prolactin and dopamine in stimulating the release of prolactin from anterior pituitary gland has been established fewer reports are available in combating prolactin release from anterior pituitary gland in birds. It is presumed that pharmacological intervention using a D2 receptor agonist bromocriptine will inhibit the release of prolactin from the anterior pituitary. Studies conducted in white leghorn hens (Reddy *et al.*, 2002) and in backyard poultry strains developed in India *viz.*, Girirani (Reddy *et al.*, 2010) and broiler stain Punjab Brown-3 hens (Reddy *et al.*,2008) have confirmed this hypothesis. On the contrary Bedrak *et al.*, (1983) did not find any beneficial effect on circulating levels of prolactin in broody hens when administered with bromocriptine.

Studies on bromocriptine administration established that subcutaneous dose of 100µg/bird at weekly intervals between 17-36 weeks of age is sufficient to maintain the circulating levels of prolactin within physiological limits (Reddy *et al.,* 2001). It also results in 4 per cent increase in hen day egg production up to 72 weeks of age in white leg horn strain birds (Reddy *et al.,* 2002). This increase was due to the decrease in inter sequence pause days and increase in clutch size compared to control birds (David *et al.,* 2003).

In large farms subcutaneous administration of bromocriptine on a weekly basis for 20 weeks would be a labor intensive and cumbersome managemental practice. Hence, administration of bromocriptine as a feed supplement to layer flocks and its impact on egg production for better adoptability was attempted. A dose dependent increase in hen day egg production was achieved when fed with 340µg/bird/day (Reddy *et al.,* 2003) comparable with those birds that received bromocriptine subcutaneously. There were no residual effects of bromocriptine in the egg or body of the bird (Authors, unpublished observation). Birds administered with bromocriptine also had earlier age at sexual maturity compared to the control birds (Reddy *et al.,* 2001), which would have contributed to the increase in the hen day egg production.

The backyard poultry Girirani and the Punjab Brown-3 hens are characterized by maximum production of about 80 to 100 eggs per year due to the long inter sequence pause days. Administration of bromocriptine in these birds showed increased hen day egg production by a whopping 6 to 9 per cent (Reddy *et al.,* 2008) during the entire production period up to 72 weeks of age. However, Murthy *et al.* (2009) reported that in Punjab Brown-2 hens, administration of bromocriptine subcutaneously increased hen day egg production from 24 to 40 weeks of age by about 8.9% against 2.94% when fed orally.

3.2 Immunological intervention

3.2.1 Active immunization against VIP

The knowledge on the endogenous VIP on the release of prolactin and the several experiments conducted hitherto in bantam hens and turkeys (Sharp *et al.,* 1989; El-Halawani *et al.,* 1990), to reduce the circulating levels of prolactin by active immunization against VIP translating such a technique to layer hens seems ideal. Several experiments were conducted at this institute to study the effect of active immunization against VIP to increase egg production of white leghorn strain birds and also in other local strains including girirani and Punjab brown -3 hens. It has been observed that administration of VIP at a dose of 125µg (1ml) / bird / month ; 3 booster injections (25 µg (1ml)/bird/ month) was able to maintain high antibody titer to VIP throughout the production period up to 72 weeks of age (El-Halawani *et al.*,1995; Reddy *et al.*, 2005). Hen day egg production in the immunized flock was comparatively higher to that of non immunized control flock. Immunization against VIP significantly combated the negative effects of prolactin on steroidogenesis to increase egg production by 7.4 per cent in commercial white leghorn strain birds (Reddy *et al.*, 2006).

3.2.2 Active immunization against prolactin

Circulatory prolactin in domestic hen is widely assumed to play a key role in egg production in commercial poultry farms, where longer inter sequence pause days/broodiness is a common productive problem due to higher level of prolactin with concomitant decrease in egg production during the active period of egg lay. Control of its biological activity by decreasing the rate of secretion and/or preventing its effectiveness would enhance egg production by decreasing the pause days under normal husbandry practices. Immunization against chicken prolactin using hapten conjugated chicken prolactin at a dose of 125µg (1ml)/bird/1 month ; 3 booster injections (25 µg (1ml)/bird/month) was able to maintain high antibody titer to prolactin throughout the production period up to 72 weeks of age. Immunization against prolactin resulted in a non significant increase in egg production by 3.72 per cent in these birds (Reddy *et al.*, 2006).

Immunization against VIP and prolactin were also found equally efficient in backyard chicken *viz.* Girirani and Punjab brown-3 hens. In both the strains egg production was increased by 9.71 and 12.59 per cent, respectively (Reddy *et al.*, 2008). These findings clearly state that prolactin has a direct effect on subsequent ovulation of the follicles by interfering with gonadotropin secretion and thus decrease egg production by increasing the inter sequence pause days.

3.3 RNA interference of prolactin

Prolactin is a peptide hormone that is mainly synthesized in the anterior pituitary gland and is known to be involved in numerous biological actions in vertebrates. In avian species, the main documented functions of PRL are the onset and maintenance of incubation behaviour in galliformes and the production of crop-sac milk in pigeons (Horseman and Buntin, 1995). Moreover, PRL also plays important roles during embryogenesis such as the development of the immune system and the control of osmo-regulation (Sakamoto *et al.*, 1997). Prolactin is one of the abundant hormones in the anterior pituitary gland during late embryogenesis in avian species. In turkey embryos, the level of PRL and PRL mRNA increase from 5 days before hatching in the anterior pituitary gland, and the circulating level of PRL increases from

2 days before hatching. Subsequently, these levels reach a plateau between the day of hatch and 3 days of age (Gen Hiyama *et al.*, 2009). When siRNA was used to suppress PRL gene expression in cultured embryonic pituiticytes about 56% reduction of PRL mRNA was observed from embryonic day 24. Conversely, levels of growth hormone mRNA and PRL receptor (PRL-R) mRNA were not significantly altered in prolactin suppressed birds. These results may suggest that the siRNA suppresses PRL gene expression specifically, and that the level of PRLR mRNA expression is not associated with PRL in anterior pituitary (Gen Hiyama *et al.*, 2010). Using RNAi it will be possible to knockdown PRL gene and thereby keep the prolactin levels within physiological limits in layer hens and in backyard poultry will help to increase egg production.

3.4 Effects of different wave length lights

Light is an important environmental factor that influences the reproductive system of domestic avian species. Research has shown that the color of light can have many different effects on the behaviour, growth and reproduction in poultry (Lewis and Morris, 2000). Birds sense light through the retinal photoreceptors and the extra retinal photosensitive cells in the brain. It has been observed that growth and behaviour are linked to retinal photoreception of shorter wave lengths and that of reproduction to extra retinal photoreceptors at the hypothalamus (Lewis and Morris, 2000). It has also been shown that blue and green lights stimulate growth in chicken (Joseph *et al.*, 2009) while orange and red stimulates reproduction (Saldanha *et al.*, 2001). The observation that red light is more gonad stimulatory than a shorter wavelength is well established in poultry (Pyrzak *et al.*, 1986), yet, the precise mechanism has not been fully understood. Recent studies, indicate the photoreception by hypothalamic opsins (that are similar to the G protein receptors found in photoreceptor cells of the retina that mediate the conversion of a photon of light into an electrochemical signal, the first step in the visual transduction cascade thus facilitating vision) to various wavelengths *viz.*, vertebrate ancient (VA) opsin respond to 460-500 nm wave lengths (Stefen *et al.*, 2009) and opsin 5 to that of 420nm (Nakane *et al.*, 2010). Light perceived by photoreceptors within the hypothalamus is transduced into nervous impulses that initiate the synthesis and release of gonadotropin releasing hormone (GnRH; Chaiseha and El Halawani, 2005; Shimizu and Bedecarrates, 2006), thereby trigger the events of the hypothamo-pituitary-gonadal axis (Philip *et al.*, 1985) resulting in development of gonads (Sharp, 2005). Nevertheless, as observed in mammals, the relative sensitivity of the avian pituitary to GnRH stimulation and the hypothalamic GnRH content is dependent on the physiological stage, sex and age (Gumene and Williams, 1999).

Experiments with different wavelengths *viz.* 675, 475 and 450 nm of lights using monochromatic red, blue or incandescent bulbs showed increase in hen day egg production by 4.0 and 8.01 per cent in birds exposed to 650 nm wavelength compared to 475 and 450 nm wavelengths, respectively (Reddy *et al.,* 2011). Exposure to 675 nm wavelength significantly increased egg production in birds beyond 72 weeks of age by 4.68 per cent in a short term trial conducted up to 82 weeks of age. The increase in egg production happens due to the photo stimulation of the extra retinal hypothalamic photoreceptors that act directly on the mediobasal hypothalamus (Yasuo and Yoshimura, 2009) and increase GnRH I mRNA expression in the hypothalamus (Reddy *et al.,* 2012), whereas the decrease in egg production with blue spectrum of light is due to increase in GnIH secretion (El Halawani *et al.,* 2007).

4. Socioeconomic relevance and priority

At present India ranks 5th in the world production of eggs with a total production of 1.61 million tones of eggs. The decreased egg output could be attributed to the increased number of inter sequence pause days observed in commercial layer flock and to the meager annual production (80-100 eggs) of the desi bird strains developed like Girirani and Punjab Brown-3 for the benefit of the rural backyard and/or large scale poultry production system. Increasing egg production within the number of layers without additional infrastructure would improve net income of the poultry entrepreneurs. This additional income in egg production in the country will bring additional revenue to the exchequer and add to the total GDP from poultry sector.

Conclusions

Prolactin has been related to increase in the inter sequence pause days between laying cycles and thus decrease the production potential of domestic hens including commercial layer strain birds. Uses of pharmacological and immunological interventions have shown the potential to augment egg productions in birds. Most recently RNA interference has been used to minimize the prolactin production in embryonic chicks which appears to be a promising technology towards regulating the prolactin levels and hence improve the egg production potential of domestic chicken in the long run.

References

Bedrak E., Harvey S., Robinson B. (1983). Pharmacological disruption of broodiness in white rock domestic fowls. *British Poultry Science* **24:** 573-579.

Chaiseha Y., El Halawani M.E.(2005). Neuroendocrinology of the female turkey reproductive cycle. *Journal of Poultry Science* **42:** 87-100.

David C.G., Reddy I.J., Khub Singh. (2003). Oviposition patterns associated with prolactin concentration in chicken (*Gallus domesticus*). *Asian-Australian Journal of Animal Sciences* **16:** 1565-1571.

El Halawani M.E., Silsby J.L., Rozenboim I., Pitts G.R. (1995). Increased egg production by active immunization against vasoactive intestinal peptide in the turkey (*Meleagris gallopavo*) *Biology of Reproduction* **52:** 179-183.

El Halawani M.E. (2007). Domestic light spectrum and breeder hen turkeys egg production. In: Proceedings of the Midwest Poultry Federation Convention, St. Paul, Minnesota, USA, pp 43-46.

El Halawani M.E., Silsby J.L. Mauro L.J. (1990). Enhanced vasoactive intestinal polypeptide induced prolactin secretion from anterior pituitary cells of incubating turkeys (*Meleagris gallapavo*). *General and Comparative Endocrinology* **80:** 138-145.

Etches R.J. (1996). Reproduction in poultry. *CAB International*, Wallingford. University Press, Cambridge UK, pp 267-397.

Gen Hiyama G., McQuaid R., Reddy I.J., Kansaku N., Zadworny D. (2010). In vitro suppression of PRL transcription and translation in turkey embryonic pituicytes by RNAi. In: *Proceedings of the XIII European poultry conference,* pp 161-172.

Hiyama G., Kansaku N., Kinoshita M., Sasanami T., Nakamura A., Noda K., Tsukada A., Shimada K., Zadworny D. (2009). Changes in post-translational modifications of prolactin during development and reproductive cycles in the chicken. *General and Comparative Endocrinology* **161:** 238-245.

Guemene D., Etches R.J. (1990). Changes in the plasma concentration of prolactin, LH, progesterone and d-hydroxybutyrate in turkey hens during treatment of broodiness under commercial conditions. *British Poultry Science* **32:** 831-834.

Guemene, D. and Williams, J.B., (1999). LH responses to chicken luteinizing hormone-releasing hormone I and II in laying, incubating, and out of lay turkey hens. *Domestic Animal Endocrinology*. **17:** 1-15.

Horseman, N.D. and Buntin, J.D. (1995). Regulation of pigeon cropmilk secretion and parental behaviors by prolactin. *Annual Review of Nutrition*, **15:** 213-238.

Joseph, N.T., K. Morgan, R. Sellar, D. McBride, R.P. Millar and I.C. Dunn.2009. The chicken type III GnRH receptor homologue is predominantly expressed in the pituitary, and exhibits similar ligand selectivity to the type I receptor. *Journal of Endocrinology* **202:** 179–190.

Kobayashi M., Ito T., Ishii S., Wada M. (2004). Seasonal change in luteinizing hormone subunit mRNA in Japanese quail and effects of short daylength and low temperature. *General and Comparative Endocrinology* **139:** 38-47.

Lewis P.D., Morris T.R. (2000). Poultry and colored light. *World's Poultry Science Journal* **56:** 189-207.

Murthy H.N.N., Srinidhi K.P., Reddy I.J., Isloor S. (2009). Influence of route of admisnistration of 2-α- bromoergocriptine on egg production in colored broiler dam line. *Indian Journal of Poultry Science* **44:** 376-378.

Nakane, Y., Ikegami, K., Ono, H., Yamamoto, N., Yoshida, S., Hirunagi, K., Ebihara, Shizufumi, Kubo, Y., and Yoshimura, T. (2010). A mammalian neural tissue opsin

(Opsin 5) is a deep brain photoreceptor in birds. *Proceedings of the National Academy of Sciences, USA* **107:** 15264-15268.

Pyrzak R., Snapir N., Goodman G., Arnon E., Perek M. (1986). The influence of light quality on initiation of egg laying by hens. *Poultry Science* **64:** 1617-1622.

Reddy I.J., David C.G., Khub Singh (2003). Oviposition patterns associated with prolactin concentration in chicken (*Gallus domesticus*). *Asian Australasian Journal of Animal Science*, **16:** 1565-1571.

Reddy I.J.. David C.G., Khub Singh (2005). Relationship between Intersequence pauses, laying persistency and concentration of prolactin during productive period in white Leghorn hens. *Asian Australasian Journal of Animal sciences* **18:** 686-691.

Reddy I.J., David C.G., Raju S.S. (2007). Effect of suppression of plasma prolactin on luteinizing hormone concentration, intersequence pause days and egg production in domestic hen. *Domestic Animal Endocrinology* **33:** 167-175.

Reddy I.J., David C.G., Raju S.S. (2006). Inter sequence pause days, egg production , steroid and luteinizing hormone in domestic hen (gallous domesticus) immunized against cProlactin. *International Journal of Poultry Science* **5:** 420-427.

Reddy I.J., David C.G., Ravi Kiran G. (2010). Endocrine interactions and egg production in girirani birds treated with bromocriptine during early stages of laying period. *Indian veterinary Journal* **87:** 659-662.

Reddy I.J., David C.G., Ravi Kiran G., Mondal S. (2011). Pulsatile secretion of luteinizing hormone and GnRH and its relation to pause days and egg production in hens exposed to different wavelengths of light. *Indian Journal of Animal Sciences* **81:** 919-923.

Reddy I.J., David C.G, Sarma P.V., Khub Singh. (2003) Modulation of prolactin levels for increased egg production in domestic hen. *Indian Journal of Animal Science* **73:** 743-747.

Reddy I.J., David C.G., Sarma P.V., Khub Singh (2002). Influence of 2 bromo-a- ergocriptine on plasma prolactin, oestradiol-17b and progesterone levels in domestic hen. *Asian Australasian Journal of Animal Science* **15:** 1103-1109.

Reddy, I.J.. David, C.G, Sarma, P.V. and Khub Singh (2002). Possible role of prolactin on laying performance and steroid hormones in domestic hen (*Gallus domesticus*). *General and Comparative Endocrinology* **127:** 249-255.

Reddy I.J., David C.G., Sarma P.V., Khub Singh (2001). Modulation of prolactin hormone and inter sequence pause days in domestic chickens. *Veterinary Record* **149:** 590-592.

Reddy, I. J., Ravi Kiran, G., Mondal, S. and Anandan. S. (2008). Immunization against vasoactive intestinal peptide and its effects on prolactin, steroid, luteinizing hormone, and egg production during mid laying cycle in Punjab Brown (PB3) birds. *International Journal of Poultry Science* **7:** 1100-1104.

Reddy I.J., Ravi Kiran G., Mondal S., Anandan S. (2008). Pulsatile secretion of luteinizing hormone and its relation to pause days and egg production in dual purpose hens treated with antiprolatin agent. *Indian Journal of Animal Sciences* **79:** 988-991.

Reddy I.J., Ravi Kiran G., Mondal S., Anandan S. (2007). Proalctin, luteinizing hormone and steroid hormone concentration in punjab brown (PB3) birds immunized against vasoactive intestinal peptide during the early stages of egg production. *International Journal of Poultry Science* **6:** 637-641.

Sakamoto, T., Shepher, B. S., Madsen S. S., Nishioka R. S., Siharath K., Richman N.H., Bern H.A. and Grau, E. (1997). Osmoregulatory Actions of Growth Hormone and Prolactin in an Advanced Teleost. *General and Comparative Endocrinology,* **106:** 95-101.

Saldanha C.J, Silverman A.J, Silver R. (2001).Direct innervation of GnRH neurons by encephalic photoreceptors in birds. *Journal of Biological Rhythms* **16:** 39-49.

Scanes C.G., Sharp P.J., Chadwick A. (1977). Changes in plasma prolactin concentration during the ovulatory cycle of the hen. *Journal of Endocrinology* **72:** 401-402.

Sharp P.J. (2005). Photoperiodic regulation of seasonal breeding in birds. *Trends in Comparative Endocrinology and Neurobiology* **1040:** 189-199.

Sharp P.J., Dunn I.C., Cerolini S. (1992). Neuroendocrine control of reduced persistence of egg laying in domestic hens: evidence for the development of photo refractoriness. *General and Comparative Endocrinology* **94:** 221-235.

Sharp P.J., Sterling R.J., Talbout R.T., Huskinson N.S. (1989). The role of hypothalamic vasoactive intestinal polypeptide in the maintenance of prolactin secretion in incubating bantam hens. *Journal of Endocrinology* **122:** 5-13.

Shimizu M., Bedecarrats G.Y. (2006). Identification of a novel pituitary specific chicken gonadotropin-releasing hormone receptor and its splice variants. *Biology of Reproduction* **75:** 800-808.

Surai P.F., Sparks N.H.C. (2001). Designer eggs: From improvements of egg composition to functional food. *Trends in Food Science and Technology* **12:** 7-16.

Yasuo S., Yoshimura T. (2009).Comparative analysis of the molecular basis of photoperiodic signal transduction in vertebrates Integrative and Comparative Biology, **49:** 507-518.

Youngren O.M., Chaischa Y., El Halawani M.E. (1998). Serotogenic stimulation of avian prolactin secretion requires an intact dopaminergic system. *General and Comparative Endocrinology* **112:** 63-68.

❑❑❑

Chapter 8

Designer Animal Products

C.G. David, A. Thulasi, I.J. Reddy, V.Lyju Jose, S. Velusamy, S. Mathivanan, M. Bagath
National Institute of Animal Nutrition and Physiology, Adugodi, Bangalore-560 030, Karnataka, India

Summary

In the industrialized world, animal products contribute to more than 60% of total lipids, 70% saturated fats and 100% cholesterol of diet. Since, preference for animal products will likely to continue, it would be of importance to modify animal products in such a way that dietary risks are minimized. As consumers have begun to take control of their own health and are driving the market for a new category of foods with the potential for health promotion well beyond the traditional benefits. Certain paradigms to develop designer products of milk, meat and egg their merits, economics and future research are being discussed in this chapter.

Livestock systems occupy about 30% of the planet's surface area (Steinfeld *et al.,* 2006) and are a significant global asset with a value of at least Rs 70 trillion. The livestock sector is increasingly getting organized into market chains that employ around 1.3 billion people globally and directly support the livelihood of 600 million poor smallholder farmers in the developing world (Thornton *et al.,* 2006). Livestock products contribute 17% of food consumption (in kilocalories) and 33% of protein consumption globally, though there are large differences in consumption of energy and protein between the rich and poor countries (Rosegrant *et al.,* 2009). The livestock systems have both positive and negative effects on the natural resource base, public health, social equity and economic growth (World Bank 2009). Currently, livestock is one of the fastest growing agricultural subsectors in developing countries. Its share of agricultural GDP is already 33% and is increasing further. This growth is driven by the rapidly increasing demand for livestock products, this demand being driven by population growth, urbanization and increasing incomes in developing countries (Delgado, 2005).

The livestock sector is characterized by a dichotomy between developing and developed countries. The total meat production in the developing world tripled between 1980 and 2002, from 45 to 134 million tons (World Bank, 2009). Most of this growth was observed in countries that experienced rapid economic growth and revolved around poultry and pigs. In the developed countries, production and consumption of livestock products are growing slowly or stagnating, although at high levels. The livestock production and merchandizing in developed countries account for 53% of agricultural GDP (World Bank, 2009). The combination of growing demand in developing world and stagnant demand in developed countries represents a major opportunity for livestock keepers in developing countries, where most demand is met by local production. This trend is likely to continue in the near future. Simultaneously, the expansion of agricultural production needs to take place in a way that the increased demand of animal products benefits the lower strata of the human society with the least impact on the environment. In the industrialized world, animal products contribute to more than 60% of total lipids, 70% saturated fats and 100% cholesterol of diet. Since, preference for animal products will likely to continue, it would be of importance to modify animal products in such a way that dietary risks are minimized. Consumers have begun to take control of their own health. They are driving the market for a new category of foods with the potential for health promotion well beyond the traditional benefits. It is foreseeable thus that designer milk, eggs and meat would be welcomed by a population that is increasingly becoming aware of good health.

1. Designer milk

In the recent years, the advent of genetic engineering and biotechnology has changed the breeding policy from producing more milk to adding more value to milk and to study the health implications. The composition of milk can be altered by nutrition management or through the exploitation of naturally occurring genetic variation among cattle. 'Designer milk' meeting consumer preferences are developed by combining the two approaches of nutritional and genetic interventions.

The need for manipulating the composition of milk is the same as it was 25 years ago which includes improving the manufacturing, processing of dairy products, altering the nutritional value of milk to conform dietary guidelines and using milk as a delivery system for nutraceuticals. To obtain the full potential of these advantages, it would be desirable to alter milk composition in several ways. For diet and human health measures, it would be beneficial to generate a greater proportion of unsaturated fatty acids (USFA) in milk fat, to reduce lactose content in milk to cater to persons suffering from lactose intolerance and to remove beta-lacto globulin (β-lg) from milk. From a technological point of view it would be beneficial if there is an alteration of primary structure of casein, production of high protein in milk, engineering milk for cheese manufacturing, increased yield and/or more protein recovery, milk containing nutraceuticals and replacement for infant formula.

1.1. Manipulation of milk fat

Ideal milk would contain approximately 8% saturated fatty acids, less than 10% polyunsaturated fatty acids, and the remainder (82%) as monounsaturated fatty acids (Berner, 1993). The market pressures continued over the last two and a half decades to enhance the concentration of the healthy unsaturated fatty acids in milk. Increasing the oleic acid content in milk enhances the plasticity and softness of milk fat, hence improve the spreadability of butter. Recently the beneficial effects of unsaturated *trans*-fatty acids produced in the rumen, paired way to several research attempts to enhance their concentration in meat and milk. Nutritional control of milk fatty acid profile has received considerable attention over the last three decades. Manipulation of milk fat has to be taken up with the objective of increasing one or few polyunsaturated fatty acids whereby the beneficial effects of such milk is translated into useful effects to humans.

Attempts have been made to determine the ability of different dietary formulations to reduce milk fat content or enhance the concentration of unsaturated fatty acids (Jenkins and McGuire, 2005). Dietary factors receiving the most attention were the amounts of grain and fat fed to cows. The control of milk fat and fatty acid composition by fat supplements is very complex phenomenon. The transfer of dietary unsaturated fatty acids to milk can be significantly lessened by several factors such as biohydrogenation by ruminal microorganisms, poor rates of intestinal absorption and their deposition in adipose tissue rather than in mammary fat.

1.1.1 Decreasing the level of saturation in milk fat

Feeding of unsaturated fats in an encapsulated or protected form, result in a prompt rise in the degree of unsaturation of serum lipids, tissue fat and milk fat. Feeding highly unsaturated oils (*e.g.*, soybean oil) led to depression in milk fat, but increased the proportion of unsaturated fatty acids to saturated fatty acids in milk (Jenkins and McGuire, 2005). Feeding canola oil in the encapsulated form (to protect it from biohydrogenation by the rumen microorganisms) led to higher increases in linoleic (18:2) and linolenic (18:3) acid than feeding unprotected oil seeds. As the melting point of milk fat containing unsaturated fatty acids is more, the spreadability of butter made from this milk improved tremendously (Mason, 2001). Feeding a blend of canola and soybean meal in the protected form resulted in doubling in the spreadability of butter. Clinical trials also established that consumption of dairy products made from this milk led to decrease in low density lipoprotein (LDL) levels in the blood of the consumers. Studies were carried out on the desaturase gene focusing on the production of milk with decreased saturated fatty acid (SFA) and to conclude if genetic differences among breeds and individual animals are translated into ratios of SFA and USFA.

1.1.2 Increasing conjugated linoleic acid levels in milk fat

Conjugated dienoic derivatives of linoleic acid are a series of positional and geometric isomers of linoleic acid (*cis*-9, *cis*-12 octadecadienoic acid). Conjugated linoleic acid (CLA) occurs naturally in foods. The principal dietary sources are dairy products and other foods derived from ruminant animals (Murthy and Kanawjia 2002). The primary isomer of CLA is *cis*-9, *trans*-11 octadecadienoic acid. It accounts for more than 82% of the total CLA isomers in dairy products (Murthy and Kanawjia, 2002). The *cis*-9, *trans*-11 CLA isomer is an intermediate product of biohydrogenation of linoleic acid by the rumen bacterium, *Butyrivibrio fibrisolvens*. Biohydrogenation in the rumen is affected by the type and amount of fatty acid substrate, forage to grain ratio, and nitrogen content of the diet. Changes in substrate supply and extent of biohydrogenation affects the supply of intermediate and end products of biohydrogenation, thereby influencing the CLA content of milk and meat from ruminants.

Dairy products are rich in CLA, a product synthesized in the rumen during the biohydrogenation of linoleic acid. Research has shown that it is possible to influence the extent of ruminal biohydrogenation and the concentration of CLA absorbed and incorporated into milk fat. A diet rich in linoleic acid led to increasing the CLA levels in milk fat by two fold. Incorporating CLA along with soy oil in the diet of cows increased the CLA levels; simultaneously decreasing the SFA in milk fat. Moreover, milk from a grass-fed cow can have five times as much CLA as milk from a grain-fed animal (Robinson, 2003, *www.eatwild.com*).

The average CLA content of milk varies between 3 and 5.5 mg/g of fat. Typical consumption of CLA by humans is lower than the dose that has been shown to be effective in reducing tumors in animal models. The intake of CLA can be increased by increasing the consumption of foods of ruminant origin or by increasing the CLA content of milk and meat. Increasing the CLA content of milk and meat is more practical and has the potential of increasing the nutritive and therapeutic value of the animal product especially milk.

Incorporation of fish oil in reminant diet effectively increased the contents of eicosapentaenoic acid (EPA), docosahexaenoic acid (DHA) and conjugated linoleic acid (CLA) Nelson and Martini (2009).

CLAs are the only natural fatty acids exhibiting consistent antitumor properties (Ha *et al.*, 1987, 1990; Ip *et al.*, 1991, Parodi, 1997). It inhibits proliferation of leukemia and cancers of the colon, prostate and breast. The other reported beneficial health effects of CLA as supported by biomedical studies with animal models are antiatherogenic effect in hamsters (Nicolosi and Lattinen, 1996) and rabbits (Lee *et al.*, 1994) altered nutrient partitioning and lipid metabolism, antidiabetic action (type II diabetes), immunity enhancement and improved bone mineralization.

1.1.3 Reducing fat content in milk

In changing the milk fat composition, it is necessary to target enzymes that influence the synthesis of fat. Acetyl Co-A carboxylase regulates the rate of fat synthesis within the mammary gland. Reduction of this enzyme would translate to a drastic reduction in the fat content of milk and reduce the energy required by the animal to produce milk (Ntambi *et al.*, 1999). Wall *et al.* (1997) suggested that modifying the cow's genetic makeup to enable it to produce milk with 2% fat would reduce the cost of feed per kg milk by 22%.

1.1.4 Type of fatty acids vs product quality

The type of fatty acids present in milk fat can influence the flavor and physical properties of dairy products. Butter produced from cows fed with high oleic sunflower seeds and regular sunflower seeds were equal or superior in flavor (Middaugh *et al.*, 1988). The butter was softer, more unsaturated and exhibited acceptable flavor, manufacturing, and storage characteristics. Extruded soybean and sunflower diets yielded Cheddar cheese that had higher concentration of USFA while maintaining flavor, manufacturing and storage characteristics. The accumulation of fatty acids, namely C12, C14, and C18:1 and C18:2 enhanced the safety of cheese against *Listeria monocytogenes* and *Salmonella typhimurium* bacteria (Schaffer *et al.*, 1995).

1.2 Modification of protein

The second major products of the mammary gland is protein which provide exciting research and technology opportunities for better protein supplementation to human. Transgenic cows secreting elevated levels of beta (8–20%) and kappa caseins (two fold) have been produced by genetic engineering. Beta-casein, which is the most abundant milk protein, is involved in binding calcium phosphate and thus controlling milk calcium levels. Higher k-casein content in milk is linked to smaller micelles, better heat stability, and improved cheese-making properties. This has a positive influence on the cheese yield and also on the casein and milk protein concentrate industry. Edible casein is used in vitamin tablets, instant drinks and infant formulas. Caseins being easily digestible are quite sensitive to plasmin, a serine protease occurring naturally in milk along with plasminogen. Plasmin activity leads to limited proteolysis in milk leading to decrease in the curd yield while cheese processing and inducing organoleptic defects and gelation of ultra high temperature treated milk. Milk augmented with specific inhibitors of either plasmin or plaminogen activator would therefore be a boon to the process industry.

1.3 Modification of lactose

Milk is a major component in the human diet. Hence, lactose intolerance limits the use of valuable nutritional source for many people. As, milk provides the required calcium for maintaining bone health; lactose intolerance can lead to osteopaenia in later life which is an issue of increasing importance in old people. The consequences of intolerance can be limited by dietary management strategies. The pre-harvest methodologies of reducing lactose involve :

- The removal of α-lactalbumin and gene 'knock-out' methodologies or
- Introducing the lactase enzyme in milk via mammary gland-specific expression.

These approaches provided valuable tools to alter milk physiology. They reduce the overall sugar content of milk, resulting in highly viscous milk, which is not a desireable characteristies of milk for dairy industry. Therefore, it is likely that postharvest technology will be required to reduce lactose content of milk.

1.4 Milk with human therapeutic proteins

Global interest has focused on the production of high value, low volume therapeutic proteins in the milk of domestic animals. Several human proteins have been expressed with considerable success. Both goats and cows have been used to produce more than 60 therapeutic proteins, including plasma proteins, monoclonal antibodies and vaccines. Recombinant human anti-thrombin III, an anti-coagulant protein found in blood has been produced in goat milk. Work has been undertaken to develop a malaria vaccine from goat milk. It is understood that a litre of goat milk can contain up to 9 g of the transgenic protein and that eight goats can produce enough vaccine to inoculate 20 million people. The cost to produce a transgenic protein in goat milk can be 3 to 30 times cheaper than the current method using mammalian cell culture. Research is also being carried out with rabbits and sheep to produce antitrypsin, fibrinogen, and a lipase to treat pancreatic insufficiency in digesting dietary lipids. Products such as insulin and growth hormone have also been obtained from the milk of transgenic cows, sheep or goats. Transgenic animals can also secrete proteins such as blood clotting factors needed by human haemophilia-sufferers. Mice that produce milk with 33% more total solids (40–50% TS) and 17% less lactose than normal control mice have been generated by transgenesis (Sabikhi, 2004). The increase in the total solids (TS) expand during first use is associated with a decrease in total milk volume and hence, the same amount of total milk fat and protein is being produced in a lesser total milk volume. If this technology could be propagated in dairy animals, milk that contains 6.5% protein, 7% fat, 2.5% lactose and 50% less water is not an improbable accomplishment. The advantages would be skim milk with twice protein content and half the lactose content of normal milk, easier to produce low lactose or lactose-free dairy products, better product yields due to concentration, reduction in total whey output because of low milk volume and lactose content and decrease in mastitis as less lactose available for organisms.

2. Designer eggs

Egg has been used for food by man since antiquity. Unlike egg no other single food of animal origin has been eaten by many people all over the world and served in such a variety of ways. Its popularity has been justified mostly because of its nutritive quality (Stadelman and Colterill, 1995). Eggs play an important role in our everyday food. In 2007 total egg production in the world was ca. 62.6 million tons (FAO, 2009).

2.1 Nutritive values of egg

Chicken eggs are one of the most versatile foods. They contain high-quality proteins, carbohydrates, easily digestible fats and minerals, as well as valuable vitamins (Huopalahti, *et al.*, 2007). Egg proteins are highly digestible, containing most important essential amino acids in a profile, providing the ideal balance of amino acids needed by human beings and companion animals *viz.* dogs, cats. Egg also supply various minerals, some in significant amounts and contain major vitamins. In a study in the USA, it has been shown that eggs contribute about 10-20% of daily intake of folate and total saturated and poly unsaturated fat and 20-30% of daily intake of vitamins A, E and B_{12} (Song and Kerver, 2000). The per cent value of nutrients can be received from the egg per day is presented in Table 1. Albeit, several of those nutrients in the egg can be manipulated by dietary means, a real value for improvement of human diet could have only those nutrients which are usually in short supply or have a beneficial effect on health when consumed in excess. Amongst, this n-3 fatty acids vitamin E, carotenoids and selenium have attracted a lot of attention in nutritional sciences.

Table 1 : Daily value of an egg for a nutrient

Nutrient	% daily value
Protein	10
Riboflavin	15
Vitamin B12	8
Vitamin A	6
Vitamin D	6
Folate	6
Vitamin B6	4
Vitamin E	3
Thiamin	2
Zinc	4
Iron	4

Adapted from : Surai and Sparks, 2001

Egg has been considered a wholesome food owing to its unique composition thus supplying excellent quality proteins along with balanced supply of most nutrients in addition to its low caloric content (Hu *et al.*, 2001). Egg is comprised of yolk (29%) albumen (61.5%) and shell (9.5%) and is ranked second richest source of vitamin D but ranked very poor source of vitamin C (Shrimpton, 1987). The various nutrients present in the egg are listed in Table 2.

Table 2 : Composition of whole and different compartments of the egg

	Whole egg (/100g edible portion)	Yolk (%)	Albumen (%)	Egg content (%)	Shell and shell membrane (%)
Total egg weight (g)	56.8				
Energy (MJ)	0.66	1.456-1.498	0.172-0.213	0.728-0.82	Negligible
Water (%)	74.57	49.2-50.1	87.6-89.3	73.7-75.3	Negligible
Protein (g)	12.14	16-16.4	9.4-10.9	12.0-12.9	6.4
Carbohydrates (g)	1.2	0.6-0.7	0.8	0.7-0.9	Traces
Lipids (g)	11.12	3.0-3.1	Traces	6.1-6.6	0.45
Ash (g)	0.94	1.7	0.6-0.7	1.0	92.0

Adapted from : Etches, 1996 ; Ocherman,1978

To mention a few myths about eggs are, the belief that brown shelled egg is more nutritious than a white shelled egg. The yolk colour is believed to be an indication of vitamin A content by some people. The lower demand for eggs during summer months in India is due to the misconception that "*eggs are heat*" so, they increase the body temperature. In fact, eggs are the best food for summer months since during these periods there is a decrease in food intake and thus the requirement of minerals and vitamins are more. Consumption of low energy eggs supply the required vitamin and minerals for better functioning. It is clear that this rapidly emerging area of designer egg production has enormous market potential. The egg industry has been very responsive in seeking new technology to improve negative perception on the egg associated cholesterol, salmonella and even allergy problems attached to egg products. The desire to alter composition of an egg is not due to an innate flaw, but to produce an egg with unique features. These include increased mineral and/or vitamin content, lower lipid and cholesterol concentration and altered fatty acid profile.

2.2 Egg: A functional food

Functional foods may be defined as foods or food ingredients that may enhance health through their production of a physiological benefit beyond traditional nutrients. Modification of nutrient content of the egg has led to a number of designer eggs. Modifying egg quality can be accomplished by inducing metabolic changes in the hen that can result in synthesis of compounds that essentially end up in the egg. Another way is to change the characteristics of membrane transport to facilitate movement of compounds into the egg. One of the most common acceptable way to modify egg quality is to manipulate the diet of the hen such that the desired compounds eventually find their way into the egg. If a food, such as the egg, is nutritionally modified it is referred to as a designer or functional food (American Dietetic Association, 1995).

According to the concept and strategies of functional food science six major targets have been identified (Roberfroid, 2000): Gastro-intestinal function, redox and antioxidant system, metabolism of the macronutrient, development in fetal and early life, xenobiotic metabolism, or cognition and physical performance. Designer eggs can contribute to several mentioned categories.

a) *Redox and antioxidant system*: An egg delivers three anti oxidant components *viz.*, vitamin E, selenium and lutetium.
b) *Development in fetal and early life*: Egg delivers minimum recommended daily allowance for DHA, which is an essential element for development of brain in infants.

c) *Mood improvement*: An egg delivers 50 % of required daily allowance of selenium, which is considered to have an negative effect of human mood.

Besides several bioactive peptides in the egg have been characterized with anti-hypertensive, phagocytosis stimulating and opioid properties that are beneficial for humans (Kato *et al.*, 1998), in addition to being important sources to nutraceuticals and pharmaceutical (Stadelman, 1999) such as immunoglobulin Y production.

2.3 Mineral and vitamin enriched eggs

2.3.1 Iodine

The best way to combat iodine deficiency in endemic areas is through supplementation of iodine in diet for instance, iodized salts. However, depending up on the time of storage iodine is lost from iodized salt, which can be up to 50%. The other source for supplying sufficient amount of dietary iodine could be marine fishes, yet it is not enough. The daily requirement of iodine for growing population is about 150-200μg, which is not met from the common diets as they does not supply sufficient quantity; hence there exists a negative balance of iodine.

Several experiments have been done in order to produce designer eggs enriched with higher concentration of iodine, by adding potassium iodide in the feed mixtures or by adding larger amounts of fish meal in feed composition. Amount of iodine in yolk enriched slowly, reaching the highest level one month after supplementation of potassium iodide in the layer ration (Gjorgovska and Kiril, 1996). Iodine enriched yolk enable the supply of daily requirement of adult people with iodine on the level of about 5-7% if they consume 3 eggs per week.

2.3.2 Chromium

In recent years there has been considerable research interest in utilization of chromium in animal feed. Beneficial effects of chromium in human health are well documented and include a role in maintenance of normal blood sugar and cholesterol levels. Chromium, as an integral component of the glucose tolerance factor, helps control appetite, hypoglycemia and protein uptake and plays a protective role against heart disease and diabetes (Mertz, 1993). The hormone insulin regulates energy metabolism, muscle tissue deposition, fat metabolism and cholesterol utilization. If glucose cannot be utilized by body cells due to low insulin activity, it is converted into fat cells. Furthermore, if adequate amino acids cannot enter the cells, muscle cannot be built (Anderson, 1988).

Chromium is involved in maintenance of the normal physical state of egg albumen. The possible mechanism by which chromium could work to maintain egg quality are: (1) as a structural component of egg albumen or in the cross linking of proteins, (2) chromium is necessary for the synthesis of ovomucin which is responsible for gel structure of albumen, and (3) facilitate transfer of cations (possibly magnesium) into the albumen of eggs during the plumping process in the uterus.

In the field of animal nutrition, there is emerging evidence to suggest that pigs and poultry may have a greater dietary requirement for chromium than that supplied from a corn-soybean meal diet. Recent findings (Jacela *et al.*, 2009; Sales and Janèík, 2011) on the positive effects of chromium supplementation for pigs on carcass leanness and on reproductive parameters have been quite impressive. Published data on the effect of chromium supplementation on poultry performance and meat and egg quality is more limited.

Anderson *et al.* (1989), supplemented diets of turkey breeders with 25 and 100 ppm chromium from chromium chloride. The results indicated that supplemental chromium led to a significant linear increase in chromium concentration of the egg yolk but not the egg white. Addition of 100 ppm chromium led to an approximate doubling of chromium in the egg yolk but not egg white. Chromium concentration of the yolk was approximately 10 fold greater than that of the egg white when expressed on a wet weight basis and two to three fold greater on a dry weight basis for control eggs as well as for eggs from turkeys supplemented with either 25 or 100 ppm chromium.

2.3.3 Selenium

Most of the biological functions of selenium are due to its incorporation into selenoproteins such as glutathione peroxidases. Inclusion of organic selenium in the chicken diet could substantially increase its accumulation in the egg. A supplementation of 0.4 mg of selenium enriched yeast per kilogram of diet yield 30 μg selenium in the egg. This is about 50% or the daily requirement. This could be used to improve the selenium content of diet meets only 50% of the requirement (Rayman, 2000).

2.3.4 Folate

The term folate encompasses a number of different water soluble compounds based on the structure of folic acid or pteroylmonoglutamate but differing in oxidation state and number of additional glutamase residues (Selhub and Rosenberg, 1996). Folic acid does not occur naturally in appreciable amounts in foods; hence, supplemented through vitamin supplements, fortified foods and vitamin premixes. Poor to marginal folate status is linked to increased formation of homocysteine as folate acts as a cofactor in re-methylation of homocysteine to methionine (House *et al.*, 1999). Homocysteine has been shown to as a risk factor for development of cardiovascular disease (Boushey *et al.*, 1995). Eggs are natural source of folate containing approximately 22 μg folate per large egg (USDA, 2001), which is equivalent to 6 % of the adult daily requirement daily requirement for folate (Institute of Medicine, 1998). Folate can be enriched in eggs through supplementation in layer chicken ration with crystalline folic acid. Since the folate transport across the intestinal epithelia has been shown as a saturable process, the intestinal uptake of folate could play an important role in the regulation of egg yolk folate concentrations (Said *et al.*, 2000). One large folate enriched egg provides approximately 45 to 50μg folate or roughly 25% of the recommended nutrient requirement for adult (180μg/day and 220μg/day for males and females, respectively). Folate enriched eggs remain stable up to 4 weeks of storage at 4°C (House *et al.*, 1999).

2.4 Modulation of egg lipids

Yolk consists of the major proportion of egg lipids comprising of 5.5 to 6 g of fat in a standard sized egg of 60 g weight (Cherian, 2002). Yolk lipids are present primarily as triacyl glycerols, phospholipids and free cholesterol. Of the total fatty acids consists of mono unsaturated fatty acids (44%), saturated fatty acids (29%) and poly unsaturated fatty acids (11%) (Sparks, 2000). The dietary source of lipids and *de novo* lipid synthesis influences the composition of egg's lipids (Sim and Sunwoo, 2002).

Cruickshank (1934) demonstrated for the first time the ability to change the nutrient profile of the egg, the polyunsaturated fatty acid profile through dietary manipulation. The nutritional importance of this discovery was not fully appreciated until the 1970s, when health conscious Americans began to shun eating eggs. In the recent past, amongst the nutrients lipids have attracted the attention of consumer's and researchers due to the link between high dietary fat composition and coronary heart disease and some forms of cancer (Simopoulous and Salem, 1992). They believed if they consumed eggs the cholesterol and saturated fatty acids contained in the egg would immediately put them at the death's door. The rapid decline in the per capita consumption of eggs over the past five decades is one of the problems the industry is facing even today. Hence, modification of egg cholesterol and to decrease the ratio of saturated to unsaturated fatty acid content became the goal of numerous research efforts (Table 3).

Table 3 : Nutritive value of enriched and conventional eggs

Component	Enriched egg	Standard egg
Calories (MJ)	75	75
Protein (g)	6	6
Carbohydrates (g)	0.6	0.6
Total fat (g)	6	6
Saturated FA (g)	1.5	2.2
PUFA (g)	1.35	0.9
ù- 6 FA (mg)	750	800
ù- 3 FA (mg)	350	60
18:3 n-3 (mg)	250	40
22:6 n-3 (mg)	100	20
ù- 6: ù- 3 ratio	2.6	13.0
MUFA (g)	2.8	2.4
Cholesterol (mg)	180	210

Adapted from : Gill, 2001

2.4.1 Omega-3 enriched eggs

Efforts have been made to enrich eggs with polyunsaturated fatty acids (PUFA) to get the health benifits associated with its consumption (van Elswyk *et al.*, 1992). The major PUFAs of nutritional importance fall under two categories *viz.*, n-6 and n-3 fatty acids. Alpha linolenic (C18:3) and Arachidonic (C20:4) acids belongs to n-6 fatty acids where as the n-3 acids are eicosapentonoic (EPA; C20:5) and decosahexnoic (DHA; C22:6) acids. Since animals cannot synthesis EPA and DHA *de novo* they have to be supplemented in the diet. These essential fatty acids have a positive effect on human health especially in cognition and developmental stages of brain of infants, platelet aggregation, lowering systolic and diastolic blood pressure and lower the plasma triglycerides and cholesterol levels.

Commercial table eggs are rich source of n-6 but not that of n-3 fatty acids. Therefore, the best way is to produce an egg enriched with alpha linolenic acid (van Elswyk, 1997) the precursor of DHA. Supplementation of chicken ration with flax seed, linseed and their corresponding oils leads to the enrichment of alpha linolenic acid in yolk with a corresponding increase in the level of DHA (Ferrier *et al.*, 1995). Feeding of flax seed to laying chicken has shown to increase the omega 3 fatty acid content of the egg by 6-8 times (Yannakopoulos *et al.*, 2005). The DHA content of eggs can be increased by feeding fish meal in the diet of hens or supplementation with marine algae. It has been shown that fatty acid profile of eggs enriched with n-3 the PUFAs were not lost during cooking (van Elswyk, 1992) and were stable up on storage for 7 weeks at 25°C (Oku *et al.,* 1996).

The major disadvantage of omega-3 enriched eggs is the development of off flavors due to flax seed in the chicken diet (Ahn *et al.,* 1995) or the formation of fishy odor in these eggs due to rancidity of the n-3 enriched diet (Coughley *et al.,* 1997). It has been suggested that use of combinations of antioxidants in the hen's diet would suppress these off flavors (Farrell, 1998). However yet high levels of vitamin E failed to prevent formation of off-flavors in hens fed on a >10% flax diet (Leeson *et al.,* 1998).

Over the past decades several omega 3 enriched eggs are being widely available on the shelves of the supermarkets. Of the various brands available across the European markets, Columbus eggs claim enrichment with alpha linolenic acid by 12.6% and that of DHA by 2% (Surai and Sparks, 2001). Consumption of ω-3 enriched eggs have been shown to improve the circulating cell membrane fatty acid composition by favourably altering the ω-6:ω-3 ratio (DeMeester *et al.,* 1998). On the other hand, eggs produced by England's Best Inc. claim to have increased ω-3 fatty acid level by 3 folds with a reduction of 25% in the saturated fat compared to standard egg (Michella and Slaugh, 2000).

2.4.2 Low cholesterol eggs

Cholesterol facilitates four major functions of in the mammalian body *viz.,* maintaining the structural homeostasis of cell membrane, act as precursor for the synthesis of bile acids thus facilitating fat digestion, provide substrate for synthesis of steroid hormones and in the synthesis of vitamin D from cholesterol derivative 7-dehydrocholesterol. Despite being beneficial depending on its concentration, circulation, accumulation and abnormal deposition it is one of the culprits and hence used as a general indicator for heart health. The increased level of cholesterol in the chicken egg has caused decline in the per capita consumption of eggs in the western world over the past decades. Henceforth several researches attempted to produce eggs with low cholesterol and succeeded (Clarenburg *et al.,* 1971; Elkin and Rogler, 1990; Chowdhury *et al.,* 2002; Ginzberg *et al.,* 2003; Salma *et al.,* 2007).

Egg yolk of chickens fed with algae tended to have reduced cholesterol levels by 10% and increased linoleic acid and arachidonic acid levels by 29% and 24%, respectively; (Ginzberg *et al.,* and 2003). Inclusion of garlic at 1% level to layer chicken has resulted in a 10% reduction in yolk cholesterol (Gorti, 2012 *personal communication*), this is in contradiction to the observation of Lim *et al.* (2006) where garlic power at 1% level failed to decrease the egg yolk cholesterol levels when fed to 50 week old layer hens.

The mechanism of action of most of these cholesterol lowering functional foods act through one of the following mechanisms: 3-Hydroxy 3 methyl glutaryl CoA (HMG-CoA) reductase inhibition thus preventing *de novo* synthesis of cholesterol from acetate (garlic, polidosanols, soybean *etc.*), sterol regulatory element binding protein 2 (SREBP 2) activation (grape seed polyphenols), Niemann-Pick C1 like protein (NPC1L1) inhibition thus prevent absorption of cholesterol from circulation into the enterocytes (phytosterols and phytostanols), bile acid sequestrants that increases bile acid excretion (oats).

2.5 Designer eggs: Economics and future

The production of designer eggs involves extra cost and they are usually sold at premium prices. Consumer preference decides the pricing of these eggs; still we have to go a long way before consumer awareness and acceptance for designer eggs get popular in countries like India. The cost of egg depends on the additional cost incurred by feeding additional sources of vitamins or minerals and/or other feed ingredients to manipulate lipids in the egg. Enriching eggs with alpha linolenic acid is much cheaper compared to enrichment of DHA due to usage of stabilized source of fresh fish oil. Usage of algal sources to enrich DHA will also be inexpensive. Therefore, there is a need to differentiate DHA enriched eggs from alpha linolenic acid enriched eggs at retail outlets.

The modification of nutrient content of the egg has led to a number of designer eggs and several can be on the pipeline. Research reports from around the world have indicated that the level of almost any vitamin or mineral can be influenced by modifying the diet of the hen (Stadelman and Pratt, 1989), since an over dose is impossible. It is not far away that a fluoride enriched egg for children to improve tooth structure or a vitamin D enriched egg for the senior citizen is made available across the counter.

The egg yolk is a reservoir of antibodies with many proven uses as well as many theoretical applications and several specific antibodies have been isolated purified from the egg yolk. Feeding of eggs enriched with antibodies against an enteric microorganism has shown to minimize mortality in piglets (Marquardt, 1998; Mime, 1998). Dried yolk from hens hyper immunized against *Staphylococcus aureus* and *Streptococcus agilata* fed @ 200ppm for three weeks to cows significantly minimized somatic cell count in milk.

3. Designer meat

3.1 Manipulation of fatty acid composition of meat

There has been an increased interest in recent years to manipulate the fatty acid composition of meat. This is because meat is seen to be a major source of fat in the diet and especially of saturated fatty acids, which have been implicated in diseases associated with modern life. These include various cancers and especially coronary heart disease. The recommended ratio of polyunsaturated fatty acids (PUFA) to saturated fatty acids (P:S) should be increased to above 0.4. Since some meats naturally have a P:S ratio of around 0.1, meat has been implicated in causing the imbalanced fatty acid intake. For this reason, ways to improve the P:S ratio during meat production is required. More recently, nutritionists have focused on the type of PUFA and the balance in the diet between n-3 PUFA formed from α-linolenic acid (C18:3) and n-6 PUFA formed from linoleic acid (C18:2). The ratio of n-6: n-3 PUFA is also a risk factor in cancers and coronary heart disease, especially the formation of blood clots leading to a heart attack. The recommendation is for a ratio of less than 4 and again some meats are higher than this. As with the P:S ratio, meats can be manipulated towards a more favorable n-6: n-3 ratio. In pigs, by feeding sources such as linseed in the diet the n-3 PUFA in meat can be increased. Adverse effects on meat quality, in terms of shelf life (lipid and myoglobin oxidation) and flavor are noticed when the concentration of linolenic acid (C18:3) approach 3% of neutral lipids or phospholipids. Ruminant meat is a relatively good source of n-3 PUFA due to the presence of 18:3 in grass. Further increases can be achieved with animals fed grain-based diets by including whole linseed or linseed oil, especially if this is protected from rumen biohydrogenation (Scollan *et al., 2001*). Long-chain (C20–C22) n-3 PUFA is synthesized from C18:3 in the animal although docosahexaenoic acid (DHA, 22:6) is not increased. DHA can be increased by feeding sources such as fish oil, but high levels cause adverse flavor and color changes. Grazing provides antioxidants including vitamin E which maintain PUFA levels in meat and prevent quality deterioration during processing and display. In pork, beef and lamb the melting point of lipid and the firmness/hardness of carcass fat is closely related to the concentration of stearic acid (C18:0) (Wood *et al.*, 2008).

There have been suggestions that dietary fatty acids influence tenderness and juiciness of the meat. However, these are more likely to be affected by the total amount of fatty acids rather than individual ones. The effect of fatty acids on firmness is due to the different melting points of the fatty acids in meat. In the 18C fatty acid series, stearic acid (C18:0) melts at 69.6°C, oleic acid (C18:1) at 13.4°C, C18:2 at 15°C and C18:3 at 11°C. Therefore with an increase in the unsaturation, it has been found that there is a decline in the melting point. Variations in the structure of the molecule are also important. For example, trans-fatty acids melt at a higher temperature than their *cis*-isomers and branched chain fatty acids have lower melting points than the straight chain fatty acids with the same number of carbon atoms. The effect of fatty acids on shelf life is explained by the propensity of unsaturated fatty acids to oxidize, leading to the development of rancidity as display times increases. The colour change is due to the oxidation of red oxymyoglobin to brown metmyoglobin, this reaction on generally proceeding in parallel to that of rancidity. Several studies have shown that lipid oxidation products can promote pigment oxidation and vice versa although the strength of the relationship between these two aspects of shelf life is sometimes low. Antioxidants, especially α-tocopherol (vitamin E) have been used to delay lipid and color oxidation and to extend shelf life. The effect of fatty acid on meat flavor is due to the production of volatile, odorous, lipid oxidation products during cooking and the involvement of these with Maillard reaction products to form other volatiles which contribute to odour and flavor. The unsaturated phospholipid fatty acids are particularly important in flavor development.

3.1.1 Fatty acids and pork quality

Fat tissue consists not only of fatty acids contained in fat cells but also the connective tissue matrix associated with water. In pigs, the concentration of water in thin back fat is very high as in collagen. These constituents are also good predictors of tissue firmness along with the concentrations of 18:0 and 18:2 and the thickness of the fat tissue. Fat tissue development in the pig is an extremely ordered process with all the major constituents closely interrelated. As subcutaneous fat tissue develops and changes in composition, it becomes more cohesive. Studies have shown that cohesiveness is closely related to water, collagen, C18:0 and C18:2 fatty acid concentrations, just as is firmness.

The total fatty acid content (*i.e.*, neutral lipid plus phospholipid fatty acids) of muscle is termed marbling fat. This fat has long been recognized as a factor in eating quality, especially juiciness and tenderness although the strength of the relationship has been questioned (Wood *et al.*, 2008). There are several possible explanations for a positive effect of lipid on tenderness, including the location of neutral lipid in fat cells within the perimysium which could have a physical effect in separating muscle fibre bundles, beginning the process of tenderisation by "opening up the muscle structure". Lipids could also trap moisture in muscle, improving juiciness. There are clear genetic effects on the concentrations of total fatty acids in muscle. It was found that Duroc and Berkshire pure bred pigs had higher concentrations of both neutral lipids and phospholipids in longisimus and psoas muscles than Large Whites and Tamworths. The two traditional breeds (Berkshire and Tamworth) had by far the fattest carcasses so the results indicated a big genetic effect on "fat partitioning" between intramuscular and carcass fat depots.

3.1.2 Fatty acids and beef quality

Ruminant fat tissue is naturally firmer than that of pigs, because the fatty acid profile is more saturated. In the first stages of fattening in cattle, the concentration of saturated fatty acids relative to unsaturated fatty acids increases as in pigs, but beyond a certain fat levels in the animal these ratio then declines. In very fat cattle, fat is soft and oily, mainly due to an increase in C 18:1 relative to C 18:0 and 16:0. A value of 14.7% of C 18:0 in the total fatty acids in a young heifer and 2.7% in an 11-year-old fat steer was recorded. In 1000 lambs selected and studied it was found that the concentration of 18:0, as with pigs, showed the highest correlation with melting point. The average melting point of subcutaneous fat was 39.5°C (range 30 to 49°C) and correlations were 0.89, 0.42 and 0.31 for C 18:0, C 18:1 and C 18:2 fatty acid concentrations, respectively. It was calculated that only 35% of these fat samples would melt in the mouth of the consumer, confirming the hard nature of lamb fat and its tendency to feel sticky in the mouth. In lambs, especially ram lambs, soft fat develops in animals fed grain-based (concentrate) diets. This is due not only to a lower concentration of C 18:0 but also to an increased deposition of medium to long-chain (C10 – C17) branched chain fatty acids formed from methylmalonate, a metabolite of propionate. As the concentration of branched chain fatty acids increased, that of C 18:0 fell, perhaps by direct inhibition.

The presence of the rumen makes fatty acid composition in beef and sheep more difficult to manipulate by changing diet than in pigs. Nevertheless, there are some clear effects of diet on tissue fatty acid composition. Studies with beef and lamb have shown that the concentrations of C 18:3 and C 20:5 in muscle phospholipids are higher when animals have consumed grass than when they have been fed grain-based (concentrate) diets. In the latter case, (C 20:4 n-6) fatty acids (linoleic aiach donic) are increased relative to n-3 fatty acids (linoleic acid C 18:3, Sanudo *et al.*, 2000). There exists a preference for grain finished products in the western world and consumers are more used to the taste of beef and lamb produced in feedlot conditions and prefer it to grass-fed beef and lamb. It has also been shown that lipid oxidation and color development of ruminant meats is influenced by both fatty acid composition and the concentration of the tissue antioxidant and vitamin E.

3.2 Broiler carcass quality

Increasing consumer concern regarding quality of chicken meat has encouraged poultry producers to focus on the production of high quality chicken. There is a growing need to provide nutrition, environment, health and management programs to improve the end product that meets the consumer requirements for fat content, nutritional value, color, taste and texture. In addition to the end product attributes, consumers must be aware of what birds are fed so that they can make choices in selection of the final product.

3.2.1 Growth and development

One of the major challenges is to provide the environment, management, and nutrition to allow the bird to express its genetic potential for growth. Presently there is demand for lean meat which has resulted in a need for understanding the manner in which bird's partition energy and nutrients for maintenance and tissue growth. Bone, muscle and fat have different rates of growth and maturation and the proportion of these three tissues in the body largely determines carcass value. Muscle and fat ratios within the carcass are of greater economical interest than bone deposition, although adequate skeletal development is not unimportant. As the bird matures, the digestive organs of the bird are gradually reduced as a percentage of the body, while the proportions of edible meat increase. Birds attempt to adjust feed consumption to achieve a target energy intake, given that the diet is balance for all nutrients. At elevated dietary energy concentrations, overall body weight increases. This is due to increased fat deposition rather than greater protein and lean tissue deposition. The extra fat is laid down as abdominal fat, which is costly to producers and processors and undesirable to the consumer. Thus, it is important to optimize daily energy intake, growth rate and feed efficiency without promoting excessive fat deposition.

3.2.2 Amino acid intake

Amino acid nutrition plays a central role in protein deposition and muscle tissue growth. Studies have demonstrated that the amino acid requirements for maximum breast meat yield may exceed those for optimal growth and feed efficiency. Therefore, the amino acid specifications should be based on specific economic objectives. Presently, synthetic forms of the essential amino acids-lysine, methionine, threonine, and tryptophan - are commercially available and can be used in conjunction with knowledge of the amino acid content of feedstuffs to formulate diets which closely match the requirements of the bird. The availability of a growing number of synthetic amino acids would make feed formulation more complex and precise over the coming years.

3.2.3 Minerals and vitamins

Feedstuffs make a significant contribution to the mineral and vitamin content of commercial diets. Knowledge of the growing bird's requirements for macro minerals such as calcium and phosphorus is essential to ensure adequate bone mineralization. Whether the end product is boneless or bone-in, bone breakage creates processing problems and a deterioration of end product quality. These nutrients need to be provided in the correct amounts and in a bio-available form to meet the needs of today's fast growing birds. Although micro minerals and vitamins represent a relatively small proportion of diet cost, the provision of adequate micro mineral and vitamin levels is vital for optimum growth, development and immune status.

3.2.4 Effect of health on carcass quality

Effective disease prevention and control strategies are needed to create an attractive retail product. Within flock variation of final body weight increased drastically in the presence of a disease challenge, resulting in greater proportions of birds failing to meet food service specifications. In addition, infectious diseases can have a detrimental effect on final carcass quality. This is because acute infections can elicit a febrile response that results in an increase in basal metabolic rate from 10 to 15% for each 1°C increase in body temperature. They can cause a loss of appetite and growth depression. There is a net protein loss during infection but of more interest is the fact that acutely infected birds lose proportionately more body protein than they do body weight. Thus, infectious disease has a greater negative impact on lean tissue and carcass quality than on live weight.

3.2.5 Designer meat with balanced nutrients

There are two main strategies for manipulating the composition and quality of poultry meat through nutritional means. The first involves the manipulation of dietary nutrients to affect bird composition at various stages of maturity. When the energy level of the diet increases relative to dietary protein, fat deposition also increases. This results in an undesirable carcass with proportionately more fat than protein. It has been shown recently that increasing the levels of lysine or methionine above the levels required for optimal growth and feed efficiency has a positive impact on breast meat yield. Similar work with threonine, the third limiting amino acid, indicates that requirements for maximum breast meat yield are at least as high as those for optimal performance.

The second strategy employed in the manipulation of carcass composition involves the direct incorporation of dietary nutrients into tissues in order to enhance the nutritional attributes of poultry meat. Omega-3 fatty acids found in fish, shellfish and flaxseed, for example, can be protective against cardiovascular diseases in humans. The relative ease with which these polyunsaturated fatty acids can be transferred to the fatty acid profile of the bird's tissues allows poultry producers to tailor their product to meet the demands of consumers.

The problem however, is that these unsaturated fatty acids result in an oily carcass which will be more susceptible to oxidation and will result in off flavors. Thus it is important that dietary fats be properly stabilized and that antioxidants such as vitamin E, be included in the diet. This helps to prevent lipid oxidation and odours while increasing shelf life. Research is also being carried out on the incorporation of other fat-soluble vitamins and trace minerals into the diet to improve meat quality. In summary the production of a high quality, cutting edge retail product requires excellence and innovation in all parts of the broiler chicken productions chain, from genetics right through to feeding, management, environment and health.

Conclusions

Despite all these promising prospects, there is a tendency among human beings to resist change, especially those that trouble their feeling and instincts. As all changes that arise as a consequence of biological research would fall into these categories, there is bound to be tremendous resistance to topics such as transgenics. The future of biotechnologically derived foods is, therefore, at crossroads even after two decades of positive results. Hi-tech milk processing may be more acceptable to consumers than transgenesis for altering milk composition. Controversy will inevitably tint all biotechnological manipulations aimed at increasing milk production or altering milk composition. Ultimate acceptability will depend on the four key factors of animal welfare, demonstrable safety of the product, enhanced health properties of the product and increased profitability compared with conventional practices. Various ethical, legal and social aspects of biotechnological research need to be addressed before we would see designer transgenic herds similar to the organic herds that thrive in the current economic and social climate. With all the research being conducted on designer food the best is yet to come and it will certainly be a breakthrough for all the sustained efforts put forth.

References

Ahn D.U., Sunwoo H.H., Wolfe F.H., Sim J.S. (1995). Effects of dietary alpha-linolenic acid and strain of hen on the fatty acid composition, storage stability and flavor characteristics of chicken eggs' in American Dietetic Association. *Poultry Science* **74:** 1540-1547.

Anderson R.A. (1988). Chromium. In: *Trace minerals in foods.* Marcel Dekker Inc. New York, p 231.

Anderson R.A., Bryden N.A., Planski M.M., Richards M.P. (1989). Chromium supplementation of turkeys: effects on tissue chromium. *Journal of Agriculture and Food Chemistry* **37:** 131-134.

Berner L.A. (1993). Roundtable discussion on milkfat, dairy foods, and coronary heart disease risk. *Journal of Nutrition* **123:** 1175-1184.

Boushey C.J., Beresford S.A., Omenn G.S., Motulsky A.G. (1995). A quantitative assessment of plasma homocysteine as a risk factor for vascular disease. Probable benefits of increasing folic acid intakes. *Journal of American Medical Association* **274:** 1049-1057.

Bremel R.D., Yom H.C., Bleck G.T. (1989). Alteration of milk composition using molecular genetics. *Journal of Dairy Science* **72:** 2826-2833.

Cherian G. (2002). Lipid modification strategies and nutritionally functional poultry foods. In: *Food science and product technology,* (T. Nakano, L. Ozimek, eds), Research Sign Post, Trivandrum, India, pp 77-92.

Chowdhury S.R., Chowdhury S.D., Smith T.K. (2002). Effects of dietary garlic on cholesterol metabolism in laying hens. *Poultry Science* **81:** 1856-1862.

Clarenburg R., Kim Chung I.A., Wakefield L.M. (1971). Reducing the egg cholesterol level by including emulsified Sitosterol in standard chicken diet. *Journal of Nutrition* **101:** 289-298.

Cloughley J., Noble R., Speake B., Sparks N. (1997). Manipulation of docosahexaenoic (22:6n-3) acid in chicken's egg. *Prostaglandins, Leucotrienes and Essential Fatty Acids* **57:** 222-226 .

Cruikshank E.M. (1934). Studies in fat metabolism in the fowl: The composition of the egg fat and depot fat of the fowl as affected by the ingestion of large amounts of fats. *Biochemical Journal.* **28:** 965-971.

De Meester F., Stannard J., Remacle C., D'Hollander F., Goerminne X., Erpicum T. (1998). Columbus, the natural original egg a model for healthy animal-derived food. *Leatherhead Food Research Association Food Industry Journal* **1:** 289-300.

Delgado C. (2005). Rising demand for meat and milk in developing countries: implications for grasslands-based livestock production in Grassland: a global resource (D.A. McGilloway, ed.), Wageningen Academic Publishers, The Netherlands, pp 29-39.

Elkin R.G., Rogler J.C. (1990). Reduction of the cholesterol content of the eggs by oral administration of Lovastatin to laying hens. *Journal of Agriculture and Food Science* **38:** 1635-1641.

Etches R.J. (1996). Reproduction in poultry. CAB International, Wallingford. University Press, Cambridge, UK.

Farrell D.J. (1998). Manipulation of the fatty acid composition of poultry meat and eggs to meet consumer demands. In: *Proceedings of the 6th Asia Pacific Poultry Congress* Nagoya, Japan. 4–7 June, pp 58-63.

Food and Agriculture Organization of United States (FAO) (2009). FaoStat. Livestock primary.

Gill C. (2001). Formulation of nutraceutical eggs. *Feed International* **22:** 16-19.

Ginzberg A., Merav Cohen M., Sod-Moriah U.A., Shany S., Rosenshtrauch A., Arad S. (2000). Chickens fed with biomass of the red microalga *Porphyridium* sp. have reduced blood cholesterol level and modified fatty acid composition in egg yolk. *Journal of Applied Phycology* **12:** 325-330.

Gjorgovska N., Kiril F. (1996). Enriching table eggs with iodine (I). *Lucrari Stiintifice Seria Zootechnie* **53:** 722-725.

Ha Y.L., Grimm N.K., Pariza M.W. (1987). Anticarcinogens from fried ground beef: heat-altered derivatives of linoleic acid. *Carcinogenesis* **8:** 1881-1887.

Ha Y.L., Storkson J., Pariza M.W. (1990). Inhibition of benzo (á) pyrene-induced mouse forestomach neoplasia by conjugated dienoic derivatives of linoleic acid. *Cancer Research* **50:** 1097-1101.

House J.D., Jacobs R.L., Stead L.M., Brosnan M.E., Brosnan J.T. (1999). Regulation of homocysteine metabolism. *Advances in Enzyme Regulation.* **39:** 69-91.

House J.D., Braun K., Ballance D.M., O'Connor C.P., Guenter W. (2002). The enrichment of eggs with folic acid through supplementation of the laying hen diet. *Poultry Science* **81:** 1332-1337.

Hu F.B., Manson J.E., Willett W.C. (2001). Types of dietary fat and risk of coronary heart disease: A critical review. *Journal of the American College of Nutrition* **20:** 5-19.

Huopalahti R., López F.R., Anton M., Schade R. (2007). Bioactive egg compounds. Springer-Verlag, Heidelberg, pp 298.

Institute of Medicine. (1998). Folate. In: *Dietary reference intakes for Thiamin, Riboflavin, Niacin, Vitamin B6, Folate, Vitamin B12, Pantothenic Acid, Biotin, and Choline.* National Academy Press, Washington, DC. pp 196-305.

Ip C., Chin S.F., Scimeca J.A., Pariza M.W. (1991). Mammary cancer prevention by conjugated linoleic acid. *Cancer Research* **51:** 6118-6124.

Jacela J.Y., DeRouchey J.M., Tokach M.D., Goodband R.D., Nelssen J. L., Renter D.G. and Dritz, S.S. (2009). Feed additives for swine: Fact sheets – carcass modifiers, carbohydrate-degrading enzymes and proteases, and anthelmintics. *Journal of Swine Health Production* **17:** 325-332.

Kato A. (1998).Chemistry of functional substances in poultry eggs and its applications to human health. In: *Proceedings of the 6th Asian pacific poultry congress,* Nagoya, June 4 - 7, 1998 pp 52-57.

Sabikhi L. (2004). Designer milk – An imminent milestone in dairy biotechnology. *Current Science* **87:** 1530-1535.

Lee K.N., Kritchevsky D., Pariza M.W. (1994). Conjugated linoleic acid and atherosclerosis in rabbits. *Atherosclerosis* **108:** 19-25.

Leeson S., Caston L., MacLaurin T. (1998). Organoleptic evaluation of eggs produced by laying hens fed diets containing graded levels of flaxseed and vitamin E. *Poultry Science* **77:** 1436-1440.

Lim K.S., You S.J., An B.K., Kang C.W. (2006). Effects of dietary garlic powder and copper on cholesterol content and quality characteristics of chicken eggs. *Asian Australasian Journal of Animal Sciences* **19:** 582-586.

Marquardt R.R. (1998). Antibody-loaded eggs for piglets: Prevention of mortality of baby pigs from diarrhea. *In*: Second international symposium on Egg nutrition and newly emerging Ovo-biotechnologies, Banff, AB, Canada. (Abstr.) p 39.

Mertz W. (1993). Chromium in human nutrition: A review. *Journal of Nutrition* **123:** 626-633.

Michella S.M., Slaugh B.T. (2000). Producing and marketing a specialty egg. *Poultry Science* **79:** 975-976.

Mime Y., Yoshimasu M. (1998). Production of hens' immunoglobulin against an enzymatic cross linked human insulin for immunodiagnosis using a microbial transglutaminase. In: *Second international symposium on egg nutrition and newly emerging Ovo- Biotechnologies*. Banff, AB, Canada, p 56 (Abstr.).

Murthy G.L.N., Kanawjia S. K. (2002). Designer milk: Nutritional and technological significance. *Indian Dairyman* **54:** 49-58.

Nelson K.A., Martini S. (2009). Increasing omega fatty acid content in cow's milk through diet manipulation: effect on milk flavor. *Journal of Dairy Science* **92:** 1378-1386.

Nicolosi R.J., Laitinen L. (1996). Dietary conjugated linoleic acid reduces aortic fatty streak formation greater than linoleic acid in hypercholesterolemic hamsters. *Federation of American Societies for Experimental Biology* **10:** (Abstr. 2751), A 477.

Ntambi J.M., Kim Y.C. (2001). Regulation of stearoyl-CoA desaturase gene expression: Role of polyunsaturated fatty acids. In: Nutrition and Gene Expression, CRS Press, pp 49-61.

Ockerman H.W. (1978). Source book for food scientists. AVI Publishing Co. Inc., p 89.

Oku T., Kato H., Kunishige-Taguchi T., Hattori M., Wada K., Hayashi M. (1996). Stability of fat soluble components such as N-3 polyunsaturated fatty acids and physicochemical properties in EPA- and DHA-enriched eggs. *Japanese Journal of Nutrition* **54:** 109-119.

Parodi P.W. (1997). Cow's milk fat component as potential anticarcinogenic agents. *Journal Nutrition* **127:** 1055-1060.

Rayman M.P. (2000). The importance of selenium to human health. *Lancet* **366:** 233-241.

Roberfroid M.B. (2000). Concepts and strategy of functional food science: The European Perspective'. *American Journal of Clinical Nutrition* **71:** 1660S-1664S.

Rosegrant M.W., Fernandez M., Sinha A., Alder J., Ahammad H., de Fraiture C., Eickhout B., Fonseca J., Huang J., Koyama O., Omezzine A., M. Pingali P., Ramirez R., Ringler C., Robinson S., Thornton P., van Vuuren D., Yana-Shapiro H., Ebi K., Kruska R., Munjal P., Narrod C., Ray S., Sulser T., Tamagno C., van Oorschot M., Zhu T. (2009). Looking into the future for agriculture and AKST (Agricultural Knowledge Science and Technology). In: *Agriculture at a crossroads* (B. D. McIntyre, H. R. Herren, J. Wakhungu and R. T. Watson, eds), Washington DC, Island Press, pp 307–376.

Said H.M., Chatterjee N., Haq R.U., Subramanian V.S., Ortiz A., Matherly L.H., Sirotnak F. M., Halsted C., Rubin S. A. (2000). Adaptive regulation of intestinal folate uptake: Effect of dietary folate deficiency. *American Journal of Physiolology A: Cell Physiology* **279:** C1889-1895.

Sales J., Janèík F. (2011). Effects of dietary chromium supplementation on performance, carcass characteristics, and meat quality of growing-finishing swine: A meta-analysis. *Journal of Animal Science* **89:** 4054-4067.

Salma U., Miah A.G., Tareq K.M.A., Maki T., Tsujii H. (2007). Effect of dietary *Rhodobacter capsulatus* on egg-yolk cholesterol and laying hen performance. *Poultry Science* **86:** 714-719.

Sanudo C., Enser M.E., Camp M.M., Nute G.R., Maria G., Sierra L., Wood J.D. (2000). Fatty acid composition and sensory characteristics of lamb carcasses from Britian and Spain. *Meat Science* **54:** 339-346.

Schaffer S.M., Tatini S.R., Bear R.J. (1995) Microbiological safety of blue and cheddar cheese containing naturally modified milk fat. *Journal of Food Protection* **58:** 132-138.

Scollan N.D., Dhanoa M.S., Choi N.J., Maeng W.J., Enser M., Wood J.D. (2001). Biohydrogenation and digestion of long chain fatty acids in steers fed on different sources of lipid. *Journal of Agricultural Science,* **136:** 345-355.

Selhub J., Rosenberg I.H. (1996). Folic acid. In: *Present knowledge in nutrition.* 7th ed., (E. E.Ziegler and L. J. Filer, eds.) ILSI Press, Washington DC, pp 206-219.

Shrimpton D.H. (1987). The nutritive value of eggs and their significance. Egg quality current problems and recent advances. Butterworth and Co., Ltd. London.

Sim J.S., Sunwoo H.H. (2002). Designer Eggs: Nutritional and Functional Significance, In: *Egg and health promotion.* (R. R. Watson, ed.) 1st ed. Iowa State Press, Iowa, USA, pp 19-35.

Simopolous A.P., Salem N. (1992). Egg yolk as a source of long chain polyunsaturated fatty acids in infant feeding. *American Journal of Clinical Nutrition* **55:** 411-415.

Song W.O., Kerver J.M. (2000). Nutritional contribution of eggs to American diets. *Journal of the American Collage of Nutrition* **19** (Suppl): 556S-562S.

Stadelman W.J. (1999). The incredibly functional egg. *Poultry Science* **78:** 807-811.

Stadelman W.J., Cotterill W.J. (1995). Egg science and technology. (4th ed), Food Products Press, New York, pp 213-235.

Stadelman W.J., Pratt D.E. (1989). Factors influencing composition of the hen's egg. *World's Poultry Science* **75:** 247-266.

Steinfeld H., Gerber P., Wassenaar T., Castel V., Rosales M., de Haan C. (2006). Livestock's long shadow: environmental issues and options. Rome, Italy: FAO.

Surai P.F., Sparks N.H.C. (2001). Designer eggs: from improvements of egg composition to functional food. *Trends in Food Science and Technology* **12:** 7-16.

USDA, Agricultural Research Service. (2001). USDA Nutrient database for standard reference, Release14, Nutrient data laboratory, Home page.

http//www.nal.usda.gov/fnic/foodcomp.

Van Elswyk M.E. (1997). Nutritional and physiological effects of flax seed in diets for laying fowl. *World's Poultry Science Journal* **53:** 253-264.

Wall R.J., Keer D.E., Bondioli K.R. (1997). Transgenic dairy cattle: Genetic engineering on a large scale. *Journal of Dairy Science* **80:** 2213-2224.

Wood J.D., Enser M.B., Fisher A.V., Nute G.R., Richardson R.I., Hughes S.I., Whittington F.I. (2008). Fat deposition fatty acid composition and mead quality; A review. *Meat Science* **78:** 343-358.

World Bank (2009). Minding the stock: bringing public policy to bear on livestock sector development. Report no. 44010-GLB.Washington, DC.

Yannakopoulos A., Tserveni-Gousi A., Christaki E. (2005). Enhanced egg production in practice: The case of Bio-Omega-3 egg. *International Journal of Poultry Science* **4:** 531-535.

❑❑❑

Chapter 9

Probiotics in Livestock and Poultry Production

S. Senani, A.K. Samanta, A.P. Kolte, M. Sridhar
National Institute of Animal Nutrition and Physiology, Adugodi, Bangalore-560 030, Karnataka, India

Summary

It has been claimed, over a century ago, that intestinal microflora has a beneficial influence on host health. In the gut live about 10^{14} bacterial cells, including up to 2000 species of anaerobic bacteria. These intestinal bacteria play a key role in maintenance of health. The lactic acid bacteria in fermented milk products are capable to increase longevity and maintenance of vigor in humans, and consumption of fermented milk was closely related with longevity of Bulgarian peasants. The probiotics have been considered as live microbial supplements which beneficially affect the host by improving its intestinal microbial balance. The use of antibiotics is being discouraged in many countries of the world due to their residues in milk, meat and possible resistance in bacteria of human and animal origin. A probiotic is usually defined as a live commensal microorganism that, when consumed in adequate quantities, confers a health benefit to the host. Criteria for designating a commensal strain as a probiotic include a nonpathogenic, human origin; acid and bile resistance; survival of gastrointestinal transit; production of antimicrobial substances; and immune modulator activity. Recent studies have demonstrated that beneficial effects were achieved not only by live bacteria but also by heat-inactivated or gamma-irradiated not viable bacteria, isolated bacterial DNA or even probiotic-cultured media. More elaborate efforts to elucidate mechanism of probiotic action have recently made. Studies were able to demonstrate that probiotics can 'talk' to immune cells recognizing directly specific receptors or that are otherwise sensitive to probiotic-derived products. Many of the beneficial effects are the manifestation of this cross talk at molecular and cellular level.

Intestinal micro-flora has been first claimed to have a beneficial influence on human health over a century ago, and the ensuing research has by now soundly confirmed this concept. In the gut live about 10^{14} bacterial cells, including up to 2000 species dominated by anaerobic bacteria (Neish, 2009). Intestinal micro-flora benefits from a constant nutrient flow, a stable temperature and appropriate niches for various metabolic requirements provided by the intestinal environment. Likewise, the host benefits from the ability of the intestinal micro-flora to synthesize vitamin K, exert trophic effects on intestinal epithelial cells, salvage energy from unabsorbed food by producing short-chain fatty acids (SCFA), inhibit the growth of pathogens, sustain intestinal barrier integrity, maintain mucosal immune homeostasis and participate to the xenobiotic metabolism system (Ekberg *et al.*, 2005). Probiotics are beneficial microorganism or combination of such microorganisms, which would quickly establish in the gut to suppress colonization and growth of harmful bacteria. The term 'probiotics' is derived from Greek word '*pro bios*' meaning 'for life.' Probiotics improve the health and well being of animals, birds or human beings. In animal production systems, probiotics are frequently used for improving the health status as well as production performances, feed conversion efficiency and immune responses especially in cattle, swine and poultry.

1. History of probiotics

The idea that intestinal bacteria plays a key role in maintenance of health was originated by Elie Metchnikoff (1908) when he found that lactic acid bacteria in fermented milk products are capable to increase longevity and maintenance of vigor in humans, and noted that consumption of fermented milk was closely related with longevity of Bulgarian peasants (Fuller, 1992). Later, Lilly and Stillwell coined the term 'probiotics' in 1965 derived from Greek word '*pro bios*', meaning 'for life'. Probiotics as per World Health Organization (WHO) and Food and Agriculture Organization (FAO), are 'live microorganisms', which when supplemented in adequate amounts affect the host intestinal microbial ecosystem by providing a favorable balance between beneficial and harmful microbes in the intestinal microbial environment, help prevent the growth of pathogens resulting in improved health and prolonged life, which altogether confers a health benefit on the host. Probiotics may contain only one or a consortium of different bacterial species, and the mechanisms of action of different bacterial strains may differ. The commonly used microorganisms as probiotics are the strains of lactic acid producing bacteria which have specificity of adhering to the intestinal epithelium. Besides, other microbes *viz., Bacillus, Saccharomyces, Aspergillus oryzae* and many more along with their products are also classified as probiotics (Hajati and Rezaei, 2010). The importance of probiotics as an appropriate alternative has increased more than ever due to the possible hazards and risks of antibiotics in animal production.

As compared to antibiotics, probiotics as a feed additive have been acclaimed to be a safe growth promoter in animals (Sabatkova *et al.*, 2008; Bansal *et al.*, 2011). A variety of microbial species *viz.*, *Bacillus, Bifidobacterium, Enterococcus, Escherichia, Lactobacillus, Lactococcus, Streptococcus* and *Saccharomyces* and their undefined mixed cultures have been generally regarded as safe (GRAS) have been used as probiotics.

Criteria for designating a commensal strain as a probiotic include a nonpathogenic, human origin; acid and bile resistance; survival of gastrointestinal transit; production of antimicrobial substances; and immune modulator activity (Jijon *et al.*, 2004). The lactobacilli, streptococci belong to a large group of bacteria designated as LAB (Monterose and Floch, 2005). The LAB is described as Gram positive, nonsporing, anaerobic cocci or rods, and traditionally has become associated with the genera *Lactobacillus, Leuconostoc, Pediococcus* and *Streptococcus* (Aguire and Collins, 1993). This denomination emphasizes the commercially important aspect of their metabolism, since they produce lactic acid as the major end product during the fermentation of carbohydrates. The genus Bifidobacterium is unrelated to LAB phylogenetically, and the Bifidobacterium species use a unique metabolic pathway for sugar metabolism. However, they are often considered to be LAB and probiotics because of their documented health-promoting effects (Stiles and Holzapfel, 1997). Recent studies have demonstrated that beneficial effects were achieved not only by live bacteria but also by heat-inactivated or gamma-irradiated not viable bacteria, isolated bacterial DNA or even probiotic-cultured media (Dotan, and Rachmilewitz, 2005), presuming that probiotics can 'talk' to immune cells recognizing directly specific receptors or that are otherwise sensitive to probiotic-derived products (e.g., metabolites, cell wall components, DNA).

2. Characteristics of a good probiotics and probiotic criteria

Through various studies in the field of probiotics and variability encountered in the effects of the live microbial supplementation, following criteria have been decided for a good probiotics.

- Should be acid and bile resistance
- Be strain specific and possess high ability to multiply in the GIT
- Should not have any side effect; should neither be pathogenic nor toxic to the host
- Culture should have strong adhesion capability with the digestive tract of the host
- Be durable enough to duress of commercial manufacturing, processing and distribution
- Should have the ability to reduce pathogenic microorganisms

A probiotic should contain sufficient number of viable microorganisms which can withstand the regours of gut environment like pH variations, and higher bile salt tolerance. It should be stable in large numbers, and be non-pathogenic, non-toxic and preferably host-specific strain(s) of beneficial microbes. Probiotics must be having a short generation time. These should adhere to intestinal epithelium, have the ability to rapidly and efficiently colonize the intestine and exclude the pathogenic microbes, and be persistently present among gut micro flora. In addition to these they should have the ability to produce antimicrobial compounds and modulate immune responses. Probiotics need to be free of diffusible antibiotic resistant genes, be sufficiently stable while manufacturing, processing and storage, should not undergo recombination with pathogenic strains and should not produce any side effects. These should preferably able to survive processing be compatible with most feed additives and should have good sensory properties (Hajati and Rezaei, 2010).

3. Commonly used microbes as probiotics

Generally, live non pathogenic bacterial strains belonging to genus *Lactobacillus, Streptococcus, Bacillus* or *Enterococcus* and the yeast *Saccharomyces* are used in livestock and poultry. The strains of lactic acid producing bacteria, which have specificity of adhering to the intestinal epithelium, and *Aspergillus oryzae,* which confers beneficial effect on performance of poultry were frequently used in poultry industry. *Lactobacillus* and *Bifidobacterium* species have been used most exhaustively in humans. Since probiotics may also include fungi and yeast, besides bacteria, therefore the use of term 'Direct Fed Microbials' (DFM) has been suggested. The most commonly used probiotics contain one or a mixture of harmless microbes. The microbes generally considered for developing probiotic growth promoters are presented in Table 1. Most commonly used among these are *Lactobacillus*-based probiotics. Yeast and *Lactobacillus sporogens* are highly resistant to pelleting temperatures and storage at different environmental conditions.

4. Synbiotics

The term synbiotic is used 'when a product contains both probiotics and prebiotics' (Quigley and Quera 2006). For example, the symbiotic combination of a specific oligofructose-enriched inulin and *Lactobacillus rhamnosus* GG and *Bifidobacterium lactis* Bb12 for 12 weeks caused a 16% and 18% increase in the numbers of Lactobacillus and Bifidobacterium, respectively, and a 31% decrease in the numbers of *Clostridium perfringens* (Kolida and Gibson, 2007). Recent in vitro studies have confirmed that symbiotic was more effective than prebiotics or probiotics in modulating the gut microflora (Saulnier *et al.,* 2008).

Table 1 : Main probiotics used in commercial preparations

Types of bacteria	Names
Lactobacilli	*L. acidophilus, casei, delbrueckii subsp. bulgaricus, reuteri, brevis, cellobiosus, curvatus, fermentum, plantarum, paracasei, rhamnosus (GG), salivarius, gasseri, johnsonii, helviticus, farciminis, sporogenes, animalis*
Bacillus	*Bacillus subtilis, Bacillus coagulans,*
Cocci	*Pediococcus acidilactici, Pediococcus pentosaceus, Lactococcus* spp.,
Bifidobacteria	*B. bifidum, infantis, longum, thermophilum, adolescents, lactis, animalis, breve , Bacillus clausii, Bacillus oligonitrophilis*
Fungi	*Saccharomyces cerevisiae and s boulardii , Aspergillus oryzae,*
Others	*Streptococcus thermophilus, Streptococcus faecium, Streptococcus cristatus, Enterococcus faecium, Lactococcus lactis, Propionibacterium freudenreichii, Escherichia coli Nissle 1917, Pediococcus pantosaceus, Hawaiian spirulina, Torulopsis* spp.

Sources: Vegad (2004); Patterson and Burkholder (2003); Czerucka *et al.* (2007); Dhama *et al.*, (2008); Hajati and Rezaei (2010).

5. Mechanism of action

To explain exact mechanism of action of probiotics several hypotheses have been put forwarded (Ahmad, 2003; Ng *et al.*, 2009). Probiotics improve the microbial environment of a bird's intestinal tract by displacing harmful bacteria. Probiotics compete for receptors on the gut mucosa necessary for the attachment and proliferation of the microorganisms, thus rapid colonization of these beneficial microorganisms prevents the pathogens getting established in the gut. Its inhibitory action against pathogens is also mediated by competition for nutrients, the production of primary and secondary metabolites (antibacterial substances) and the stimulation of immunity (Bal *et al.*, 2004; Rowghani *et al.*, 2007). Probiotics include bacteria, fungi and yeasts as live microbes (Russell and Grimes, 2009) that may be supplemented in feed to improve host intestinal microbial balance and growth performance. There are two population of microorganisms that are found within the gastrointestinal (GI) tract of poultry: the autochthonous bacteria colonising gut by environmental exposure and normal feeding activities of the bird (Gusils *et al.*, 1999a; Shome et. al., 2002; Chichlowski *et al.*, 2007a), and allochthonous bacteria introduced as a dietary supplement through feed or drinking water as direct fed microbial (DFM) or probiotics (Patterson and Burkholder, 2003; Chichlowski, *et al.*, 2007c). These may be anaerobes and facultative anaerobes.

The selection of probiotic microorganisms and their administration and usage recommendations like preparation, dosages and condition of animals are very crucial for getting the desired health and production impact (Huang *et al.*, 2004). Numerous *in vivo* and *in vitro* studies have shown that the commensal intestinal microbiota inhibit pathogens but sometimes their disturbances may lead to susceptibility to infection; addition of probiotics may help fighting against establishment of such infection (Stavric and Kornegay, 1995; Rolfe, 2000). Thus the use of defined probiotic cultures in the poultry industry has recently become more common for obtaining better productivity and health benefits (Singh and Chauhan, 2002; Torres-Rodriguez *et al.*, 2007; Hajati and Rezaei, 2010).

6. Probiotic colonization in the gastrointestinal (GI) tract

In newly hatched chicks, the gut is sterile and starts acquiring microflora from environment from day one. Since pathogenic microbes may multiply faster than the beneficial bacteria, chicks may get infected at this time. The establishment of a healthy gut microflora helps in improving the gut environment and thwarts pathogens. However, as the days progress post-hatch, the micro flora stabilizes and attains balance between the 'favorable' and 'harmful'. As the balance between these two gets affected or influenced by the surrounding environment like infectious pressure or internal factors like stress, the concept of probiotics supplementation emerges which is highly helpful. Successful colonization of probiotics depends on the survival and stability of the microbial strain used their relationship with the host, dose and usage frequency, and host health, nutritional status, age, stress and genetics (Tortuero, 1973; Mason *et al.*, 2005). Measured as colony forming units (CFU), colonization increases at the beak and progresses distally to the colon (Simon *et al.*, 2004). The small intestine is a reservoir of various bacteria including anaerobes with population ranging from 10^4 to 10^8 CFU/ ml (Lactobacilli, Streptococci and Enterobacteria). The maximum bacterial population, accounting to 10^{10} to 10^{13} CFU/ml, has been recorded in the colon and caecum, (Heczko *et al.*, 2000). Some probiotic bacteria may be found attached to individual feed particles (such as starch granules) while others simply exist within the aqueous matrix of the digesta. An important microenvironment where microbes exist abundantly is the mucous blanket of the GI tract, covering the epithelial lining of intestinal villi and caecal and colonic surfaces, and which also acts as a source of nutrients for bacteria (Jacobsen *et al.*, 1999). Ability to adhere to the mucus and epithelial cell surfaces is one of the main selection criteria for a candidate probiotic (Rojas and Conway, 1996). The adhesion and colonization of probiotic bacteria occurring to the complexity of the intestinal enterocytes and the extensive interaction amongst cell types within the intestinal tract need further studies (Henriksson *et al.*, 1995). Lactobacilli, shed from epithelial surfaces or multiplying in ingested food, occur in all parts of digestive tract (Lonnermark, 2010).

6.1 Modulation of intestinal microflora composition and antibacterial activity

Probiotic can limit the role of bacterial pathogens in non alcoholic fatty liver disease (NAFLD) through at least two mechanisms: the exclusion or inhibition of invading bacteria and the production of antimicrobial factors. Nonspecific antimicrobial substances include short chain fatty acids (SCFAs) (Carr *et al.,* 2002), hydrogen peroxide (Eschenbach *et al.,* 1989) bacteriocins, bacteriocin-like inhibitory substances and bacteriophages (Tagg and Dierksen, 2003). The SCFA are produced during the anaerobic metabolism of carbohydrates, especially by strains of lactobacilli, and have an important role in decreasing pH and inhibiting the growth of a wide range of Gram negative pathogenic bacteria. The inhibition of microbial growth by organics may be due to the ability of these acids to pass across the cell membranes, dissociate in the more alkaline cell environment and acidify the cytoplasm (Terracciano *et al.,* 1987). Alternatively, fermentation acid dissociation in the more alkaline interior causes an accumulation of the anionic species, and this accumulation is dependent on the pH gradient (delta pH) across the membrane and may cause osmotic stress (Diez-Gonzalez and Russell, 1997). In microbial fermentor systems, pH modification may lead to a shift in the composition of the microbiota community (Walker *et al.,* 2005), limiting the populations of certain gut pathogens (Diez-Gonzalez *et al.,* 2007). Bacteriophages are highly specific and can be active against a single strain of bacteria. The two component lantibiotics, a class of bacteriocins produced by Gram-positive bacteria, such as *Lactococcus lactis,* are small antimicrobial peptides (Cotter *et al.,* 2005). These peptides have been found to be active at nanomolar concentrations to inhibit multidrug-resistant pathogens by targeting the lipid II component of the bacterial cell wall (Morgan *et al.,* 2005). Other non-lanthionine-containing bacteriocins are small antimicrobial peptides produced by lactobacilli. These peptides have a relatively narrow spectrum of activity and are mostly toxic to Gram-positive bacteria, including *Lactococcus, Streptococcus, Staphylococcus,* Listeria and mycobacteria. The main mechanisms of bacteriocin action are based on forming pores in the cytoplasmic membrane of sensitive bacteria and interfering with essential enzyme activities. In addition, several strains of Bifidobacteria have been found to produce bacteriocin-like compounds toxic to both Gram-positive and Gram-negative bacteria (Collado *et al.,* 2005). *Bifidobacteria* and lactobacilli can adhere to intestinal epithelial cells through surface-expressed proteins (Bernett *et al.,* 1993, 1994). In particular, *Lactobacillus casei* binds to extracellular matrix components, such as collagen, fibronectin or fibrinogen (Munoz-Provencio *et al.,* 2009). Moreover, apart from their antimicrobial effects, some secreted probiotic factors are also able to inhibit the binding of pathogenic bacteria to the specific receptors expressed on the epithelium surface (Bernett *et al.,* 1993). Several strains of lactobacilli and bifidobacteria are capable to compete with and displace pathogenic bacteria, including *Bacteroides vulgatus, Clostridium histolyticum, Clostridium difficile, Enterobacter aerogenes, Listeria monocytogenes, Staphylococcus aureus, Salmonella enterica, Yersinia enterocolitica* (Candella *et al.*, 2005), enterotoxigenic *Escherichia coli* (Collado *et al.*, 2007) and enteropathogenic *Escherichia coli* (Sherman *et al.*, 2005), even if the pathogens have attached to intestinal epithelial cells prior to probiotic treatment (Candella *et al.*, 2005).

In this context, recent studies regarding proteinase treatment and carbohydrate competition have confirmed that the probiotic binding to intestinal epithelial cells is mediated by lectin-like adhesion and proteinaceous cell surface components (Mukai *et al.*, 2004), which are the same receptors mediating pathogenic bacteria binding to intestinal epithelial cells. For example, lactobacilli and bifidobacteria establish mannose and Galβ1-3GalNAc-specific adhesions to attach to intestinal epithelial cells and mucus (Mukai *et al.*, 2004), competing with pathogens for lectin binding sites of glycoconjugate receptors for intestinal adherence.

Therefore, the capability of probiotics to improve gut ecology and microbial composition, in inhibiting pathogenic bacteria growth and/ or competing with and displacing pathogenic bacteria, is likely to prevent small intestinal bacteria overgrowth.

6.2 Interference with corum sensing signaling agents

From the recent research it has been concluded that the quorum sensing regulate the virulence expression in probiotics which may interfere with the signaling system avoiding the onset of virulence in the pathogenic bacteria (Vila *et al.*, 2010). Bacteria communicate with each other as well as with their surrounding environment through chemical signaling molecules called autoinducers (Vila *et al.*, 2010). This phenomenon is called quorum sensing. The probiotics bacteria *Lactobacillus, Bifidobacterium* and *B. cereus* strains degrade the autoinducers of the pathogenic bacteria by enzymatic secretion or production of autoinducer anatagonists which renders the quorum sensing bacteria mute and deaf. Medllin-Pena *et al.* (2007) demonstrated that Lactobacillus acidophilus secretes a molecule that inhibits quorum sensing signaling or directly interacts with bacterial transcription of *E. coli* 0157 gene, involved in colonization and thus, bacterial toxicity is thwarted. Medina-Martinez *et al.* (2007) and Cerda-Cuellar *et al.* (2009) recorded similar conclusions *using B. cereus* and *B. toyoi* probiotics bacteria.

6.3 Competitive exclusion

The stress or pathogenic microbes existing in any animal or poultry rearing unit create an imbalance in the intestinal microflora by impairing defense mechanisms. This gives an opportunity to proliferation of pathogens, leading to physiological disturbances like diarrhea, loss of appetite, improper digestion and poor absorption of nutrients in host (Dhama *et al.*, 2008). The disturbances in balance of natural microflora results in proliferation of harmful bacteria which in turn affect production performance and immuno-competence, causing heavy economic loss to poultry producers (Vegad, 2004). Application of probiotic may help to maintain a healthy balance of microbes and help maintain health and productivity. Probiotics compete with harmful bacteria/ pathogens for intestinal adhesion receptors that are necessary for the attachment and proliferation of the microorganisms. Thus rapid colonization of probiotics blocks the mucosal sites for the pathogen attachment and getting established in the gut. Another mechanism by which pathogen exclusion is attained is by way of secretion of antibacterial substances like bacteriocins, lactocin, lactocidin, acidolin, acidophilin, nisin, reuterin, organic acids (lactic and acetic acid), lactoferrin, hydrogen peroxide and lactoperoxidase which inhibit pathogenic microbes. By releasing anti-enterotoxin substances (acidolin, acidophilin and lactin), probiotics help neutralize enterotoxins released by pathogenic bacteria. Probiotics are also proved to bind mycotoxins present in feed.

Probiotics also make nutrients non-available to pathogens, by becoming successful colonizers in the intestine that efficiently utilize the available substrates. By antagonistic action towards ammonifying bacteria and reducing urease activity, probiotics decreases ammonia formation in litter and thus prevents keratoconjunctivitis which is a common problem as a result of excess ammonia in litter. Recently, an increased apoptosis has been suggested to be a mechanism by which the probiotic culture reduces Salmonella infection (Higgins *et al.*, 2011). Thus the intestinal microbiota, epithelium, and immune system provide passive and active resistance to enteric pathogens in birds (Patterson and Burkholder, 2003; Czerucka *et al.*, 2007; Dhama *et al.*, 2008; Hajati and Rezaei, 2010).

The exact mechanism of action associated with the beneficial effects of probiotics is still unclear (Chichlowski *et al.*, 2007). The single most frequently described mechanism is "competitive exclusion" or "bacterial antagonism" (Mack *et al.*, 1999) which refers to the physical blocking of opportunistic pathogen colonization and altering the environmental niches within the intestinal tract (such as intestinal villus and colonic crypts which are favorite sites of enteric pathogens) by the probiotics bacteria (Duggan *et al.*, 2002). Probiotic organisms compete with pathogens for nutrients thus preventing them from acquiring energy to grow and function in the gut environment (Cummings and Macfarlane, 1997). A variety of primary and secondary metabolites *viz.*, organic acid, volatile fatty acid (VFA) and lactic acid (Gibson, 1999) lower the gut pH that is detrimental for the survival of pathogenic bacteria such as *E. coli* and *Salmonella* (Marteau *et al.*, 2004). Antimicrobial molecules, collectively known as bacteriocins, kill pathogenic bacteria or impede their colonization, while other nonbacteriocin compounds also inhibit the growth of pathogens (Madsen *et al.*, 2001; Chichlowski, 2007). Piperidine inhibits the binding and internalisation of *Salmonella* and *Shigella* to intestinal epithelial cells *in vitro* (Gusils *et al.*, 2003).

Probiotic supplementation significantly enhances the intestinal immunity of birds and plays a vital role in fighting against infectious diseases and providing resistance especially to enteric bacterial infections and the coccidian parasites. In poultry, probiotics have been reported to inhibit pathogens such as *Staphylococcus aureus*, *E. coli*, *Salmonella* Enteritidis, *S.* Typhimurium, *Clostridium perfringens*, *Listeria monocytogenes*, *Campylobacter jejuni*, *Yersinia enterocolitica*, *Candida albicans* and coccidian (*Eimeria sp.*). (Singh and Chauhan, 2002; Patterson and Burkholder, 2003; Vegad, 2004; Dalloul *et al.*, 2005, Dhama *et al.*, 2008). Lactobacilli, isolated from chicken gastrointestinal tract, were found having potential probiotics properties and inhibitory activity against enteropathogenic bacteria like *Salmonella*, *E. coli* and *Clostridium perfringens*. *Pediococcus*, *Lactobacillus* and *Saccharomyces* strains significantly lowered incidences of coccidiosis (Dalloul *et al.*, 2005). Few selected probiotic organisms are able to reduce idiopathic diarrhea in commercial turkey brooding houses and *Salmonella* colonisation in turkeys and broilers. For safety from food-borne pathogens like *Salmonella*, *Campylobacters*, *Escherichia* and *Listeria*, probiotics need to be paid due attention.

6.4 Enhancing digestion and nutrient utilization

Probiotics help improving digestion, nutrient metabolism and utilization of nutrients by offering digestible proteins, vitamins, enzymes and other important co-factors and by decreasing gut pH by production of lactic acids (Senani *et al.*, 1997, 2000 and 2004; Saha *et al.*, 1998, 1999). As *'live enzyme factory'* (amylase, protease, lipase) enhances digestion and absorption of carbohydrates, proteins and fats, which also increases the feed conversion efficiency. Probiotics help in metabolism of minerals and synthesis of vitamins (Biotin, Vitamin-B1, B2, B12 and K), which are responsible for proper growth and metabolism. The facultative anaerobes (*Bifidobacterium* and *Ljptobacillus*) included in probiotics bacterial consortium reduce the redox potential in the gut and render the environment suitable for obligate anaerobes (Chichlowski, 2007). An increase in digestibility of dry matter is closely related to enzymes released by yeast (Lee *et al.*, 2006). The effect of *Aspergillus oryzae* on macronutrient metabolism in laying hens might be of practical relevance (Han *et al.*, 1999). It is imperative to evaluate the interaction between indigenous digestive enzymes and the microbial metabolites used as probiotics, to better understand the mechanism of action with respect to improvement in the digestion process.

6.5 Modification of intestinal epithelial permeability and function

Probiotics are able to improve the nonspecific intestinal barrier defense mechanism, modulating tight junctional protein mucins and stimulating their production. These effects limit small intestinal bacterial overgrowth and bacterial translocation. Both events are observed in humans and in animal models and are responsible for a reduced endotoxemia (Ramakrishna, 2009). The mucus layer covering the gastrointestinal mucosa is considered the first line of defense against mechanical, chemical or microbiological aggressions arising from the luminal contents. Indeed, the break of the mucus barrier in an inflamed colon has been shown to allow bacterial adherence to the epithelial tissue (Swidsinski *et al.*, 2007), and the removal of the mucus layer favors the penetration of high molecular weight probes in the mucosa (Khan *et al.*, 1999). It has been demonstrated that lactobacilli up-regulate the MUC2 and MUC3 mucins and inhibit attachment of entero-hemorrhagic *Escherichia coli in vitro* (Kim *et al.*, 2008) and that a probiotic mixture of lactobacilli and bifidobacteria increase the secretion of mucin, stimulating MUC2 gene expression in the rat colon in vivo (Caballero-Franco *et al.*, 2007). Probiotics stimulate the production of SCFAs (Sakata *et al.*, 2003)., which, in turn, are able to modulate intestinal permeability as demonstrated under several conditions, including antibiotic-associated colitis, inflammatory bowel disease, colon cancer and hepatic encephalopathy. Probiotic administration may potentially reduce bacterial metabolites, which may be toxic to the intestinal epithelium, for instance hydrogen sulfide and extracellular superoxide (Attene-Ramos *et al.*, 2007). The *Lactobacillus GG, Bifidobacterium infantis, Bifidobacterium lactis* and *Escherichia coli* Nissle 1917, increase tight junction integrity, preventing tight junction disruption. The biochemical pathways mediating the probiotic effect on tight junction functions include protein kinase C and mitogen-activated protein kinase pathways, and involve both the redistribution and altered expression of the tight junction proteins occludin, ZO-1 and ZO-2, and claudins 1, 2, 3 and 4 (Johnson-Henry *et al.*, 2008; Zyrek *et al.*, 2007).

6.6 Immune system modulation by probiotics

Among the beneficial effects of probiotics use, probiotics has been reported to tweek the immune system *viz.*, stimulation of both humoral and cell mediated immunity through enhanced production of natural interferons/ cytokines, increased macrophage, lymphocyte and natural killer (NK) cell activity, up regulated oxidative burst in heterophils, and increased immunoglobulin (IgG, IgM and IgA) (Koenen *et al.*, 2004). The administration of probiotics bacteria leads to an increase in the levels of pathogen-specific

IgA (Cross, 2006), and IgA responses are enhanced in formula-fed infants supplemented with probiotics as compared with infants receiving placebo (Rautava *et al.,* 2006). Noteworthy is the induction of IgA in the gut being heavily dependent on TGF-β, and also closely involved in the maturation of regulatory T cells (Fantini *et al.,* 2004). In agreement with these studies, a recent randomized, double-blind, placebo-controlled trial has demonstrated that the administration of two probiotic bacteria, Lactobacillus gasseri CECT5714 and *Lactobacillus coryniformis,* increased the proportion and activity of phagocytic and NKT cells, as well as the levels of IgA in healthy adults (Sheikh *et al.,* 2001).

Probiotics produce a gut-stabilizing effect; and immune regulation, particularly through balanced control of pro-inflammatory and anti-inflammatory cytokines. Probiotics increases the number of lymphocytes and lymphoid cells in lamina propria and intra-epithelial lymphocytes (IEL) in the small intestine and is found to inhibit the growth of infectious organisms. Commensal bacteria can modulate the immune system at both local and systemic levels. Signals mediated by these bacteria are essential for optimal mucosal and immune development, and to maintain or restore gut integrity (Fukata *et al.,* 2005). In the intestinal tract, immunocytes, such as enterocytes, M cells and dendritic cells (DCs), are constantly responding to intestinal bacteria. These cells express pattern recognition receptors, such as toll like receptors (TLRs), that engage bacterial signals (LPS, lipotechoic acid, bacterial DNA and flagellin) and contribute to the activation of transcription factors and pro-inflammatory cascade. Immune engagement and systemic immunologic changes are associated with oral consumption of probiotics (McCarthy *et al.,* 2003), which share the same host–microbial signaling pathways of commensal microbiota. In the intestine, probiotic bacteria are internalized by M cells to interact with DCs and follicle-associated epithelial cells, initiating responses mediated by macrophages and T and B lymphocytes (Winkler *et al.,* 2007).

Dendritic cells initiate immune responses in vivo by presenting antigens to T cells and influence polarization of T-cell responses (Th1, Th2, Th3 or regulatory T cells) through secretion of immuno-regulatory cytokines.

Moreover, DCs contribute to oral tolerance induction by generating regulatory T cells and IgA-producing B cells through production of cytokines, such as IL-10 and transforming growth factor (TGF)-β (Iwasaki and Kelsall, (1999). Regulatory T cells produce high levels of IL-10 and suppress the proliferation of effecter T cells in an IL-10-dependent manner. Different strains of lactobacilli and other probiotic bacteria can modulate DCs function modulating cell maturation and the expression of regulatory cytokines, such as IL-10 (Christensen *et al.,* 2002; Hart *et al.,* 2004). DCs from different lymphoid compartments exhibit divergent cytokine responses to probiotic and pathogenic bacteria (O'Mahony *et al.,* 2006). Some strains of probiotic bacteria, such as *Lactobacillus casei* or *Lactobacillus reuteri,* but not *Lactobacillus plantarum,* can promote DCs to induce tolerance driving the development of regulatory T cells (Mohamadzadeh *et al.,* 2005). Similarly, VSL#3 can ameliorate Th1 cell-mediated murine colitis, by restoring cytokine balance through the induction of IL-10- and TGF-β-bearing regulatory T cells (Di Giacinto *et al.,* 2005). Probiotics can interact either directly with DCs or indirectly, via the action of M cells. Very recently, the ability of three lactobacilli strains (plantarum, LGG and paracasei B21060) to activate DCs has been evaluated. Lactobacillus paracasei B21060 has been identified as the more immunomodulatory among the three strains, being able to inhibit the inflammatory potential of pathogenic Salmonella and to protect against experimental colitis (Mileti *et al.,* 2009).

Intestinal enterocytes monitor surface area of epithelial cells for the presence of potential pathogens, as a result there is a constant interaction amongst different cell types, including members of the innate and adaptive immune systems and bacteria in the gut lumen, epithelium or lamina propria (Mueller and Macpherson 2006; Kim *et al.,* 2011).

Probiotics may influence the inflammatory response elicited by pathogens by declining specific signaling pathways including those utilizing MAP kinase and *NFkappa-beta* pathways for activation of immune response in microflora or when cells are infected by a variety of pathogens (Yurong *et al.,* 2005; Chichlowski, 2007). Modulation of the expression of various pro- and anti-inflammatory cytokines is one suggested mechanism. The information in this regard is limited in chickens in comparison to mammals.

The use of probiotics increases the amount of IgA found in the lumen, the numbers of IgA, IgM and IgG producing cells as well as the number of T cells in the cecal tonsils (Yurong *et al.,* 2005). Oral administration of probiotics increases natural antibodies against different antigens in both the gut and the serum (Haghighi *et al.,* 2005). An increased antigen-specific antibody response following probiotic treatment and Newcastle disease vaccination has been documented (Zulkifli *et al.,* 2000). Apart from the potential effects on systemic immunity regarding enhancement of antibody responses, probiotic supplementation have been found to significantly increase the oxidative burst and degranulation of heterophils (Farnell *et al.,* 2006). The inclusion of probiotics at 100 to 150 mg/ kg diet did not show any impact on carcass like dressing percent or weight of liver, heart, gizzard, giblet and abdominal fat (Kannan *et al.,* 2005), however, dietary supplementation of *L. sporogenes* enhanced the immune status against "Ranikhet" disease in broilers at 28 days of post vaccination.

There is still much to understand about how these organisms interact with the host or the factors which decide their efficacy. Haghighi *et al.,* (2005) indicated that difference in the antigen used to test the immune stimulatory responses of probiotics could affect the significance of the results. Koenen *et al.,* (2004) and Janardhana *et al.,* (2009) described that the same strain of bacteria had different effects on the gastrointestinal tract and immune system of birds depending on their genetics and age, suggesting that the different types of birds (layer versus broiler) may require different doses of probiotics at different intervals. Lactobacilli can have a positive effect on humoral and cellular immune responses, but the strain to be used and effective doses to be administered need to be optimized (Koenen *et al.,* 2004). A commercial Lactobacillus-based probiotic clearly underlined its positive impact on cellular immune responses to *Eimeria sp.,* as assessed by the cytokine and oocyst production, in infected broilers (Dalloul *et al.,* 2005). A synbiotic consisting of *L. casei* and dextran elicited an enhanced humoral immune response, which can be useful in developing an oral immuno-adjuvant in birds to protect against infectious diseases (Ogawa *et al.,* 2006).

7. Probiotics as growth promoter

As a group of growth promoters, the addition of probiotics to the diet of livestock (especially cattle and swine) and poultry has been found to improve growth performance, increase feed conversion efficiency and improve immune responses (Mountzouris *et al.,* 2007; Rowghani *et al.,* 2007; Awad *et al.,* 2009; Saadia *et al.,* 2010; Bansal *et al.,* 2011). Many studies undertaken to test the effect of probiotics on the production efficiency of broiler chickens have shown positive response (Senani *et al.,* 2004; Saha *et al.,* 1999, Shome *et al.,* 2000 and O'Dea *et al.,* 2006). Huang *et al.,* (2004) has also reported that some inactivated probiotics, similar to live ones has also been shown to have the beneficial effects on production performance and immune response in broiler chickens. A multispecies and chicken-specific probiotic preparation in fluid form, consisting of seven *Lactobacillus* species isolated from the digestive tract of chickens was recently developed for application in broiler production (Timmerman *et al.,* 2006). The *Lactobacillus* strains showed modulating effects on the immune system of layer and broiler chickens.

8. Benefits of use

Specifically, the use of probiotics is recommended in the newly hatched chicks, stressful conditions, during antibiotic therapy, and as alternatives to antibiotic growth promoters. These could prevent diseases like early chick mortality, gastro-intestinal disturbances like scouring, loss of appetite, improper digestion and poor absorption of nutrients, pathogenic/infectious conditions by fighting against pathogenic microbes especially the enteric pathogens.

Thus these can alleviate reduced production performance and prevent heavy economic loss to the poultry producers (Anandakumar and Lakshminarayan, 1997; Patterson and Burkholder, 2003).

Probiotics improves intestinal microbial balance, absorption of nutrients, increases digestibility, improves feed conversion and growth rate, efficiency inhibits growth of pathogenic microbes and especially prevents digestive disorders due to bacterial invasions, checks digestive upsets and diarrhea, significantly help lowering of chick mortality, improves egg production and quality, fertility and hatchability of eggs, egg albumen quality and reduces yolk cholesterol concentration; nullifies effects of enterotoxins, helps in quicker detoxification of mycotoxins, reduces ammonia in faecal contents, stimulates immunity and improves disease resistance, thus making birds less vulnerable to diseases; reduces stress after vaccination, antibiotic therapy, change of accommodation, transportation, change of feed *etc.* synthesise B-vitamins; strengthens skeletal system of birds, reduces carcass contamination, can augment effects of drugs and vaccines, helps to maintain healthy gastrointestinal tract after antibiotic therapy (Fuller, 2001). Antibiotics are often used as feed additives to suppress or eliminate harmful organisms in the intestine, and to improve growth, feed efficiency and production performances. However, illegitimate and prolific use of sub-therapeutic levels of antibiotics may result in residues in poultry products and the development of drug resistant microorganisms; which calls for the use of probiotics (Dhama *et al.,* 2008; Yang *et al.,* 2009). Also the antibiotics administered in disease conditions not only kill the targeted pathogenic bacteria but also destroy the general microflora of host which sometimes result in bacterial dysbiosis leading to diarrhea and secondary infection that are even difficult to treat (Sulakvelidze *et al.,* 2001). Using probiotics in conjunction with antibiotics maintains the required intestinal balance of microflora and reduces diarrhea, without affecting the efficacy of antibiotics. Failure of antibiotics to effectively treat human diseases has led the European Union to ban the use of low doses of antibiotics in animal feeds and encouraged government officials to, seriously consider restricting the use of antibiotics in animal production in the United States. Probiotics must be given right from 1 day old on a regular basis for optimum benefits. Since under intensive rearing system, the birds are always under stress and amidst of high infectious pressure, so, it would be better to supplement probiotics continuously. It is healthier if given before the infection challenge occurs to the bird.

During periods of stress it is necessary to give booster doses. Probiotics must follow after any antibiotic therapy for balanced beneficial results, rejuvenating the healthy microflora. Probiotics are available commonly as powder/liquid feed supplements. Commercial probiotics available in the market may comprise of single strain of yeast or/ and a single strain of bacteria or a mixture of these. The number of organisms in an ideal multi-strain probiotics should be in sufficient number, generally in an order of 10^7 to 10^9 or even higher $1x10^9$ to 2×10^{11} CFU guaranteed levels of beneficial microbes like *Lactobacillus acidophilus, L. casei, L. bulgaricus, Streptococcus faecium, Aspergillus oryzae, Sacchromyces cerevisiae etc.* in one kg pack and the mixing ratio for the poultry flocks should be as directed by the manufacturer. Usually the dose for chicks/ layers/broilers is 0.5-1 kg/ tonne of feed and for breeders it is 1 kg/ tonne of feed. *Bacilli.* Probiotics should be given in feed or water by the oral route; and need be applied via drinking water or as a top dressing in case of already pelleted feed (Vegad, 2004; Dhama and Singh, 2010).

9. Adverse effect of probiotics

Probiotics are generally regarded as safe. Side effects are rarely reported and generally amount to little more than flatulence or changes in bowel habits. A review outlining the safety of current probiotic compounds has been published recently (Borillo *et al.,* 2003). The use of probiotics in immune-compromised or in critical ill patients should be carefully evaluated to limit the risk of endocarditis or sepsis. However, cases of infection caused by lactobacilli and bifidobacteria are extremely rare and are estimated to occur in approximately 0.05–0.4% of all cases of infective endocarditis and bacteremia (Borillo *et al.,* 2003). One important clinical characteristic of lactobacilli is their resistance to antibiotic vancomycin, empirically used against Gram-negative bacteremia. Lactobacilli are considered as emerging pathogens in high-risk patients with neutropenia induced by chemotherapy (Cooper *et al.,* 1998), in neonates submitted to surgery on a count of cardiovascular disorders in pediatric patients submitted to gastrojejunostomy (Land *et al.,* , 2005). No increase in bacteremia caused by *Lactobacillus* species was seen in Finland over the period of 1990–2000 despite an increased consumption of *Lactobacillus rhamnosus* GG. A study on a long-term consumption of *Bifidobacterium lactis* and *Streptococcus thermophilus* supplemented formula in children aged less than two years showed that the product was well tolerated (Saavadra *et al.,* 2004). Complications of treatment with probiotics have been observed in patients who are immune-compromised or in the intensive care setting. *Saccharomyces cerevisiae* fungemia (Riquelme *et al.,* 2003) and *Lactobacillus* bacteremia (Land *et al.,* 2005) have been reported in patients with severe underlying illnesses. Nevertheless, case reports have identified fungemia in two immune-suppressed patients (Riquelme *et al.,* 2003) and exacerbation of diarrhea in two patients with ulcerative colitis who consumed *S. boulardii* (Candelli *et al.,* 2003).

Conclusions

The study of intestinal microbiota composition and role in different pathological conditions helps in understanding on the potential use of probiotics in liver diseases, from simple steatosis to cirrhosis. What is now clear is that not all probiotics may have the same effect. High-quality preclinical studies and few randomized controlled trials support the therapeutic use of probiotics in liver diseases. The rationale of the use of mixtures of bacteria is based on the possible combination of different mechanisms of action of individual strains. Additional carefully designed, mechanistic-based laboratory and clinical studies need to be undertaken to provide scientific evidence for the efficacy of probiotics alone or in appropriate synergistic combination between strains or with some prebiotics.

Probiotics are currently used in dairy products as a means to improve health. In livestock and poultry industry they have a greater role in promoting health, growth and reduce enteric pathogens and to provide a antibiotic residue free milk meat and egg for human consumption.. From a practical point of view, knowledge of the potentials and application of probiotics to optimize the balance of microflora in gut, act as growth promoters, immuno-stimulants, and inhibiting pathogenic microbes is essential. Probiotics provide a cost-effective alternative to antibiotic growth promoters and are generally regarded as safe without any reported side effects.

Through probiotics supplementation, the gut environment of the host is altered resulting in more favorable gut microbiome responsible for developing natural resistance and a myriad of other benefits. The area of probiotic research is exciting opportunity to have concerted and focused effort to search novel probiotics and to elucidate their beneficial effects and mechanism of action.

References

Aguirre M., Collins M.D. (1993). Lactic acid bacteria and human clinical infection. *Journal of Applied Bacteriology* **75:** 95-107.

Ahmad F.E. (2003). Genetically modified probiotics in foods. *Trends in Biotechnology* **21:** 491-497.

Anandakumar K., Lakshminarayan N.G. (1997). Probiotics: Importance in poultry production. *Poultry Advisor*. April Issue, pp: 7-9.

Attene-Ramos M.S., Wagner E.D., Gaskins H.R., Plewa M.J. (2007). Hydrogen sulfide induces direct radical-associated DNA damage. *Molecular Cancer Research* **5:** 455-459.

Awad W.A., Ghareeb K., Abdel-Raheem S., Böhm J. (2009). Effects of dietary inclusion of probiotics and synbiotic on growth performance, organ weights, and intestinal histomorphology of broiler chickens. *Poultry Science* **88:** 49-56.

Bal A.P., Ouyang Q., Zhang W., Wang C.H., Li S.F. (2004). Probiotics inhibit TNF-α-induced interlukin- 8 secretion of HT29 cells. *World Journal of Gastroenterology* **10:** 455-457.

Bansal G.R., Singh V.P., Sachan N. (2011). Effect of probiotic supplementation on the performance of broilers. *Asian Journal of Animal Science* **5:** 277-284.

Bernet M.F., Brassart D., Neeser J.R., Servin A.L. (1993). Adhesion of human bifido-bacterial strains to cultured human intestinal epithelial cells and inhibition of enteropathogen- cell interactions. *Applied Environmental Microbiology* **59:** 4121-4128.

Bernet M.F., Brassart D., Neeser J.R., Servin A.L.(1994) Lactobacillus acidophilus LA 1 binds to cultured human intestinal cell lines and inhibits cell attachment and cell invasion by enterovirulent bacteria. *Gut* **35:** 483-589.

Borriello S.P., Hammes W.P., Holzapfel W., Marteau P., Schrezenmeir J., Vaara M. (2003). Safety of probiotics that contain lactobacilli or bifidobacteria. *Clinical Infection and Diseases* **36:** 775-780.

Caballero-Franco C., Keller K., De Simone C., Chadee K. (2007). The VSL#3 probiotic formula induces mucin gene expression and secretion in colonic epithelial cells. *American Journal of Physiology- Gastrointestinal and Liver Physiology* **292:** G315-322.

Candela M., Seibold G., Vitali B., Lachenmaier S., Eikmanns B.J., Brigidi P. (2005). Real-time PCR quantification of bacterial adhesion to Caco-2 cells: competition between bifido-bacteria and enteropathogens. *Research in Microbiology* **156:** 887-895.

Candelli M., Nista E.C., Nestola M., Armuzzi A., Silveri N.G., Gasbarrini G. (2003). *Saccharomyces cerevisiae*-associated diarrhea in an immunocompetent patient with ulcerative colitis. *Journal of Clinical Gastroenterology* **36:** 39-40.

Carr F.J., Chill D., Maida N. (2002). The lactic acid bacteria: a literature survey. *Critical Review on Microbiology* **28:** 281-370.

Cerda-Cueliar M., Badiola I., Castillo M. (2009). *In vitro* degradation of N-acyl-L-homoserine lactones by *Bacillus cereus* var toyoi. In: *Proc. 9th International Symposium on "Digestive physiology of pigs"*, May 20-22, Montbrio del Camp, Costa Daurada, Spain, pp 2-36.

Chichlowski M, Croom J., McBride B. W., Daniel L., Davis G. and Koci M. D. (2007a). Direct-fed Microbial primalac and salinomycin modulate whole-body and intestinal oxygen consumption and intestinal mucosal cytokine production in the broiler chick. *Poultry Science* **86:** 1100-1106.

Chichlowski M., Croom J., Edens F.W., McBride B.W., Qiu R., Chiang C.C., Daniel L.R., Havenstein G.B., Koci M.D. (2007c). Microarchitecture and spatial relationship between bacteria and ileal, cecal and colonic, primalac and salinomycin. *Poultry Science* **86:** 1121-1132.

Christensen H.R., Frokiaer H., Pestka J.J. (2002). Lactobacilli differentially modulate expression of cytokines and maturation surface markers in murine dendritic cells. *Journal of Immunology* **168:** 171-178.

Collado M.C., Hernandez M., Sanz Y. (2005). Production of bacteriocin-like inhibitory compounds by human fecal Bifidobacterium strains. *Journal of Food Protection* **68:** 1034-1040.

Collado M.C., Meriluoto J., Salminen S. (2007). Role of commercial probiotic strains against human pathogen adhesion to intestinal mucus. *Letters in Applied Microbiology* **45:** 454-460.

Cooper C.D., Vincent A., Greene J.N., Sandin R.L., Cobian L. (1998). Lactobacillus bacteremia in febrile neutropenic patients in a cancer hospital. *Clinical Infection and Diseases* **26:** 1247-1248.

Cross M.L. (2006). Microbes versus microbes: immune signals generated by probiotic lactobacilli and their role in protection against microbial pathogens. *FEMS Immunology and Medical Microbiology* **34:** 245-253.

Dalloul R.A., Lillehoj H.S., Tamim N.M., Shellem T.A., Doerr J.A. (2005). Induction of local protective immunity to *Eimeria acervulina* by a *Lactobacillus*based probiotic. *Comparative Immunology Microbiology and Infectious Diseases* **28:** 351-361.

Dhama, K., Mahendran M., Tomar S., Chauhan R.S. (2008). Beneficial effects of probiotics and prebiotics in livestock and poultry: the current perspectives. *Intas Polivet* **9:** 1-13.

Di Giacinto C., Marinaro M., Sanchez M., Strober W., Boirivant M. (2005). Probiotics ameliorate recurrent Th1-mediated murine colitis by inducing IL-10 and IL-10-dependent TGF-beta-bearing regulatory cells. *Journal of Immunology* **174:** 3237-3246.

Diez-Gonzalez F., Belina D., Labuza T.P., Pal A. (2007). Modeling the growth of Listeria monocytogenes based on a time to detect model in culture media and frankfurters. *International Journal of Food Microbiology* **113:** 277-283.

Dotan I., Rachmilewitz D. (2005) Probiotics in inflammatory bowel disease: possible mechanisms of action. *Current Opinion in Gastroenterology* **21:** 426-430.

Eckburg P.B., Bik E.M., Bernstein C.N., Purdom E., Dethlefsen L., Sargent M.(2005). Diversity of the human intestinal microbial flora. *Science* **308:** 1635-1638.

Eschenbach D.A., Davick P.R., Williams B.L., Klebanoff S.J., Young-Smith K., Critchlow C.M. (1989). Prevalence of hydrogen peroxide-producing Lactobacillus species in normal women and women with bacterial vaginosis. *Journal of Clinical Microbiology* **27:** 251-256.

Fantini M.C., Becker C., Monteleone G., Pallone F., Galle P.R., Neurath M.F. (2004). Cutting edge: TGF-beta induces a regulatory phenotype in CD4+CD25- T cells through Foxp3 induction and down-regulation of Smad7. *Journal of Immunology* **172:** 5149-5153.

Farnell M.B, Donoghue A.M., Solis de los Santos F., Blore P.J., Hargis B.M., Tellez G., Donoghue D.J. (2006). Upregulation of oxidative burst and degranulation in chicken heterophils stimulated with probiotic bacteria. *Poultry Science* **85:** 1900-1906.

Fukata M., Michelsen K.S., Eri, R., Thomas L.S., Hu B., Lukasek K. (2005). Toll-like receptor-4 is required for intestinal response to epithelial injury and limiting bacterial translocation in a murine model of acute colitis. *American Journal of Physiology Gastrointestinal & Liver Physiology* **288:** G1055-1065.

Fuller R. (1992). History and development of probiotics. In: *Probiotic, the scientific basis.* (R. Fuller, ed), Chapman and Hall, London, pp 1-8.

Gaskins H.R. (2003). The commensal microbiota and developments of mucosal defense in the mammalian intestine. 9th International Synposium on Digestive Physiology in pigs (OB Ronald, eg, University of Alberta, Banff, Canada, May 14-18, pp. 57-71.

Gusils C., Perez C.A., Gonzalez S., Oliver G. (1999a). Lactobacilli isolated from chicken intestines: potential use as probiotics. *Journal of Food Protection* **62:** 252-256.

Haghighi H.R., Gong J.H., Gyles C.L., Hayes M.A., Sanei B., Parvizi P., Gisavi H., Chambers J.R., Sharif S. (2005). Modulation of antibody-mediated immune response by probiotics in chickens. *Clinical and Diagnostic Laboratory Immunology* **12:** 1387-1392.

Han S.W., Lee K.W., Lec B.D., Sung C.G. (1999). Effect of feeding *Aspergillus oryzae* cultare on fecal microflora, egg qualities and nutrient metabolizabilities in laying hens. *Asian Australasian Journal of Animal Science* **12:** 417-421.

Hajati H., Rezaei M. (2010). The application of probiotics in poultry production. *International Journal of Poultry Science* **9:** 298-304.

Hart A.L., Lammers K., Brigidi P., Vitali B., Rizzello F., Gionchetti P. (2004). Modulation of human dendritic cell phenotype and function by probiotic bacteria. *Gut* **53:** 1602-1609.

Heczko U., Abe A., Finlay,B.B. (2000). Segmented filamentous bacteria prevent colonization of enteropathogenic *Escherichia coli* O103 in rabbits. *Journal of Infection and Disease* **181:** 1027-1033.

Henriksson A., Andre L., Conway P.L. (1995). Distribution of lactobacilli in the porcine gastrointestinal tract. *FEMS Microbiology and Ecology* **16:** 55-60.

Huang M.K., Choi Y.J., Houde R., Lee J.W., Lee B., Zhao X. (2004). Effects of Lactobacilli and an acidophilic fungus on the production performance and immune responses in broiler chickens. *Poultry Science* **83:** 788-795.

Iaconoa A., Rasoa G.M., Cananib R.B., Calignanoa A., Melia R. (2011). Probiotics as an emerging therapeutic strategy to treat NAFLD: focus on molecular and biochemical mechanisms. *Journal of Nutritional Biochemistry* **22:** 699-711.

Iwasaki A., Kelsall B.L. (1999). Freshly isolated Peyer's patch, but not spleen, dendritic cells produce interleukin 10 and induce the differentiation of T helper type 2 cells. *Journal of Experimental Medicine* **190:** 229-239.

Jacobsen C.N., Rosenfeldt Nielsen V., Hayford A.E., Moller P.L., Michaelsen K.F., Parregaard A., Sandstrom B., Tvede M., Jakobsen M. (1999). Screening of probiotic activities of forty-seven strains of *Lactobacillus* spp. by *in vitro* techniques and evaluation of the colonization ability of five selected strains in humans. *Applied Environmental Microbiology* **65:** 4949-4956.

Janardhana V, Broadway M.M, Bruce M.P., Lowenthal J.W., Geier M.S., Hughes R.J., Bean A.G. (2009). Prebiotics modulate immune responses in the gut associated lymphoid tissue of chickens. *Journal of Nutrition* **139:** 1404-1409.

Jijon H., Backer J., Diaz H., Yeung H., Thiel D., McKaigney C. (2004) DNA from probiotics bacteria modulates murine and human epithelial and immune function. *Gastroenterology* **126:** 1358-1373.

Johnson-Henry K.C., Donato K.A., Shen-Tu G., Gordanpour M., Sherman P.M. (2008). *Lactobacillus rhamnosus* strain GG prevents enterohemorrhagic *Escherichia coli* O157: H7-induced changes in epithelial barrier function. *Infection and Immunity* **76:** 1340-1348.

Kannan D., Viswanathan K. and Mohan B. (2005). Effect of feeding antibiotics and probiotic on the immune status and carcass characteristics of broiler. *Indian Journal of Poultry Science* **40:** 93-95.

Khan J., Iiboshi Y., Cui L., Wasa M., Okada A. (1999). Role of intestinal mucus on the uptake of latex beads by Peyer's patches and on their transport to mesenteric lymph nodes in rats. *Journal of Parenteral Enteral Nutrition* **23:** 19-23.

Kim G.B., Seo Y.M., Kim C.H., Paik I.K. (2011). Effect of dietary prebiotic supplementation on the performance, intestinal microflora and immune response of broilers. *Poultry Science* **90:** 75-82.

Kim Y., Kim S.H., Whang K.Y., Kim Y.J., Oh S.(2008). Inhibition of Escherichia coli O157:H7 attachment by interactions between lactic acid bacteria and intestinal epithelial cells. *Journal of Microbiology and Biotechnology* **18:** 1278-1285.

Koenen M.E., Kramer J., van der Hulst R., Heres L., Jeurissen S.H., Boersma W.J. (2004). mmunomodulation by probiotic lactobacilli in layer and meat-type chickens. *British Poultry Science* **45:** 355-366.

Kolida S., Gibson G.R. (2007).Prebiotic capacity of inulin-type fructans. *Journal of Nutrition* **137** (11 Suppl): 2503S-2506S.

Land M.H., Rouster-Stevens K., Woods C.R., Cannon M.L., Cnota J., Shetty A.K. (2005). Lactobacillus sepsis associated with probiotic therapy. *Pediatrics* **115:** 178-181.

Lee S., Lillehog H.S., Park D.W., Hong Y.H., Lin J.J. (2007). Effect of Pediocoecus and Sacharomyees based probioties (Mito Max) on coccidiosis in broiler chickens. *Comparative Immunology and Microbiology of Infectious Diseases* **30:** 261-268.

Lilly D.M., Stillwell R.H. (1965). Probiotics. Growth promoting factors produced by micro-organisms. *Science* **147:** 747-748.

Lonnermark E. (2010). Lactobacilli in the normal microbiota and probiotic effects of *Lactobacillus plantarum*. University of Gothenburg, Printed by Intellecta Infolog AB, Västra Frölunda, Sweden, pp 1-101.

Mason C.K., Collins M.A., Thompson K. (2005). Modified electroporation protocol for lactobacilli isolated from the chicken crop facilitates transformation and the use of genetic tool. *Journal of Microbiological Methods* **60:** 353-363.

McCarthy J., O'Mahony L., O'Callaghan L., Sheil B., Vaughan E.E., Fitzsimons N. (2003). Double blind, placebo controlled trial of two probiotic strains in interleukin 10 knockout mice and mechanistic link with cytokine balance. *Gut* **52:** 975-980.

Medellin- pena M.J., Wang H., Johnson R., Anand S., Griffiths M.W. (2007). Probiotics affect virulence-related gene expression in Escherichia coli O157:H7. *Applied Environmental Microbiology* **73:** 4259-4267.

Medina- Martinez M.S., Uyttendaele M., Rajkovic A., Nadal P., Debevere J. (2007). Degradation of N-acyl-L-homoserine lactones by Bacillus cereus in culture media and pork extract. *Applied Environmental Microbiology* **73:** 2329-2332.

Metchnikoff E. (1908). Prologation of life. (R D and Bootwala F.M. eds) National Food Ingredient Association, West Des Moines, Iowa, U.S.A., pp 117-132. (Originally published in 1908 and later reprinted in English in 1991).

Mileti E., Matteoli G., Iliev I.D., Rescigno M. (2009). Comparison of the immunomodulatory properties of three probiotic strains of lactobacilli using complex culture systems: prediction for in vivo efficacy. *PLoS One* **4:** e7056.

Mohamadzadeh M., Olson S., Kalina W.V., Ruthel G., Demmin G.L., Warfield K.L. (2005). Lactobacilli activate human dendritic cells that skew T cells toward T helper 1 polarization. *Proceedings of National Academy of Science, USA* **102:** 2880-2885.

Montrose D.C., Floch M.H. (2005). Probiotics used in human studies. *Journal of Clinical Gastroenterology* **39:** 469-484.

Morgan S.M., O'Connor P.M., Cotter P.D., Ross R.P., Hill C. (2005). Sequential actions of the two component peptides of the lantibiotic lacticin 3147 explain its antimicrobial activity at nanomolar concentrations. *Antimicrobial Agents and Chemotherapy* **49:** 2606-2611.

Mountzouris K.C., Tsirtsikos P., Kalamara E., Nitsch S., Schatzmayr G., Fegeros K. (2007). Evaluation of the efficacy of a probiotic containing *Lactobacillus, Bifidobacterium, Enterococcus* and *Pediococcus* strains in promoting broiler performance and modulating cecal microflora composition and metabolic activities. *Poultry Science* **86:** 309-317.

Mueller C., Macpherson A.J. (2006). Layers of mutualism with commensal bacteria protect us from intestinal inflammation. *Gut* **55:** 276-284.

Mukai T., Kaneko S., Matsumoto M., Ohori H. (2004). Binding of Bifidobacterium bifidum and Lactobacillus reuteri to the carbohydrate moieties of intestinal glycolipids recognized by peanut agglutinin. *International Journal of. Food Microbiology* **90:** 357-362.

Munoz-Provencio D., Llopis M., Antolin M., de Torres I., Guarner F., Perez-Martinez G., (2009). Adhesion properties of *Lactobacillus casei* strains to resected intestinal fragments and components of the extracellular matrix. *Archives in Microbiology* **191:** 153-161.

Neish A.S. (2009). Microbes in gastrointestinal health and disease. *Gastroenterology* **136:** 65-80.

Netherwood T., Gilbert H. J., Parker D. S., O'Donnell A.G. (1999). Probiotics shown to change bacterial community structure in the avian gastrointestinal tract. *Applied Environmental Microbiology* **65:** 5134-5138.

Ng S.C., Hart A.L., Kamm M.A., Stagg A.J., Knight S. C. (2009). Mechanisms of action of probiotics: recent advances. *Inflammatory Bowel Disease.* **15:** 300-310.

Ogawa T., Asai Y., Sakamoto H., Yasuda K. (2006). Oral immuno-adjuvant activity of *Lactobacillus casei* subsp. *casei* in dextran-fed layer chickens. *British Journal of Nutrition* **95:** 430-434.

O'Mahony L., O'Callaghan L., McCarthy J., Shilling D., Scully P., Sibartie S. (2006). Differential cytokine response from dendritic cells to commensal and pathogenic bacteria in different lymphoid compartments in humans. *American Journal of Physiology- Gastrointestinal and Liver Physiology* **290:** G839-845.

Patterson J.A., Burkholder K.M. (2003). Application of prebiotics and probiotics in poultry production. *Poultry Science* **82:** 627-631.

Quigley E.M., Quera R. (2006). Small intestinal bacterial overgrowth: roles of antibiotics, prebiotics and probiotics. *Gastroenterology* **130** (2 Suppl1): S78-90.

Ramakrishna B.S. (2009). Probiotic-induced changes in the intestinal epithelium: implications in gastrointestinal disease. *Tropical Gastroenterology* **30:** 76-85.

Rautava S., Arvilommi H., Isolauri E. (2006). Specific probiotics in enhancing maturation of IgA responses in formula-fed infants. *Pediatric Research.* **60:** 221-224.

Riquelme A.J., Calvo M.A., Guzman A.M., Depix M.S., Garcia P., Perez C. (2003). *Saccharomyces cerevisiae* fungemia after *Saccharomyces boulardii* treatment in immunocompromised patients. *Journal of Clinical Gastroenterology* **36:** 41-43.

Rojas M., Conway P.L. (1996). Colonisation by *Lactobacillus* of piglet small intestinal mucus. *Journal of Applied Bacteriology* **81:** 474-480.

Rolfe R. (2000). The role of probiotic cultures in the control of gastrointestinal health. *Journal of Nutrition* **130:** 396S-402S.

Rowghani E., Arab M., Akbarian A. (2007). Effects of probiotic and other feed additives on performance and immune response of broiler chicks. *International Journal of Poultry Science* **6:** 261-265.

Russell S.M., Grimes J.L. (2009). The effect of a direct fed microbial (Primalac) on turkey live performance. *Journal of Applied Poultry Research* **18:** 185-192.

Saadia M.H., Soliman N.K. (2010). Effect of probiotics (*Saccharomyces cerevisiae*) adding to diets on intestinal microflora and performance of hy-line layers hens. *Journal of Animal Science* **6:** 159-169.

Saavedra J.M., Abi-Hanna A., Moore N., Yolken R.H. (2004). Long-term consumption of infant formulas containing live probiotic bacteria: tolerance and safety. *American Journal of Clinical Nutrition* **79:** 261-267.

Saha S.K, Senani S., Padhi M.K., Rai R.B. (1998). Manipulation of rumen fermentation by feeding *Saccharomyces cerevisiae* and its effect on nutrient uilization in goat. *Journal of Andaman Science Association* **14:** 55-57.

Saha S.K., Senani S., Padhi M. K., Shome B.R., Rajeswari S., Ahlawat S.P.S. (1999). Microbial manipulation of rumen fermentation using *Saccharomyces cerevisiae* as probiotics. *Current Science* **77:** 696-697.

Sakata T., Kojima T., Fujieda M., Takahashi M., Michibata T. (2003). Influences of probiotic bacteria on organic acid production by pig caecal bacteria *in vitro*. *Proceedings of Nutrition Society* **62:** 73-80.

Saulnier D.M., Gibson G.R., Kolida S. (2008). In vitro effects of selected synbiotics on the human faecal microbiota composition. *FEMS Microbiology and Ecology* **66:** 516-527.

Senani S., Saha S.K., Padhi M.K., Rai R.B. (2000). Efficacy of various *lactobacillus* strains on broiler production. *Indian Journal of Animal Science.* **70:** 845-846.

Senani S., Rai R, B., Padhi M. K. and Saha S. K. (1997). Studies on the Lactobacillus incorporation in the ration of broiler chicks. *Indian Veterinary Journal* **74:** 808-810.

Senani S., Jai Sunder, Ahlawat S.P.S., Saha S.K., Kundu A., Chatterjee R.N., Rai R.B., Singh A.K., Yadav S.P. (2004) Effect of dietary supplementation of Lactobacillus in Japanese Quail. *Indian Journal of Poultry Science* **39:** 136-141.

Sheih Y.H., Chiang B.L., Wang L.H., Liao C.K., Gill H.S. (2001). Systemic immunity-enhancing effects in healthy subjects following dietary consumption of the lactic acid bacterium *Lactobacillus rhamnosus* HN001. *Journal of American College of Nutrition* **20**(Suppl2): 149-156.

Sherman P.M., Johnson-Henry K.C., Yeung H.P., Ngo P.S., Goulet J., Tompkins T.A.(2005). Probiotics reduce enterohemorrhagic *Escherichia coli* O157:H7- and enteropathogenic *E. coli* O127:H6-induced changes in polarized T84 epithelial cell monolayers by reducing bacterial adhesion and cytoskeletal rearrangements. *Infection and Immunity* **73:** 5183-5188.

Shome B.R., Senani S., Shome R., Padhi M.K., Kumar A., Verma N.D., Saha S.K. (2000). Effect of probiotics on performance of native chicken of Andaman. *Indian Journal of Poultry Science* **33:** 258-261.

Simon O., Vahjen W., Taras D. (2004). Interaction of nutrition with intestinal microbial communities. In: *Interfacing Immunity, Gut Health and Performance,* (LA Tucker, JA Taylor-Pickard, eds.) Nottingham: University Press, 33-46.

Singh B.P., Chauhan R.S. (2002). Role of probiotics in control of poultry diseases. *Pashudhan* **17:** 3.

Stavric S., Kornegay E.T. (1995). Microbial probiotics for pigs and poultry. In: *Biotechnology in Animal Feeds and Animal Feeding.* (R. J. Wallace, and A. Chesson, eds.) VCH, New York, pp 205–231.

Stiles M.E., Holzapfel W.H. (1997). Lactic acid bacteria of foods and their current taxonomy. *International Journal of Food Microbiology* **36:** 1-29.

Sulakvelidze A., Alavidze Z., Morris G. Jr. (2001). Bacteriophage therapy. *Antimicrobial Agents and Chemotherapy* **45:** 649-659.

Swidsinski A., Loening-Baucke V., Theissig F., Engelhardt H., Bengmark S., Koch S., (2007). Comparative study of the intestinal mucus barrier in normal and inflamed colon. *Gut* **56:** 343-350.

Tagg J.R., Dierksen K.P. (2003). Bacterial replacement therapy: adapting 'germ warfare' to infection prevention. *Trends in Biotechnology* **21:** 217-223.

Timmerman H.M., Veldman A., van den Elsen E., Rombouts F.M., Beynen A.C. (2006). Mortality and growth performance of broilers given drinking water supplemented with chicken-specific probiotics. *Poultry Science* **85:** 1383-1388.

Torres-Rodriguez A., Donoghue A.M., Donoghue D.J., Barton J.T., Tellez G., Hargis B.M. (2007). Performance and condemnation rate analysis of commercial turkey flocks treated with a *Lactobacillus* spp. based probiotic. *Poultry Science* **86:** 444-446.

Tortuero F. (1973). Influence of implantation of *Lactobacillus acidophilus* in chicks on the growth, feed conversion, malabsorption of fats syndrome and intestinal flora. *Poultry Science* **52:** 197-203.

Vegad J.L. (2004). Poultry diseases: A guide to farmers and poultry professionals. International Book Distributing Co., Lucknow,UP, India, pp 343-346 & 674-683.

Vila B., Steve-Garcia E., Brufau J. (2010). Probiotic microorganisms: 100 years of innovation and efficacy, mode of action. *Worlds Poultry Science Journal* **65:** 369-380.

Winkler P., Ghadimi D., Schrezenmeir J., Kraehenbuhl J.P. (2007).Molecular and cellular basis of microflora–host interactions. *Journal of Nutrition* **137**(*Suppl* 2): 756S-772S.

Yang Y., Iji P.A., Choct M. (2009). Dietary modulation of gut microflora in broiler chickens: a review of the role of six kinds of alternatives to in-feed antibiotics. *World's Poultry Science Journal* **65:** 97-114.

Yurong Y, Ruiping S, Shimin Z and Yibao J. (2005). Effect of probiotics on intestinal mucosal immunity and ultrastructure of cecal tonsils of chickens. *Archives of Animal Nutrition* **59:** 237-246.

Zulkifli I., Abdullah N., Azrin N.M., Ho Y.W. (2000). Growth performance and immune response of two commercial broiler strains fed diets containing *Lactobacillus* cultures and oxytetracycline under heat stress conditions. *British Poultry Science* **41:** 593-597.

Zyrek A.A., Cichon C., Helms S., Enders C., Sonnenborn U., Schmidt M.A. (2007). Molecular mechanisms underlying the probiotic effects of *Escherichia coli* Nissle 1917 involve ZO-2 and PKCzeta redistribution resulting in tight junction and epithelial barrier repair. *Cell Microbiology* **9:** 804-816.

❏❏❏

Chapter 10

Prebiotics in Livestock Production

A.K. Samanta, S. Senani, A.P. Kolte, M. Sridhar, A. Dhali
National Institute of Animal Nutrition and Physiology, Adugodi, Bangalore-560 030, Karnataka, India

Summary

During the last few decades, attempts for improving livestock productivity, are focusing on ways for modulating rumen or hindgut microflora by supplementation of oligosaccharides, now called 'prebiotics'. Prebiotics are plant derived compounds or produced through microbial enzymes. Owing to the presence of osidic bonds, these are indigestible by the livestock's own enzymes and are utilized by the selective group of gut microflora. As a result short chain fatty acids are produced and pH alters in the gut microenvironment; which is unsuitable for growth and multiplication of pathogenic microflora. Further the prebiotics also exhibits their beneficial effects through immune modulation, cholesterol reduction, enhanced villi length and mineral absorption. As it possess several beneficial roles, these are thought to be the future feed additives to replace conventional feed additives for improving livestock production.

In keeping with the pace for demands of livestock products by ever increasing human population, the Indian livestock industry has made a long journey from its informal farmyard activity to modern factory style involving improved nutrition, management, housing, stress amelioration and quality control. Along with the regular supply of diversified animal products to the consumer, the industry also supports millions for their livelihood as the sector is jointly contributed by the big enterprises as well as small and marginal farmers. The visible growth witnessed during the past century is the fruit of untiring efforts made by all the people associated with one or other activities pertaining to the industry. However, the major driving forces for rapid growth and development of livestock could be: (1) Improved breed, (2) Advanced practices of housing and management, (3) Progressive knowledge on veterinary medicine and vaccination, (4) Development in the sciences of nutrition, (5) Willingness of stakeholders to apply advance knowledge of scientific development and (6) Likings of Indian people who prefer milk, meat or eggs instead of other protein sources. The primary aim of the livestock industry is to deliver the safe and high quality animal products for human consumption after considering the welfare of the animals and concern to the environment. In livestock sector, feed is the major component of the total cost of production. During the previous century, several antibiotics have been included in animal feeds at sub-therapeutic levels to promote higher growth and to prevent infectious diseases (Singer and Hofacre, 2006). These antibiotic feed additives resulted in improved feed conversion efficiency and body weight gain by modulating the composition and activities of gut microflora. However, worldwide concern about the development of antimicrobial resistance and transfer of antibiotic resistance gene from animal to human have led to the ban on using antibiotics as growth promoters in European Union since January, 2006. Moreover, many other countries are also in the way to gradually stopping the use of antibiotics as a feed additive for livestock. The removal of antibiotics from feeds of the ruminants and non-ruminants is expected to put tremendous pressure on the livestock itself as well as the whole industry because it will make livestock vulnerable to several diseases namely enteritis, coccidiosis and salmonellosis. In such situation, there is an urgent need for using viable alternatives that would look after the activities of antibiotic growth promoters without compromising the productivity and quality of livestock products. Considerable efforts are being made throughout the world for developing such alternatives and prebiotics seem to be the frontrunner in this respect as these are of plant origin and satisfies the consumers concerns (Samanta *et al.,* 2010).

1. Prebiotics

During the past two decades, researchers have revealed that some segments of the gastrointestinal (GI) tract are the most metabolically active organs in both ruminants and non-ruminants which harbor an extremely complex microbial consortium (microbiome) that plays multifaceted roles. The microbiome is responsible for salvaging energy from ingested fibrous feeds that animal's own enzyme system is unable to do. Additionally it is involved in many other unique activities such as barrier function, immune development and angiogenesis. The concept of prebiotic has emerged out as a nutrient for balancing the gut microflora to ensure better gut health and functionality. Unlike probiotics, the theory of prebiotics is much more recent and has been introduced in 1995 by Gibson and Roberfroid as an alternative approach that would overcome the survivability issues of probiotics during storage, distribution and passage through the GI tract. Accordingly, the definition of a prebiotic has been given as 'a non-digestible dietary ingredients that beneficially affect the host by selectively stimulating the growth and or activity of a limited number of bacteria in the colon, thus improving the host health'. However, with the growing interests and intense research and development activities on prebiotic, it has been proposed to revisit its definition and suggested to exclude the word 'non-digestible'. The updated definition of prebiotic encompasses as 'a selectively fermented ingredient that allows specific change, both in the composition and or activity in the GI microflora that confers benefits upon host well being and health' (Gibson *et al.*, 2004). In 2007, further attempts have been made to incorporate whole foods and dietary supplements under the umbrella of 'prebiotic' nomenclature. Therefore, prebiotics may be considered as 'non-viable food components, ingredients or supplements that selectively modulate the microbiota of the digestive ecosystem, thus conferring benefits upon host well being and health' (Roberfroid, 2007). Considering the importance of prebiotic on overall human health, Food and Agricultural Organisation (FAO) in 2007 constituted a technical committee to revisit the definition of prebiotic. According to FAO, a prebiotic is a non-viable food component that confers a health benefit on the host associated with modulation of microbiota. FAO has suggested three criteria for qualifying a substrate as prebiotic: (1) Component: not an organism or drug; a substance that can be characterized chemically and in most cases these will be of food grade (2) Health benefits: measurable and that does not due to absorption of the component in the blood or due to the component acting alone and (3) Modulation: deliver changes in the composition or activities of microbiota of the target host including fermentation, receptor blockage or others. Therefore, a prebiotic could be fiber but all fibers need not be prebiotic. Further, attempt has been made to broaden the site of action of prebiotics such as skin, oral cavity and female genital tract in addition to its fundamental action at the GI tract (Pineiro *et al.,* 2008). Recently, the proposers of prebiotic concept have opposed the philosophy of broadening its application sites such as vagina and skin and wanted to restrict once again to the gastrointestinal microflora. Therefore, the accepted definition remains closer to the 1995 concept: a prebiotic is a selectively fermented ingredient that results in specific changes in the composition and/or activity of the gastrointestinal microbiota thus conferring benefit(s) upon host health (Gibson *et al.,* 2010). Looking towards the developmental changes in the definition of prebiotics, it appears that emphasis is given only after keeping in mind the prospects of prebiotics on human GI microflora (Samanta *et al.,* 2011). However, irrespective of the different concepts, an ideal prebiotic should have the following criteria.

- Selective fermentability (evident from *in vitro* or *in vivo* experiments)
- Changes in the gut microflora composition (should be a selective substrate for one or more beneficial bacteria resulting an increase in their population or metabolic activities)
- Ensures host health and well being
- Originated from plant or synthesized by microorganism or their enzymes
- Remains intact while passing through different parts of the digestive tracts in ruminants and non-ruminants
- No residues problem
- Ideally to be used as a food/feed additive
- Compatibility with other feed ingredients or premix
- No adverse affects on productivity or product quality
- Should increase nutrient digestibility and reduce enteric methane emission in ruminants

2. Types of prebiotics

Prebiotics are non-digestible short chain oligosaccharides manufactured either by enzymatic reactions or synthesized from plant biomass through a series of processes including extraction, precipitation, isomerization, hydrolysis and catalysis (Table 1). In poultry, these oligosaccharides either enhance the growth of beneficial microflora in the GI tract or attach competitively to pathogenic bacteria. Currently several prebiotics of diverse nature are available and most popular among them are frutooligosaccharides, inulin, galactooligosaccharides, xylooligosaccharides, soya-oligosaccharides, pectin oligosaccharides, mannan oligosaccharides and arabinogalactans (Samanta *et al.,* 2007).

3. Gut health

Although the term gut health is very popular and widely used both in animal and human medicine, it lacks clear definition (Choct, 2009, Bischoff, 2011). According to WHO definition of 'health', the 'gut health' in respect to livestock could be defined as 'state of physical status in the absence of GI disturbances that requires attention of veterinary doctor'. Feedstuffs ingested by the domestic animals contain nutrients, non-nutrients, beneficial and harmful microorganisms. Thereby, the GI tract is exposed to potential pathogens, which is a matter of concern to the livestock sector as well as to the researchers. A lot of emphasis has been given on the large intestine microflora composition and their activities, but gut health encompasses the entire GI tract. The relevance of gut health is underlined by the fact that today intestinal tract is not considered as a mere organ for digestion and absorption, but it has immense role on protection against disease, angiogenesis, immune stimulation, detoxification of toxic principles, synthesis of nutrients and finally delivering the quality animal products. There are two functional entities that are keys for achieving and maintaining gut health; namely GI barrier and GI microflora. The GI barrier is a complex entity as it encompasses epithelial defense and metabolic functions, mucosal immune system and enteric nervous system. In ruminants, rumen microflora encompassing bacteria, protozoa, fungi and archaea occupy significant niche for entrapping energy and nitrogen from the plant macronutrients and their further transformation into short chain fatty acids and microbial proteins.

Table 1 : List of prebiotics and their source

Name of prebiotic	Source/ raw materials	Method of production
Inulin	Chicory root, onion, garlic, bamboo shoots, Jerusalem artichoke, banana, leek etc.	Extraction
Fructooligosaccharides	Sucrose	Enzymatic catalysis (fructosyltransferase)
	Inulin	Enzymatic hydrolysis (Inulinase)
Galactooligosaccharides	Lactose	Enzymatic (Beta galactosidase)
Xyloo-ligosaccharides	Corn cobs, corn husks, wheat bran, rice bran, sugarcane bagasse, wheat straw, rice straw, almond shell, peanut shell etc.	Auto hydrolysis, mild acid hydrolysis, enzymatic (xylanase)
Pectino-ligosaccharides	Cell walls of fruits and vegetables like apple pomace, citrus peels, sugar beet pulp, potato fibers, sunflower head	Mild acid hydrolysis, enzymes (endo-polygalacturonase, exopolygalacturonase etc.)
Arabino-galactans	Leek seeds, carrots, ryegrass, radish, black gram beans, pears, wheat, tomato, ragweed, sorghum, bamboo grass, coconut meat and milk, larch tree etc.	Natural secretion of Acacia plants, water extraction, enzyme application.
Mannano-ligosaccharides	Guar seed, locust bean, tara gum, tuber of konjac, copra meal, coffee seed, yeasts cell walls etc.	Steam, microwave irradiation, thermal hydrolysis, mild acids, enzymatic (mannase).
Tagatose	D-galactose	Enzymatic (L-arabinose isomerase)

4. Rumen development and microflora establishment

The rumen of a newborn calf is similar to that of the monogastric animals with simple undivided sterile stomach completely free of anaerobic microorganism. Nevertheless, as the calf grows, all the four chambers *viz.*, rumen, reticulum, omasum and abomasum are developed into functional form. The physical and functional development of the rumen is grouped into three phases: (1) 0 to 3 weeks of age, non-ruminant, (2) 3 to 8 weeks of age, transition phase and (3) more than 8 weeks of age, adult ruminant. The new born animals acquire the microflora through contact with previously faunated older animals. The microflora transfers among animals by direct contact with saliva containing viable organisms. During rumen development, the organ increases in size, ruminal papillae increases in length and epithelial lining becomes keratinized. The microflora detected during the birth belongs to aerobic or facultative anaerobes (Samanta and Walli 1994). The strict anaerobic bacteria may appear two days after birth, but their survival is not guaranteed as the anaerobic conditions are not created by this time. At the age of 4 weeks, the predominating bacteria are *Selenomonas ruminantium* and *Bacteroides ruminicola* (Muller *et al.*, 1984). Total viable anaerobic bacteria population ranges from 5.89×10^{10}/ml to 6.0×10^{10}/ml of rumen contents at the age of 7 to 8 weeks (Rai, 2007). Faunation occurs in young animals when their mother licks and grooms them. When the newborn animals are kept in close proximity of the adults, protozoa is detected in the stomach of calves at 2 weeks of age. Although this inoculation is frequent but the protozoa are not able to establish because foregut is too acidic and protozoa cannot tolerate acidity. As the animals start consuming solid feed and twigs, the pH increases due to salivary secretions and thus conditions become favourable for establishment of protozoa. In case of goats the order of protozoa establishment is *Entodinia*>*Polyplastron*>*Eudiplodinium*>*Ophryoscolex*>*Dasytricha*>*Isotricha* (Rai, 2007).

Fungi may appear in the foregut of young lambs by 8 to 10 days after birth, though their survival is not guaranted. The fungal population increases from 0.21×10^2 to 8.27×10^3/ml of foregut contents during the 1 to 3 weeks of age in kids and peak population (14.63×10^3/ml) reaches at the age of 8 weeks.

5. Gastrointestinal tract development in poultry

At the time of incubation of fertilized egg, the weight of embryonic intestine increases at a faster rate compared to body weight. The weight ratio of small intestine to whole body increases from 1% to 3.5% on 17th day at the time of hatching (Uni *et al.*, 2003). Administration of exogenous nutrients into the amniotic fluid at 17 to 18th day of incubation leads to enhanced intestinal development of chicks by increasing the villi length as well as digestion capacities (Tako *et al.,* 2004). During the initial 48 h after hatching, the chicks are exposed to the transition from utilizing lipids of yolk to the carbohydrate rich external feed. During the post hatch periods as well, the increase in the weight of small intestine is faster than rest of the body mass. The development of intestinal segments is accompanied by increasing activities of enzymatic secretions as well as absorption capacities. Similar to the neonatal mammals, the small intestine of poultry undergoes morphological, biochemical and molecular changes during the first 2 weeks after hatching (Geyra *et al.,* 2001). As the chick begins to consume exogenous feed, rapid development takes place in the GI tract for ensuring efficient digestion, absorption and utilization. The predominance of saccharolytic bacteria namely *Bifidobacterium* and *Lactobacillus* in the GI tract of poultry is thought to be desirable as they do not contain any known pathogens unlike the proteolytic bacteria, such as *Bacteroides* and *Clostridium*. The fermentative activity of saccharolytic microflora leads to the generation of short chain fatty acids, while proteolytic bacteria generate ammonia, phenols, indoles, thiols, amines and sulphides representing the breakdown of GI microbial homeostasis and development of pathogenesis. Further, *Bifidobacterium* and *Lactobacillus* are believed to play critical role in maintenance of colonization resistance.

The early days of post-hatch period is very important for the establishment of the gut microbial communities as it begins from sterile gut environment and approaching towards stable microflora habitat with the advancement of age. Factors influencing the composition of microflora in the gut are diet, breed and geographic location. The microbial densities in broiler chicks has been found to be 10^8 cells/g of digesta at ileum and 10^{10} cells/g of digesta at caecum after 24 h of hatching (Yegani and Korver, 2008). On the day-3 post-hatch, the microflora densities reaches up to 10^{10} cells/g of ileal digesta and 10^{11} cells/g of caecal digest (Apajalahti *et al.,* 2002) and remain relatively stable for remaining period of the life. Using the 16S rRNA based molecular tools at least 640 species of microbes representing 140 genera have been identified in the caecum of poultry. Among these, only 10% microbes have been found to belong to the previously known phylotypes (Apajalahti *et al.,* 2004). Establishment of microflora in the newly hatched chick and their survivability during later periods of life results in protection against intestinal infections including different types of *Salmonella* and also exerts positive influence on growth rate (Yegani and Krover, 2008).

6. Homeostasis of the gut microflora in poultry

The whole set of gut microflora inhabited at the GI tract of livestock could be considered as metabolically active organ with its diversity in terms of species and cell densities. They salvage the energy that escapes enzymatic digestion of the host, synthesize vitamins, exclude pathogens, stimulate immunity and upkeep the health for sustaining desired production (meat, milk or eggs) level. The major microbial groups in poultry are *Bacteroides, Clostridium, Bifidobacterium, Eubacteriium, Lactobacillus, Enterobacteriaceae, Streptococcus, Fusobacterium, Peptostreptococcu* and *Propionibacterium* (Gaggia *et al.,* 2010). Based on their contributions to GI ecosystems, the microbes are broadly grouped into two categories, potentially pathogenic and beneficial. An intricate balance (homeostasis) exists between the beneficial and harmful bacteria, which ensure the healthy status of gut and production performance. The major beneficial bacteria are *Lactobacillus* and *Bifidobacterium*. The harmful bacteria include *Clostridium, E. coli, Campylobacter* etc. Any deviation in the homeostasis of the gut microflora composition owing to physiological or environmental stressors leads to the development of subclinical or acute pathological symptoms that impedes the productivity. The various stressors (feed changes or imbalances, transportation, processing at the hatchery, high stocking densities) may weaken the immune functions and thus predispose the birds for colonization of GI tract by bacterial pathogen, posing a threat to birds' health and food safety. Obviously under such circumstances, the population of beneficial gut microflora dramatically decreases leading to poor growth rate and loss of productivity in poultry farms (Si *et al.,* 2004).

7. Gut microflora in livestock health and production

A close relationship exists between the development of normal intestinal microflora population and resistance against enteric pathogens. It is now well accepted that the gut microbiota plays a significant role in digestion, nutrient utilization, absorption, detoxification and overall health in ruminants as well as non-ruminants. Since the anaerobic environment coupled with high redox potential is conducive for both beneficial and harmful microflora belonging to all classes of life, the GI tract represents an ecosystem of the highest complexity. In fact the GI tract of newly hatched chick is not only sterile, but also relatively immune-incompetent (Lee *et al.,* 2010). Thereby, the newly hatched chicks are highly susceptible to pathogen colonization compared to the adult birds. The ingested microflora from the habitat mainly pass through the intestine and unable to colonize in any compartment of the GI tract except the ones having competency to thrive at the anaerobic, high redox potential, competitive environment. The communities that thrive under the symbiotic environment of the gut become members of the residential community for interaction and playing roles to the host. Bacterial communities are metabolically versatile mixtures of numerous species whose relative abundance is governed by environmental factors such as substrate flows, feed composition, structure and function of epithelium etc. (Apajalahti, 2005).

7.1 In ruminants

The application of prebiotics in ruminants is limited due to their utilization by rumen microflora before it could be utilized by the microflora inhabiting the large intestine. Therefore, rumen protection technology should be applied in order to prevent utilization of prebiotics by the rumen microflora. Nevertheless, inulin has been used to modulate the rumen fermentation for enhancing the digestibilities of nutrients from total mixed ration (Samanta *et al.*, 2012). Addition of mannan oligosaccharides (MOS) in the diets of Holestein calves improved fecal score (Gaggia *et al.*, 2010). All the rumen hemicellulose utilizing bacteria (*Butyrivibrio fibrisolvens, Eubacterium ruminantium, Ruminococcus albus* etc.) are capable to utilize xylooligosaccharides and ferment it into short chain fatty acids (Cotta, 1993). The rumen pH remains unaltered (6.7) when galactooligosaccharides (GOS) is fed to Holestein cows maintained on silage diets (Santoso *et al.*, 2003). The rumen ammonia nitrogen concentration is slightly lower in GOS supplemented cows, sheep and steers which might be due to faster utilization of ammonia by rumen microflora or suppression of ammonia producing bacteria (Santoso *et al.*, 2003, Mwenya *et al.*, 2004, 2005). Methane production reduced by 11% in dairy cows receiving GOS in the diets due to a decline in acetate to propionate ratios in the rumen. The inclusion of inulin in the milk replacer of preruminat calves significantly improved body weight gain and fecal consistency (Kaufhold *et al.*, 2000).

7.2 In non-ruminants

7.2.1 Swine

Swine experiences many stressors during their entire life out of which weaning is most important. During this phase, often there is breach in the gut microbial homeostasis as a result of changes in gut microflora composition. Under such circumstances prebiotics are useful for improving the gut health. Newborn piglets consuming oligofructose exhibit higher number (1.68×10^{10} vs. 4.85×10^{9} CFU/g fecal contents) of *Bifidobacterium* on 6th day of consumption (Howard *et al.*, 1995).

Effort has been made in 3-week old piglets to investigate the potentiality of inulin on recovery from diarrhoea induced by cholera enterotoxin. It has been found that the population of *lactobacillius* was increased significantly in caecum (9.3 vs. 7.7 $\log_{10}$ CFU per gram) and colon (9.3 vs. 8.3 $\log_{10}$ CFU per gram) following daily consumption of 9.5 g of oligofructose. In contrast, the population of harmful bacteria (*Enterobacteriace*) was significantly decreased at both caecum (6.2 vs. 7.4 $\log_{10}$ CFU per gram) and colon (6.2 vs. 8.5 $\log_{10}$ CFU per gram) in piglets received oligofructose compared to that not received prebiotics (Oli *et al.*, 1998). When oligofructose was given in combination with probiotic, a significant increase in the population of total anaerobes,

Bifidobacterium and *Lactobacillius* with concomitant decrease in the number of *Enterococcius* and *Clostridium* population were observed (Nemcova *et al.*, 1999). Supplementation of chickory inulin in the diets of pig has resulted in a significant decrease of ammonia concentration in caecum and colon. Consumption of prebiotics has also enhanced dry matter and organic matter digestibility at ileum (Houdijk *et al.*, 1999).

7.2.2 Dogs

Intake of oligofructose (1% of diet) for a period of 50 days has significantly reduced the population of total gut aerobes, facultative aerobes in duodenal fluid and mucosa of German shepherd dogs suffering from intestinal bacterial overgrowth (Williard *et al.*, 1994). Oligofructose are preferentially fermented and utilized by *Enterobacterium* and *Eubacteria* strains which in turn prevent adhesion and survival of pathogenic bacteria in the colon of Beagles (Kearns *et al.*, 1998). When graded levels of oligofructose were incorporated in the diets of female hounds, the fecal concentration of *Clostridium perfringens* was decreased and total aerobes and *Bifidobacterium* were increased significantly (Flickinger *et al.*, 2003). *In vitro* fermentation of oligofructose in the presence of microflora of dog fecal matter leads to rapid production of short chain fatty acids including acetate, butyrate and propionate (Sunvold *et al.*, 1995). Short chain fatty acids are believed to possess trophic effect on the colonic epithelium (Flickinger *et al.*, 2003). The dogs consuming oligofructose exhibit longer and heavier small intestine with greater available surface areas for absorption (Buddington *et al.*, 1999). Fecal concentration of ammonia, putrescine, cadaverine, total phenols are found to be reduced following supplementation of oligofructose in the diet of dogs (Flickinger *et al.*, 2003). These are the metabolites usually produced by the harmful bacteria community inhabited at the GI tract and are responsible for bad odour of feces or other detrimental consequences. Plasma cholesterol concentration in dogs has been reduced significantly following regular consumption of oligofructose for a period of 6 weeks (Diez *et al.*, 1998).

7.2.3 Rabbit

In rabbit, caecum is the primary site of fermentation, which is carried out by several anaerobic genera. To achieve higher performances, rabbits are usually fed diets rich in protein and starch and low in fiber. Therefore, it appears that the diet of rabbit should be enriched with sufficient quantities of fermentable carbohydrates (prebiotic) to maintain the homeostasis and functionality of gut microflora. Therefore, oligofructose is routinely added (1 to 3 g/kg) in rabbits' diet in Europe. Higher body weight and daily weight gain were evident in rabbits consuming oligosaccharides (Mul and Perry, 1994, Mul, 1997).

7.2.4 Poultry

The importance of a well balanced gut microflora to promote and maintain livestock health is widely recognized. Dietary additives that selectively enrich particular intestinal bacterial population such as *Lactobacillus* and *Bifidobacterium* are regarded as beneficial since these microorganisms are found to be desirable saccharolytic microbiota of the GI tract (Table 2). Feeding of chicory fructan to the broilers results an increase in *Lactobacillus* cell counts, but substantially decreases *Campylobacter* and *Salmonella* populations (Yusrizal and Chen, 2003). Administration of 0.5% fructan rich (derived from Jerusalem artichoke) syrup to broilers is capable to reduce the population of *Clostridium perfringens* along with decreased levels of bacterial endotoxin in the GI tract. Isomaltooligosaccharides have been found to significantly reduce the pathogens load with concomitant increase in the *Bifidobacterium* population at caecum of young chicks. Administration of 2.5% mannan oligosaccharides through drinking water reduces *Salmonella typhimurium* colonization in the GI tract of broilers. Diet containing mannan oligosaccharides (0.4%) derived from yeast cell walls reduces the intestinal salmonella by 26% in broiler chicks (Spring *et al.,* 2000). As the name implied, mannan oligosaccharides are comprised of mannose that binds with the receptor present in certain enteric pathogens. *Salmonella typhimurium,* a common enteric pathogen of poultry, possesses type 1 fimbriae, which allows the particular pathogenic bacteria to attach at the receptors of intestinal epithelial cells. Mannan oligosaccharides also posses same kind of binding site by virtue of the presence of mannose where pathogenic bacteria (*Salmonella*) binds and get excreted through feces. Other school of thought suggests that mannan oligosaccharides cause aggregation or clump formation of enteric pathogen (*Salmonella enteritidis* and *Salmonella typhimurium*) and thus bring them out of the solution for excretion through feces (Spring *et al.,* 2000, Hajati and Rezaei, 2010). Administration of xylooligosaccharides (0.25%) increases the population of *Bifidobacterium* in the GI tract after one week of feeding, while the same dose of arabinoxylooligosaccharides exhibits similar response after 2 weeks of feeding in broilers (Courtin *et al.,* 2008). The delayed prebiotic effects of arabinoxylooligosaccharides might be due to more complex structure that delays the bifidogenic response. This implies that less substituted prebiotics are more efficiently utilized by *Bifidobacterium* than their highly substituted analogues. Similarly, galactooligosaccharides also exhibit increased *Bifidobacterium* population in the GI tract of poultry (Jung *et al.,* 2008).

Table 2 : Effect of prebiotics on gastrointestinal microflora of birds

Name of prebiotic	Inclusion levels	Response	Reference
Fructo-oligosaccharides	0.4% of diet	↑ *Bifidobacterium* ↑ *Lactobacillus* ↓ *E. coli*	Xu *et al.* (2003)
	0.375% of diet	↓ *Salmonella*	Bailey *et al.* (1991)
	0.375% of diet	No response	Waldroup *et al.* (1993)
Chicory fructans	-	↑ *Lactobacillus* ↓ *Campylobacter* ↓ *Salmonella*	Yusrizal and Chen (2003a)
Mannan oligosaccharides	2.5% of diet	↓ *Salmonella*	Oyofo *et al.* (1989)
Isomalto-oligosaccharides	-	↑ *Bifidobacterium* ↓ *Salmonella*	Thitaram *et al.* (2005)
Xylo-oligosaccharides	0.25% of diet	↑ *Bifidobacterium*	Courtin *et al.* (2008)
Galacto-oligosaccharide	-	↑ *Bifidobacterium*	Jung *et al.* (2008)

Therefore, currently, poultry industry is reluctant to use conventional antibiotic growth promoters. The industry is now interested to use plant derived feed additives like prebiotics in order to enhance product quality as well as productivity. Supplementation of diet with 0.4% fructooligosaccharides significantly improves the average daily gain and feed conversion efficiency in broilers (Xu *et al.*, 2003). Lower inclusion level of fructooligosaccharides to 0.2% only improves the feed conversion efficiency without affecting the daily gains in broiler. Administration of prebiotics derived from chicory roots is found to improve weight gain, feed conversion efficiency and carcass weight, and reduce cholesterol in broilers (Yusrizal and Chen, 2003). Supplementation of mannan oligosaccharide increases the feed conversion efficiency and body weight gain in turkeys (Sims *et al.*, 2004). Meta-analysis also confirmed the improved growth performance of birds following dietary supplementation of mannan oligosaccharides (Hooge, 2004). Histological evidences reveal an increase in the number of goblet cells at the epithelial lining of duodenum and jejunum in birds receiving mannanoligosaccharides (Savage *et al.*, 1997). In contrast, addition of arabino-xylooligosaccharides (2.5 g/kg diet) does not make any significant difference in final body weight of broilers (Courtin *et al.*, 2008). Some of the studies involving supplementation of prebiotics fail to elicit response on either body weight gain or feed conversion efficiency, which might be due the lower doses or the ineffective forms of prebiotics.

8. Advantages of prebiotics

Diet is the important determinant of the livestock industries as it shares major expenditure of a firm. Ban has been imposed over the application of antibiotics in the animal diets since 2006 by several countries. This has created a huge vacuum in the feed additive market which can be safely and effectively overcome by using several functional feeds and prebiotic is one among them. As most of the prebiotics are originated from the plant biomass, these are safe and possibly carry no side or residual effects. Unlike probiotics, there is also no question of viability of prebiotics during the time of processing. The important advantages of using prebiotics are mentioned below.

- Plant origin
- Enhances beneficial bacterial population in the gastrointestinal tract
- Exerts beneficial effects even at lower doses
- Antioxidant properties
- Anticarcinogenic effects
- Healing properties
- Reduces pathogenic bacteria loads in the GI tract
- Viability is not a concern unlike probiotics
- Mixing ability with other feed ingredients
- Reduces cholesterol levels
- Having energy values unlike antibiotics
- Enhances mineral absorption
- Improves GI tract health

Conclusions

The different segments of the GI tract of livestock are inhabited by microorganisms of diverse nature. Although several plant derived compounds are being examined around the world for matching the efficacy of antibiotic growth promoters, prebiotics seem to occupy the top position among those phytonutrients. The major factor that makes prebiotics advantageous over other nutraceuticals is its ability to exhibit the potency through several physiological activities beginning from gut microflora modulation to cholesterol reduction, immune stimulation, enhanced mineral absorption, antioxidant activities etc. unlike other functional foods that target only one or few physiological functions.

References

Apajalahti J. (2005). Comparative gut microflora, metabolic challenges and potential opportunities. *Journal of Applied Poultry Research* **14:** 444-453.

Apajalahti J.H., Kettunen H., Kettunen A., Holben W.E., Nurminen P.H., Rautomen N., Mutanen M. (2002). Culture independent microbial community analysis reveals that inulin in the diet primarily affects previously unknown bacteria in the mouse cecum. *Applied and Environmental Microbiology* **68:** 4986-4995.

Apajalahti J.H.A., Kettunen A., Graham H. (2004). Characteristics of the gastrointestinal microbial communities with special reference to the chicken. *World Poultry Science* **64:** 4084-4088.

Bailey J.S., Blankenship L.C., Cox N.A. (1991). Effect of fructooligosaccharides on Salmonella colonization of the chicken intestine. *Poultry Science* **70:** 2433-2438.

Bischoff S.C. (2011). Gut health: a new objective in medicine? *BMC Medicine* **9:** 24 (doi:10.1186/1741-7015-9-24).

Buddington R.K., Buddington K.K., Sunvold G.D. (1999). Influence of fermentable fiber on small intestinal dimensions and transport of glucose and proline in dogs. *American Journal of Veterinary Research* **60:** 354-358.

Choct M. (2009). Managing gut health through nutrition. *British Poultry Science* **50**: 9 - 15.

Cotta M.A. (1993). Utilization of xylooligosaccharides by selected ruminal bacteria. *Applied and Environmental Microbiology* **59:** 3557-3563.

Courtin C.M., Swennen K., Broekaert W.F., Swennen Q., Buyse J., Decuypere E., Michiels C.W., Ketelaere B.D., Delcour J.A. (2008). Effect of dietary inclusion of xylooligosaccharides, arabinoxylooligosaccharides and soluble arabinoxylan on the microbial composition of cecal contents of chickens. *Journal of the Science Food and Agriculture* **88:** 2517-2522.

Diez M., Hornick J.L., Baldwin P., Van Eenaeme C., Istasse I. (1998). Etude des fibres alimentaires chez le chien: Presentation des resultants decssais experimentaux. *Annales de Medicine Veterrinaire* **142:** 185-201.

Flickinger E.A., Van Loo J., Fahey G.C.Jr. (2003). Nutritional responses to the presence of inulin and oligofructose in the diets of domesticated animals: a review. *Critical Reviews in Food Science and Nutrition* **43:** 19-60.

FAO. (2007). Food and Agriculture Organization technical meeting on prebiotics. www.fao.org/ag/agn/agns/index_en.stm.

Gaggia F., Mattatelli P., Biavati B. (2010). Probiotics and prebiotics in animal feeding for safe food production. *International Journal of Food Microbiology* **141:** 515-528.

Geyra A., Uni Z., Sklan D. (2001). Enterocyte dynamics and mucosal development in the posthatch chick. *Poultry Science* **80:** 776-782.

Gibson G.R., Roberfroid M.B. (1995). Dietary modulation of the human colonic microbiota: introducing the concept of prebiotics. *Journal of Nutrition* **125:** 1401-1412.

Gibson G.R., Probert H.M., Van Loo J., Rastall R.A., Roberfroid M. (2004). Dietary modulation of the human colonic microbiota: updating the concept of prebiotics. *Nutrition Research Review* **17:** 259-275.

Gibson G.R., Scott K.P., Rastall R.A., Tuohy K.M., Hotchkiss A., Dubert-Ferrandon A., Gareau M., Murphy E.F., Saulnier D., Loh G., Macfarlane S., Delzenne N., Ringel Y., Kozianowski G., Dickmann R., Lenoir-Wijnkoop I., Walker C., Buddington R. (2010). Dietary prebiotics: Current status and new definition. *IFIS Functional Foods Bulletin* **7:** 1-19.

Hajati H., Rezaei M. (2010). The application of prebiotics in poultry production. *International Journal of Poultry Science* **9:** 298-304.

Hooge D. (2004). Meta-analysis of broiler chicken pen trials evaluating dietary mannan-oligosaccharide 1993-2003. *International Journal of Poultry Science* **3:** 163-174.

Houdijk J.G.M., Hartemink R., Van Laere K.M.J., Williams B.A., Bosch M.W., Verstagen M.W.A., Tamminga S. (1999). Fructooligosaccharides and transoligosaccharides in weaner's pig diets. In: *Proc. International symposium on "Non-digestible Oilgosaccharides: healthy food for the colon"*, Wageningen, The Netharlands, pp 69-78.

Howard M.D., Gordon D.T., Pace L.W., Garleb K.A., Kerley M.S. (1995). Effects of dietary supplementation with fructooligosaccharides on colonic microbiota population and epithelial cell proliferation in pigs. *Journal of Pedeatric Gastroenterology and Nutrition* **21:** 297-303.

Jung S.J., Houde R., Baurhoo B., Zhao X., Lee B.H. (2008). Effects of galacto-oligosaccharides and a *Bifidobacteria lactis*-based probiotic strain on the growth performance and fecal microflora of broiler chickens. *Poultry Science* **87:** 1694-1699.

Kaufhold J.N., Hammon H.M., Blum J.W. (2000). Fructooligosaccharides supplementation effects on metabolic, endocrine and hematological traits in veal calves. *Journal of Veterinary Medicine (Series A)* **47:** 17-29.

Kearns R.J., Hayek M.G., Sunvold G.A. (1998). Microbial changes in aged dogs. In: *Recent advance in canine and feline nutrition: 1998 IAMS Nutritional Symposium Proceedings,* (G.A. Reinhart and D.P. Carey, Eds) Orange Frazer Press, Wilmington, OH, pp 337-351.

Lee K., Lillehoj H.S., Soragusa G.R. (2010). Direct fed microbials and their impact on the intestinal microflora and immune system of chickens. *Journal of Poultry Science* **47:** 106-114.

Morisse J.P., Maurice R., Boiletot E., Cotte, J.P. (1993). Assessment of the activity of fructooligosaccharide on different cecal parameters in rabbits experimentally infected with *E.coli* O103. *Annales de Zootechnie* **42:** 81-87.

Mul A.J. (1997). Application of oligofructose in animal feeds. In: *Proceedings of International Symposium "Non-digestible oligosaccharides: healthy food for colon?"* Wageningen, The Netharlands.

Mul A.J., Perry F.G. (1994). The role of fructooligosaccharides in animal nutrition. In: *Recent advances in animal nutrition.* (P.C. Garnsworthy and D.J.A. Cole, Eds), Nottingham University Press, Nottingham, UK, pp 57-79.

Muller R.E., Annotti E.L., Asplund J.M. (1984). Isolation and identification of adherent epithelial bacteria during succession in young lambs. *Applied and Environmental Microbiology* **47:** 724-730.

Mwenya B., Santoso B., Sar C., Gamo Y., Kobayashi T., Arai I., Takahashi J. (2004). Effects of including â- 1, 4 galactooligosaccharides, lactic acid bacteria or yeasts culture on methanogenesis as well as energy and nitrogen metabolism in sheep. *Animal Feed Science and Technology* **115:** 313-326.

Mwenya B., Sar C., Santoso B., Gamo Y., Kobayashi T., Morikawa R., Takura K., Umetsu K., Kogawa S., Kimura K., Mizukoshi H., Takahashi J.(2005). Comparing the effects of beta 1,4 -galactooligosaccharides, and L-cysteine to monensin on energy and nitrogen utilization in steers fed a very high concentrate diets. *Animal Feed Science and Technology* **118:** 19-30.

Nemcova R., Bomba A., Gancarikova S., Herich R., Guba P. (1999). Study of the effect of Lactobacillus paracasei and fructooligosaccharides on the fecal microflora in weanling piglets. *Berl. Munch Teraarzil Wschr.* **112:** 225-228.

Oli M.W., Petschow B.W., Buddington R.K. (1998). Evaluation of fructooligosaccharides supplementation of oral electrolyte solutions for treatment of diarrhea. *Digestive Disease Science* **43:** 138-147.

Oyofo B.A., DeLoach J.R., Corrier D.E., Norman J.O., Ziprin R.L., Mollenhauer H.H. (1989). Prevention of *Salmonella typhimurium* colonization of broilers with D-mannose. *Poultry Science* **68:** 1357-1356.

Pineiro M., Asp N.G., Reid G., Macfarlane S., Morelli L., Brunser O., Tuohy K. (2008). FAO technical meeting on prebiotics. *Journal of Clinical Gastroenterology* **42:** S156-S159.

Rai S. (2007). Establishment of rumen protozoa, fungi and their fermentative role in goats of Bundelkhand. Ph.D. Thesis submitted to Bundelkhand University, Jhansi, Uttar Pradesh.

Roberfroid M.B. (2007). Prebiotics: The concept revisited. *Journal of Nutrition* **137:** 830S-837S.

Samanta A.K., Walli, T.K. (1994). Rumen anaerobic fungi and their role on fiber degradation. *Indian Journal of Dairy Science* **48:** 179-184.

Samanta A.K., Kolte A.P., Chandrasekhariah M., Thulasi A., Sampath K.T., Prasad, C.S. (2007). Prebiotics: The rumen modulator for enhancing the productivity of dairy animals. *Indian Dairyman* **59:** 58-61.

Samanta A.K., Senani S., Kolte A.P., Sridhar M., Jayapal N. (2010). Potentiality of prebiotics in poultry diets. *Agrovet Buzz.* Vol. **III (3)**: 39-42.

Samanta A.K., Kolte A.P., Senani S., Sridhar M, Jayapal N. (2011). Prebiotics in ancient Indian diets. *Current Science* **101:** 43-46.

Samanta A.K., Senani S., Kolte A.P., Sridhar M, Bhatta R., Jayapal N. (2012). Effect of prebiotic on digestibility of total mixed ration. *Indian Veterinary Journal* **89:** 41-42.

Santoso B., Kume S., Nonaka K., Gamo Y., Kimura K., Takashi J. (2003). Influence of beta galactooligosaccharide supplementation on nitrogen utilization, rumen fermentation, and microbial nitrogen supply in dairy cows fed silage. *Asian Australian Journal of Animal Sciences* **26:** 1137-1142.

Savage T.E., Zakrzewska E.I., Andreasen J.R. (1997). The effects of feeding mannan oligosaccharides supplemented diets to poults on performance and the morphology of the small intestine. *Poultry Science* **76** (suppl 1): 139.

Si J.M., Yu Y.c., Fan Y.J., Chen S.J. (2004). Intestinal microbiology and quality of quality of life in irritable bowel syndrome patients. *World Journal of Gastroenterology* **10:** 1802-1805.

Sims M.D., Dawson K.A., Newman K.E., Spring., Hoogell D.M. (2004). Effects of dietary mannan oligosaccharide, bacitracin methylene disalicylate, or both on the live performance and intestinal microbiology of turkeys. *Poultry Science* **83:** 1148-1154.

Singer R.S., Hofacre C.L. (2006). Potential impacts of antibiotic use in poultry production. *Avian Disease* **50:** 161-172.

Spring, P., Wenk, C., Dawson, K.A., Newman K.E. (2000). The effects of dietary mannoligosaccharides on cecal parameters and the concentration of enteric bacteria in the ceca of Salmonella challenged broiler chicks. *Poultry Science* **79:** 205-211.

Sunvold G.D., Fahey G.C., Jr. Merchen N.R., Titgemeyer E.C., Bourquin I.D., Baur L.L., Reinhart G.A. (1995). Dietary fiber for dogs; IV. In vitro fermentation of selected fiber sources by dog fecal inoculums and in vivo digestion and metabolism of fiber supplemented diets. *Journal of Animal Science* **73:** 1099-1109.

Tako E., Ferket P.R., Uni Z. (2004). Effects of *in ovo* feeding of carbohydrates and beta hydroxyl beta methyl butyrate on the development of chickens intestine. *Poultry Science* **45:** 55-60.

Thitaram S.N., Chung C.H., Day D.F., Hinton A., Bailey J.S., Siragusa G.R. (2005). Isomalto-oligosaccharides increase caecal *Bifidobacterium* population in young broiler chickens. *Poultry Science* **84:** 998-1003.

Uni Z., Tako E., Gal garber O., Sklan D. (2003). Morphological, molecular and functional changes in the chicken small intestine of the late term embryo. *Poultry Science* **82:** 1747-1754.

Waldroup A.L., Skinner J.T., Heierholzer R.E., Waldroup P.W. (1993). An evaluation of fructooligosaccharides in diets for broiler chickens and effects on Salmonella contamination. *Poultry Science* **72:** 643-650.

Williard M.D., Simpson R.P., Delles E.K., Coben N.D., Fossum T.W., Kolp D., Reinhart, G. (1994). Effects of dietary supplementation of fructooligosaccharides on small intestinal bacterial overgrowth in dogs. *American Journal of Veterinary Research* **55:** 654-659.

Xu Z.R., Hu C.H., Xia M.S., Zhan X.A., Wang M.Q. (2003). Effect dietary fructooligosaccharides on digestive enzyme acticities, intestinal microflora and morphology of male broilers. *Poultry Science* **82:** 1030-1036.

Yegani M., Korver D.R. (2008). Factors affecting intestinal health in poultry. *Poultry Science* **87:** 2052-2063.

Yusrizal X., Chen T.C. (2003). Effect of adding chicory fructans in feed on broiler growth performance serum cholesterol, and intestinal length. *International Journal of Poultry Science* **2:** 214-219.

Yusrizal X., Chen T.C. (2003a). Effect of adding chicory fructans in feed on fecal and intestinal microflora and excreta volatile ammonia. *International Journal of Poultry Science* **2:** 188-190.

❏❏❏

Section - 2

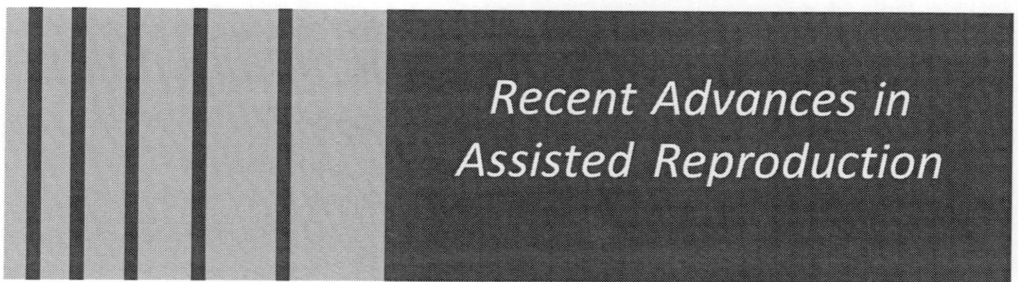

Chapter 11

Ovarian Follicle Development in Ruminants and its Modulation

J.P. Ravindra, S. Selvaraju
National Institute of Animal Nutrition and Physiology, Adugodi, Bangalore 560 030, Karnataka, India

Summary

The primordial follicles, each with an oocyte surrounded by a single layer of pregranulosa cells, form the resting pool of the nongrowing follicles in the ovary. These follicles continuously leave the resting pool and are progressively depleted during the life span of the female animal. Once the primordial follicle enters the growth phase, it end up either with atresia, which is the fate of most of them or with ovulation, which is limited to only a few numbers during the lifespan. In addition to the urge to know how the follicle's growth and regression are controlled, the interest in elucidating this process grew with the introduction of techniques of multiple ovulation and embryo transfer for faster genetic improvement and enhancing productivity of animals. Rescue of follicles from atresia was the need. The ultrasound imaging technique, along with the ultrasound guided follicle fluid/oocyte aspiration and the molecular biological techniques have aided in gaining much deeper insight into the phenomenon of follicular waves, follicle selection and dominance, and the apoptotic demise of the subordinate follicles including the factors and genes involved in them. The balance between several promoting or inhibiting hormones, protein/peptide (growth) factors acting through autocrine, paracrine and endocrine routes, their receptors, all determine the fate of the follicle and chronobiology is of utmost importance in the events. A comprehensive look at these would help in modulation of the follicle development for improving reproductive efficiency and better success in assisted reproductive techniques.

Since the time Rajakoski (Rajakoski, 1960) published his work, interest in the follicular development, especially in monoovulators gained momentum. Of interest has been while many follicles begin to develop as a cohort, why only one, as in case of monoovulators and a few as in case of multiple ovualators, go on to ovulate in each sexual cycle. Investigations took a surge with the introduction of multiple ovulation and embryo transfer techniques for faster genetic improvement and enhancing productivity of animals. Initial studies involved examination of ovarian follicles from animals slaughtered at known stages of the oestrous cycle, or limited to repeated laparotomic observation on ovaries of live animals with India ink marking for identification of the follicles on repeated observations. Introduction of B-mode realtime ultrasound imaging technique brought in more of a revolution in follicle dynamic studies, since it allowed non-invasive, repeated visualization of ovaries and monitoring follicular growth in live animals. Ultrasound guided follicular fluid and oocyte aspiration, Doppler method for assessing blood flow, all adjuncts to the ultrasonographic technique gave further boost to the studies on ovarian follicle dynamics in detail to understand and to improve reproductive efficiency in animals. Adoptions of the molecular biological techniques have given further insight into the factors regulating follicle growth, the mechanism of atresia by apoptosis and possible ways of modulating the process.

1. Ovarian follicle development

The primordial follicles, each with an oocyte surrounded by a single layer of pregranulosa cells, form the resting pool of the follicles that are progressively depleted during the life span of a female animal. The primordial follicles continuously leave the resting pool to go through the stages of primary, secondary and tertiary or the antral follicles. Once the primordial follicle enters the growth phase, it end up either with atresia, which is the fate of most of them or ovulation. Ovulation is limited to only a few numbers during the lifespan of the animal. In ruminants and primates, the formation of primordial follicles begins during fetal development and occurs over a long period of time, so that some primordial follicles are activated before other follicles have been formed (Fortune *et al.,* 2000). The duration of folliculogenesis from primordial follicle to ovulation is remarkably consistent between sheep and cattle at approximately 4-6 months (Cahill *et al.,* 1981; Lussier *et al.,* 1994). The antral cavity begins to form in sheep ovarian follicles of about 0.2 to 0.5 mm diameter (Brand and DeJong, 1973). Further, from this stage, it takes about four weeks for the follicle to reach preovualtory size (Turnbull *et al.,* 1977; Cahill and Mauleon, 1980). The following terms have been suggested by Goodman and Hodgen (1983) in describing the process of follicular development: *recruitment*- a gonadotropin dependent event during which a group of follicles gain the ability to respond to gonadotrpoins and require gonadotropins for their continued growth; *selection*- a process whereby only a few of the recruited follicles are selected to escape atresia and survive to ovulate; and *dominance*- the mechanism a follicle(s) uses to escape atresia. These terms are used, along with the use of growth and regression rates and size (diameter) and number of follicles, as characteristics, for describing follicular dynamics during the oestrous cycle. With interest in understanding the phenomenon of selection and dominance using the ultrasonograhic monitoring of growth and regression of follicles, another important term 'the point of deviation' in growth of follicle came into use. The point of deviation is the beginning of the greatest difference in growth rates (diameter changes between adjacent examinations) when the second largest follicle reached its maximum diameter. Identification of the day of deviation and analysing the differences between the follicles gives insight into the mechanism of dominance and methods to overcome this to rescue more follicles from atresia or in other words increase the superovulatory response. Another term used is the *wave emergence*, which is the mark of the beginning of the final stage of follicular growth before ovulation or atresia of the follicle as identified by the ultrasonic or direct visualization of the ovarian follicle.

The ovary of a newborn calf contains approximately 150,000 primordial follicles (Erickson, 1966). In buffalo, the total number of primordial and Graafian follicles is about 50% less than in cattle (Aboul-Ela, 2000). The number of primordial follicles has been reported to be approximately 12,000-19,000 in riverine buffalo heifers (Samad and Nasseri, 1979; Danell 1987), and in swamp buffaloes, the number of antral follicles equal to only 20 percent of those observed in cattle under similar conditions (Le Van Ty *et al.*, 1989). The ovary of an adult ewe contains between 12,000 and 86,000 small follicles and between 100 and 400 large developing follicles, of which 10 to 40 are visible on the surface of the ovary at any one time (Cahill *et al.*, 1979; McNatty *et al.*, 1982). Despite the large number of follicles growing at any stage in the mono-ovulators, such as cattle, buffalo and most breeds of sheep, only one follicle completes growth and maturation to ovulate during each estrous cycle. The mechanism involved in such strict control over the number of follicles ovulating, has been subject of intense investigations. An understanding of this has major implication in modulating and enhancing reproduction including success rate in superstimulation of ovary for multiple follicle development/ovulation and oocyte/embryo recovery as well as in other assisted reproductive technologies.

Reviewing the results of several studies on ovarian follicular dynamics, Webb *et al.* (1992) explained the characteristics of follicular wave pattern in cattle. Each wave of follicular development is characterised by the simultaneous emergence of a cohort of follicles from the pool of small follicles (5 - 7mm), to form a pool of larger, growing follicles of >5mm in diameter.

One of these cohorts rapidly establishes itself as the dominant follicle and continues to develop, while the other follicles become atretic and regress. The dominant follicle developed during luteal phase normally reaches a maximum diameter of 10-15 mm and remains dominant for a few days, until it too becomes atretic and regresses, to be replaced within approximately five days by a further dominant follicle grown from the next wave of follicles. If luteal regression occurs during the growth phase or early period of dominance, then the dominant follicle, free from a restrictive hormonal milieu, will continue to develop to preovulatory size and will eventually trigger the hormonal cascade leading to ovulation.

In bovines, follicular waves are reported at 2 weeks of age (Evans *et al.*, 1994). Numbers of follicles (small, medium and large follicles) and diameter of the largest follicle increase from 2 to 14 weeks of age. Between 6 and 24 weeks of age, there is a marked but transient increase in blood concentrations of both LH and FSH in bovine (Evans *et al.*, 1992; Honaramooz *et al.*, 1999). In cows, the follicles become gonadotropin dependent at the follicle size of 3 to 4mm (Driancourt *et al.*, 1995; Miller *et al.*, 1999) and the diameter of the follicles in which the granulosa cells first display LH receptors is 9 to10 mm (Lucy *et al.*, 2001).

2. Regulators of folliculogenesis

Ovarian follicle development in mammals is primarily orchestrated by endocrine factors, mainly gonadotropins (FSH and LH), their receptors (FSHR and LHR) and ovarian steroids. The growth factors are essential for the initial stages of follicle growth, whereas gonadotropins are essential for the final stages of follicle growth (for review Webb *et al.*, 2004). Any alterations in secretion of FSH and LH are related to follicle recruitment and growth in cattle. The follicular recruitment is mainly controlled by the FSH surge and LH appears to be minimally involved in this process (Evans *et al.*, 1997). There is a minimal threshold of FSH concentration necessary for the follicular recruitment and this threshold level varies between animals (Picton *et al.*, 1991).

The action of FSH on the granulosa and LH on the theca cells is very important particularly in the 'fast' growth phase of antral follicle development. While attaining dominance, the dominant follicle survives even during declining and nadir phases of plasma FSH by virtue of its enhanced responsiveness to gonadotropins relative to that of subordinate follicles (Ginther *et al.*, 1996, 2001). Certain factors mainly, estradiol and inhibin are also critical in increasing responsiveness of the dominant follicle to gonadotropins at the time of follicle selection (Mihm *et al.*, 2000; Austin *et al.*, 2001; Ginther *et al.*, 2003). Along with this, intraovarian complex regulatory mechanisms mainly growth factors are involved in the control of folliculogenesis (Adashi and Roban, 1992). Ovarian follicles are known to produce a range of locally acting peptide/protein growth factors. These can either interact directly with the same cell (autocrine action) or with other cells of the follicle (paracrine action) to stimulate or attenuate the cellular response to gonadotropins. Responsiveness of the follicle to gonadotropin involves expression of the appropriate receptor mainly FSH and LH in the follicular cells and maturation of the post-receptor signal transduction systems. The follicular development is also dependent on angiogenesis (Koos, 1989), while follicular atresia is often associated with a decrease in vascularisation. The vasculature then develops to form two connected capillary networks in the theca interna and externa layers, but do not penetrate the basement membrane and consequently the granulosa cell layer remains avascular until ovulation. The follicle cannot proceed to the gonadotropin-dependent stage without the responsiveness of FSH (Findlay *et al.*, 2002) and the responsiveness of the dominant follicles to LH alters the fate of dominant follicle (Webb *et al.*, 1992; Campbell *et al.*, 1995).

The survival factors derived from oocytes, such as growth differentiation factor, IGFs and BMP's determine the fate of primordial and primary follicles (Webb *et al.*, 2004), while granulosa cell products are the major determining factors in late pre-antral and larger follicles development (Johnson, 2003). The key factors secreted by follicular somatic cells regulating the oocyte and follicular growth are estradiol, epidermal growth factor, transforming growth factor-β (activin, BMP-2,-4,-6), fibroblast growth factor, meiosis-activating sterols, inhibin, and activin (Driancourt *et al.*,1998). Similarly, oocytes also control follicular growth and development by secreting various oocyte-secreted factors (Webb *et al.*, 2004).

Though the indispensable role of LH pulses in dominant follicle development is established (Gong et al. 1996), the role of LH receptor in follicular selection and dominance is being explored till today. Some studies suggest that the acquisition of LH receptor on granulosa cells is the primary determinant of selection for dominance (Bao *et al.*, 1997), whereas other studies could not confirm such findings (Hampton *et al.*, 2004). In cattle, atresia was associated with reduced expression of gonadotropin receptor mRNAs (Henderson *et al.*, 1984). Similar to the cattle, LH receptor mRNA was detected in buffalo granulosa cells only in healthy dominant follicles with >8mm diameter and was not detected or low in the regressing dominant follicles (Anand, 2011). There is a short period from the start of deviation to the expression of LHR on granulosa cells, other factors influence the survival of the follicle leading to dominance of the follicles. Various intra-ovarian growth factors may play an important role in selection of dominant follicle. The IGFs and insulin like growth factor binding proteins (IGFBPs) in association with gonadotropins play a critical role in selection and steroidogenesis of ovarian follicles (Bao and Garverick, 1998). The IGF-I and IGF-II increase production of P450-17α-hydroxylase (Magoffin and Weitsman, 1993), progesterone (Veldhuis and Furlanetto, 1985) and synergize with FSH to enhance aromatase activity (Adashi *et al.*, 1985). In a dominant follicle, an increase of free IGF, synergizes with FSH to increase follicular estradiol production, which exerts negative feedback to decrease FSH secretion, preventing further development of the other follicles of the cohort (Fortune *et al.*, 2004). In a cohort of the follicles, the follicles with the lowest concentration of IGFBP-4 always became dominant even though they don't always have the highest amounts of follicular fluid estradiol (Mihm *et al.*, 2000).

Members of the transforming growth factor-β (TGF-β) have been shown to play an important role in folliculogenesis in a stage dependant manner (Knight and Glister, 2003). Some of the important TGF-β family molecules expressed in the ovary are (Knight and Glister, 2003): anti-mullerian hormone (AMH), inhibins, activins, BMP (-2,-4,-6,-7,-15) and growth/differentiation factors-9 (GDF). The major regulatory process in ovarian steroidogenesis by BMPs is the control of FSH receptor signaling, leading to normal follicular development in the ovary with prevention of immature ovulation there by acting as luteinization inhibitors (Otsuka *et al.*, 2001; Shimasaki *et al.*, 2004). The BMPs play crucial roles in female reproduction not only by regulating ovarian steroidogenesis and mitogenesis but also by activating pituitary gonadotropin secretion in an autocrine/paracrine manner (Otsuka and Shimasaki, 2002). Studies from ruminant support a potential positive local role for BMP-2 in folliculogenesis (Selvaraju *et al.*, 2009; Vinodkumar, 2011). The BMP-4, -6, and -7 could potentially affect the FSH and dominant follicle selection process (Knight and Glister, 2006) by promoting granulosa cell proliferation, while suppressing progesterone secretion (Glister *et al.*, 2004). In cattle, GDF-9 promotes granulosa cell proliferation, and inhibits estradiol and progesterone production induced by FSH and IGF-I together, but not the production induced by FSH alone (Spicer *et al.*, 2006). Though GDF9 and BMP15 affect the expression/activity of FSH receptor in granulosa cells (Knight and Glister, 2006), the role of these two proteins in dominant follicular selection is not clear.

The changes in follicular fluid may influence steroidogenesis, oocyte maturation, ovulation, oocyte transport in the oviduct and corpus luteum function (Peters and McNatty, 1980). Follicular fluid is a complex component of serum and follicular-synthesized secretions (Bellin and Ax, 1984). It contains steroids (Anand, 2011), gas and electrolyte (Shalgi *et al.*, 1972), growth factors (Nakatani *et al.*, 1991; Yuan *et al.* 1998) and protein components (Mette *et al.*,

1976; Anand, 2011) and all these regulate fertility of the animal. Proteomic studies in bovine follicular fluid protein revealed the possible role of 40-45 kDa protein in atresia of the follicle of 5-8mm diameter (Anand, 2011). Such proteins could be of the nature of either IGFBP or inhibin or follistatin (Armstrong *et al.*, 1996). On the other hand presence of around 25 kDa protein in >8mm healthy follicle may influence final follicular growth and ovulation (Anand, 2011).

3. Follicular atresia

The development of an activated primordial follicle to the preovulatory size is considered to be continuous unless a follicle undergoes atresia during the course of its development. The majority of these growing follicles (99%) will be lost as a result of atresia, unless they are rescued by follicle-stimulating hormone (FSH). This rescue by FSH starts after puberty when the pituitary-gonadal endocrine axis has been activated. Among the cohort of rescued follicles, only one follicle is selected to become the dominant follicle and ovulates under the influence of LH. The atretic process of the follicle happens by the process of apoptosis, the programmed cell death. The balance between the survival and death genes determines the success of the follicular development and ovulation or atresia (Amsterdam *et al.*, 2003; Quirk *et al.*, 2004). The atretic rate at various stages of follicle development has been established in cattle and buffalo.

3.1 Follicular atretic pathways

Many internal and external signals operate in the atretic pathways to influence follicular growth. Internal signals, such as the withdrawal of growth factors usually induce the perturbation of mitochondria to release cytochrome-c, activate proapoptotic proteins such as Bad and Bax. These will lead to the activation of a caspase cascade and cause cell death (Bridgham *et al.*, 2003). This caspase cascade starts from the release of cytochrome-c from mitochondria, followed by the formation of apoptosome (cytochrome c, Apaf1, procaspase-9), the activation of caspase-9, then caspase-3 and-7, and finally caspase-6. There are also apoptotic signals, such as activation of granzyme-B that could bypass the mitochondrial signals for apoptosis (Amsterdam *et al.*, 2003). External signals, such as Fas ligand, TNF-related apoptosis-inducing ligand, tumor necrosis factor-α, interleukin-1, *etc.*, will bind to the corresponding death receptors and initiate another caspase cascade (from caspase 8 and 10 to caspase 3 and 7, then caspase 6), leading to cell death (Bridgham *et al.*, 2003). The changes in these gene expression levels seem to coordinate with the changes in other genes, such as LH receptor, FSH receptor, *etc.*, to determine the fate of the follicle (Quirk *et al.*, 2004).

In the antral follicles, atresia is associated with a decrease in estrogen synthesis and increase in production of progesterone (Anand 2011). This change of estrogen to progesterone ratio is attributed to decrease in $C_{17, 20}$-lyase activity, leading to a decrease in androgen substrate for granulosa cell aromatization and a loss of aromatase activity (Tilly, 1992). Although several intracellular molecules such as B-cell lymphoma-2 (Bcl-2, Tilly *et al.*, 1995), Bcl-2-associated X protein (Bax, Tilly *et al.*, 1995), caspases (Bridgham *et al.*, 2003) and DNase-I (Boone *et al.*, 1995) have been implicated in the atretic process, recent studies on the cellular and molecular events leading to granulosa cell apoptosis have suggested that Fas antigen may be central in the induction of follicular atresia.

In humans, rats, cows and sows, both FasL and Fas are expressed in ovary (Quirk *et al.*, 1995; Porter *et al.*, 2001). Granulosa cells express Fas mRNA and protein, and Fas expression is elevated in atretic follicles of bovine (Sunil *et al.*, 2012). Under certain conditions, bovine granulosa cells undergo apoptosis when treated with soluble Fas-L *in vitro* (Rahila, 2011). Addition of IGF-I could overcome the effect of Fas-L mediated granulosa cell apoptosis in buffalo (Ravindra *et al.*, 2011). This effect of IGF-I was more in medium and large size follicles as compared to small size follicles (Rahila, 2011).Though BMP-2 has been proposed to influence the follicular survival, addition of BMP-2 could not improve granulosa cell apoptosis (Vinodkumar, 2011).

The protein kinase-A (PKA) signaling pathway is the major survival pathway in the follicular function. This pathway can be activated by FSH, LH, VIP (vasoactive intestinal peptide), or PACAP (pituitary adenylate cyclase-activating polypeptide). Downstream of PKA pathway, upregulation of the some of the genes such as Bcl-2, Bcl-xL, induced myeloid leukemia cell differentiation protein (Mcl-1) and inhibitor of apoptosis proteins (IAPs) occurs. These either directly promote survival, or suppress the expression of proapoptotic factors such as Bax, apoptotic protease activating factor 1(Apaf1, caspase 3), or inhibit the activities of the proapoptotic factors (Johnson, 2003).

Besides the PKA pathway, there is also evidence that FSH activates other pathways, including PKB (protein kinase B, also known as Akt), PKC, *etc.* PKB is activated through phosphorylation by PDK-1 (phospho-phosphoinositide-dependent protein kinase-1). Besides FSH, IGF-1 and TGF-β are known to activate PKB and to promote granulosa cell survival (Westfall *et al.*, 2000; Johnson and Bridgham, 2001). Other main factors involved in follicular survival include EGF (epidermal growth factor), FGF (fibroblastic growth factor), prolactin, laminin, leptin, glucocorticoid and estradiol (Amsterdam *et al.*, 2003).

4. Major factors influencing ovarian function and fertility

4.1 Heat stress on ovarian function

Heat stress is a major factor that influences fertility in dairy animals. The conception rates drop from about 40 to 60% in cooler seasons to 10 to 20% in warm seasons (Cavestany *et al.,* 1985). Heat stress activates the hypothalamo pituitary–adrenal axis and the sympathoadrenal system which in turn leads to irregular estrous cycle, abnormal gamete quality, poor expression of oestrus and failure to establish successful pregnancy. Heat stressed cow produces low oestradiol from the preovulatory follicles, affecting ovarian feed-back on hypothalamo-hypophyseal axis. Early atresia in medium sized follicles may be associated with low oestradiol production by granulosa cells and increased progesterone concentrations in the follicular fluid of heat-stressed cows (Roth *et al.,* 2000).

Heat stress in dairy cows resulted in decreased concentrations of LH and reduced dominance of the selected follicle (Wilson *et al.,* 1998). Heat stress can also cause an increase in peripheral concentrations of estradiol-17β between day 1 and 4 of the estrous cycle (Wolfenson *et al.,* 1995) and a reduction from day 4 through 8 (Wolfenson *et al.,* 1995) and day 11 through 21 of the cycle (Wilson *et al.,* 1998).

The mechanisms by which heat stress alters the concentrations of circulating reproductive hormones are not known. Heat stress can cause increased cortisol secretion (Wise *et al.,* 1988; Elvinger *et al.,* 1992). Adrenocortico tropic hormone has been reported to block estradiol- induced sexual behavior (Hein and Allrich, 1992). Increased corticosteroid secretion during heat stress may also inhibit GnRH and thus, LH secretion (Gilad *et al.,* 1993). Heat stress could also act directly on the ovary to decrease its sensitivity to gonadotropin stimulation (Wolfenson *et al.,* 1997). The theca and granulosa cells are also damaged by heat stress and affects steroid production (Roth *et al.,* 2001).

Embryo death due to heat stress occurs mainly between the period of fertilization and maternal recognition of pregnancy. One of the reasons for the death of embryo during heat stress may be the luteal insufficiency. Low plasma progesterone concentrations during the luteal phase of the estrous cycle can compromise embryo survival and also follicular development in the subsequent cycle leading to abnormal oocyte maturation and early embryonic death (Ahmad *et al.,* 1995). Asynchronous development of the embryo coupled with delayed or advanced development of the corpus luteum lead to higher rates of implantation failure in animals (Lamming and Royal, 2001).

4.2 Nutrition: energy levels and post partum fertility

Decline in postpartum fertility in dairy cattle is a world-wide problem. Management, nutrition, production, and genetics are the main reasons for the decline in post partum fertility in dairy cow. Resuming ovulatory cyclicity and successful breeding within a reasonable period during 45–60 days and 60–90 days postpartum, respectively are essential to maintain sustainable productivity and economy of the farmer. Nearly half of the postpartum dairy cattle fail to ovulate and many have abnormal oestrous cycles, with anovulatory anoestrus, cystic ovarian disease or extended luteal phases. In some animals, induced ovulation is usually followed by a short cycle and a return to acyclicity. Even when animals return to ovarian cyclic activity, many high milk-yielders have limited estrus expression compared with cows studied 40 years ago (Sheldon *et al.,* 2011). Numerous follicular waves precede the first postpartum ovulation that occurs between days 30 and 65 post partum in cattle. Understanding resumption of ovarian follicular activity in postpartum dairy cow and modulating it has a major impact on augmenting fertility. An understanding of follicular dynamics and their hormonal basis made was possible mainly by the adaptation of ultrasound scanning and radioimmunoassay technologies. These technologies have prompted attempts to manipulate ovarian function to optimize reproduction in dairy cattle.

Optimal concentrations of metabolic hormones, mainly IGF-1 and insulin along with glucose are crucial for optimal follicular development (Beam and Butler, 1999) and oocyte quality (Adamiak *et al.,* 2005). Both IGF-1 and glucose are generally stimulatory to follicular growth, whereas, glucose is a primary fuel for the ovary (Rabiee *et al.,* 1997). Importantly, antral follicles respond to dietary manipulation in the absence of an alteration in circulating patterns of the gonadotropins. Instead, the follicular responses are correlated with changes in peripheral concentrations of metabolic hormones including growth hormone (GH), insulin, IGF-I and leptin (Webb *et al.,* 2004).

High producing dairy cows are highly susceptible to negative energy balance (NEB) during postpartum. Negative energy balance may prohibit the development of pulsatile GnRH and LH patterns required for the establishment of ovulatory cycles (Butler and Canfield, 1989). In dairy cows, as the energy balance on day 15 postpartum increased, plasma LH concentration and size of the largest follicle on the ovary also increased (Lucy *et al.,* 1991). Insulin and/or IGF-I concentrations are greater in cows whose first dominant follicle ovulated (Beam and Butler, 1997) and are positively related to CL development and progesterone concentrations (Spicer *et al.,* 1990), and to energy status and follicular growth rate (Lucy *et al.,* 1992). Insulin also acts as a metabolic signal that may influence LH secretion in postpartum animals (Butler and Canfield, 1989).

4.3 Repeat breeding

Repeat breeding may be either due to fertilization failure or early embryonic mortality. In mammals, fertilization occurs in most of the cases (upto 90-98%), but early embryonic mortality has been proposed to affect reproductive efficiency.

4.3.1 Ovulatory defect

In domestic animals, ovulation occurs approximately 24–30 h after the onset of LH surge and the interval between the onset of oestrus and the LH surge can vary from 1 to 12 h in bovine (Hafez and Hafez, 2000). Various studies indicate that the ovulation occurs around 36 h after the onset of estrus. The conditions essential for ovulation are the presence of dominant responsive follicle at the time of estrus (Sartori *et al.,* 2001) and low or basal circulating progesterone levels. Any defect in ovulation (anovulation or delayed ovulation) that may arise either due to abnormal folliculogenesis or abnormal endocrine milieu may lead to infertility in female. Repeat breeders due to delayed ovulation, have extended follicular phase due to supra-basal progesterone concentration (Duchens *et al.,* 1995). Extended follicular growths delay LH surge, resulting in ovulation of aged oocyte and finally embryonic mortality (Bage, 2003). Some repeat breeders also are more likely to have delayed post-ovulatory rise in progesterone concentration. Luteal insufficiency is also suggested to be a cause for repeat breeding. Role of metabolic hormones in ovarian follicular function and fertility have been explored. Administration of insulin during recruitment and selection of the follicular wave improved fertility in repeat breeding dairy cattle (Selvaraju *et al.,* 2002).

4.3.2 Early embryonic mortality- luteal perspective

A major detriment to fertility in dairy cattle and buffalo is the high rate of embryonic mortality occurring during early pregnancy. About 40% of early embryos are lost in bovine pregnancy, and most of this loss occurs between 8 to 16 days of conception, referred to as the critical period. Maternal recognition of pregnancy by feto-maternal cross talk happens during this period leading to embryo survival. Signals between conceptus and maternal unit are not always successful, resulting in approximately 40% embryonic death in bovine. Corpus lutem plays an important role for maintaining pregnancy in bovine. Various methods have been proposed to improve luteal function in this species, such as decreasing the maternal response to luteolytic response or increasing antiluteolytic stimulation by the conceptus by producing interferon tau (IFN-t), increasing luteal phase progesterone and decreasing estrogen levels during critical period, administration of GnRH (Machado *et al.,* 2008), insulin (Selvaraju *et al.,* 2002), COX-2 inhibitors (Rajkumar *et al.,* 2010)., for enhancement of embryonic survival and fertility. Since the ovulated follicles get transformed into corpus luteum, knowledge on the follicular dynamics will improve predictable estrus, ovulation and high pregnancy rates. Studies on follicular selection and dominance can be applied to improve efficiency of timed artificial insemination, superovulation, CL function and conception rate (reviewed in Lucy, 2007). In cattle, some reports correlate a larger pre-ovulatory follicle with higher pregnancy rates, due a greater progesterone concentration from the newly formed corpus luteum. The higher progesterone stimulates the conceptus to produce higher concentrations of IFN-τ, which prevents luteolysis (reviewed in Binelli *et al.,* 2001; Perry *et al.,* 2007).

Changing the circulating concentrations of certain hormones may modulate ovarian function and fertility in dairy animals. In this regard, growth factors and metabolic hormones including somatotrophin, insulin and insulin-like growth factor (IGF) have received considerable attention in the regulation of ovarian function (Gong *et al.,* 1994; Selvaraju *et al.,* 2003). Growth factors, along with gonadotropins, modulate survival, proliferation and differentiation of follicular cells and ensure growth of small antral follicles by enhancing granulosa cell mitosis. The metabolic hormones influence the superovulatory response probably by increasing the population of gonadotropin-dependent follicles and conception rate (Selvaraju *et al.,* 2003).

5. Possible intervention strategies targeting ovary for modulating reproduction

5.1 Progesterone

Luteal progesterone during luteal phase is essential for the maintenance of pregnancy. The progesterone secretion can be improved during luteal phase by exogenous administration of progesterone. Alternatively the progesterone levels can be increased by administering GnRH which induces ovulation of a dominant follicle resulting in formation of accessory corpora lutea or luteinisation of the subordinate follicle. This, luteinized corpora luteal or luteinized follicle secretes progesterone resulting in improved pregnancy rate (Ryan *et al.,* 1991). Progesterone is administered early in the estrous cycle to mimic the mid-luteal phase levels which may lead to induce premature regression of the corpus luteum and ovulation of the 1st wave dominant follicle (Taylor and Rajamahendran, 1994). In cycling cows, low plasma progesterone concentrations associated with endogenous or exogenously induced luteolysis result in increased LH pulse frequency, persistent dominant follicle, elevated estradiol concentrations and depression of subsequent conception rates (McDougall *et al.,* 2004). The negative effects of subluteal progesterone concentration at periestrus period can be overcome, either by increasing the progesterone dose so that the LH pulse frequency is controlled or by inducing atresia or ovulation of the existing dominant follicle by injection of progesterone, estradiol benzoate (ODB) or GnRH at the commencement of treatment with chronic exogenous progesterone (Savio *et al.,* 1993; Kindler *et al.,* 1996).

5.2 GnRH and GnRH analogues

GnRH has been used extensively in animal reproduction to initiate follicular wave, induce ovulation and also to improve progesterone secretion from the corpus luteum. Since GnRH releases both FSH and LH, administration of GnRH has been advocated to reduce postpartum anestrous period in bovine. The GnRH induces ovulation at the end of superovulation programs. In estrus synchronization programs and fixed time insemination protocols GnRH has been used to synchronize follicular emergence and ovulation. In buffaloes, with administration of 100 μg gonadorelin, a dominant follicle ovulated within 48 h and this was followed by the emergence of a new follicular wave within 72 h.

5.3 Bovine somatotropin

Treatment with recombinant bovine somatotropin (BST) increases the number of antral follicles of 2-5 mm in diameter in mature heifers (Gong *et al.,* 1991). Since the population of healthy ovarian follicles >1.7 mm in diameter present at the time of gonodotropin treatment may play a very important part in determining the subsequent superovulatory response in cattle (Monniaux *et al.,* 1983), various combination of treatments were employed to improve superovulatory response. Co-treatment with growth hormone (GH) has been shown to enhance the superovulatory response to PMSG treatment in heifers, and seemed to reduce the variability in the responses among individual animals (Gong *et al.,* 1993a). The BST affects recruitment of small follicles by increasing peripheral concentrations of IGF-1, or of insulin or both. Moreover, the effect of BST on the small follicle population was not mediated through the mechanism(s) by which the dominant follicle inhibits subordinate follicles (Gong *et al.,* 1993b).

5.4 Follistatin and inhibin immunization

In bovine, immunization against follistatin increases the mean number of small follicles (3–5 mm) and causes greater response to superovulatory treatment (Singh *et al.,* 1999). The improved response in the growth or static phase of small subordinate follicles in follistatin immunized cows is due to prevention of direct paracrine or autocrine actions of follistatin (Shukovski *et al.,* 1993) or from reduced neutralization of activin. Immunisation against inhibin stimulated development of ovarian follicles. In buffaloes, following superovulation and artificial insemination, inhibin-immunisation resulted in more developing follicles. The heifers immunised against inhibin had higher plasma concentrations of activin, estradiol and progesterone (Li *et al.,* 2011). Similar to the improvement in the superovulatory response, inhibin-immunized heifers also produced more transferable embryos (Li *et al.,* 2009).

5.5 Synchronization of estrus

Synchronization makes the animal to have a follicular wave and ovulation at a predetermined time. Progesterone is used to extend the cycle and promote follicular growth, whereas $PGF_{2\alpha}$ shortens the cycle and makes the follicle to ovulate. The GnRH -$PGF_{2\alpha}$ based synchronization methods are reported to give high conception rate (Twagiramungu *et al.*, 1994; Pursely *et al.*, 1995). The administration of first GnRH induces the release of LH and FSH. In response to LH and depending on their stage of development, large follicles disappear either by ovulation and formation of new CL or by atresia. If the CL is present at the time of GnRH treatment, LH increases the number of large luteal cells. The FSH increases the turnover of follicles from <3mm (small) to >3mm (medium), but increases atresia in medum size follicles and limits further growth to larger-sized classes of follicles in cattle (Twagiramungu *et al.*, 1994). After GnRH treatment, a new dominant follicle is selected from the newly synchronized follicular wave within 3–4 days. Injection of $PGF_{2\alpha}$ on day 6 causes complete luteolysis. Subsequently, estradiol concentrations and LH pulses increase, estrus and the LH preovulatory surge occur, and the selected dominant follicle becomes the ovulatory follicle. This improves the synchronization rate and the precision of estrus between day 7 and 10 and results in normal fertility in GnRH- $PGF_{2\alpha}$ treated cows (Twagiramungu *et al.*, 1994; Pursely *et al.*, 1995). In a minority of cows however, estrus does not occur because PGF-induced luteolysis is incomplete, and the selected dominant follicle becomes persistent. This protocol has been modified by various ways and is used extensively for improving fertility in dairy animals.

Present systems of estrus synchronization need to take account of both synchronization of follicle development and corpus luteal regression in order to optimize fertility. With current ways of manipulating follicle development, the potential to implement a timed insemination program to improve reproductive management exists. Ovulation of the 1st-wave dominant follicle with hCG provides a means to markedly increase the concentration of plasma progesterone in the luteal phase and improves fertility in the subsequent estrus.

5.6. Superovulation

The objective of superstimulatory treatments in the cow is to obtain a maximum number of fertilized and transferable embryos with a high probability of producing pregnancies (Armstrong, 1993). Though superovulation has been practiced over two decades, variability in ovarian response between animals is very high. Only one third of the animal responds to superovulatory treatments. This has been related to differences in superovulatory treatments, gonadotropin preparation and inherent capacity of the animal to respond to superovulatory treatment. The follicular status of the animal mainly, follicular wave dynamics, presence of dominant follicle influences the responsiveness of the ovary to FSH and LH (Adams, 1994). Various hormonal and non-hormonal methods are tried as a pre- or co-treatment with standard superovulatory schedule (FSH and PMSG treatment) to improve superovulatory response in domestic animals (Adams, 1994; Selvaraju *et al.,* 2003).

5.7. Nutritional intervention

Various micro and macro minerals are involved in essential processes of reproduction like folliculogenesis, ovulation, fertilization and embryo survival. The energy balance in an animal can be improved by increasing dry matter intake, increasing energy density of the diet or both. Increasing energy density of diets fed to early lactation cows can be difficult. Energy density can be increased by substituting high energy concentrates such as cereal grains for forage or by supplementing fat. Since feeding cereal grain may induce acidosis, propylene glycol, a glucose precursor supplementation has been examined as an alternative way to enhance reproduction. Fats in the diet can influence reproduction positively by altering both ovarian follicle and corpus luteum function via improved energy status and by increasing precursors for the synthesis of reproductive hormones such as steroids and prostaglandins (Mattos *et al.,* 2000). Specific fatty acids may influence reproductive performance by influencing folliculogenesis and $PGF_{2\alpha}$ production by the uterus. Fat supplementation increases total number of follicles and the size of preovulatory follicles (Wehrman *et al.,* 1991; Lammoglia, 1997). The increase in size of preovulatory follicles in fat supplemented animals may be due in part to increased concentrations of plasma LH, which stimulates the latter stage of follicular growth (Mattos *et al.,* 2000). A recent study indicated that supplementing fish meal decreased the concentrations of $PGF_{2\alpha}$ without alterations in the size of CL and plasma progesterone concentrations in dairy buffaloes (Malik *et al.,* 2011). The evidences above indicate that manipulation of animal diet with the inclusion of fatty acid may improve fertility in cattle.

Conclusions

Ovarian follicle development is a complex process involving several factors both promoting and inhibiting ones. Elucidating the time relationships or the chronology of the events is of utmost importance to clearly explain the phenomenon of follicle growth and atresia and their modulation. While the techniques of ultrasound monitoring of follicle development, analysis of aspirated follicle fluid, follicle cells and the oocyte have shed some light on the gross and molecular processes, the real insight into the genomic regulation is to be pursued further for newer approaches to modulate the ovarian function and optimize reproduction.

Application of functional genomics in reproduction helps identify genes or even gene networks involved in regulating fertility. The microarray, whole genome sequencing, metabolomics and proteomics technologies help to delineate the functional genomics of the female reproduction in general and ovary in particular. Knowledge on genes and gene networks might be important for the development of new management practices and tools like the development of biomarkers and sensors to identify animals in estrus, pregnant versus non-pregnant, or cycling versus non-cycling animals. Studies in cattle have focused on oocyte maturation (Vallee *et al.,* 2005), folliculogenesis, corpus luteum development (Casey *et al.,* 2005), oviductal cell function (Bauersachs *et al.,* 2004), the endometrium during the estrous cycle (Bauersachs *et al.,* 2005), pre-implantation embryonic development (El-Halawany *et al.,* 2004) and embryo-induced transcriptome changes of the endometrium in the pre- and peri-attachment period (Ishiwata *et al.,* 2003). Apart from these various glands, organs and systems interactions in relation to ovarian function can also be elucidated (Review on Beerda *et al.,* 2008).

References

Aboul-Ela M.B. (2000). Super ovulation in the buffalo: constraints and manipulation. *Buffalo Journal* **1:** 1-20.

Adamiak S.J., Mackie K., Watt R.G., Webb R., Sinclair K.D. (2005). Impact of nutrition on oocyte quality: cumulative effects of body composition and diet leading to hyperinsulinaemia in cattle. *Biology of Reproduction* **73:** 918-926.

Adams G.P. (1994). Control of ovarian follicular wave dynamics in cattle: Implications for synchronization and superstimulation. *Theriogenology* **41:** 19-24.

Adashi E.Y., Resnick C.E., D'Ercole J.A., Svoboda M.E., Van Wyk J.J. (1985). Insulin-like growth factors as intraovarian regulators of granulosa cell growth and function. *Endocrinology Reviews* **6:** 4W-420.

Adashi E.Y., Roban R.M. (1992). Intraovarian regulation: peptidergic signalling systems. *Trends in Endocrinology and Metabolism* **3:** 243-248.

Ahmad N., Schrick F.N., Butcher R.L., Inskeep E.K. (1995). Effect of persistent follicles on early embryonic losses in beef cows. *Biology of Reproduction* **52:** 1129-1135.

Amsterdam A., Sazo´ n R., Keren-Tal I., Aharoni D., Dantes A., Rimon E., Land A., Cohen T., Dor Y., Hirsh L. (2003). Alternative pathways of ovarian apoptosis: death for life. *Biochemistry and Pharmacology* **66:** 1355-1362.

Anand (2011). Characterization of growth and atresia of buffalo ovarian follicle by biochemical analysis and expression studies. *MVSc thesis,* Veterinary, Animal and Fisheries Sciences University, Karnataka, India.

Armstrong D.G., Gutie´rrez C.G., Hogg C.O., Campbell B.K., Webb R. (1996). The expression of insulin-like growth factor binding protein (IGFBP) mRNA in primary cultures of bovine granulosa and theca cells. *Journal of Reproduction and Fertility (Abstract Series)* **17:** 31.

Armstrong D.T. (1993). Recent advances in superovulation of cattle. *Theriogenology* **39:** 7-24.

Austin E.J., Mihm M., Evans A.C.O., Knight P.G., Ireland J.L.H., Ireland J.J., Roche J.F. (2001). Alterations in intrafollicular regulatory factors and apoptosis during selection of follicles in the first follicular wave of the bovine estrous cycle. *Biology of Reproduction* **64:** 839-848.

Båge R., Petyim S., Larsson B., Hallap T., Bergqvist A.S., Gustafsson H., Rodriguez-Martinez H. (2003). Oocyte competence in repeat-breeder heifers: effects of an optimized ovum pick-up schedule on expression of oestrus, follicular development and fertility. *Reproduction Fertility and Development* **15:** 115-123.

Bao B., Garverick H.A., Smith G.W., Smith M.F., Salfen B.E., Youngquist R.S. (1997). Changes in messenger ribonucleic acid encoding luteinizing hormone receptor, cytochrome P450-side chain cleavage, and aromatase are associated with recruitment and selection of bovine ovarian follicles. *Biology of Reproduction* **56:** 1158-1168.

Bao B., Garverick H.A. (1998). Expression of steroidogenic enzymes and gonadotropin receptor genes in bovine follicles during ovarian follicular waves: a review. *Journal of Animal Science* **76:** 1903-1921.

Bauersachs S., Rehfeld S., Ulbrich S.E., Mallok S., Prelle K., Wenigerkind H., Einspanier R., Blum H., Wolf E. (2004). Monitoring gene expression changes in bovine oviduct epithelial cells during the oestrous cycle. *Journal of Molecular Endocrinology* **32:** 449-466.

Bauersachs S., Ulbrich S.E., Gross K., Schmidt S.E.M., Meyer H.H.D., Einspanier R., Wenigerkind H., Vermehren M., Blum H., Sinowatz F., Wolf E. (2005). Gene expression profiling of bovine endometrium during the oestrous cycle: detection of molecular pathways involved in functional changes. *Journal of Molecular Endocrinology* **34:** 889-908.

Beam S.W., Butler W.R. (1997). Energy balance and ovarian follicle development prior to the first ovulation postpartum in dairy cows receiving three levels of dietary fat. *Biology of Reproduction* **56:** 133-142.

Beam S.W., Butler W.R., (1999). Effects of energy balance on follicular development and first ovulation in postpartum dairy cows. *Journal of Reproduction and Fertility (Suppl.)* **54:** 411-424.

Beerda B., Wyszynska-Koko J., de Pas M.F.W., de Wit A.A.C., Veerkamp R.F. (2008). Expression profiles of genes regulating dairy cow fertility: recent findings, ongoing activities and future possibilities. *Animal* **2:** 1158-1167.

Belin M.E., Ax R.L. (1984). Chondroitin sulfate: an indicator of atresia in bovine follicles. *Endocrinology* **114:** 428-434.

Binelli M., Thatcher W.W., Mattos R., Baruselli P.S. (2001). Antiluteolytic strategies to improve fertility in cattle. *Theriogenology* **56:** 1451-1463.

Boone D.L., Yan W., Tsang B.K. (1995). Identification of a deoxyribonuclease I-like endonuclease in rat granulosa and luteal cell nuclei. *Biology of Reproduction* **53:** 1057-1065.

Brand A., de Jong W.H.R. (1973). Qualitative and quantitative micromorphological investigations of the tertiary follicle population during the oestrous cycle in sheep. *Journal of Reproduction and Fertility* **33:** 431-439.

Bridgham J.T., Wilder J.A., Hollocher H., Johnson A.L. (2003). All in the family: evolutionary and functional relationships among death receptors. *Cell Death and Differentiation* **10:** 19-25.

Butler W.R., Canfield R.W. (1989). Interrelationships between energy balance and postpartum reproduction. In: *Proc. Cornell Nutrition Conference for Feed Manufacturers,* Cornell University, Ithaca.

Cahill L.P., Mariana J.C., Mauleon P. (1979). Total ovarian follicular population in ewes of high and low ovulation rate. *Journal of Reproduction and Fertility* **55:** 27-36.

Cahill L.P. (1981). Folliculogenesis in the sheep as influenced by breed, season and oestrous cycle. *Journal of Reproduction and fertility Supplement* **30:** 135-142.

Cahill L.P., Mauléon P. (1980). Influences of season, cycle and breed on follicular growth rates in sheep. *Journal of Reproduction and fertility* **58:** 321-328.

Campbell B.K., Scaramuzzi R.J., Webb R. (1995). Control of antral follicle development and selection in sheep and cattle. *Journal of Reproduction and Fertility (Suppl.)* **49:** 335-350.

Casey O.M., Morris D.G., Powell R., Sreenan J.M., Fitzpatrick R. (2005). Analysis of gene expression in non-regressed and regressed bovine corpus luteum tissue using a customized ovarian cDNA array. *Theriogenology* **64:** 1963-1976.

Cavestany D., El-Whishy A.B., Foote R.H. (1985). Effect of season and high environmental temperature on fertility of Holstein cattle. *Journal of Dairy Science* **68:** 1471-1478.

Choudary J.B., Gier H.T., Marion G.B. (1968). Cyclic changes in bovine vesicular follicles. *Journal of Animal Science* **27:** 468-471.

Danell B. (1987). Oestrus behaviour, ovarian morphology and cyclical variation in follicular system and endocrine pattern in Water Buffalo Heifers. *Ph.D.Thesis,* Uppsala. Swedish University of Agricultural Sciences, Sweden.

Driancourt M.A., Locatelli A., Prunier A. (1995). Effects of gonadotrophin deprivation on follicular growth in gilts. *Reproduction Nutrition Development* **35:** 663-673.

Driancourt M.A., Thuel B. (1998). Control of oocyte growth and maturation by follicular cells and molecules present in follicular fluid: A review. *Reproduction Nutrition Development* **38:** 345.

Duchens M., Maciel M., Gustafsson H., Forsberg M., Rodriguez-Martinez H., Edqvist L.E. (1995). Influence of perioestrous suprabasal progesterone levels on cycle length, oestrous behaviour and ovulation in heifers. *Animal Reproduction Science* **37:** 95-108.

El-Halawany N., Ponsuksili S., Wimmers., Gilles M., Tesfaye D., Schellander K. (2004). Quantitative expression analysis of blastocyst-derived gene transcripts in preimplantation developmental stages of in vitro-produced bovine embryos using real-time polymerase chain reaction technology. *Reproduction Fertility and Development* **16:** 753-762.

Elvinger F., Natzke R.P., Hansen P.J. (1992). Interactions of heat stress and bovine somatotropin affecting physiology and immunology of lactating cows. *Journal of Dairy Science* **75:** 449-462.

Erickson B.H. (1966). Development and senescence of the post natal bovine ovary. *Journal of Animal Science* **25:** 800-805.

Evans A.C.O., Adams G.P., Rawlings N.C. (1994). Follicular and hormonal development in prepuberal heifers from 2 to 36 weeks of age. *Journal of Reproduction and Fertility* **102:** 463-470.

Evans A.C.O., Currie W.D., Rawlings N.C. (1992). Effects of naloxone on circulating gonadotrophin concentrations on prepubertal heifers. *Journal of Reproduction and Fertility* **96:** 847-855.

Evans A.C.O., Komar C.M., Wandji S.A. (1997). Changes in androgen secretion and luteinizing hormone pulse amplitude are associated with the recruitment and growth of ovarian follicles during the luteal phase of the bovine oestrous cycle. *Biology of Reproduction* **57:** 394-401.

Findlay J.K., Drummond A.E., Dyson M.L., Baillie A.J., Robertson D.M., Ethier J.F. (2002). Recruitment and development of the follicle: role of the transforming growth factor-â superfamily. *Molecular and Cellular Endocrinology* **191:** 35-43.

Fortune J.E., Cushman R.A., Wahl C.M., Kito S. (2000). The primordial to primary follicle transition. *Molecular and Cellular Endocrinology* **163:** 53-60.

Fortune J.E., Rivera G.M., Yang M.Y. (2004). Follicular development: the role of the follicular microenvironment in selection of the dominant follicle. *Animal Reproduction Science* **82-83:** 109-126.

Gilad E., Meidan R., Berman A., Graber Y., Wolfenson D. (1993). Effect of heat stress on tonic and GnRH-induced gonadotrophin secretion in relation to concentration of oestradiol in plasma of cyclic cows. *Journal of Reproduction and Fertility* **99:** 315-321.

Ginther O.J., Beg M.A., Kot K., Meira C., Bergfelt D.R. (2003). Associated and independent comparisons between the two largest follicles preceding follicle deviation in cattle. *Biology of Reproduction* **68:** 524-529.

Ginther O.J., Beg M.A., Bergfelt D.R., Donadeu F.X., Kot K. (2001). Follicle selection in monovular species. *Biology of Reproduction* **65:** 920-927.

Ginther O.J., Wiltbank M.C., Fricke P.M. (1996). Selection of the dominant follicle in cattle. *Biology of Reproduction* **55:** 1187-1194.

Glister C., Kemp C.F., Knight P.G. (2004). Bone morphogenetic protein (BMP) ligands and receptors in bovine ovarian follicle cells: actions of BMP-4,-6 and -7 on granulosa cells and differential modulation of Smad-1 phosphorylation by follistatin. *Reproduction* **127:** 239-254.

Gong J.G., Bramley T.A., Webb R. (1993b). The effect of recombinant bovine somatotrophin on ovarian follicular growth and development in heifers. *Journal of Reproduction and Fertility* **97:** 247-254.

Gong J.G., Bramley T.A., Wilmut I., Webb R. (1993a). Effect of recombinant bovine somatotropin on the superovulatory response to pregnant mare serum gonadotropin in heifers. *Biology of Reproduction* **48:** 1141-1149.

Gong J.G., McBride D., Bramley T.A., Webb R. (1994). Effects of recombinant bovine somatotrophin, insulin-like growth factor-I and insulin on bovine granulosa cell steroidogenesis in vitro. *Journal of Endocrinology* **143:** 157-164.

Gong J.G., Bramley T., Webb R. (1991). The effect of recombinant bovine somatotropin on ovarian function in heifers: follicular populations and peripheral hormones. *Biology of Reproduction* **45:** 941-949.

Gong J.G., Campbell B.K., Bramley T.A., Gutierrez C.G., Peters A.R., Webb R. (1996). Suppression in the secretion of follicle-stimulating hormone and luteinizing hormone, and ovarian follicle development in heifers continuously infused with a gonadotropin-releasing hormone agonist. *Biology of Reproduction* **55:** 68-74.

Goodman A.L., Hodgen G.D. (1983). The ovarian triad of the primate menstrual cycle. *Recent Progress in Hormone Research* **39:** 1-73.

Hafez B., Hafez E.S.E. (2000). Reproduction in farm animals. (B. Hafez, and E.S.E. Hafez, eds). Wiley-Blackwell publication, Philadelphia, USA.

Hampton J.H., Bader J.F., Lamberson W.R., Smith M.F., Youngquist R.S., Garverick H.A. (2004). Gonadotropin requirements for dominant follicle selection in GnRH agonist-treated cows. *Reproduction* **127:** 695-703.

Hein K.G., Allrich R.D. (1992). Influence of exogenous adrenocorticotropic hormone on estrous behavior in cattle. *Journal of Animal Science* **70:** 243-247.

Henderson K.M., Kieboom L.E., McNatty K.P., Lun S., Heath D.A. (1984). ^{125}I-hCG binding to bovine thecal tissue from healthy and atretic follicles. *Molecular and Cellular Endocrinology* **34:** 91-98.

Honaramooz A., Cook S.J., Beard A.P., Bartlewski P.M., Rawlings N.C. (1999). Nitric oxide regulation of gonadotrophin secretion in prepubertal heifers. *Journal of Neuroendocrinology* **11:** 667-676.

Ishiwata H., Katsuma S., Kizaki K., Patel O.V., Nakano H. Takahashi T., Imai K., Hirasawa A., Shiojima S., Ikawa H. (2003). Characterization of gene expression profiles in early bovine pregnancy using a custom cDNA micro array. *Molecular Reproduction and Development* **65:** 9-18.

Johnson A.L. (2003). Intracellular mechanisms regulating survival in ovarian follicles. *Animal Reproduction Science* **78:** 185-201.

Johnson A.L., Bridgham J.T. (2001). Regulation of steroidogenic acute regulatory protein and luteinizing hormone receptor messenger ribonucleic acid in hen granulosa cells. *Endocrinology* **142:** 3116-3124.

Kinder J.E., Kojima F.N., Bergfeld E.G.M., Wehrman M.E., Fike K.E. (1996). Progestin and estrogen regulation of pulsatile LH release and development of persistent ovarian follicles in cattle. *Journal of Animal Science* **74:** 1424-1440.

Knight P.G., Glister C. (2003). Local roles of TGF-beta superfamily members in the control of ovarian follicle development. *Animal Reproduction Science* **78:** 165-183.

Knight P.G., Glister C. (2006). TGF-β superfamily members and ovarian follicle development. *Reproduction* **132:** 191-206.

Koos R.D. (1989). Potential relevance of angiogenic factors to ovarian physiology. *Seminars in Reproductive Endocrinology* **7:** 29-40.

Lamming G.E., Royal M.D. (2001). Ovarian hormone patterns and subfertility in dairy cows. In: Fertility in the high producing dairy cow (M.G. Diskin, ed), *BSAS Endiburgh: Occasional Publication* **26:** 105-118.

Lammoglia M.A., Willard S.T., Hallford D.M., Randel R.D. (1997). Effects of dietary fat on follicular development and circulating concentrations of lipids, insulin, progesterone, estradiol 17β, 13,14-dihydro-15-ketoprostaglandin F2, and growth hormone in estrous cyclic Brahman cows. *Journal of Animal Science* **75:** 1591-1600.

Le Van T.Y., Chupin D., Driancourt D.A. (1989). Ovarian follicular population in buffaloes and cows. *Animal Reproduction Science* **19:** 171-178.

Li C., Zhu Y.L., Xue J.H., Zhang S.L., Ma Z., Shi Z.D. (2009). Immunization against inhibin enhances both embryo quantity and quality in Holstein heifers after superovulation and insemination with sex-sorted semen. *Theriogenology* **71:** 1011-1017.

Li D.R., Qin G.S., Wei Y.M., Lu F.H., Huang Q.S., Jiang H.S., Shi D.S., Shi Z.D. (2011).Immunisation against inhibin enhances follicular development, oocyte maturation and superovulatory response in water buffaloes. *Reproduction and Fertility Development* **23:** 788-797.

Lucy M.C. (2007). Fertility in high-producing dairy cows: reasons for decline and corrective strategies for sustainable improvement. *Society of Reproduction and Fertility (Suppl.)* **64:** 237-254.

Lucy M.C., Liu J., Boyd C.K., Bracken C.J. (2001). Ovarian follicular growth in sows. *Reproduction* **58:** 31-45.

Lucy M.C., Savio J.D., Badinga L., de la Sota R.L., Thatcher W.W. (1992).Factors affecting ovarian follicular dynamics in cattle. *Journal of Animal Science* **70:** 3615-3626.

Lucy M.C., Staples C.R., Michel F.M., Thatcher W.W. (1991). Effect of feeding calcium soaps to early post-partum dairy cows on plasma prostaglandin $F_{2\alpha}$, luteinizing hormone, and follicular growth. *Journal of Dairy Science* **74:** 483-489.

Lussier J.G., Matton P., Guilbault L.A., Grasso F., Mapletoft R.J., Carruthers T.D. (1994). Ovarian follicular development and endocrine responses in follicular-fluid-treated and hemi-ovariectomized heifers. *Journal of Reproduction and Fertility (Suppl.)* **102:** 95-105.

Machado R., Bergamaschi M.A.C.M., Barbosa R.T., Oliveira C.A., Binelli M. (2008). Ovarian function in Nelore (*Bos taurus indicus*) cows after post-ovulation hormone treatments. *Theriogenology* **69:** 798-804.

Magoffin D.A., Weitsman S.R. (1993). Differentiation of ovarian theca-interstitial cells in vitro: regulation of 17á-hydroxylase messenger ribonucleic acid expression by luteinizing hormone and insulin-like growth factor-I. *Endocrinology* **132:** 1945-1951.

Malik A.A., Gandotra V.K., Brar P.S., Ghuman S.P.S., Dhaliwal G.S., (2011). Attenuation of luteolytic response following fish meal supplementation in dairy buffaloes (*Bubalus bubalis*). *Animal Reproduction Science* **126:** 45-49.

Mattos R., Staples C.R., Thatcher W.W. (2000). Effects of dietary fatty acids on reproduction in ruminants. *Reviews of Reproduction* **5:** 38-45.

McDougall S., Compton C.W.R., Anniss F.M. (2004). Effect of exogenous progesterone and oestradiol on plasma progesterone concentrations and follicle wave dynamics in anovulatory anoestrous post-partum dairy cattle. *Animal Reproduction Science* **84:** 303-314.

McNatty K.P., Gibb M., Dobson C., BaU K., Custer J., Heath D., Thurley D.C. (1982). Preovulatory follicular development in sheep treated with PMSG and/or prostaglandin. *Journal of Reproduction and Fertility* **65:** 111-123.

Mette M., Andersen J., Krøll A.G., Byskov., Faber M. (1976). Protein composition in the fluid of individual bovine follicles. *Journal of Reproduction and Fertility* **48:** 109-118.

Mihm M., Austin E.J., Good T.E.M., Ireland J.L.H., Knight P.G., Roche J.F., Ireland J.J. (2000). Identification of potential intrafollicular factors involved in selection of dominant follicles in heifers. *Biology of Reproduction* **63:** 811-819.

Miller A.T., Picton H.M., Hunter M.G. (1999). Suppression of ovarian activity in the gilt and reversal by exogenous gonadotrophin administration. *Animal Reproduction Science* **54:** 179-189.

Monniaux D., Chupin D., Saumande J. (1983). Superovulatory responses of cattle. *Theriogenology* **19:** 55-81.

Nakatani A., Shimasaki S., Erickson G.F. (1991). Tissue-specific expression of four insulin-like growth factor-binding proteins (1, 2, 3, and 4) in the rat ovary. *Endocrinology* **129:** 1521-1529.

Otsuka F., Moore R.K., Shimasaki S. (2001). Biological function and cellular mechanism of bone morphogenetic protein-6 in the ovary. *Journal of Biological Chemistry* **276:** 32889-32895.

Otsuka F., Shimasaki S. (2002). A negative feedback system between oocyte bone morphogenetic protein 15 and granulosa cell kit ligand: Its role in regulating granulosa cell mitosis. *Proceedings of National Academic Sciences, USA* **99:** 8060-8065.

Perry G.A., Smith M.F., Roberts A.J., MacNeil M.D., Geary T.W. (2007). Relationship between size of the ovulatory follicle and pregnancy success in beef heifers. *Journal of Animal Science* **85:** 684-689.

Peters H., Mc Natty K.P. (1980). The ovary: A correlation of strucure and function in Mammals. Granda Publishing, London, Toronto, Sydney and New York.

Picton H.M., McNeilly A.S. (1991). Effect of basal and pulsatile LH release on FSH-stimulated follicle growth in ewes chronically treated with gonadotrophin-releasing hormone agonist. *Journal of Endocrinology* **128:** 449-456.

Porter D.A., Harman R.M., Cowan R.G., Quirk S.M. (2001). Relationship of Fas ligand expression and atresia during bovine follicle development. *Reproduction* **121:** 561-566.

Pursley J.R., Mee M.O., Wiltbank M.C. (1995). Synchronization of ovulation in dairy cows using $PGF_{2\alpha}$ and GnRH. *Theriogenology* **44:** 915-923.

Quirk S.M., Cowan R.G., Joshi S.G., Henrikson K.P. (1995). Fas antigen-mediated apoptosis in human granulosa/luteal cells. *Biology of Reproduction* **52:** 279-287.

Quirk S.M., Cowan R.G., Harman R.M. (2004). Progesterone receptor and the cell cycle modulate apoptosis in granulosa cells. *Endocrinology* **145:** 5033-5042.

Rabiee A.R., Lean I.J., Gooden J.M, Miller B.G., Scaramuzzi R.J. (1997). An evaluation of transovarian uptake of metabolites using arterio-venous difference methods in dairy cattle. *Animal Reproduction Science* **48:** 9-25.

Rahila G. (2011). Immunohistochemical and in-vitro studies on stage dependent Fas mediated apoptosis in ovarian follicles of Buffalo (bubalus bubalis). *MVSc thesis* Karnataka Veterinary, Animal and Fisheries Sciences University. Karnataka, India.

Rajakoski E. (1960).The ovarian follicular system in sexually mature heifers with special reference to seasonal, cyclical and left-right varaiations. *Acta Endocrinologica (Suppl.)* **52:** 1-68.

Rajkumar R., Singh S.K., Agarwal S.K., Mahmood S., Shankar U. (2010). Effect of selective COX-2 inhibitor on conception rate, progesterone and PGFM profile in buffalo (*Bubalus bubalis*). *Journal of Applied Animal Research* **38:** 209-212.

Ravindra J.P., Sunil K.P., Jamuna K.V., Dhanya J., Raghavendra B.S., Selvaraju S. (2011). IGF-I prevents Fas ligand induced apoptosis in granulosa cells of buffalo (*Bubalus bubalis*) ovarian follicles *in vitro*. 44th SSR annual meeting, in Portland, Oregon, USA. July 31 - August 4, 2011, (*Abstr. No* 657) p 154.

Roth Z., Meidan R., Braw-Tal R., Wolfenson D. (2000). Immediate and delayed effect of heat stress on follicular development and its association with plasma FSH and inhibin concentration in cows. *Journal of Reproduction and Fertility* **120:** 83-90.

Roth Z., Meidan R., Shaham-Albalancy A., Braw-Tal R., Wolfenson D. (2001). Delayed effect of heat stress on steroid production in medium-sized and preovulatory bovine follicles. *Animal Reproduction Science* **121:** 745-751.

Ryan D.P., Kopel E., Boland M.P., Godke R.A. (1991). Pregnancy rates in dairy cows following the administration of a GnRH analogue at the time of artificial insemination or at mid-cycle post insemination. *Theriogenology* **36:** 367-377.

Samad H.A., Nasseri A.A. (1979). A quantitative study of primordial follicles in buffalo heifers ovaries. *Compendium 13th FAO/SIDA International Course* on *Animal Reproduction* (Abstr No. 197).

Sartori R., Fricke P.M., Joao Ferreira C.P., Ginther O.J., Wiltbank M.C. (2001). Follicular deviation and acquisition of ovulatory capacity in bovine follicles. *Biology of Reproduction* **65:** 1403-1409.

Savio J.D., Thatcher W.W., Badinga L., de la Sota R.L., Wolfenson D. (1993). Regulations of dominant follicle turn over during the oestrous cycle in cows. *Journal of Reproduction and Fertility* **97:** 197-203.

Selvaraju S., Agarwal S.K., Karche S.D., Majumdar A.C. (2003). Ovarian response, embryo production and hormonal profile in superovulated goats treated with insulin. *Theriogenology* **59:** 1459-1468.

Selvaraju S., Agarwal S.K., Karche S.D., Srivastava S.K., Majumdar A.C., Shanker U. (2002). Fertility responses and hormonal profiles in repeat breeding cows treated with insulin. *Animal Reproduction Science* **73:** 141-149.

Selvaraju S., Folger J.K., Ireland J.J., Smith G.W. (2009). Temporal changes in granulosa cell BMP-2 mRNA at specific stages of a follicular wave in beef heifers and effects of BMP-2 on granulosa cell function *in vitro. In: Compendium of the XXV Annual Convention of ISSAR and International Symposium on "Expanding the horizons of reproductive technologies for augmenting fertility in farm and pet animals in the global scenario"* held at Namakkal, Tamilnadu, India.

Shalgi R., Kraicer P.F., Soferman N. (1972). Gases and electrolytes of human follicular fluid. *Journal of Reproduction and Fertility* **28:** 335-340.

Sheldon I.M., Cronin J., Borges A. (2011). The postpartum period and dairy cow fertility. Part 2: Ovarian function. *Livestock* **16:** 20-24.

Shimasaki S., Moore R.K., Otsuka F., Erickson G.F. (2004). The bone morphogenetic protein system in mammalian reproduction. *Endocrinology Reviews* **25:** 72-101.

Shukovski L., Dyson M., Findlay J.K. (1993). The effects of follistatin, activin and inhibin on steroidogenesis by bovine thecal cells. *Molecular and Cellular Endocrinology* **97:** 19-27.

Singh J., Brogliattil G.M., Christensen C.R., Adams G.P. (1999). Active immunization against follistatin and its effect on FSH, follicle development and superovulation in heifers. *Theriogenology* **52:** 49-66.

Spicer L.J., Aad P.Y., Allen D., Mazerbourg S., Hsueh A.J. (2006). Growth differentiation factor-9 has divergent effects on proliferation and steroidogenesis of bovine granulosa cell. *Journal of Endocrinology* **189:** 329-339.

Spicer L.J., Tucker W.B., Adams G.D. (1990). Insulin-like growth factor-I in dairy cows: relationships among energy balance, body condition, ovarian activity, and estrous behavior. *Journal of Dairy Science* **73:** 929-937.

Sunil K.P., Ravindra J.P., Jamuna K.V., Dhanya J., Raghavendra B.S., Prasad R.V., Selvaraju S. (2012). Assessment of immuno-localization of Fas antigen in the ovarian follicle and the role of IGF-I in Fas-L induced granulosa cell apoptosis in water buffalo (*Bubalus Bubalis*). *Indian Journal of Animal Science* (In press).

Taylor C., Rajamahendran R. (1994). Effect of mid-luteal phase progesterone levels on the first wave dominant follicle in cattle. *Canadian Journal of Animal Science* **74:** 281-285.

Tilly J. L., Kowalski K. A., Shomberg D. W., Hsueh A.J.W. (1992). Apoptosis in atretic ovarian follicles is associated with selective decreases of messenger ribonucleic acid transcripts for gonadotropin receptors and cytochrome P450 aromatase. *Endocrinology* **131:** 1670-1676.

Tilly J.L., Tilly K.I., Kenton M.L., Johnson A.L. (1995). Expression of members of the *bcl-2* gene family in the immature rat ovary: equine chorionic gonadotropin-mediated inhibition of granulosa cell apoptosis is associated with decreased bax and constitutive bcl-2 and bcl-xlong messenger ribonucleic acid levels. *Endocrinology* **136:** 232-241.

Turnbull K.E., Braden A.W.H., Mariner P.E. (1977). The pattern of follicular growth and atresia in the ovine ovary. *Australian Journal of Biological Sciences* **30:** 229-241.

Twagiramungu H., Guilbault L.A., Proulx J.G. (1994). Influence of corpus luteum and induced ovulation on ovarian follicular dynamics in postpartum cyclic cows treated with buserelin and cloprostenol. *Journal of Animal Science* **72:** 1796-1805.

Vallee M., Gravel C., Palin M.F., Reghenas H., Stothard P., Wishart D.S., Sirard M.A. (2005). Identification of novel and known oocyte-specific genes using complementary DNA subtraction and microarray analysis in three different species. *Biology of Reproduction* **73:** 63-71.

Veldhuis J.D., Furlanetto R.W. (1985). Trophic actions of human somatomedin C/insulin-like growth factor I on ovarian cells: In vitro studies with swine granulosa cells. *Endocrinology* **116:** 1235-1242.

Vinodkumar D. (2011). Immunohistochemical and in-vitro studies on the role of BMP-2 on buffalo ovarian follicular function. *MVSc thesis* Karnataka Veterinary, Animal and Fisheries Sciences University. Karnataka, India.

Warriach H.M., Ahmad N. (2007). Follicular waves during the oestrous cycle in Nili-Ravi buffaloes undergoing spontaneous and $PGF_{2\alpha}$-induced luteolysis. *Animal Reproduction Science* **101:** 332-337.

Webb R., Garnsworthy P.C., Gong J.G., Armstrong D.G. (2004). Control of follicular growth: local interactions and nutritional influences. *Journal of Animal Science* **82** (*E. Suppl.*): E63-E74.

Webb R., Gong J.G., Law A.S., Rusbridge S.M. (1992). Control of ovarian function in cattle. *Journal of Reproduction and Fertility (Suppl.)* **45:** 141-156.

Wehrman M.E., Welsh T.H. Jr Williams G.L. (1991). Diet-induced hyperlipidemia in cattle modifies the intrafollicular cholesterol environment, modulates ovarian follicular dynamics, and hastens the onset of postpartum luteal activity. *Biology of Reproduction* **45:** 514-522.

Westfall S.D., Hendry I.R., Obholz K.L., Rueda B.R., Davis J.S. (2000). Putative role of the phosphatidylinositol 3-kinase – Akt signaling pathway in the survival of granulosa cells. *Endocrine* **12:** 315-321.

Wilson S.J., Marion R.S., Spain J.N., Spiers D.E., Keisler D.H., Lucy M.C. (1998). Effect of controlled heat stress on ovarian function in dairy cattle: I. Lactating cows. *Journal of Dairy Science* **1:** 2124-2131.

Wise M.E., Armstrong D.V., Huber J.T., Hunter R., Wiersma F. (1988). Hormonal alterations in the lactating dairy cow in response to thermal stress. *Journal of Dairy Science* **71:** 2480-2485.

Wolfenson D., Lew B.J., Thatcher W.W., Graber Y., Meidan R. (1997). Seasonal and acute heat stress effects on steroid production by dominant follicles in cow. *Animal Reproduction Science* **47:** 9-19.

Wolfenson D., Thatcher W.W., Badinga L., Savio J.D., Meidan R., Lew B.J. (1995). The effect of heat stress on follicular development during the estrous cycle dairy cattle. *Biology of Reproduction* **52:** 1106-1113.

Yuan W., Bao B., Garverick H.A., Youngquist R.S., Lucy M.C. (1998). Follicular dominance in cattle is associated with divergent patterns of ovarian gene expression for insulin-like growth factor (IGF)-I, IGF-II and IGF binding protein-2 in dominant and subordinate follicles. *Domestic Animal Endocrinology* **15:** 55-63.

❑❑❑

Chapter 12

Laboratory Production of Bovine Embryo: Present Status, Limitations and Out Look

S. Nandi, P.S.P. Gupta
National Institute of Animal Nutrition and Physiology, Adugodi, Bangalore-560 030, Karnataka, India

Summary

Techniques of IVF and the related technologies have been vastly improved in bovines with the birth of viable offspring. However, still high maturation rates of oocytes, moderate fertilization rates and low blastocysts production are recorded. The success rates in buffalo are comparatively low than cattle. This chapter discusses the techniques involved in laboratory production of embryos, related problems and other technologies associated with IVF technology. Substantial work need to be done to bring all these assisted reproductive technologies at the field level.

Poor genetic makeup and reproductive failure limit the productivity of our livestock. Assisted reproductive technologies like artificial insemination (AI), superovulation, *in vitro* fertilization (IVF), embryo transfer (ET) have been introduced to overcome these problems, to increase the number of offspring from selected females and to reduce the generation intervals in farm animals. Laboratory production of embryos (IVF technology) provides an excellent and cheap source of embryos for carrying basic research on developmental physiology, farm animal breeding and for commercial application of the emerging biotechniques like cloning and transgenesis. During the past two decades, considerable advancements have been made and more are still to come as a result of continuous scientific efforts. Despite technological progress in the last two decades, the practical application of invitro fertilization

(IVF) technology is still less than anticipated because of low efficiency and high cost. The efficiency of *in vitro* embryo production in buffalo is much lower than in cattle.

1. Application of *in vitro* fertilization technology

The common scheme of *in vitro* production (IVP) of embryos involves maturing primary oocytes from tertiary follicles in culture (IVM), fertilizing the now secondary oocytes with frozen thawed semen (IVF) and then placing resulting cleaved embryos in culture (IVC) until a portion of it form morulae and blastocyst which can be transferred surgically/ non surgically to recipients (ET) or cryopreserved for future use.

In vitro fertilization technology (IVFT) has an excellent potential, both for practical applications on the farm and for basic research. The IVF coupled with embryo transfer has a wide potential for genetic improvement in livestock. Production of identical twin, sexed calves, cattle hybrid and heat tolerant embryos are the other commercial applications. The IVFT is instrumental in the progress of some related area research such as developmental biology (embryology, organogenesis), sperm and embryo sexing, cryopreservation of gametes and embryos, sperm injection, gene transfer, maternal recognition of pregnancy, disease transmission research and in emerging biotechniques like transgenesis, nuclear transfer, chimera production and cloning.

2. Present status of IVF technology

Despite technological progress in the last two decades, the practical application of IVF technology is still less than anticipated because of high cost and low success rate (Wilmut *et al.,* 2000). Overall success rate and reliability of growing bovine IVP embryos has improved and is being extended to other domestic animals (Pope, 2000). However it has been observed that *in vitro* produced embryos may produce developmentally compromised blastocysts as compared to the *in vivo* counterpart (Leibfried-Rutledge *et al.,* 1999). Though biomedical companies can accept increased cost of *in vitro* technologies, immediate implementation of this and other high end technologies on a large scale is limited for agricultural purposes as both current and future uses of gamete and culture systems become increasingly more sophisticated.

Recent data in IVF studies indicate high rate of meiotic maturation (> 85% in cattle, >80% in buffalo), fertilization (>80% in cattle, >70% in buffalo) and cleavage (>70% in cattle, >50% in buffalo) but low rates of blastocyst formation (~30% in cattle, ~25% in buffalo) and development to term (10-15%) (Blanco *et al.,* 2011, Suresh *et al.,* 2010). Newborns resulting from *in vitro* produced embryo showed severe anomalies like high birth weight, congenital malformations, impaired growth and development in cattle (Boerjan *et al.* 2000). These results provide the basis for the following conclusions: First, approximately 70% of oocytes fail to develop to blastocyst. Secondly, a high percentage of IVM/ IVF blastocysts are incapable of developing to term. Thirdly, the gamete and embryo culture conditions are still need to be optimized. One question remains pertinent: why many oocytes fail to acquire developmental competence when cultured *in vitro* whether it is due to inefficiency in competence of gametes used or inadequacies in culture systems?

3. Oocyte retrieval

In conventional IVF technology, immature oocytes are harvested from antral follicles. Follicle enclosed oocytes are arrested at the deplotene stage of prophase of 1st meiotic division. Oocytes are generally retrieved from slaughtered house ovaries, from live animals by 'Ovum pick up technique' or from preantral follicles cultured *in vitro*.

3.1 Oocyte from abattoir house ovaries

Abattoir ovaries provide a cheap and abundant source of oocyte. Though several techniques like aspiration of follicles, slicing of ovaries, puncture and dissection of follicles are available in recovering oocyte from slaughter house ovaries, aspiration is the most widely accepted technique for its speed of operation. Overall yield of acceptable oocytes in cattle (10 per ovary, Gordon and Lu, 1990) were much higher as compared to buffalo (0.4/ovary , Madan *et al.,* 1994, 0.6/ovary, Nandi *et al.,* 2000a, 1.76/ovary, Samad *et al.,* 1998). This discrepancy may be due to a) considerable low number of primordial follicle, about 12,000-19,000 (Samad and Nasseri, 1979) reserve in buffalo as compared to 150,000 in cattle (Erickson, 1966), b) low number of antral follicles at all stages of estrous cycle in buffaloes (Kumar *et al.,* 1997, c) a high incidence of deep atresia, ranging from 82% (Ocampo *et al.,* 1994) to 92% (Palta *et al.,* 1998) and d) buffaloes are slaughtered in unproductive state due to sub fertility, aging and detrimental body condition (Dominguez, 1995).

Oocytes retrieved in cool season from ovaries without any corpus luteum yield more total and acceptable quality oocytes with higher developmental potential (in cattle: Rocha *et al.,* 1998; in buffaloes: Nandi *et al.,* 2000a,b, 2001). Morphological classification of the ovaries prior to follicle aspiration could be used as an indicator of developmental competence of the collected oocytes and that the presence of a dominant follicle in either one or both ovaries of a pair has a negative effect on the IVF produced bovine embryos (Hagemann 1999). Current research aims at mimicking the effects of follicular dominance on 'oocyte capacitation' (Hyttel *et al.,* 1997) by blocking nuclear oocyte maturation in order to allow for cytoplasmic capacitation before nuclear maturation is resumed. Moreover, the possibility of allowing a routine period of follicular dominance prior to ultrasound guided ovum pick up for IVP should be considered. Molecular clock of ooplasmic maturation involving in its biochemistry is yet another unexplored area.

3.2 From live animals

'Ovum pick up' or transvaginal oocyte recovery by ultrasonographic and endoscopic instruments is an emerging technique that allows for the repeated non-surgical collection of oocytes from superior donor cows (Bungartz *et al.*, 1995), heifers (Beckers *et al.*, 1996), calves (Majerus *et al.*, 1999), pregnant (Meinjtes *et al.*, 1993) and buffaloes (Manjunatha *et al.*, 2008) without any noticeable effects on the future reproductive performances of the animals. The advantages of this technique are that genetic potential is known and disease transmission which is possible in slaughter house ovaries can be avoided (Chauhan *et al.*, 1999).

3.3 From cultured primordial and preantral follicles

Cows are born with millions of primordial and preantral follicles, of which only 0.1% ovulates in the reproductive life (Ireland 1987). Harvesting oocytes only from antral follicles limits the number of offspring per animal and the optimal exploitation of the genetic material and propagation of valuable animal stock.

Primordial and preantal follicles can be isolated (in cattle: Gutierrez *et al.*, 2000; in buffalo: Gupta *et al.*, 2000) by mechanical slicing and filtration, enzyme (trypsin, hyalaronidase, collagenase, DNAase) digestion and micro dissection of cortical species. Using all these techniques preantral follicles ranging from 50mm to 180mm in size has been isolated. Culture systems for preantral follicles in bovines are still in a very early stage of development (Telfer, 1999). Unlike in cattle where large preantral follicles (>150mm) develop more (>50mm vs. >20mm) than small preantral follicles (30-70mm) (Telfer, 1999), large buffalo preantral follicles grow faster than small preantral follicles in buffaloes and culture conditions used in cattle preantral follicles culture may not be applicable in buffalo. It can be suggested that bovine preantral follicles will require months to reach the final fertilizable stage.

4. Selection of oocytes for *in vitro* studies

Oocytes are selected on the basis of compaction of cumulus -corona investment and the granulation of ooplasm. Oocytes with more than three layers of cumulus cells and homogenous granular ooplasm are selected for IVF studies. The developmental competence of denuded oocytes is very low and cannot be improved by addition of cumulus cells to the culture medium during IVM (Das *et al.*, 1997). Recent findings demonstrated a clear relationship between oocyte diameter and developmental competence (Hyttel *et al.,* 1997). Cattle oocytes have acquired full meiotic competence at a diameter of 115 μm and full developmental competence at a diameter of 120 μm (Otoi *et al.,* 1997), whereas it is 144 μm where an buffalo oocytes gained full developmental competence (Raghu *et al.,* 2002). Trypan blue (0.05%) staining of oocytes for 2 min could be used to differentiate live and dead oocytes with no deleterious effect on maturation rate (Gupta *et al.,* 2002).

5. *In vitro* maturation of oocytes

Maturation of oocytes is a complex biological process where the primary oocytes resumes meiosis, progress from the deplotene stage of prophase of 1st meiotic division to metaphase of second meiotic division with breakdown of germinal vescicle, formation of meiotic spindle, extrusion of first polar body and expansion of surrounding cumulus cells. In conventional IVM studies, oocytes were matured in TCM199 supplemented with 10% fetal calf serum in the presence of gonadotrophins at 38.5°C in 5% CO_2 for 24 h. Maturation rate *in vitro* of oocytes are assessed by various methods like staining the oocytes (M II stage), identification of extruded first polar body in the perivitteline space and degree of expansion of cumulus cell mass, the later is routinely employed for evaluating oocyte maturation for its ready use in fertilization studies. Large variation in the timing of extrusion of first polar body and occurrence of cumulus cells expansion *in vitro,* ranging from 20 to 31h (Gordon 1994) were reported in cattle. Cumulus expansion and extrusion of first polar body commenced at 16 and 17 h respectively of buffalo oocyte culture and these events mainly exhibited during 22-24 h of culture (Nandi *et al.,* 2002).

The focus of the present research is to develop a suitable medium which will be effective but economic. Keeping this in view, attempts have been made for partial or complete replacement of basic medium with normal and cystic follicular fluid, fetal calf serum with easily proccessable and inexpensive steer serum, imported pure follicle stimulating hormone (FSH) with locally available pregnant mare serum gonadotrophin (PMSG) and replacement of both hormones and sera with somatic cells support and growth factors like insulin like growth factor I and II (IGF-I and II), epidermal growth factor (EGF), fibroblast growth factor (FGF). Current IVM technology needs further improvement to better assist those oocytes which are developmentally challenged.

6. *In vitro* fertilization of oocytes

Fertilization involves activation of oocyte by the sperm which results in the union of male and female gametes, formation of pronuclei and zygote. In most of the *in vitro* fertilization studies, *in vitro* matured oocytes are co-incubated with frozen thawed *in vitro* capacitated spermatozoa in fertilization medium for 24-48 h at 38.5°C in 5% CO_2. Though the present success rate in fertilization rate is over 80%, various hurdles are still to be overcome. Considerable variability exists among different bulls in terms of the ability of their spermatozoa to fertilize oocytes *in vitro*. The spermatozoa used for IVF may be separated by various means: swim up technique (Nandi *et al.*, 1998) and percoll gradient technique (Totey *et al.*, 1996). Use of haparin and various sperm motility enhancer like caffein, glutathione, mixture of penicillamine, hypotaurine and epinephrine (PHE), 2-cyclo-adenosine, 2-cyclo- adenosine, platelet activating factor (PAF), theothylline, pentotoxifylline have been tried to increase the fertilization and cleavage rate. Sperm concentration, volume of fertilization medium and sperm-oocytes incubation must be optimized for efficient embryo production. Attempts have been made to remove the cumulus cells prior to IVF which have particular relevance for cloning, sperm injection and other forms of gamete micromanipulation with conflicting reports such as positive effect (Hawk *et al.*, 1992) negative effect (Chian *et al.*, 1995, Nandi *et al.*, 1998) or no effect (Beholova and Greve, 1993). The fertilization rate is assessed by examination of cleavage rate which obviates the death of presumptive zygotes or embryos. For accurate analysis, including polyspermic fertilization, it is necessary to fix some oocytes 18-24h after insemination. Oocytes are fixed in 3:1 ethanol: acetic acid for 24h stained with orcein or lacmoid and observed under phase contrast microscope.

7. Culture of embryos

The weakest aspect of the *in vitro* fertilization technology is the culture of embryos to transferable stage, as the proportion of cleaved embryos developed to blastocyst was only 25-30%, though our understanding of the requirements for the development of embryos to blastocyst stage has progressed enormously in the final decade of the last millennium. Three system of culturing embryos *in vitro* are commonly used. First, cleaved embryos are transferred to the ligated oviduct of sheep or rabbit. Five or seven days later the embryos are recovered, evaluated and frozen or transferred. Second, cleaved embryos are cultured *in vitro* in basic medium (TCM199 etc.) supplemented with serum along with somatic cells (oviductal epithelial cells, granulosa cells, buffalo rat liver cells etc.) at 38.5°C in 5% CO_2 or in medium conditioned by somatic cells for 7-10 days. Somatic cells like cumulus and oviductal cells are reported to secrete proteins, growth factors etc. besides removed inhibitory components from *in vitro* culture environment of oocytes/embryos thereby providing conducive culture environment. Third, cleaved embryos are cultured in simple defined media where components are in accordance to the needs of embryos without any somatic cell support. The most common defined medium for *in vitro* culture is synthetic oviductal fluid, SOF (Tervit *et al.*, 1972) or a modified form of SOF

(Takahashi and First, 1992). The *in vitro* embryo production is now moving towards serum free defined media (Kruip *et al.,* 2000, Nandi *et al.,* 2008) for its simple procedures, reduced the in between and within laboratory variations and to ensure biosafety. Morphologically normal blastocysts after thawing and their survivability were significantly higher in blastocysts obtained from embryos cultured in mSOF than those cultured in complex co-culture system (Nandi et al. 2003). Another concept of *in vitro* culture system is the regulation of energy metabolism (Thompson *et al.,* 2000). Subtle difference exists at the cellular level in terms of metabolic profiles and morphology (Leese *et al.,* 1998) and in the gene expression (Wrenzychi *et al.,* 1999). As suboptimal culture conditions may lead to production of embryos with developmental abnormalities and reduced viability, a renewed research focus on the relationship between embryo development and sub-optimal culture environment and greater understanding of the regulation of expression of the genes related to blastocyst formation (Huang *et al.,* 2010) is necessary if an improvement in embryo production is to occur.

Embryos produced *in vitro* are either transferred or cryopreserved for further use. Two well known cryopreservation techniques are vitrification and programmable freezing. Vitrification, a recently developed technique without the use of expensive freezing machine, involves a physical process by which a highly concentrated solution of cryoprotectants solidifies during cooling without the formation of ice crystals. Vitrification has been used successfully for oocytes (cow: Saha *et al.,* 1996; buffalo: Dhali *et al.,* 2000) and embryos (Delval *et al.,* 1996, Ravindranatha *et al.,* 2001). Comparison of vitrification and programmable freezing for cattle *in vivo* and *in vitro* produced embryos revealed that vitrification though inflict significantly more cryoinjury compared to programmable freezing without any significant difference in conception and calving rates (Ravindranatha *et al.,* 2001). Vitrification having advantage in terms of speed of operation and low cost may be useful for embryo transfer in the field level. *In vivo* cultured embryos frozen and transferred give 60-70% pregnancy rate. In contrast, pregnancy rate is only 20-40% following transfer of frozen *in vitro* produced embryos. However, when *in vitro* embryos are transferred as fresh, then a reasonable pregnancy rate (50-60%) can be achieved.

8. Open problems

In spite of tremendous potential, the practical application of IVF technology is still limited. A number of problems have to be overcome to make these technologies farmers friendly. These problems are causing disillusionment with the promises this technology once held.

8.1 Fertilization abnormalities

Of the various fertilization abnormalities which limits the success of IVF polyspermy, parthenogenesis, polygyny, acynchronous development of male and female pronuclei, preactivation of cytokinesis and abnormal karyotype are the most important ones. Polyspermy is a major problem as polyspermic oocytes cleave but do not develop beyond blastocyst stage. Parthenogenesis is the development of oocytes without the intervention of the male gametes. Parthenogenesis may produce blastocyst but they will not progress to term. In buffalo, 2% of oocytes were found to be cleaved due to parthenogenesis (Chauhan 2012 personal communication). Polygyny is characteristics by the presence of more than two pronuclei, or two pronuclei and one decondensing sperm head which may be due to the failure of the first or second polar body to be extruded, or from parthenogenetic activation (Xu and Greve, 1988). Preactivation of cytokinesis compromises symmetrical division of the ooplasm, similar to normal cytokinesis but pronuclei may be found in one or each of the two cellular components (Xu and Greve, 1988). Incidence of karyotypically abnormal embryo is another problem as these embryos tends to die in early embryonic period. The embryos are mixoploid, polyploid (3n or 4n) or haploid (n). In cattle, 72% of embryos produced *in vitro* were mixoploid which was significantly higher than the 25% mixoploid embryos after superovulation and *in vivo* growth (Viuff *et al.*, 1999).

8.2 Quality of embryos

Anything against the normal procedures bound to have some abnormalities. Question is how viable are embryos that are manipulated *in vitro* as compared to embryos *in vivo*? Manipulation of oocytes and embryos can interfere with normal embryonic development (Wright and Ellington, 1995). A large proportion of *in vitro* embryos possessed square and swollen blastomeres and compaction of morulae are not clear. Embryos cultured *in vivo* develop faster than that cultured *in vitro* for example in cow: 6 days vs 7 days (Galli and Lazzari, 1996), in buffalo 7 days vs 7-8 days (Chauhan *et al.*, 1998). *In vitro* derived embryos accumulate lipids (Pollard and Leibo, 1994) thus make more sensitive to freezing.

8.3 Efficiency of calf production

Since the birth of first cattle (Brackett *et al.*, 1982), buffalo (Madan *et al.*, 1991) calf from IVF oocytes and most recently in sheep, the first somatic cell cloned animal "Dolly" (Wilmut *et al.*, 1997), so much advancement have been made, thus, by now , there should be thousands of calves born following IVP of preimplantation embryos. The efficiency of the *in vitro* system is significantly poorer than the *in vivo* system (55 versus 8 calves born per 100 oocytes after *in vivo* (AI) or IVP of embryos, respectively) Approximately twice as many transfer were needed per pregnancy for embryos produce *in vitro* as for those produced *in vivo*.

8.4 Quality of offspring produced

Quality of offspring is adversely affected by IVP of embryos. The IVP embryos result in skewed sex ratio towards increased male birth (Gutierrez-Adan *et al.*, 1996) heavier and less vigorous calves (Leibfried-Rutledge, 1999), overgrown fetus ("large calf syndrome", Farin and Farin, 1995, Young *et al.*, 1998), longer gestation periods (Van Wagtendonk-de Leeuw *et al.*, 1998), increased abortion rates, perinatal and neonatal calf losses (Hasler *et al.*, 1995), dystocia (Kruip and den Daas, 1997), increased incidence of congenital malformations like gastroschisis, hypospadias (Silver *et al.*, 1999), hydronephrosis, fused digits, untestes, pigmented naevus (check spell) and umbilical hernia (Boerjan *et al.*, 2000), more hydroallantois (Hasler *et al.*, 1995, van Wagtendonk-de Leeuw *et al.*, 1998), disproportionate growth of different vital organs like liver , kidney and heart (Farin and Farin, 1995) compared to calves born after AI or after multiple ovulation and embryo transfer (MOET). Upon cloning by nuclear transfer and transgenesis, these problems are more pronounced. 3.7% of calves born after IVP co-culture show malformation in contrast to only 0.8% in normally conceived (Boerjan *et al.*, 2000). The factors causing "large calf syndrome" are not clear. It may be due to use of the complex culture media having serum and co-cultured cells (Jacobson *et al.*, 2000) which secrete embryonic growth factors in an attempt to mimic *in vivo* circumstances, thus making them undefined, high oxygen tension in embryo culture system, the static culture system and the high ammonium concentrations (waste product of protein metabolism). The skewed sex ratio (more male: female) may be due to the fact that male embryos develop faster than female embryos in presence of exogenous glucose (Bredbacka and Bredbacka, 1996) or due to oxidative stress as a result of oxidation-induced gene expression (Sohal and Allen, 1990). Male embryos are more advanced (Avery *et al.*, 1991) and survive micro-manipulation better than female embryos (King *et al.*, 1992). Combination of this entire situation could lead to an artificial sex shift in the offspring (Galli and Lazzari, 1996). As suggested by Wagtendonk-de Leew *et al.*, 1998, the "metabolic setting" concept of Hales and Barker (1992) might apply to the *in vitro* production of bovine embryos. The *in vitro* culture environment is still sub-optimal by unbalanced with an oversupply of certain nutrients and lacking of others and the resulting effects are manifested at pre and post natal life.

8.5 Disease transmission

Great risk in transmission of bacterial and viral diseases through transfer of IVP embryos exist where abattoir ovaries are used as oocytes sources

(Stringfellow and Givens, 2000). Out of various disease transmission, bovine herpes virus, bovine rhinotrachietes, infectious pastular vaginitis, bovine viral diarrhoea, vesicular stomatitis, Brucellosis, *E. coli* , *Mycobacterium, Mycoplasma, Streptococci* infections are most common.

8.6 Ethical issues

Anything involving manipulation of embryos or that causing stress to animals invites ethical concerns. Ethical concerns relates to animal health and welfare, integrity of animal or the interrelationship between two (Christiansen and Sandoe, 2000). Reproductive technologies such as ovum pick up, ET cause stress to animals and oversized offspring, physical abnormalities due to IVF, cloning and transgenesis pose a risk to animal welfare. Many ethical consideration need to be addressed before implementing the technology at the field levels.

9. Overcoming the problems

To solve the problems and to improve the present status of bovine IVP there are some measures:

a) Use of low cost indigenous components and replacement of imported chemicals, to make the technology economical and farmer friendly.

b) Utilization of various selection criteria of ovaries and oocytes, correlation of these criteria with performance of blastocyst generated after transfer and developing culture system that support completion of oocyte "biological program" is required.

c) Defined media like SOF, CRI, CZB, KSOM without serum or only with non-dialysable fraction and with a low oxygen tension (5-10%) might be an ideal oocyte and embryo culture media. Use of serum is not recommended as it is an important disturbing factor, either via effects on the genome imprinting (Young *et al.*, 2000) or directly on mitochondria (Bavister *et al.*, 2000) or on the other organelles and membrane (Kruip *et al.*, 2000).

d) Quality control is a must for culture media, sera, additives used and transferable embryos obtained through IVP system must be free of pathogens by washing, antibiotic and enzyme (trypsin) treatment.

e) Emphasis should be given on development of an efficient *in vitro* embryo production system without any side effects on health and welfare of the offspring.

10. Looking to the future

Purposes of IVF technology are not only to produce embryos for genetic manipulation and/or embryo transfer and for basic research in gamete biology and developmental physiology but also it is the only means for commercial utilization of emerging biotechnologies like embryo sexing, transgenic livestock production and cloning.

10.1 *In vitro* culture of primordial, preantral and early-antral follicles for the production of embryos

Harvesting oocytes from primordial and preantral follicles not only tremendously increase in the production of a uniform population of genetically superior animals, i) it would shorten the generation interval of valuable animals, ii) avoid exposure of oocytes to undesirable environmental influences, iii) function as a new model for investigating the complex mechanisms involved in early folliculogenesis, iv) favourably impact on assisted reproduction in endangered species and in humans (Van der hurk *et al.,* 1997). Research has been focused recently in this aspect; clear understanding of the metabolic, substrate and hormonal requirements for each stage of development is yet to be established. Practical application of preantral follicles for IVP of livestock species may not be far away after the success of production of embryos from oocytes derived from in vitro grown buffalo preantral follicles (Gupta *et al.,* 2008).

10.2 Gamete manipulation

Four approaches of gamete manipulation are available under conditions of reduced sperm number or when sperm motility is compromised or even non-existent: i) Zona thinning by enzymatic (pronase) digestion, ii) Zona drilling in which a hole is made in the zona surface mechanically, by laser ablation or by localized application of a zona solvent (acid Tyrode) which facilitates access of sperm to the oocyte surface, iii) subzonal sperm insertion (SUZI) in which one or more sperm are placed under the zona pellucida, iv) intracytoplasmic sperm injection (ICSI) in which a sperm of any type (sperm head, immotile sperm, dead sperm, defective sperm, round spermatids) is microinjected into the ooplasm. Though popular in human, ICSI is not successfully applied in a production setting for domestic mammalian species. The ICSI is controversial due to its putative genetic implications (Menezo *et al.,* 2000). Other technologies are "*in vitro* spermatogenesis" (Tesarik *et al.,* 1999) and sperm sexing (Johnson *et al.,* 2000). These are new areas of research in farm animal reproductive technology waiting further in depth investigations.

10.3 Embryo splitting and sexing

Embryo splitting or quartering is used to produce identical twin, facilitating embryo sexing and increase the number of transferable embryos (Rho *et al.*, 1998). Direct transfer of embryos yielded around 60 calves per 100 embryos; transfer of split embryos typically produced 105 calves per 100 embryos (Wilmut, 2000). Preselection of offspring sex has long been an objective for animal breeder. However, extensive use require the methods of sexing to be effectively accurate, non-invasive, rapid, simple and most importantly to have minor or no detrimental effects on the embryos (Agca *et al.*, 1998). Sexing of embryos prior to transfer is now possible using PCR. Although accuracy is 95% and 50-70% of biopsied grade I embryos establish pregnancy, the technology is not applicable as a routine procedure (Wilmut, 2000). One economic factor is that usually half the embryos are to be discarded as the breeder only wants calves of female sex thus making the cost of embryo transfer double.

10.4 Nuclear transfer, transgenesis and cloning

In vitro embryo production techniques have facilitated and enabled the success of large scale efforts to generate, evaluate and breed nuclear transfer, cloned and transgenic cattle. Nuclear transfer involves the introduction of the nucleus from a totipotent donor cell into a matured enucleated oocyte. The resulting embryo is transferred to a surrogate mother for development into a calf. Key to overall success of nuclear transfer is the requirement for totipotency, defined as the potential to initiate and direct normal development (Polejaeva and Campbell, 2000). Transgenesis technology permits modifications of phenotype by introducing subtle changes in genotype. Cloning can be done either by embryo splitting or nuclear transplantation. Though these technologies produce viable calves (Cibelli *et al.*, 1998, Niemann and Kues, 2000; George *et al.*, 2011) application in animal selection scheme at present is not very much practicable because of the low efficiency in particular the late and pre- and perinatal losses.

Conclusions

Laboratory production of embryo provides enormous benefit to biotechnology, biomedicine, farm animal breeding and research. It improves to design and test future therapies for managing reproduction with application for agriculture, transgenesis, endangered species and provide the model for human diseases. Laboratory production of embryos may be applicable with its current limitations for application related to biotechnology. A lot of challenges will need to be overcome before the technology is used on a broad scale for agricultural applications.

References

Agca Y., Monson R.L., Northley D.L., Peschel D.E., Schaefer D.M., Rutledge J.J. (1998). Normal calves from transfer of biopsied, sexed and vitrified IVP bovine embryos. *Theriogenology* **50:** 129-145.

Avery B., Madison V., Greve T. (1991). Sex and development in bovine *in vitro* fertilised embryos. *Theriogenology* **35:** 953-953.

Bavister B.D. (2000). Interactions between embryos and the culture milleu. *Theriogenology* **53:** 619-626.

Beckers F., Kanitz W., Nurnberg G., Kurth J., Spitschak M. (1996). Comparision of repeated tranvaginal ovum pick up in heifers by ultrasonographic and endoscopic instruments. *Theriogenology* **46:** 999-1007.

Behalova E., Greve, T. (1993). Penetration rate of cumulus enclosed versus denuded bovine eggs fertilized *in vitro*. *Theriogenology* **39:** 186 (Abstract).

Boerjan M.L., den Daas J.H.G. and Dieleman S.J. (2000). Embryonic origins of health:long term effects of IVF in humans and livestock. *Theriogenology* **53:** 537-547.

Blanco M. R., Demyda S., Moreno Millán M., Genero E. (2011). Developmental competence of *in vivo* and *in vitro* matured oocytes: A review. *Biotechnology and Molecular Biology Review* **6:** 155-165.

Brackett B.G., Bousquet D., Boice M.L., Donawick W.J., Evans J.F. and Dressel M.A. (1982). Normal development following *in vitro* fertilization in the cows. *Biolology of Reproduction* **27:** 147-158.

Bredbacka K., Bredbacka P. (1996). Glucose controls sex-related growth rate differences of bovine embryos produced *in vitro*. *Journal of Reproduction and Fertility* **106:** 169-172.

Bungartz L., Lucas-Haln A., Rath D., Niemann H. (1995) Collection of oocytes from cattle via follicular aspiration aided by ultrasound with or without gonadotrophin pretreatment and in different reproductive stages. *Theriogenology* **43:** 667-675.

Chauhan M.S., Singla S.K., Palta P., Manic R.S., Tomer O.S. (1998). Development of *in vitro* produced buffalo (*Bubalus bubalis*) embryos in relation to time. *Asian Australasian Journal of Animal Sciences* **11:** 398-403.

Chauhan M.S., Nadir S., Bailey T.L., Pryor A.W., Butler S.P., Notter D.R., Valender W.H., Gwazdauskas F.C. (1999). Bovine follicular dynamics, oocyte recovery, and the development of oocytes microinjected with a green fluroscent protein construct. *Journal of Dairy Sciences* **82:** 918-926.

Chian R.C., Okuda K., Niwa K. (1995). Influence of cumulus cells on *in vitro* fertilization of bovine oocytes derived from *in vitro* maturation. *Animal Reproduction Sciences* **38:** 37-38.

Christiansen S.B., Sandoe P. (2000). Bioethics: limits to the interference with life. *Animal Reproduction Sciences* **60-61:** 15-29.

Cibelli J.B., Stice S.S., Golueke P.J., Kane J.J., Jerry J., Blackwell C., Ponce de leon F.A., Robl J.M. (1998). Cloned transgenic calves produced from non-quiscent fetal fibroblast. *Science* **280:** 1256-1258.

Das S.K., Chauhan M.S., Palta P., Tomer O.S. (1997). Influence of cumulus cells on *in vitro* maturation of denuded buffalo oocytes. *Veterinary Record* **141:** 522-523.

Delval A., Ectors F.J., Touati K., Beckers J.F., Ectors F. (1996). Vitrification of bovine embryos produced *in vitro*: survival, hatching and pregnancy rates. *Theriogenology* **45:** 178.

Dhali A., Manic R.S., Das S.K., Singla S.K., Palta P. (2000). Vitrification of buffalo (*Bubalus bubalis*) oocytes. *Theriogenology* **53:** 1295-1303.

Dominguez M.M. (1995). Effects of body condition, reproductive status and breed on follicular population and oocyte quality in cows. *Theriogenology* **43:** 1405-1418.

Erickson, B.H. (1966). Development and senescence of post-natal bovine ovary. *Journal of Animal Sciences* **25:** 800-805.

Farin P.W., Farin C.E. (1995). Transfer of bovine embryos produced *in vivo* or *in vitro*: Survival and fetal development. *Biology of Reproduction* **52:** 676-682.

Galli C., Lazzari, G. (1996). Practical aspects of IVM/IVF in cattle. *Animal Reproduction Science* **42:** 371-379.

George, A, Sharma, R, Singh, K.P, Panda, S.K., Singla, S.K., Palta, P., Manik, R., Chauhan, M.S. (2011). Production of cloned and transgenic embryos using buffalo (Bubalus bubalis) embryonic stem cell-like cells isolated from in vitro fertilized and cloned blastocysts. *Cell Reprograming* **13:** 263-272.

Gordon I. (1994). Laboratory production of cattle embryo. *CAB International*, Wallington, Oxon, U.K.

Gordon I., Lu K.H. (1990). Production of embryos *in vitro* and its impact on livestock production. *Theriogenology* **33:** 77-87.

Gupta P.S.P., Nandi S., Ravindranatha B.M., Sarma P.V. (2000). Isolation of preantral follicles from buffalo ovaries. *Veterinary Record* **148:** 580-581.

Gupta P.S.P., Nandi S., Ravindranatha B.M., Sarma P.V. (2002). Trypan blue staining to differentiate live and dead buffalo oocytes and its effect on embryodevelopment *in vitro*. *Buffalo Journal* **18:** 321-330.

Gupta, P.S.P., Ramesh, H.S., Manjunatha, B.M., Devaraj, M. Nandi, S. and Ravindra, J.P., (2008). Production of buffalo embryos using oocytes from *in vitro* grown preantral follicles. *Zygote* **16:** 57-63.

Gutierrez-Adan A., Behboodi E., Anderson G.B., Medrano J.F., Murray, J.D. (1996). Relationship between stage of development and sex of bovine IVM-IVF embryos cultured *in vitro* versus in the sheep oviduct. *Theriogenology* **46:** 515-525.

Gutierrez C.G., Ralph J.H., Telfer E.E., Wilmut I., Webb, R. (2000). Growth and antrum formation of bovine preantral follicles in long term culture *in vitro*. *Biology of Reproduction* **63:** 267-273.

Hagemann L.J. (1999). Influence of the dominant follicle on oocytes from subordinate follicles. *Theriogenology* **51:** 449-59.

Hales, C.N., Barker D.J.P. (1992). Type 2 (non-insulin-dependent) diabetes millitus: the thrifty phenotype hypothesis. *Diabetologia* **35:** 595-601.

Hasler J.F., Handerson W.B., Hurtgen P.J., Jin Z.Q., Mccauley A.D., Mower S.A., Neely B., Shuey L.S., Stokes J. E., Trimmer, S.A. (1995). Production, freezing and transfer of bovine IVF embryos and subsequent calving results. *Theriogenology* **43:** 141-152.

Hawk H.W., Nel N.D., Waterman R.A., Wall R.J. (1992). Investigation of means to improve rates of fertilization in *in vitro* matured/*in vitro* fertilized bovine oocytes. *Theriogenology* **38:** 989-998.

Huang, W., Yandell, B.S., Khatib H. (2010) Transcriptomic profiling of bovine IVF embryos revealed candidate genes and pathways involved in early embryonic development. BMC Genomics 11:23 (http://www.biomedcentral.com/1471-2164/11/23).

Hyttel, P., Fair, T., Callesen, H., Greve, T. (1997). Oocyte growth, capacitation and final maturation in cattle. *Theriogenology* **47:** 23-32.

Ireland J.J. (1987). Control of follicular growth and development. *Journal of Reproduction and Fertility* **34:** 39-44.

Jacobson H., Schmidt M. P., Holm P., Sangild P.T., Vajta G., Greve T., Callesen, H. (2000). Body dimension and birth weight of calves derived from *in vitro* produced embryos cultured with or without serum and oviductal epithelial cells. *Theriogenology* **53:** 1761-1769.

Johnson, J.A. (2000). Sexing mammalian sperm for production of offspring in the state-of-the-art. *Anim. Reprod. Sci.* **60-61:** 93-107.

King W.A., Picard L., Bousquet D., Goff, A.K. (1992). Sex-dependent loss of bisected bovine morulae after culture and freezing. *Journal of Reproduction and Fertility* **96:** 453-459.

Kruip T.A.M., den Daas, J.H.G. (1997). *In vitro* produced and cloned embryos: effects on pregnancy, parturition and offspring. *Theriogenology* **8:** 43-52.

Kruip T.A.M., Bevers M.M., Kemp B. (2000). Environment of oocyte and embryo determines health of IVP offspring. *Theriogenology* **53:** 611-618.

Kumar A., Solanki V.S., Jindal S.K., Tripathi V.N., Jain, G.C. (1997) Oocyte retrieval and histological studies of follicular population in buffalo ovaries. *Animal Reproduction. Science* **47:** 189-195.

Leese H.J., Donnary I., Thompson J.H. (1998). Human assisted conception: a cautionary tale, lessons from domestic animals. *Human Reproduction* **13** *(Suppl. 4):* 184-202.

Leibfried-Rutledge M.L. (1999). Factors determining competence of *in vitro* produced cattle embryos. *Theriogenology* **51:** 473 – 485.

Madan M.L., Singla S.K., Jailkhani S., Ambrose, J.D. (1991). *In vitro* fertilization and birth of first ever IVF buffalo calf. *Proc. Third World Buff. Cong.* **7:** 11-17.

Madan M.L., Singla S.K., Chauhan M.S., Manik, R.S. (1994). *In vitro* production and transfer of embryos in buffaloes. *Theriogenology* **41:** 139-143.

Majerus V., deRoover R., Etienne D., Kaidi S., Massip A., Dessy F., Donnay, I. (1999). Embryos production by ovum pick up in unstimulated calves before and after puberty. *Theriogenology* **52:** 1169-1179.

Manjunatha B.M., Ravindra J.P., Gupta P.S.P., Devaraj M., Nandi, S. (2008). Oocyte recovery by ovum picks up and embryo production in river buffaloes (*Bubalus bubalis*). *Reproduction in Domestic Animals* **43:** 477-480.

Massip A., Mermillod P., Van Longendonckt A., Reichenbach H.D., Lonergan P., Roy U., Carolan C., De Ronnen R., Bren G. (1996). Calving outcome following transfer of embryos produced *in vitro* in different conditions. *Animal Reproduction Science* **44:** 1-10.

Meinjtes M., Bellow M.S., Broussard J.R., Paul J.B., Godke R.A. (1993). Tranvaginal aspiration of bovine oocytes from hormone treated pregnant beef cattle for IVF. *Theriogenology* **39:** 266.

Nandi S., Chauhan, M.S., Palta P. (1998). Influence of cumulus cells and sperm concentration on cleavage rate and subsequent embryonic development of buffalo (*Bubalus bubalis*) oocytes matured and fertilized *in vitro. Theriogenology* **50:** 1251-1262.

Nandi S., Chauhan M.S., Palta, P. (2000a). Quantity and quality of aspirated buffalo oocytes: Effect of a presence of a Corpus luteum in the ovary. *Indian Journal of Animal Sciences* **70:** 486-487.

Nandi S., Chauhan M.S., Palta P. (2000b). Effect of a corpus luteum on the recovery and developmental potential of buffalo oocytes. *Veterinary Record* **147:** 580-581.

Nandi S., Chauhan M.S., Palta, P. (2001). Effect of environmental temperature on quality and developmental competence *in vitro* of buffalo oocytes. *Veterinary Record* **148:** 278-279.

Nandi S., Ravindranatha B.M., Gupta P.S.P., Sarma P.V. (2002). Timing of sequential changes in cumulus cells and first polar body extrusion during *in vitro* maturation of buffalo oocytes. *Theriogenology* **57:** 1151-1159.

Nandi S., Raghu H.M., Ravindranatha B.M., Gupta P.S.P., Sarma P.V. (2003). Developmental competence and post-thaw survivability of buffalo embryos produced *in vitro*: Effect of growth factors in oocyte maturation medium and embryo culture system. *Theriogenology* **60:** 1621-1631.

Nandi S., Girish Kumar V., Manjunatha B.M., Ramesh H.S., Gupta, P.S.P. (2008). Follicular fluid concentrations of glucose, lactate and pyruvate in buffalo and sheep, and their effects on cultured oocytes, granulosa and cumulus cells. *Theriogenology* **69:** 186-196.

Niemann, H., Kues, W.A. (2000). Transgenic livestock: premises and promises. *Animal Reproduction Science* **60-61:** 277-293.

Ocampo M.B., De Asis A. T., Ocampo L.C., Kanagawa H. (1994). Histological observation of follicular atresia in swamp buffalo. *Buffalo Bulletin* **13:** 51-55.

Otoi T., Yamamoto K., Koyama N., Tachikawa S., Suzuki T. (1997). Bovine oocyte diameter in relation to developmental competence. *Theriogenology* **48:** 769-774.

Palta P., Chauhan, M.S. (1998). Laboratory production of buffalo (*Bubalus bubalis*) embryos. *Reprod, Fertil. Dev.* **10:** 379-391.

Polejaeva I.A., Campbell K.H.S. (2000). New advances in somatic cell nuclear transfer: application in transgenesis. *Theriogenology* **53:** 117-126.

Pollard J.W., Leibo S.P. (1994). Chilling sensitivity of mammalian embryos. *Theriogenology* **41:** 101-106.

Pope C.E. (2000). Embryo techniques in conservation efforts for endangered fields. *Theriogenology* **53:** 163-174.

Ravindranatha B.M., Nandi S., Reddy, S.M. (2001). Vitrification and programmable freezing of different stages of bovine embryos-pregnancy and calving following transfer. *Indian Journal of Dairy Science* **54:** 75-79.

Rho G.J., Johnson W.H., Betteridge, K.J. (1998). Cellular composition and viability of demi- and quarter -embryos made from bisected bovine morulae and blastocyst produced *in vitro*. *Theriogenology* **50:** 885-895.

Rocha A., Randel R.D., Broussard J.R., Lim J.M., Blair R.M., Roussel J.D., Godke R.A., Hansel W. (1998). High environmental temperature and humidity decrease oocyte quality in *Bos taurus* but not in *Bos indicus* cows. *Theriogenology* **49:** 657-665.

Saha S., Boediono A., Sumantri E., Murakami M., Kikkawa Y., Suzuki T. (1996). Vitrification of bovine *in vitro* matured and pronuclear oocyte with different vitrification solution. *Theriogenology* **45:** 179.

Samad H.A., Nasseri A.A. (1979). A quantitative study of primordial follicles in buffalo heifer ovaries. In: *Comp. 13th FAO/SIDA Int. Course Anim. Reprod.*

Sansone, G., Nastri, M.J.F. and Fabbrocini, A. (2000). Storage of buffalo (*Bubalus bubalis*) semen. *Animal Reproduction Science* **60-61:** 55-76.

Silver R.I., Rodriquez R., Chang T.S.K., Gearhart J.P. (1999). In vitro fertilization is associated with a risk of hypospadias. *Journal of Urology* **161:** 1954-1957.

Sohal R.S., Allen R.G. (1990). Oxidative stress as a causal factor in differentiation and aging: a unifying hypothesis. *Experimantal Gerontology* **25:** 499-522.

Suresh, K.P., Nandi, S., Mondal S. (2010). Factors affecting laboratory production of buffalo embryos: A meta-analysis *Theriogenology* **72:** 978-985.

Stringfellow D.A., Givens M.D. (2000). Preventing disease transmission through transfer of *in-vivo*-derived bovine embryos. *Livestock Production Science* **62:** 237-252.

Takahashi Y., First, N.L. (1992). *In vitro* development of bovine one cell embryos: influence of glucose, lactate, pyruvate, amino acids & vitamins. *Theriogenology* **37:** 963-978.

Telfer E.E., Webb R., Moor R.M., Gosden, R.G. (1999). New approaches to increase in oocyte yield from ruminants. *Animal Science* **68:** 285-298.

Tervit H.R., Whittingham D.G., Rowson L. E. A. (1972). Successful culture *in vitro* of sheep and cattle ova. *Journal of Reproduction and Fertility* **30:** 493-497.

Tesarik J., Bahceci M., Ozcan C., Greco E., Mendoza C. (1999). Restoration of fertility by *in vitro* spermatogenesis. *Lancet* **353:** 555-556.

Thompson J.G. (2000). *In vitro* culture and embryo metabolism of cattle and sheep embryos a decade of achievement. *Animal Reproduction Science* **60-61:** 263-275.

Totey S.M., Daliri M., Appa Rao K.B.C., Pawshe C.H., Taneja M., Chiller, R.S. (1996). Differential cleavage and developmental rates and their correlation with cell numbers and sex ratios in buffalo embryos generated *in vitro*. *Theriogenology* **45:** 521-533.

Van den Hurk R., Bevers M.M., Beckers J.F. (1997). *In-vivo* and *In-vitro* development of preantral follicles. *Theriogenology* **47:** 73-82.

Viuff D., Rickords L., Offenberg H., Hyttel P., Avery B., Greve T., Olsaker I., Williams J.L, Callesen H., Thomson P.D. (1999). A high proportion of bovine blastocysts produced *in vitro* are mixoploid. *Biology of Reproduction* **60:** 1273-1278.

Wagtendonk-de Leeuw van A.M., Aerts B.J.G., Den Daas J.H.G. (1998). Abnormal offspring following *in vitro* production of bovine pre-implantation embryos: a field study. *Theriogenology* **49:** 883-894.

Wilmut I., Schnieke A.E., McWhir J., Kind A.J., Campbell K.H.S. (1997). Viable offspring derived from fetal and adult mammalian cells. *Nature* **385:** 810-813.

Wilmut I., Young L., deSousa P., King T. (2000). New opportunities in animal breeding and production - an introductory remark. *Animal Reproduction Science* **60-61:** 5-14.

Wrenzychi C., Herman D., Carnwarth J.W., Nieman H. (1999). Alternation in the relative abundance of gene transcripts in pre-implantation bovine cultured in media supplemented with either serum or PVA. *Molecular Reproduction. and Development* **53:** 8-18.

Wright R.W. Jr., Ellington J.E. (1995). Morphological and physiological difference between *in vivo* and *in vitro* produced preimplantation embryo from livestock species. *Theriogenology* **44:** 1167-1189.

Xu K.P., Greve T. (1988). A detailed analysis of early events during in vitro fertilization of bovine follicular oocytes. *Journal of Reproduction and Fertility* **82:** 127-134.

Young L.E., Sinclair K.D., Wilmut I. (1998). Large offspring syndrome in cattle and sheep. *Reviews of Reproduction* **3:** 115-163.

Young L.E., Fairburn H.R. (2000). Improving the safety of embryo technologies: Possible role of genomic imprinting. *Theriogenology* **53:** 627-648.

❑❑❑

Chapter 13

Cryopreservation of Oocytes and Embryos

A. Dhali, J. Ghosh, S.C. Roy, K.S. Roy, A. Mech
National Institute of Animal Nutrition and Physiology, Adugodi, Bangalore-560 030, Karnataka, India

Summary

Cryopreservation is the method for preserving living cells to the temperature of liquid nitrogen (-196°C) at genetically stabilized condition. Cryobanking of oocytes and embryos in domestic livestock species is important for conserving and propagating the superior genome. The current advances in the field are made through extensive contributions by the scientists worldwide during the last few decades. The oocytes and embryos are cryopreserved basically through two different methods, slow freezing (oocytes and embryos are subjected to controlled slow cooling at different stage of preservation) and vitrification (oocytes and embryos are subjected to a high cooling rate by exposing them directly to liquid nitrogen vapor/liquid nitrogen). Concept of the modified ultra-rapid vitrification is introduced recently. This technique involves a very high cooling rate and small volume of vitrification medium that ensure a highly efficient vitrification process and high post-vitrification recovery of oocytes and embryos. Due to structural differences, cryopreservation of oocytes and early-stage embryos is more difficult compared to the embryos of later development stage. Future challenges are ahead to develop suitable protocols for preserving oocytes and early-stage embryos for better post-preservation survivality.

Cryopreservation is a technique for preserving living cells at genetically stabilized condition to the temperature of liquid nitrogen (-196°C). Currently this technique is used to preserve biological samples such as oocytes, embryos, stem cells, tissue slices and many more. The effect of low temperature on living cells is complex due to the changes associated with physical structure and biophysical processes. Super cooling of a living cell allows its preservation for a long time, theoretically for an indefinite time period. All biochemical or metabolic activities of the cells are virtually stopped at an extremely low temperature. Thus, the cryopreserved cells enter into a suspended animation state and can be preserved for a very long period if maintained properly. Cryopreservation of oocytes and embryos is a fascinating aspect of the assisted reproductive technology (ART). Substantial advances in this technology now allow us to successfully freeze, store and later thaw and fertilize oocytes or transfer embryos. Using the standardized cryopreservation techniques that have been developed over many years from worldwide cryobiology research, we can now preserve valuable germplasms for future use. Cryopreservation of reproductive cells permits the preservation of intact genome and thus can maximize the distribution of favorable genes or superior genotype. Oocyte and embryo cryopreservation in mammals has many potential applications. There is a need for cryobanking of oocytes and embryos from the domestic livestock species with greater genetic merits to enhance the efficacy of improved breeding programmes. It is important as well for preserving endangered species or valuable laboratory animals. The cryobanking can ensure a steady supply of oocytes and embryos for many research applications including genetic engineering, embryo cloning and epigenetic investigations.

The availability of commercially produced standard media, automated freezing machines and precisely determined parameters have transformed the cryopreservation procedure to a routine laboratory technique. Even, without understanding the underlying biological processes, a person can easily perform the steps of cryopreservation following a brief technical training. Several alternative protocols have been developed during the last three decades for preserving oocytes and embryos. Some of these methods are real breakthrough in the field. In this chapter, we will be discussing in details the principals and techniques of cryopreservation of mammalian oocytes and embryos.

1. History of cryopreservation

It was believed since long that ultra low temperature exerts negative effects on living cells and tissues. During those early days, people could not perceive the beneficial effects of cryopreservation. Currently, with substantial advances in the field, it has become one of the standardized methods of ART. The history of cryopreservation is dated back to the late 1600s (Luster, 2004). Henry Power froze a jar of vinegar eels in salt water. Surprisingly he found that after thawing they were still as active as they were prior to freezing. Power was the first to give the theory that cold does not have so-called killing properties that are possessed by heat. In 1683, the monograph "New Experiments and Observations Touching Cold" was written by Robert Boyle in which the effects of freezing on living animals were described. During late 1700s, Lazzaro Spallanzani, a pioneer in cryobiology, conducted extensive studies on the reaction of tissues to low temperatures in several species. B. J. Luyet and P. M. Gehenio published a book in 1940 entitled "Life and Death at Low Temperatures" in which they described the basic components for the study of cryobiology (Luyet and Gehenio, 1940). Christopher Polge and his colleagues at the University of Cambridge accidentally discovered the cryoprotective capabilities of glycerol in late 1940s. This unintended discovery subsequently led to the successful cryopreservation of cattle and poultry spermatozoa (Polge *et al.*, 1949). The discovery of the cryoprotective ability of glycerol led to the origin of a new branch of biological science, which is now formally known as cryobiology. Since late 1970s, remarkable success stories were made in the field of cryopreservation of mammalian embryos (Table 1) and oocytes (Table 2).

Table 1 : First reported birth in different species from the cryopreserved mammalian embryos (Luster, 2004)

Species	References
Mouse	Whittingham *et al.* (1972)
Cow	Wilmut and Rowson (1973)
Rabbit	Bank and Maurer (1974)
Rat	Whittingham (1975)
Sheep	Willadsen *et al.* (1976)
Goat	Bilton and Moore (1976)
Horse	Yamamoto *et al.* (1982)
Human	Zeilmaker *et al.* (1984)
Antelope	Kramer *et al.* (1983)
Baboon	Pope *et al.* (1984)
Cynomolgus monkey	Balmaceda *et al.* (1986)
Marmoset monkey	Summers *et al.* (1987)
Cat	Dresser *et al.* (1988)
Pig	Hayashi *et al.* (1989)
Buffalo	Kasiraj *et al.* (1993)

Table 2 : First reported birth in different species from the cryopreserved mammalian oocytes (Luster, 2004)

Species	Method	Author
Mouse	Slow-cooling	Parkening *et al.* (1976)
	Vitrification	Kono *et al.* (1991)
Rabbit	Slow-cooling	Al-Hasani *et al.* (1989)
	Slow-cooling	Vincent *et al.* (1989)
Cattle	Slow-cooling	Fuku *et al.* (1992)
	Vitrification, OPS*	Vajta *et al.* (1998)
Human	Slow-cooling	Chen (1986)
	Vitrification	Kuleshova *et al.* (1999)
Horse	Vitrification, Cryoloop	Maclellan *et al.* (2002)

* Open pulled straw

2. Factors influencing cryopreservation process

It is not fully understood why every cells do not survive and withstand the process of cryopreservation. During the process, cells experience dehydration, cooling, rehydration and exposure to extreme low temperature. It is inconclusive whether the changes in temperature, cryopreservation process itself or both are responsible for damage and death of the preserved cells (Mazur, 1970). The causes and different types of damages to cells and cell organelles during the cryopreservation are described in Table 3.

Table 3 : Causes and different types of damages to cells and cell organelles during the cryopreservation process (Shaw *et al.*, 2000).

Particulars	Causes/ types of damage
Cell	Intra and extracellular ice formation, apoptosis, toxicity, calcium imbalance, free radical, ATP levels, general metabolism, fertilization failure, cleavage failure, altered transcriptional activities
Membrane	Rupture, leakage, fusion, altered bio-functional properties
Chromosomes	Loss/gain, polyspermy, polygny (failure to extrude polar body), tertraploidy
DNA	Apoptosis, fusion, rearrangements
Cytoskeleton	Ruptured/dissolved actin microtubules
Ultrastructure	Microvilli mitochondria, vesicles, cortical granules
Zona pellucida	Hardening, fracture

2.1 Cooling and warming rates

The rates of cooling and warming during the process are crucial for survivability of the preserved cells. A too slow cooling can kill cells due to the toxicity of cryoprotectants. In contrast, an improper rapid cooling may cause cell death due to intracellular ice crystal formation. Cooling of cells suspended in cryopreservation solution (CPS) to subzero temperatures causes the formation of extracellular ice crystals and the cell cytoplasm supercools. As the cooling proceeds towards a temperature below -10 to -15°C, intracellular ice crystals form. The intracellular ice crystals are not always lethal as damage can be prevented if such cells are warmed very rapidly (Mazur, 1970). In the vitrification process, cells are cooled in highly viscous CPS so rapidly (several thousand °C/min) that entire mass including the cells and solution transformed into a glass like state and ice crystals do not form. During thawing, the warming rate is crucial for cell survivability. The warming rate may vary according to the type of cells and depends on the cooling rate that cells experience during the freezing procedures. It has been shown that embryos cryopreserved by slow-cooling had greater post-thaw survival when they were warmed slowly (Whittingham *et al.*, 1972). Similarly, in case of vitrification that involves a very high cooling rate, frozen oocytes and embryos are warmed quickly by placing them into warming solutions at 20° to 37°C. It is reported that warming rate can reach to 4,460°C/min, when frozen (-196°C) oocytes are directly plunged into warming solution at 37°C (Libermann *et al.*, 2002).

2.2 Cryoprotective agents

Two different types of cryoprotective agents (CPAs) are used in CPS. These are membrane permeating (*e.g.*, glycerol, ethylene glycol, dimethyl sulfoxide, propanediol) and membrane non-permeating (sucrose, glucose, Ficoll, proteins, lipoproteins) CPAs. During the freezing process, CPAs play many roles. The permeating CPAs play crucial roles in the cryopreservation process. They decrease freezing point of the solution and prevent damage to cells from high electrolyte concentrations. They interact with the membrane modifications occurring during the cryopreservation process. They also prevent the exposure of cells to high concentration intra and extra cellular electrolytes by linking to the electrolytes and thus acting as partial substitute to water (Rall *et al.*, 1984). In the slow freezing process, relatively low concentration (1 to 1.5 M) of CPAs is used compared to the vitrification where the concentration can be as high as 8 M (Kasai, 2002). It may be noted that if a CPS is composed of a single permeating CPA, the concentrations of the CPA would be higher in the solution. On the other hand, similar viscosity of CPS can be achieved by adding combination of permeating CPAs. In the later case, the concentration of a particular CPA would be lower in the solution. Therefore, it is believed that the toxicity to the cells can be reduced if a combination of CPAs is used for cryopreservation.

The non-permeating CPAs are added into the CPS for many beneficial effects. Their presence increases the viscosity of the CPS that generates an osmotic gradient across the cell membrane and helps to withdraw intracellular water (Orief *et al.*, 2005). The addition of non-permeating CPAs into CPS allows effective dehydration of the cells even if permeating CPAs are added into the solution at low concentration. Thus the addition of non-permeating CPAs may reduce the overall toxicity to the preserved cells. Moreover, non-permeating CPAs reduce mechanical stress which occurs during cryopreservation (Dumoulin *et al.*, 1994).

Antifreeze proteins (AFPs) are often added into CPS for modulating cell survival during cryopreservation (Carpenter and Hansen, 1992). The AFPs are extremely efficient in inhibiting ice recrystallization in frozen solution. These proteins are available in fishes, insects, centipedes, intertidal mollusks and plants from polar and north temperate regions that can survive freeze-thawing (Carpenter and Hansen, 1992). Normally, recrystallization of ice occurs rapidly when frozen samples are warmed near melting point at which there is sufficient kinetic energy for the migration of water molecules from one crystal to another (Knight and Duman, 1986). Addition of AFPs noncolligatively lowers the freezing point of fluid without affecting the melting point significantly (Carpenter and Hansen, 1992). The capacity of AFPs to inhibit ice recrystallization helps in protecting the freeze-tolerant organisms during long-term exposure to subfreezing temperatures and recurrent bouts of freezing and thawing during winter (Knight and Duman, 1986).

2.3 Dehydration

Efficient cell dehydration during the cryopreservation process is probably the most important factor for achieving greater post-thaw survival of the preserved cells. An improper dehydration causes damage to the cells due to intracellular ice formation (Ruffing *et al.*, 1993). During cryopreservation, both permeating and non-permeating CPAs cause water egress and dehydration of the cells (Li, 2005). Cell injury during the process is mediated through the excessive dehydration and exposure of the cells to high concentration of electrolytes. Therefore, changes in the cell volume during cryopreservation determine the survivability of cells. The changes in cell volume occur in two phases. In the first phase, after being suspended in the CPS, cells shrink rapidly due to osmotically driven egress of intracellular water. The cells then regain its volume as permeating CPAs enter into the cells. During the second phase, following freezing of the extracellular solution, intracellular water moves out further in response to the high concentration of extracellular electrolytes. During the thawing process, the changes in cell volume are analogous, but in reverse direction (Li, 2005).

3. Cryopreservation techniques

Cryopreservation of living cells and tissues involves five basic steps (Fig 1). These are: 1) equilibration in CPS, 2) super cooling at subzero temperature, 3) storage at the glass transition temperature of water below -130°C, 4) warming and thawing (5) removal of cryoprotectants (Luyet and Rapatz, 1970; Mazur, 1988; Leibo, 1986; Lebio and Songsasen, 2002). Currently, two fundamental procedures are available for cryopreserving oocytes and embryos *viz.*, the slow freezing technique and vitrification.

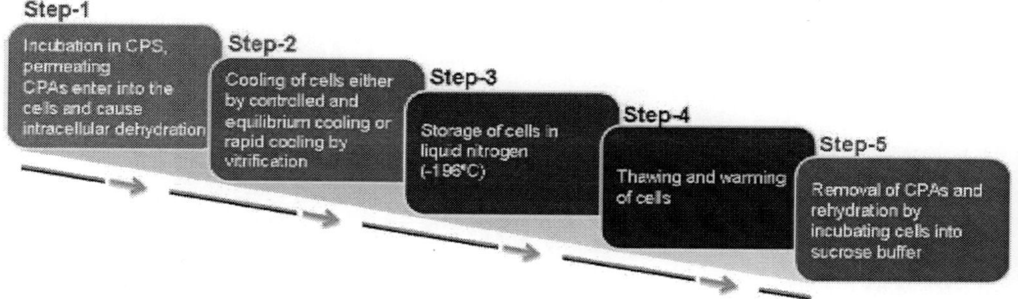

Fig. 1 : Steps of cryopreservation process

3.1 Slow freezing

The slow rate cooling technique was the first developed method for cryopreservation of oocytes and embryos. This technique was developed during the early seventies (Whittingham, 1971; Whittingham *et al.*, 1972; Wilmut, 1972). In this oocytes or embryos are exposed to a concentration gradient (from low to high concentration) of CPAs. The permeating cryoprotectants ethylene glycol (EG) or dimethyl sulfoxide (DMSO) at final concentrations of 1.0-1.5 M for oocytes or 1.3-1.5 M for embryos are generally used in this proceedure. Other preferred permeating cryoprotectants used are glycerol and propylene glycol (Chen *et al.*, 2005; *Luz et al.*, 2009). The CPS also contains non-permeating cryoprotectants such as sucrose, glucose or fructose (Diez *et al.*, 2001; Barcelo-Fimbres and Seidel, 2007). The oocytes/ embryos are incubated in the CPS and then loaded into a 0.25 ml straw along with the CPS and cooled to -5 to -7°C (~1°C/min) where they are kept for several minute to equilibrate. After equilibration, the solution is seeded to initiate extracellular freezing, and then cooled slowly (~0.5°C/min) to anywhere between -30°C and -65°C (Saragusty and Arav, 2011). Once the desired temperature of the loaded straw is reached, they are plunged into liquid nitrogen for storage. The controlled cooling of the loaded straws is done with the help of a programmable bio-freezer (Fig. 2).

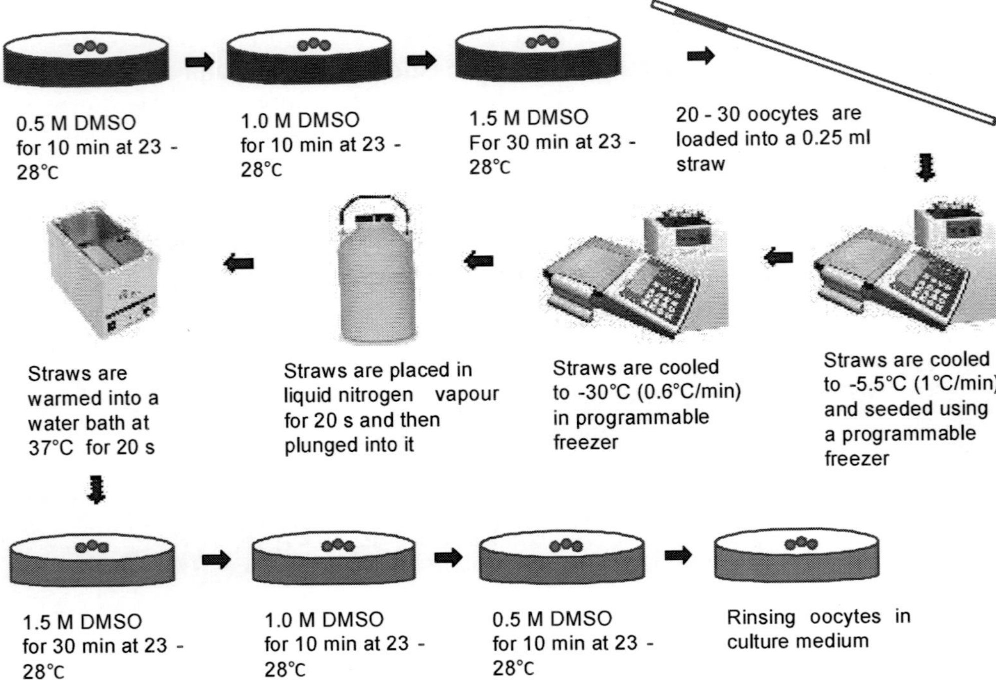

Fig. 2 : An illustration of slow rate freezing of buffalo oocytes (Gautam *et al.*, 2008)

In this technique, seeding of the extracellular solution and a very slow cooling rate ensure the freezing of the solution located outside of the oocytes/ embryos. Such procedures result in the outward movement of osmotically-active water from the cell and their gradual dehydration until they reach the temperature at which the intracellular matrix vitrifies (Mazur, 1963).

3.2 Vitrification

Vitrification is the process that induces a glass-like solidification of living cells suspended in CPS during freezing. This technique was first reported by Rall and Fahy (1985). They demonstrated the ice-free cryopreservation of mouse embryos at -196°C by vitrification. Since then a huge efforts have been made across the world to use and modify this technique for preserving oocytes/ embryos in different species. It is now considered to be a proven method for cryopreserving oocytes and embryos. The unique advantage of vitrification is the complete elimination of ice crystal formation, the most dangerous cause of cryoinjury. Vitrification can be induced when using high concentration of cryoprotectants and a rapid cooling rate. In this method, highly viscous (5-7 M) CPS and rapid cooling rates (2,000-25,000°C/min) are used. In this technique, oocytes/embryos are incubated in different solutions from low to high viscosity, loaded into a container, carrier or drop and directly plunged into liquid nitrogen (Fig. 3). It is inconclusive if vitrification is a better technique compared to slow rate freezing. Nevertheless, several reports have shown that the success of vitrification is similar to that obtained from slow rate freezing. Moreover, vitrification requires lesser time than slow rate freezing and excludes the use of a very costly biological freezer that is required for slow rate freezing.

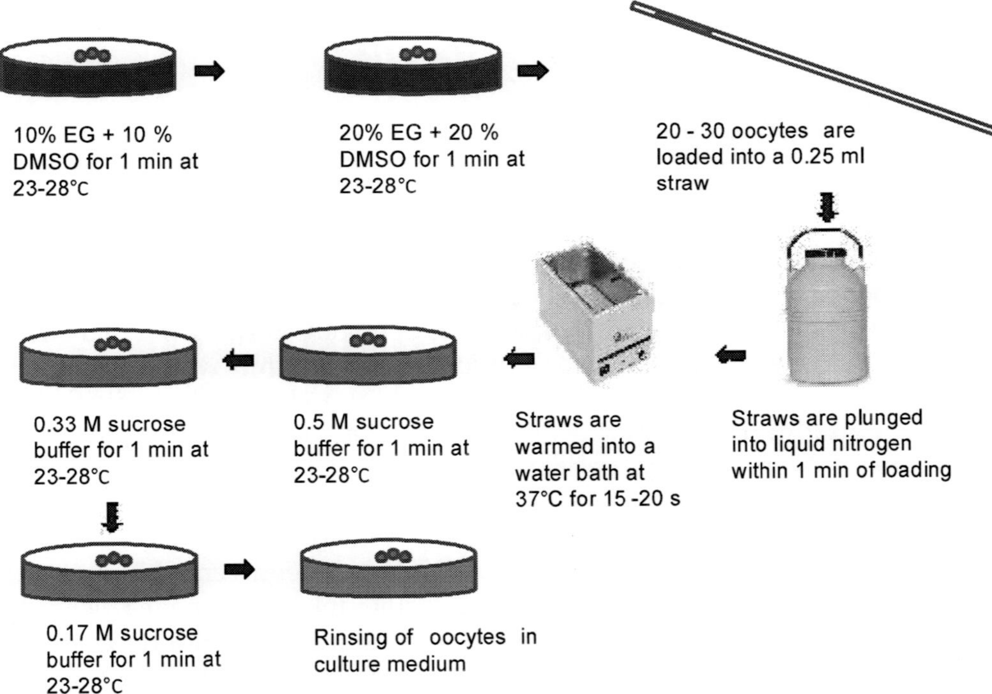

Fig. 3 : An illustration of vitrification of buffalo oocytes (Gautam *et al.*, 2008)

Three factors are important for achieving efficient vitrification: a) cooling rate during the process, b) viscosity of the medium and c) volume of the medium to be vitrified. Cooling rate is extremely high in vitrification process. Plunging the sample directly into liquid nitrogen results a cooling rate of several thousand °C/min depending on the container or carrier, volume of CPS, thermal conductivity, solution composition *etc.* (Saragusty and Arav, 2011). Viscosity of the vitrification medium in which oocytes/embryos are suspended is important. Viscosity is defined by the concentration and behavior of CPAs and other additives used in the vitrification medium. A higher concentration of CPAs in the medium ensures efficient vitrification and thus reduces the chance of ice nucleation and crystallization within the cells. Interestingly, the viscosity of the vitrification medium and cooling rate is inversely related. Thus, a medium containing lesser concentrations of CPAs and other additives can be vitrified efficiently at higher cooling rate. Different CPAs and other additives used in vitrification medium have different degree of cytotoxicity. Therefore, combinations of different cryoprotectants are often used in vitrification medium to increase viscosity and reduce the level of toxicity. Volume of the medium that is to be vitrified is another important factor. A reduction in the volume increases the efficiency of vitrification. Smaller volume allows better heat transfer and thus facilitates higher cooling rates.

3.3 Ultra-rapid vitrification

The ultra-rapid vitrification is not a different technique. It is rather a modification of the traditional vitrification procedure. This technique involves a very high cooling rate and small volume of vitrification medium that ensure a highly efficient vitrification process (Fig 4). Although the concept of ultra-rapid vitrification was introduced during early 1990s, the development of open pulled straw method (Vajta *et al.*, 1998) was the major breakthrough in the area. This method is popularly known as open pulled straw (OPS) method. In this method, oocytes/embryos are loaded into a thin wall straw along with a very small volume of vitrification medium (1-2 μl) and vitrified by directly plunging the straw into liquid nitrogen. The cooling rate in this technique is over 20,000°C/min and the post vitrification cell survival is considerably high. It is proposed that extremely high cooling and warming rates and a short contact of the cells with concentrated cryoprotective additives (less than 30 sec over -180°C) offer a possibility to circumvent chilling injury and decrease toxic and osmotic damage. Considerable efforts have been made thereafter to develop different methods of ultra-rapid vitrification (Riha *et al.*, 1991; Papis *et al.*, 2000; Chang *et al.*, 2004; Lane *et al.*, 1999; Dinnyes *et al.*, 2000). Dhali *et al.* (2009) reported that following ultra-rapid vitrification, the survival rate and expression pattern of apoptotic related genes of mouse morulae were similar to that of the non-vitrified morulae. They also demonstrated that ultra-rapid vitrification did not cause any damage to the actin cytoskeleton following vitrification, thawing and culturing.

4. Difficulties of oocyte cryopreservation

Oocytes typically have a very short fertile life that limits implementation of many assisted reproductive technologies. The problem may be solved if a regular supply of the cryopreserved oocyes can be ensured. Nevertheless, the development potential of cryopreserved mammalian oocytes is very poor compared to embryos. Despite many efforts a standardized and efficient cryopreservation protocol for oocytes, is yet to be realized (Noyes *et al.*, 2010). The cryopreservation of oocytes is quite different from the embryo

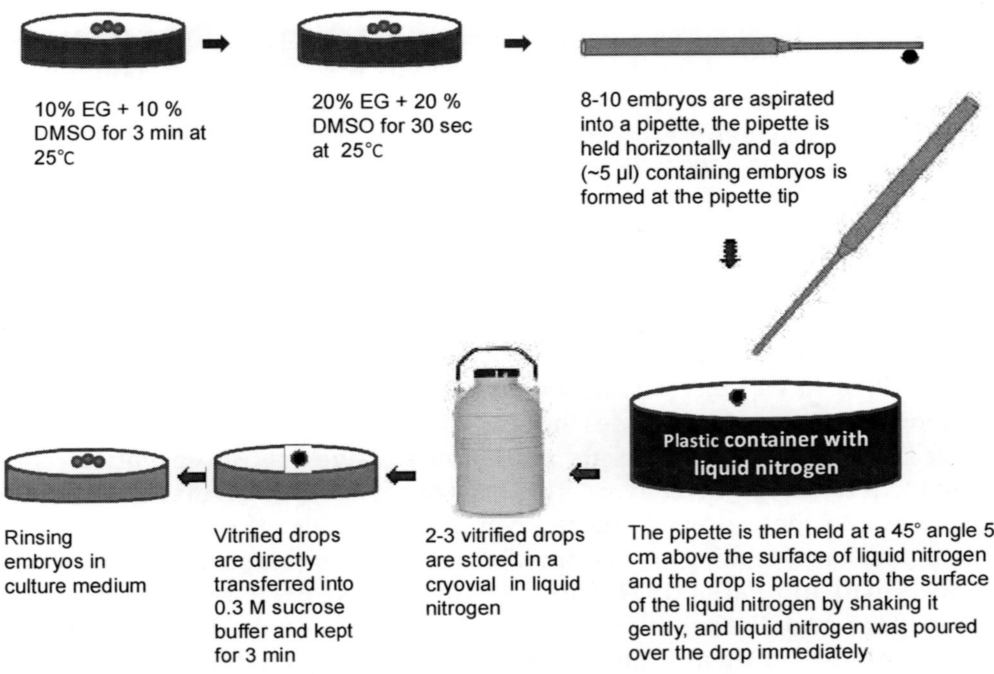

Fig. 4 : An illustration of ultra-rapid vitrification of mouse embryos (Dhali *et al.*, 2007)

cryopreservation. An oocyte requires maintaining integrity of many unique structural features to undergo fertilization and further developments. Several problems are associated with the cryopreservation of oocytes. Being a single cell, oocyte is more vulnerable to the steps of cryopreservation compared to a multi-cellular preimplantation embryo (Parks and Ruffing, 1992). The larger volume of oocyte decreases the surface/volume ratio that makes it very sensitive to chilling and intracellular ice formation (Toner *et al.*, 1990; Ruffing *et al.*, 1993; Arav *et al.*, 1996; Zeron *et al.*, 1999). The plasma membrane of oocytes at the metaphase II (MII) stage has a low permeability coefficient, thus making the movement of cryoprotectants and water slower (Ruffing *et al.*, 1993). Moreover, the zona pellucida acts as an additional barrier that restricts the movement of water and permeating molecules across it. The freeze-thaw process may cause premature cortical granule exocytosis resulting in zona pellucida hardening that makes sperm penetration and fertilization difficult (Carroll *et al.*, 1990; Mavrides and Morroll, 2005). Oocytes contain high cytoplasmic lipid that increases its sensitivity to chilling (Ruffing *et al.*, 1993). The actin cytoskeleton is less robust in oocytes (Gook *et al.*, 1993). Therefore, cryopreservation can cause cytoskeleton damage and chromosome and DNA abnormalities (Luvoni, 2000). The meiotic spindle, which is formed by the MII stage, is very sensitive to chilling and may be compromised as well (Ciotti *et al.*, 2009). Oocytes are also more susceptible to the damaging effects of reactive oxygen species (Gupta *et al.*, 2010). Many of these parameters change after fertilization that makes embryos less sensitive to chilling and cryodamage. Therefore, oocyte cryopreservation is a more challenging task compared to the cryopreservation of embryo (Gook *et al.*, 1993, Fabbri *et al.*, 2000, Ghetler *et al.*, 2005).

5. Suitable developmental stage for oocytes and embryos cryopreservation

Although many protocols, such as slow freezing (Lim *et al.*, 1992; Suzuki *et al.*, 1996), rapid cooling (Hochi *et al.*, 1998) or ultra-rapid cooling (Martino *et al.*, 1996) have been attempted to cryopreserve oocytes, no optimized method exists currently. Besides the cryopreservation protocol itself, the meiotic stage of the oocytes affects its ability to survive cryopreservation. Most researchers have focused on the cryopreservation of mature oocytes. Nonetheless, the process induces several undesirable effects such as spindle disorganization leading to disrupted chromosomes (Magistrini and Szollosi, 1980; Aman and Parks, 1994; Saunders and Parks, 1999) and microfilaments (Saunders and Parks, 1999). Further effects described are the altered distribution of cortical granules (Fuku *et al.*, 1995; Hyttel *et al.*, 2000) and increased polyploidy at fertilization (Glenister *et al.*, 1987; Carroll *et al.*, 1989; Bouquet *et al.*, 1992; Eroglu *et al.*, 1998). Immature oocytes do not have an organized meiotic spindle. Therefore, cryopreservation at this stage may be an alternative approach. Indeed, frozen immature bovine oocytes have given rise to blastocysts (Ku¨chenmeister and Kuwayama, 1997; Le and Massip, 1998), pregnancies (Otoi *et al.*, 1995; Yang *et al.*, 1998), and newborns (Suzuki *et al.*, 1996; Vieira *et al.*, 2002), but rates of *in vitro* embryo development are still very low. This could be explained by the fact that the cells immediately adjacent to the oocyte (the corona radiata) have long cytoplasmic extensions that penetrate the zona pellucida and terminate in bulbous swellings closely associated with the oocyte membrane (Heller *et al.*, 1981; Szollosi *et al.*, 1988). These processes and junctions play an important role in the metabolic cooperation that exists between oocytes and cumulus cells during the growth and final maturation of oocytes. Some studies have described irreversible structural damage to the oocyte membrane (Arav *et al.*, 1996) or impaired intercellular communication between the oocyte and cumulus cells after cryopreservation of germinal vesicle (GV) oocytes (Fuku *et al.*, 1995). Therefore, choosing an intermediate stage, such as GV breakdown (GVBD), might circumvent some of the problems associated with the cryopreservation of GV or MII oocytes (Albarraci´n *et al.*, 2005). When bovine cumulus-oocyte complexes were maturated for 0, 8, 12 or 22 h, vitrified and cultured post-thaw to complete 22 h maturation, significantly more diploid oocytes were detected after vitrification at 0 or 8 h of maturation (Luna *et al.*, 2001).

Embryos are suitable for cryopreservation at later developmental stage compared to zygote or 2-cell stage. As embryo development proceeds, the blastomere volume decreases, but the surface area increases, this in turn increases the permeability of embryos to cryoprotectants (Mazur *et al.*, 1976; Zhou *et al.*, 2005). Improved penetration of cryoprotectants into blastomeres at later developmental stages enhances freezing efficiency (Zhou *et al.*, 2005). Many researchers have reported that rapid cooling and thawing rates are more suited to later stage embryos with smaller blastomeres (Naik *et al.*, 2005; Dobrinsky *et al.*, 1990; Kobayashi *et al.*, 1990; Smorag *et al.*, 1989). Vajta *et al.* (1998) reported that in bovine, blastocyst rate was significantly low for the vitrified (OPS method) day-1 and -2 embryos compared to control, but it was not different for the vitrified day-3 through day-7 embryos. Dhali *et al.* (2009) also reported that the ultra-rapid vitrification procedure supported better survival of morulae compared to zygotes and 2-cell mouse embryos.

Conclusions

Currently, prevention of the loss of genetic resources including that of the farm animals has become a major challenge for conservation biologists worldwide. The population of many farm animal species has been reported to be critically low. *In situ* conservation is probably the best solution for safeguarding such vulnerable species. However, conserving an animal species *in situ* is a huge task that requires a lot of efforts including substantial financial involvement. Cryopreservation of oocytes and embryos is an important alternative to *in situ* conservation for preserving the germplasm of valuable livestock. Several decades of researches have established the protocols for preserving oocytes and embryos of many livestock species. Nevertheless, the quality and development of the cryopreserved oocytes and embryos have been found compromised compared to that of the fresh oocytes and embryos. Moreover, the quality and development of cryopreserved oocytes and early-stage embryos have been found lesser compared to the embryos cryopreserved at later developmental stage. Therefore, in future, research efforts will be required to develop suitable cryopreservation protocols for preserving oocytes and embryos more efficiently and consistently.

References

Albarracín J.L., Morató R., Izquierdo D., Mogas T. (2005). Vitrification of calf oocytes: effects of maturation stage and prematuration treatment on the nuclear and cytoskeletal components of oocytes and their subsequent development. *Molecular Reproduction and Development* **72:** 239-249.

Al-Hasani S., Krisch J., Diedrich K., Blanke S., van der Ven H., Krebs D. (1989). Successful embryo transfer of cryopreserved and in-vitro fertilized rabbit oocytes. Human Reproduction **4:** 77-79.

Aman R.R., Parks J.E. (1994). Effects of cooling and rewarming on the meiotic spindle and chromosomes of in vitro-matured bovine oocytes. *Biology of Reproduction* **50:** 103-110.

Arav A. Zeron Y., Leslie S.B., Behboodi E., Anderson G.B., Crowe J.H. (1996). Phase transition temperature and chilling sensitivity of bovine oocytes. *Cryobiology* **33:** 589-599.

Balmaceda J., Heitman T., Garcia A., Pauerstein C., Pool R. (1986). Embryo cryopreservation in cynamologus monkey. *Fertility and Sterility* **45:** 403-406.

Bank H., Maurer R.R. (1974). Survival of frozen rabbit embryos. *Experimental Cell Research* **89:** 188-196.

Barcelo-Fimbres M., Seidel G.E. Jr. (2007). Effects of fetal calf serum, phenazine ethosulfate and either glucose or fructose during in vitro culture of bovine embryos on embryonic development after cryopreservation. *Molecular Reproduction and Development* **74:** 1395-1405.

Bilton R.J., Moore R.W. (1976). In vitro culture, storage, and transfer of goat embryos. *Australian Journal of Biological Sciences* **29:** 125-129.

Bouquet M., Selva J., Auroux M. (1992). The incidence of chromosomal abnormalities in frozen-thawed mouse oocytes after in-vitro fertilization. *Human Reproduction* **7:** 76–80.

Carpenter J.F., Hansen T.N. (1992). Antifreeze protein modulates cell survival during cryopreservation: Mediation through influence on ice crystal growth. *Proceedings of the National Academy of Sciences of the United States of America* **89:** 8953-8957.

Carroll J., Depypere H., Matthews C.D. (1990). Freeze-thaw-induced changes of the zona pellucida explains decreased rates of fertilization in frozen-thawed mouse oocytes. *Journal of Reproduction and Fertility* **90:** 547-553.

Carroll J., Warnes G.M., Matthews C.D. (1989). Increase in digyny explains polyploidy after in-vitro fertilization of frozen-thawedmouse oocytes. *Journal of Reproduction and Fertility* **85:** 489–494.

Chang W.C., Xu J., Jiang S., Tian X.C., Yang X., Du X.L. (2004). Effect of pre-equilibration procedures on the development potential of vitrified bovine oocytes after IVF. *Reproduction Fertility and Development* **16:** 166 (*Abstr.*).

Chen C. (1986). Pregnancy after human oocyte cryopreservation. *Lancet* **1:** 884-886.

Chen S.U., Lien Y.R., Chen H.F., Chang L.J., Tsai Y.Y., Yang Y.S. (2005). Observational clinical follow-up of oocyte cryopreservation using a slow-freezing method with 1,2-propanediol plus sucrose followed by ICSI. *Human Reproduction* **20:** 1975-1980.

Ciotti P.M., Porcu E., Notarangelo L., Magrini O., Bazzocchi A., Venturoli S. (2009). Meiotic spindle recovery is faster in vitrification of human oocytes compared to slow freezing. *Fertility and Sterility* **91:** 2399-2407.

Dhali A., Anchamparuthy V.M., Butler S.P., Pearson R.E., Mullarky I.K., Gwazdauskas F.C. (2009). Effect of droplet vitrification on development competence, actin cytoskeletal integrity and gene expression in in vitro cultured mouse embryos. *Theriogenology* **71:** 1408-1416.

Dhali A., Anchamparuthy V.M., Butler S.P., Pearson R.E., Mullarky I.K., Gwazdauskas F.C. (2007). Gene expression and development of mouse zygotes following droplet vitrification. *Theriogenology* **68:** 1292-1298.

Diez C., Heyman Y., Le Bourhis D., Guyader-Joly C., Degrouard J., Renard J.P. (2001). Delipidating in vitro-produced bovine zygotes: effect on further development and consequences for freezability. *Theriogenology* **55:** 923-936.

Dinnyes A., Dai Y., Jiang S., Yang X. (2000). High developmental rates of vitrified bovine oocytes following parthenogenetic activation, in vitro fertilization, and somatic cell nuclear transfer. *Biology of reproduction* **63:** 513-518.

Dobrinsky J.R., Balise J.J., Robl J.M. (1990). Development of vitrified rabbit embryos. *Theriogenology* **33:** 213 (*Abstr.*).

Dresser B.L., Gelwicks E.J., Wachs K.B., Keller G.L. (1988). First successful transfer of cryopreserved feline (*Felis catus*) embryos resulting in live offspring. *Journal of Experimental Zoology* **246:** 180-186.

Dumoulin J.C., Janssen J.M.B., Pieters M.H., Enginsu M.E., Geraedts J.P., Evers J.L. (1994). The protective effects of polymers in the cryopreservation of human and mouse zonae pellucidae and embryos. *Fertility and Sterility* **62:** 793-798.

Eroglu A., Toth T.L., Toner M. (1998). Alterations of the cytoskeleton and polyploidy induced by cryopreservation of metaphase II mouse oocytes. *Fertility and sterility* **69:** 944-957.

Fabbri R., Porcu E., Marsella T., Primavera M.R., Rocchetta G., Ciotti P.M., Magrini O., Seracchioli R., Venturoli S., Flamigni C. (2000). Technical aspects of oocyte cryopreservation. *Molecular and Cellular Endocrinology* **169:** 39-42.

Fuku E., Kojima T., Shioya Y., Marcus G.J., Downey B.R. (1992). In vitro fertilization and development of frozen-thawed bovine oocytes. *Cryobiology* **29:** 485-492.

Fuku E., Xia L., Downey B.R. (1995). Ultrastructural changes in bovine oocytes cryopreserved by vitrification. *Cryobiology* **32:** 139-156.

Gautam S.K., Verma V., Palta P., Chauhan M.S., Manik R.S. (2008). Effect of type of cryoprotectant on morphology and developmental competence of in vitro-matured buffalo (*Bubalus bubalis*) oocytes subjected to slow freezing or vitrification. *Reproduction Fertility and Development* **20:** 490-496.

Ghetler Y., Yavin S., Shalgi R., Arav A. (2005). The effect of chilling on membrane lipid phase transition in human oocytes and zygotes. *Human Reproduction* **20:** 3385-3389.

Glenister P.H., Wood M.J., Kirby C., Whittingham D.G. (1987). Incidence of chromosome anomalies in first-cleavage mouse embryos obtained from frozen-thawed oocytes fertilized in vitro. *Gamete Research* **16:** 205-216.

Gook D.A., Osborn S.M., Johnston W.I.H. (1993). Cryopreservation of mouse and human oocytes using 1, 2-propanediol and the configuration of the meiotic spindle. *Human Reproduction* **8:** 1101-1109.

Gupta M.K., Uhm S.J., Lee H.T. (2010). Effect of vitrification and beta-mercaptoethanol on reactive oxygen species activity and in vitro development of oocytes vitrified before or after in vitro fertilization. *Fertility and sterility* **93:** 2602-2607.

Hayashi S., Kobayashi K., Mizuno J., Saitoh K., Hirano S. (1989). Birth of piglets from frozen embryos. *Veterinary Record* **125:** 43-44.

Heller D.T., Cahill D.M., Schultz R.M. (1981). Biochemical studies of mammalian oogenesis: Metabolic cooperativity between granulose cells and growing mouse oocytes. *Developmental Biology* **84:** 455-464.

Hochi S., Ito K., Hirabayashi M., Ueda M., Kimura K., Hanada A. (1998). Effect of nuclear stages during IVM on the survival of vitrifiedwarmed bovine oocytes. *Theriogenology* **49:** 787-796.

Hyttel P., Vajta G., Callesen H. (2000). Vitrification of bovine oocytes with the open pulled straw method : Ultrastructura/consequences. *Molecular Reproduction and Development* **56:** 80-88.

Kasai M. (2002). Advances in the cryopreservation of mammalian oocytes and embryos: development of ultra rapid vitrification. *Reproductive Medicine and Biology* **1:** 1-9.

Kasiraj R., Misra A.K., Mutha Rao M., Jaiswal R.S., Rangareddi N.S. (1993). Successful culmination of pregnancy and live birth following the transfer of frozen–thawed buffalo embryos. *Theriogenology* **39:** 1187-1192.

Knight C.A., Duman J.G. (1986). Inhibition of recrystallization of ice by insect thermal hysteresis proteins: A possible cryoprotective role. *Cryobiology* **23:** 256-262.

Kobayashi K., Nagashima H., Yamakawa H., Kato Y., Ogawa S. (1990). The survival of whole and bisected rabbit morulae after cryopreservation by the vitrification method. *Theriogenology* **33:** 777-788.

Kono T., Kwon O.Y., Nakahara T. (1991). Development of vitrified mouse oocytes after IVF. *Cryobiology* **28:** 50-54.

Kramer L.B., Dresser B.L., Pope C.E., Dahlhausen R.D., Baker R.D. (1983). The nonsurgical transfer of frozen-thawed eland (Tragelaphus oryx) embryos. In: *Annual Proceedings-American Association of Zoo Veterinarians*. Hills Division, Riviana Foods, Topeka, KS, pp 104-105.

Küchenmeister U., Kuwayama M. (1997). In vitro blastocysts formation, after vitrification of immature bovine oocytes. *Theriogenology* **47:** 348 (*Abstr.*).

Kuleshova L., Gianaroli L., Magli C., Ferraretti A., Trounson A. (1999). Birth following vitrification of a small number of human oocytes. *Human Reproduction* **14:** 3077-3079.

Lane M., Schoolcraft W.B., Gardner D.K. (1999). Vitrification of mouse and human blastocysts using a novel cryoloop container-less technique. *Fertility and Sterility* **72:** 1073-1078.

Le Gal F., Massip A. (1998). Development of thawed oocytes fertilized in vitro after vitrification by the open pulled straw method before or after in vitro maturation. In: *Gametes: Development and function*. (A. Lauria, F. Gandolfi, E. Enne and L. Gianaroli, eds). Serono Symposia, Rome, pp 554.

Leibo S.P. (1986). Cryobiology: preservation of mammalian embryos. *Basic life sciences* **37:** 251-272.

Leibo S.P., Songsasen N. (2002). Cryopresrevation of gametes and embryos of nondomestic animals. *Theriogenology* **57:** 303-326.

Li G. (2005). Cryopreservation of reproductive cells and tissues. *Thesis, Master of Science in Mechanical Engineering,* Submitted to the Agriculture and Mechanical College, Louisiana State University, USA.

Liebermann J., Nawroth F., Isachenko V., Isachenko E., Rahimi G., Tucker M.J. (2002). Potential importance of vitrification in reproductive medicine. *Biology of Reproduction* **67:** 1671-1680.

Lim J.M., Fukui Y., Ono H. (1992). Developmental competence of bovine oocytes frozen at various maturation stages followed by *in vitro* maturation and fertilization. *Theriogenology* **37:** 351-361.

Luna H.S., Ferrari I., Rumpf R. (2001). Influence of stage of maturation of bovine oocytes at time of vitrification on the incidence of diploid metaphase II at completion of maturation. *Animal Reproduction Science* **68:** 23-28.

Luster S.M. (2004). Cryopreservation of bovine and caprine oocytes by vitrification. *Thesis, Master of Science in Animal Sciences,* Submitted to the Agriculture and Mechanical College, Louisiana State University, USA.

Luvoni G.C. (2000). Current progress on assisted reproduction in dogs and cats: *in vitro* embryo production. *Reproduction Nutrition Development* **40:** 505-512.

Luyet B.J., Gehenio P.M. (1940). Life and death at low temperatures. Biodynamica, Normandy, Missouri, pp1-341.

Luyet B.J., Rapatz G. (1970). A review of basic research on the cryopreservation of red blood cells. *Cryobiology* **6:** 425-481.

Luz M.R., Holanda C.C., Pereira J.J., Teixeira N.S., Vantini R., Freitas P.M.C., Salgado A.E.P., Oliveira S.B., Guaitolini C.R.F., Santos M.C. (2009). Survival rate and in vitro development of *in vivo*-produced and cryopreserved dog embryos. *Reproduction Fertility and Development* **22:** 208-209.

Maclellan L.J., Carnevale E.M., Coutinho da Silva M.A., Scoggin C.F., Bruemmer J.E., Squires E.L. (2002). Pregnancies from vitrified equine oocytes collected from superstimulated and non-stimulated mares. *Theriogenology* **58:** 911-919.

Magistrini M., Szollosi D. (1980). Effects of cold and of isopropyl-Nphenylcarbamate on the second meiotic spindle of mouse oocytes. *European Journal of Cell Biology* **22:** 699–707.

Martino A., Songsasen N., Leibo S.P. (1996). Development into blastocysts of bovine oocytes cryopreserved by ultra-rapid cooling. *Biology of Reproduction* **54:** 1059-1069.

Mavrides A., Morroll D. (2005). Bypassing the effect of zona pellucida changes on embryo formation following cryopreservation of bovine oocytes. *European Journal of Obstetrics Gynecology and Reproductive Biology* **118:** 66-70.

Mazur P. (1963). Kinetics of water loss from cells at subzero temperatures and the likelihood of intracellular freezing. *Journal of General Physiology* **47:** 347-369.

Mazur P. (1970). Cryobiology: The freezing of biological systems. *Science* **168:** 939-949.

Mazur P. (1988). Stopping biological time. The freezing of living cells. *Annals of the New York Academy of Sciences* **541:** 514-531.

Mazur P., Rigopoulos N., Jackowski S.C., Leibo S.P. (1976). Preliminary estimates of the permeability of mouse ova and early embryos to glycerol. *Biophysical Journal* **16:** 232 (*Abstr.*).

Naik B.R., Rao B.S., Vagdevi R., Gnanprakash M., Amarnath D., Rao V.H. (2005). Conventional slow freezing, vitrification and open pulled straw (OPS) vitrification of rabbit embryos. *Animal Reproduction Science* **86:** 329-338.

Noyes N., Boldt J., Nagy Z.P. (2010). Oocyte cryopreservation: is it time to remove its experimental label? *Journal of Assisted Reproduction and Genetics* **27:** 69-74.

Orief Y., Schultze-Mosgau A., Dafopoulos K., Al-Hasani S. (2005). Vitrification: will it replace the conventional gamete cryopreservation techniques? *Middle East Fertility Society Journal* **10:** 171-184.

Otoi T., Yamamoto K., Koyama N., Suzuki T. (1995). In vitro fertilization and development of immature and mature bovine oocytes cryopreserved by ethylene glycol with sucrose. *Cryobiology* **32:** 455-460.

Papis K., Shimizu M., Izaike Y. (2000). Factors affecting the survivability of bovine oocytes vitrified in droplets. *Theriogenology* **54:** 651-658.

Parkening T.A., Tsunoda Y., Chang M.C. (1976). Effects of various low temperatures, cryoprotective agents and cooling rates on the survival, fertilizability and development of frozen-thawed mouse eggs. *Journal of Experimental Zoology* **197:** 369-374.

Parks J.E., Ruffing N.A. (1992). Factors affecting low temperature survival of mammalian oocytes. *Theriogenology* **37:** 59-73.

Polge C., Smith A.U., Parkes A.S. (1949). Revival of spermatozoa after vitrification and dehydration at low temperatures. *Nature* **164:** 666.

Pope C.E., Pope V.Z., Beck L.R. (1984). Live birth following cryopreservation and transfer of a baboon embryo. *Fertility and Sterility* **42:** 143-145.

Rall W.F., Fahy G.M. (1985). Ice-free cryopreservation of mouse embryos at –196 °C by vitrification. *Nature* **313:** 573-575.

Rall W.F., Reid D.S., Polge C. (1984). Analysis of slow-warming injury of mouse embryos by cryomicroscopical and physiochemincal methods. *Cryobiology* **21:** 106-121.

Riha J., Landa V., Kneissl J., Matus J., Jindra J., Kloucek Z. (1991). Vitrification of cattle embryos by direct dropping into liquid nitrogen and embryo survival after nonsurgical transfer. *Zivoèišná Vyroba* **36:** 113-120.

Ruffing N.A., Steponkus P.L., Pitt R.E., Parks J.E. (1993). Osmometric behavior, hydraulic conductivity, and incidence of intracellular ice formation in bovine oocytes at different developmental stages. *Cryobiology* **30:** 562-580.

Saragusty J., Arav A. (2011). Current progress in oocyte and embryo cryopreservation by slow freezing and vitrification. *Reproduction* **141:** 1-19.

Saunders K.M., Parks J.E. (1999). Effects of cryopreservation procedures on the cytology and fertilization rate of in vitro-matured bovine oocytes. *Biology of Reproduction* **61:** 178-187.

Shaw J.M., Oranratncachai A., Trounson A.O. (2000). Fundamental cryobiology of mammalian oocytes and ovarian tissue. *Theriogenology* **53:** 59-72.

Smorag Z., Gajda B., Wieczorek B., Jura J. (1989). Stage-dependent viability of vitrified rabbit embryos. *Theriogenology* **31:** 1227-1231.

Summers P.M., Shephard A.M., Taylor C.T., Hearn J.P. (1987). The effects of cryopreservation and transfer on embryonic development in the common marmoset monkey, Callithrix jacchus. *Journal of Reproduction and Fertility* **79:** 241-250.

Suzuki T., Boediono A., Takagi M., Saha S., Sumantri C. (1996). Fertilization and development of frozen-thawed germinal vesicle bovine oocytes by a one-step dilution method in vitro. *Cryobiology* **33:** 515-524.

Szollosi D., Desmedt V., Crozet N., Brender C. (1988). In vitro maturation of sheep ovarian oocytes. *Reproduction Nutrition Development* **28:** 1047-1080.

Toner M., Cravalho E.G., Karel M. (1990). Thermodynamics and kinetics of intracellular ice formation during freezing of biological cells. *Journal of Applied Physics* **67:** 1582-1593.

Vajta G., Holm P., Kuwayama M., Booth P.J., Jacobsen H., Greve T., Callesen H. (1998). Open Pulled Straw (OPS) vitrification: a new way to reduce cryoinjuries of bovine ova and embryos. *Molecular Reproduction and Development* **51:** 53-58.

Vieira A.D., Mezzalira A., Barbieri D.P., Lehmkuhl R.C., Rubin M.I., Vajta G. (2002). Calves born after open pulled straw vitrification of immature bovine oocytes. *Cryobiology* **45:** 91-94.

Vincent C., Garnier V., Heyman Y., Renard J.P. (1989). Solvent effects on cytoskeletal organization and in vivo survival after freezing of rabbit oocytes. *Journal of Reproduction and Fertility* **87**: 809-820.

Whittingham D.G. (1971). Survival of mouse embryos after freezing and thawing. *Nature* **233:** 125-126.

Whittingham D.G. (1975). Survival of rat embryos after freezing and thawing. *Journal of Reproduction and Fertility* **43:** 575-578.

Whittingham D.G., Leibo S.P., Mazur P. (1972). Survival of mouse embryos frozen to -196° and -269°C. *Science* **178:** 411-414.

Willadsen S.M., Polge C., Rowson L.E., Moor R.M. (1976). Deep freezing of sheep embryos. *Journal of Reproduction and Fertility* **46:** 151-154.

Wilmut I. (1972). The effect of cooling rate, warming rate, cryoprotective agent and stage of development of survival of mouse embryos during freezing and thawing. *Life Sciences* **11:** 1071-1079.

Wilmut I., Rowson LEA. (1973). Experiments in the low temperature preservation of cow embryos. *Veterinary Record* **92:** 686-690.

Yamamoto Y.N., Oguri N., Tsutsumi Y., Hachinohe Y. (1982). Experiments in the freezing and storage of equine embryos. *Journal of Reproduction and Fertility* **32:** 399-403.

Yang B.C., Ryu L.S., Kirn I.H., Yeon S.H., Choi S.S., Son D.S., Im K.S., Hwang W.S. (1998). Effect of freezing of immature and mature bovine oocytes on their development to blastocyst in vitro. In: *Proceedings 8th World Conference on Animal Production*. Seoul, Korea, vol II, pp 950-951.

Zeilmaker G.H., Alberda A.T., Gent I.V., Rijkmans C.M., Drogendijk A.C. (1984). Two pregnancies following transfer of intact frozen-thawed embryos. *Fertility and Sterility* **42:** 293-296.

Zeron Y., Pearl M., Borochov A., Arav A. (1999). Kinetic and temporal factors influence chilling injury to germinal vesicle and mature bovine oocytes. *Cryobiology* **38:** 35-42.

Zhou G.B., Hou Y.P., Jin F., Yang Q.E., Yang Z.Q., Quan G.B., Tan H.M., Zhu S.E. (2005). Vitrification of mouse embryos at various stages by open-pulled straw (OPS) method. *Animal Biotechnology* **16:** 153-163.

❑❑❑

Chapter 14

Potential of Preantral Follicle Technology for Enhancing in vitro Embryo Production

P.S.P. Gupta, S. Nandi
National Institute of Animal Nutrition and Physiology, Adugodi, Bangalore-560 030, Karnataka, India

Summary

Preantral follicles (PF) are greater in numbers compared to the antral follicles in the ovary of any species. The development of efficient ovarian preantral follicle isolation and culture systems provide a large number of oocytes for the manipulation and embryo production. It also helps for understanding the mechanisms of follicle and oocyte development. Isolation and culture protocols for PFs were developed for many domestic species like cattle, buffalo, sheep, goat, pig, horse, camel, dog and cats. However, embryo production from oocytes derived from *in vitro* grown PFs was reported only in pigs, buffalo, sheep and goat. The rate of oocyte maturation from PFs grown *in vitro* is low and requires considerable research. This chapter presents an overview of isolation and culture systems of PFs that have been developed for domestic species including cattle, buffalo, sheep, goat, pigs, horse, camel, dog and cat along with the current status of progress achieved in the direction of producing embryos using PFs as the source of oocyte in different domestic animal species.

The major hindrance for *in vitro* production of embryos is the less supply of oocytes. In dairy species like buffalo, the major dairy animal of the highest milk producing country India, this problem is more severe. Only negligible numbers of oocytes of an ovary are present in antral follicles. A large number of oocytes present in preantral follicles which would be left unutilized in the reproductive life of an animal. The number of oocytes that can be recovered from abattoir derived ovaries and from live animals by ovum pick up technique for *in vitro* fertilization (IVF) or that can be produced by super ovulation protocols in buffalo is very limited (Singh *et al.*, 2008). To come over this problem, a promising technology 'use of PF as oocyte source for IVF' has been evolved in many domestic animal species. Harvesting oocytes only from antral follicles limits the number of offspring per animal and the optimal exploitation of the genetic material and propagation of valuable animal stock (Vanderhurk *et al.*, 1997). New approaches to increase oocyte yield for manipulation *in vitro* is the current focus of research. The development of a primordial and preantral culture system not only provide a large number of homogenous oocytes for *in vitro* fertilization and embryo production but also help to decipher the regulation of follicular development and acquisition of oocyte developmental competence (Telfer, 2001). Preantral follicle culture also provides an effective and reliable method to assess the influences of environmental mutagens, pharmaceutical agents and potentially endocrine disrupting chemicals on the fidelity of female meiosis (Sun *et al.*, 2010). This technology could be used in cancer patients even who wish to preserve their fertility using ovarian tissue cryopreservation (Wang *et al.*, 2011).

Effective isolation and culture protocols for PFs were developed for many of the domestic animals *viz.*, cattle (Gutierrez *et al.*, 2000; Katska and Rinka, 1998; Telfer *et al.*, 1999), buffalo (Gupta *et al.*, 2001; Gupta *et al.*, 2002a). Embryo production from oocytes derived from *in vitro* grown PFs is reported in pigs (Wu *et al.*, 2001a, b), buffalo (Gupta *et al.*, 2008), sheep (Arunakumari *et al.*, 2010) and goat (Saraiva *et al.*, 2010; Magalhaes *et al.*, 2011a). Success has been limited to antrum formation in cultured PFs in cattle (Gutierrez *et al.*, 2000). Till date only in mice, birth of offspring is reported using oocytes from *in vitro* grown primordial /PFs (Eppig *et al.*, 1989; O'Brien *et al.*, 2003).

The basic steps in this specific technology are only two *i.e.*, isolation of PFs, and *in vitro* culture. When the PFs grow to the stage of Graafian follicle *in vitro*, the oocyte is retrieved and IVF is performed using conventional methods. Usually mechanical and enzymatic methods are employed for the isolation of PFs. Ovarian cortical pieces are incubated in collagenase, hyaluronidase and trypsin enzymes, then the PFs are isolated using micro-dissection under microscope. It is important to select only viable PFs for *in vitro* culture using vital dye exclusion techniques using trypan blue staining (Gupta *et al.*, 2002b). *In vitro* culture methods are usually the same that is used for oocytes and embryos, however, the culture medium comprises some additional components. It usually consists of serum, antibiotic, growth factors, glutamine, hypoxanthine, sodium pyruvate, insulin-transferin-selenium (ITS), and follicle stimulating hormone (FSH). Follicle stimulating hormone influences early follicular growth though there are species-related differences (Hulshof *et al.*, 1995). In a recent study, FSH receptor was found in all the size classes of buffalo PFs which indicated that FSH is involved in recruitment, growth and development of buffalo ovarian PFs (Sharma *et al.*, 2010). An overview of isolation and culture systems of PFs that have been developed for different domestic species (*viz.*, cattle, buffalo, sheep, goat, pigs, horse, camel, dog and cat) is presented below.

1. Cattle

In cattle, the mechanical method has been used for isolation of PFs from ovarian tissues (Ralph *et al.*, 1996; Itoh *et al.*, 2000; Saha *et al.*, 1999). Out of all mechanical methods used in bovine, the most common procedure has been the micro-dissection of the cortical slices of ovaries (Ralph *et al.*, 1996; Katska and Rynska, 1998). This technique is a relatively more time consuming as compared to other procedures (Telfer *et al.*, 1999) wherein either a scalpel blade or a mechanical tissue chopper adjusted to 500 μm was used to slice the ovarian cortex (Saha *et al.*, 1999). Enzymes such as collagenase and DNase have also been used in the past to isolate PFs from cattle ovaries (Figueiredo *et al.*, 1993; Wandji *et al.*, 1996). While comparing both the methods Saha *et al.*, (2002) reported that the mechanical method was more efficient compared to enzyme method. A simple, mechanical method of isolation of a large number of intact PFs from Zebu cow ovaries is reported, (Lucci *et al.*, 2002) with a high recovery rate. Based on morphometrical analysis they concluded that *Bos indicus* PFs were similar to *Bos taurus* PFs.

Attempts have been made to develop the culture systems for cattle PFs (Figueiredo *et al.*, 1993; Figueiredo *et al.*, 1994; Hulshof *et al.*, 1995; Katska and Rinka, 1998; Katska *et al.*, 2000) with varying results. Cattle PFs were cultured individually or in groups for 7-12 days. Large PFs were shown to have more growth than the small PFs in culture (Katska and Rinka, 1998). Various additives like FSH (Hulshof *et al.*, 1995), ITS (Saha *et al.*, 1999), growth factors such as epidermal growth factor (EGF) fibroblast growth factor (Wandji *et al.*, 1996), vasoactive intestinal polypeptide (Van den Hurk *et al.*, 1997) were supplemented to develop suitable culture media for cattle PFs. The development of bovine PFs up to antral stage was achieved by culturing PFs (166 μm) up to 28 days (Gutierrez *et al.*, 2000). Later Itoh *et al.* (2002) reported antrum formation by culturing bovine PFs with LH, FSH, IGF-I (Insulin like growth factor-I) and IGF-II. The regulation of IGF-I bioavailability by IGF binding proteins (IGFBPs) is necessary for the co-ordination of oocyte and follicle development *in vitro* (Thomas *et al.*, 2007). Gonadotrophins play a central role in ovarian function and various growth factors modulate the growth and development of ovarian cells. The PFs groom with 20% O_2 showed improved follicular development and survival, cellular differentiation, besides promoting an increase in the number of meiotically competent oocytes (Gigli *et al.*, 2006). There are no reports on the production of embryos using oocytes retrieved from *in vitro* grown PFs in cattle.

2. Buffalo

Use of PFs as a source of oocytes for embryo production may be more relevant for buffalo species compared to other domestic animals. This is because of the buffalo's inherent limitations in the reproductive system, such as low germ plasm reserve (Danell, 1987) and a high rate of follicular atresia (Bharadwaz *et al.*, 1999), which leads to the low availability of antral follicles that are the common source of oocytes for embryo production. The buffalo ovary contains thousands of oocytes enclosed primarily in primordial and PFs but only very few follicles eventually ovulate. The number of PFs in buffalo ovaries was estimated at 19, 819 (Mondadori *et al.*, 2010).

Effective isolation protocols for buffalo PFs employing mechanical and enzymatic methods were standardized during the last decade (Gupta *et al.*, 2001). Initially the isolation methods were focused on retrieving small PFs of <150μm size (Gupta *et al.*, 2001) and later the methods were standardized for isolating the larger PFs (>150 μm to 500 μm size) using mechanical cum enzymatic method (Fig. 1). In this method, the ovarian cortical pieces are digested in trypsin (2%) for 2 min and then the follicles are dissected out (Gupta *et al.*, 2007). The recovery rate of PFs usually had been less compared to that of cattle. When combined mechanical cum enzymatic method was used, the recovery rates of PFs of sizes categories >40–100, 101–200, 201–300, 301–400 and 401–500 μm were 5.1, 3.2, 3.1, 6.3 and 5.1 per ovary, respectively (Gupta *et al.*, 2007). The presence of corpus luteum, effect of seasons on recovery of large PFs (Gupta *et al.*, 2007), influence of cyclicity and presence of dominant follicles on recovery and growth of buffalo small and large PFs (Nandi *et al.* 2007) were reported. More large PFs could be recovered during the peak breeding season and from the ovaries having corpus luteum (Gupta *et al.*, 2007). Elaborate studies led to the classification of buffalo PFs in to small (<150μm) and large (>150 to 500 μm) PFs (Gupta *et al.*, 2007). Cyclicity of animals or follicular dominance had no effects on *in vitro* growth, survival and antrum formation rates and growth rates of oocytes in cultured PFs (Nandi *et al.*, 2009). A tool named comb-scrape, which consisted of needles, a needle fixing and a handle was designed for isolation of buffalo PFs by Ping *et al.* (2004). The comb-scrape method harvested significantly more PFs (152.35±44.81/ovary) than cutting (32.62±14.81/ovary) and micro-manipulation methods (8.95±3.44/ovary; Ping *et al.*, 2004).

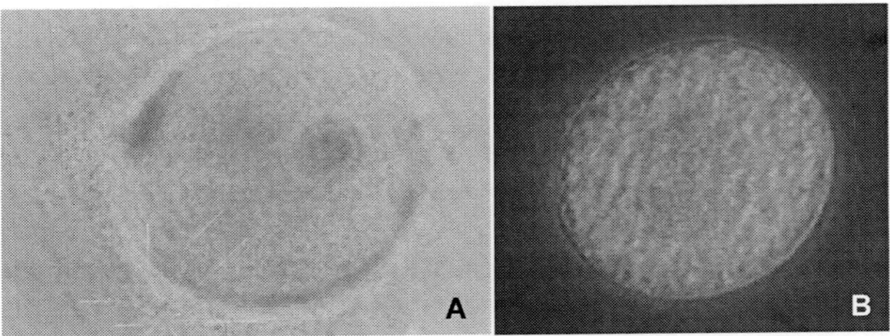

Fig. 1 : Buffalo preantral follicle after isolation from abattoir derived ovary (A) and after labeling (B) with fluorescent dye (DAPI) for detailed morphological evalution.

A culture system for buffalo PFs is first reported by Gupta *et al.* (2002a), in which different growth factors, such as EGF, fibroblast growth factor (FGF) and vasointestinal peptides (VIP), are used to promote the growth and vitality of PFs. Recently it is shown that collagen gel is a novel and efficacious 3D microenvironment for the extended culture of buffalo PFs (Sharma *et al.*, 2010). Supplementation of culture medium with growth factors is essential for antrum formation (Sharma *et al.*, 2009). A study showed that PFs of buffalo fetuses can be cultured *in vitro* and FSH is essential for follicle survival (Santos *et al.*, 2006). The growth factors (IGF and FGF) and β mercaptoethanol synergistically improved the growth (Fig. 2) and survival of large buffalo PFs (Gupta *et al.*, 2010).

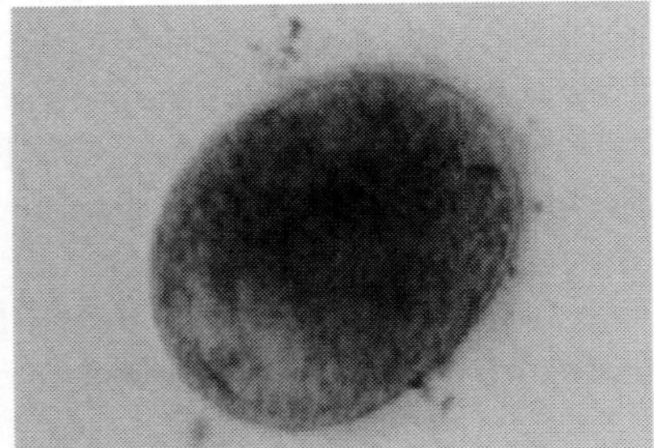

Fig. 2 : Early antral follicle during *in vitro* development of preantral follicle of buffalo

Efforts with small PFs of <150μm diameter did not yield competent oocytes for *in vitro* fertilization (Gupta *et al.*, 2002a). However, culturing large PFs results in growth of competent oocytes capable for embryo production (Gupta *et al.*, 2008). Co-culture of PFs with different somatic cells such as cumulus cells, granulosa cells and ovarian mesenchymal cells yielded success. The follicles are possible to grow 2-3 times of their initial size, from which fertilizable oocytes can be retrieved to produce transferable embryos. In an attempt to standardize the ideal culture condition buffalo PFs of 300-500 μm size were retrieved from abattoir derived ovaries by combined mechanical and enzymatic method and were grown for 100 days in five different culture conditions: (1) minimum essential medium (MEM); (2) coconut water; (3) MEM+ ovarian mesenchymal cell (OMC) co-culture; (4) MEM+ granulosa cell (GC) co-culture; or (5) MEM+ cumulus cell (CC) co-culture. Low growth rates for the PFs were observed when follicles were cultured in MEM or coconut water medium. Moderate growth rates were seen for OMC and GC co-cultures, and high rates of growth were observed when follicles were grown in CC co-culture. The survival of PFs was low in the MEM culture (< 25%), but was over 75% in the other culture systems. Oocytes were not recovered from the MEM group, while an oocyte recovery rate of 80-100% was observed when the follicles were cultured with coconut water/somatic cells. The coculture of PFS with somatic cells *i.e.*, cumulus cells, granulosa cells, ovarian mesenchymal cells and oviductal epithelial cells had shown beneficial effect on the growth. The cumulus cells supported maximum growth and survivality of PFs *in vitro* of all somatic cells tested (Ramesh *et al.*, 2008). Dispersed somatic cells from buffalo ovarian follicles were more effective in providing support for the growth and survivability of PFs in culture, compared to their mono layers (Ramesh *et al.*, 2010). *In vitro* culture of PFs in groups of 2-4 follicles was better than culturing them individually in case of both the small PFs (Gupta *et al.*, 2002a) as well as large PFs (Ramesh *et al.*, 2007). Embryos up to morulae (Fig. 3) could be produced only with the oocytes obtained from PFs grown in the OMC and CC co-culture systems (Gupta *et al.*, 2008).

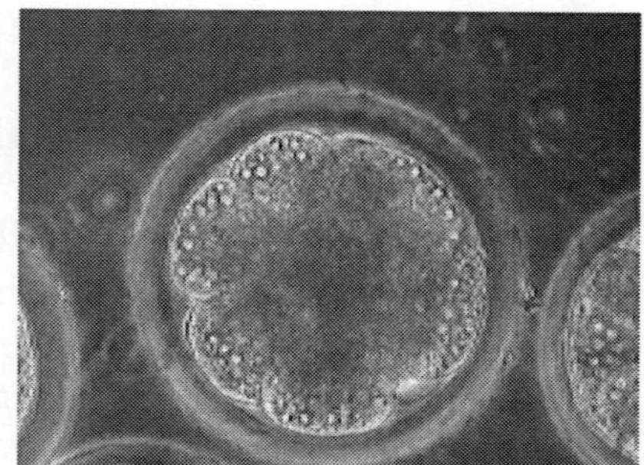

Fig. 3 : Morulae produced with the oocytes derived from *in vitro* grown buffalo preantral follicles.

3. Sheep

In sheep, the isolation of PFs was first reported by Chelikani *et al.* (1998). In their method, first the ovaries were cut into two halves and then medulla was removed. Subsequently, the ovarian cortical pieces were cut into thin slices using a surgical blade. From these cortical slices, PFs were mechanically isolated by micro dissection using two 26 ga needles fitted to 1 ml syringe barrels. A greater number of isolated PFs were obtained with serial section method using tissue chopper adjusted at 87.5μm without affecting the follicular integrity (Amorim *et al.*, 2000).

Formation of antral cavity after *in vitro* culture of sheep PFs was first reported by Cecconi *et al.* (1999). They demonstrated that 5% O_2 promoted greater rates of growth, viability, follicular antrum formation and estradiol secretion in isolated secondary follicles, than 20% O_2. Influence of TGF, IGF, EGF or FSH on *in vitro* development of PFs was studied in sheep (Hemamalini *et al.*, 2003). It was concluded that TGF α (2.5 ng/ml) supported the development of large PFs in sheep to obtain meiotically competent oocytes and PFs of > 250 μm initial diameter developed better *in vitro*. The *in vitro* development of sheep PFs could be obtained independent of gonadotropin stimulation. *In vitro* maturation of the oocytes from the cultured sheep PFs to metaphase-II (M-II) stage was achieved by Tamilmani *et al.* (2005). Later, the same group has observed the beneficial effect of thyroxin on the maturation of oocytes from cultured sheep PFs (Arunakumari *et al.*, 2007).

Finally, the same group has reported for the first time the production of embryo using the oocytes from *in vitro* cultured ovine PFs (Arunakumari *et al.*, 2010). In their study, sheep PFs measuring 250-400 μm in diameter were cultured for six days in serum-free media supplemented with growth factors (IGF-I and TGF-β) and hormones (thyroxine, growth hormone, FSH and insulin). They have reported that 1% ITS, 10 ng/ml each of IGF-I, and Insulin and 1 IU/ml of GH support the best development of sheep PFs. This was concluded based on the proportion of the PFs exhibiting growth, mean increase in diameter, proportions of PFs developing antrum, ovulations *in vitro* and oocytes maturing to M-II stage, However, the oocytes from PFs cultured in any concentration of TGF β failed to mature to M-II stage. Similarly, among the combinations studied, IGF-I+GH was found to be the best. In combination with T4 and FSH, IGF-I+GH supported the best development of the PFs. Culture of PFs in micro drops or agar gel supported high development. Magalhγes *et al.* (2011b) reported that periodic replacement of medium (every 6 days) is efficient for development of sheep PFs *in vitro*. Cyclicity of animals or follicular dominance had no effect on *in vitro* growth, survival and antrum formation rates and growth rates of oocytes in cultured PFs (Fig. 4) of sheep (Nandi *et al.*, 2009).

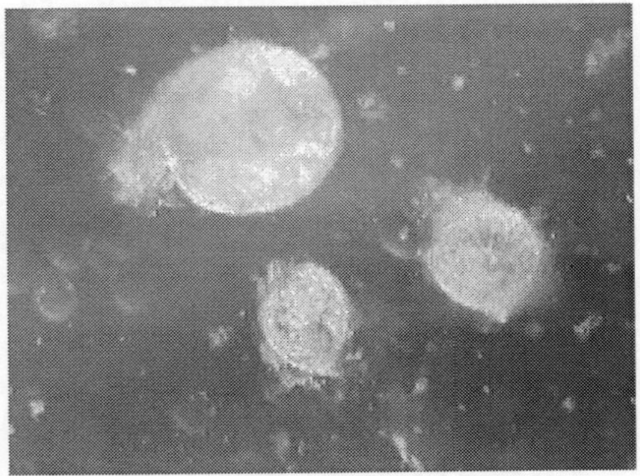

Fig. 4 : Images of different sizes ovine preantral follicles during *in vitro* culture

4. Goat

Initial report on the isolation of caprine PFs was again made by the same group who did pioneering studies on sheep PF isolation. Method of isolation as followed in sheep was used for caprine species (Chelikani *et al.*, 1998). Formation of antral cavity after *in vitro* culture of goat PFs was first reported by Huamin and Yong (2000). In their study, PFs of 50-150 μm diameter were isolated by collagenase and DNase and then cultured in agar gel in prosence of fetal calf serum, hypoxanthine, dbcAMP, FSH, ITS, IGF-I, hydrocortisone and antibiotics. A large portion of follicles entered the antral stage, and oocytes also acquired growth. The formation of theca lamina and zona pellucida was observed. It was reported that EGF was mitogenic to goat PFs, FSH was capable of inducing growth in small but not large PFs and TGF-α and IGF-II were stimulatory to goat PFs in culture (Rajarajan *et al.*, 2006). When caprine PFs of >150μm were grown for 30 days in two levels of O_2 tension *i.e.*, 5% and 20%, only the PFs, which were cultured in 20% tension resumed meiosis (Silva *et al.*, 2010). Fibroblast growth factor also stimulated the activation of primordial follicles and the growth of PFs in caprine (Matos *et al.*, 2007). The supplementation of IGF-1 and EGF to the culture medium is recommended for goat PFs. A dynamic sequential changes of culture medium containing FSH, LH and EGF promote the *in vitro* growth of PFs, their oocyte maturation and caprine embryo production (Saraiva *et al.*, 2010). Magalhães *et al.* (2011a) reported the caprine embryo production by *in vitro* fertilization of oocytes derived from PFs grown *in vitro*. The authors demonstrated that growth hormone promote *in vitro* growth and maturation of goat PF oocytes and enable the production of an embryo. Duarte *et al.* (2010) reported that follicular interactions affect the *in vitro* development of isolated goat PFs and group culture improve the growth of PFs. The frequency of medium replacement was studied in great details (Magalhães *et al.*, 2011a; Araújo *et al.*, 2011). It was suggested that the medium must be replaced every 2 days. The PF isolation and culture techniques were reviewed by Figueiredo *et al.* (2011) in details and they concluded that major achievement was accomplished in the *in vitro* development of isolated secondary PFs up to antral stages, however, subsequent efficiency of production of mature oocytes and embryos is low.

5. Pig

Both mechanical (Wu *et al.*, 2001a) and enzymatic method of isolation using trypsin (Morbeck *et al.*, 1993) and collagenese (Choi *et al.*, 2008) were adopted for the isolation of porcine PFs. Pig was the first domestic animal species in which the embryo could be produced using oocytes derived from *in vitro* grown PFs (Wu *et al.*, 2001a, b). The basic media was supplemented with L-ascorbic acid, porcine serum, insulin, transferin, FSH to culture the PFs. Another group (Shuttleworth *et al.*, 2002) observed that viable porcine PFs could be cultured for extended periods and indicated the possible role of angiotensin II in folliculogenesis and steroidogenesis in early pig follicles development. Supplementation of medium with follicular fluid collected from large follicles (LFF), rather than serum, enhance the PF and oocyte growth. Factors that enhance follicle development in LFF and factors that suppressed follicle development in media supplemented with follicular fluid collected from large follicles are proteins and these LFF factors ranged in size from 10 kDa to over 100 kDa (Metoki *et al.*, 2008). Wu *et al.* (2001b) compared intra-cytoplasmic sperm injecton (ICSI) and *in vitro* fertilization (IVF) and found no significant differences in percentage of oocyte (derived from *in vitro* grown porcine PF) fertilization, cleavage and blastocyst formation. The same group reported that the somatic cells of PFs secrete certain substances that would favor *in vitro* growth of PFs. Wu *et al.* (2007) reported that FSH is essential for the *in vitro* growth and estradiol secretion of porcine PFs and for oocytes to acquire competence to resume meiosis and undergo fertilization. The EGF with FSH treatment of porcine PFs improve the quality of oocytes, shown by a higher frequency of embryonic development (Wu and Tian, 2007).

6. Dog

Dog PFs are unique in that some of them progress to an advanced stage throughout the estrous cycle. These "advanced preantral" follicles contain fully-grown, lipid-filled oocytes with several layers of granulosa cells and contain similar populations of androgen receptors as early antral follicles. Thus, IVM of oocytes from advanced PFs may not require the preliminary *in vitro* growth period needed for PFs of other species such as the mouse, pig and human (Bolamba *et al.*, 2006). Durrant *et al.* (1998) developed PF isolation and classification protocols for the domestic dog as a model for endangered canids using collagenase/DNase methods. Dog oocytes cultured within advanced PF in vitro are competent to resume meiosis to the metaphase stage (Bolamba *et al.*, 1998). The synthetic oviductal fluid (SOF) can support nuclear maturation of a small proportion of bitch oocytes *in vitro* (Bolamba *et al.*, 2002). The sequential addition of FSH to the culture medium maintained the survival of isolated canine PFs and promoted an increased rate of follicular growth and antrum formation (Serafim *et al.*, 2010). Research has also been conducted on preservation of isolated dog PFs. Preservation of canine PFs might be better accomplished through hypothermic (4 or 20°C) storage in MEM, which ensures maintenance of morphology and viability for up to 12h (Lopes *et al.*, 2009). Powdered coconut water is shown as an appropriate medium for short-term storage of canine PFs (Lima et al., 2010). There are no published reports on the production of embryos using oocytes collected from *in vitro* grown PFs in this species.

7. Cat

In domestic cat PFs isolation and culture were mainly performed in late nineties by Jewgenow and her co-workers in Germany. The mechanical dissection of ovaries from domestic cats provide high numbers of PFs (300-24,500 per ovary, Jewgenow *et al.*, 1995). Small PFs (40 to 90 μm) of domestic cats are cultured in the presence or absence of EGF, IGF I and bFGF for 5 d. It was reported that FGF mainly induced the proliferation of granulosa cells while IGF-I was involved in cellular activation of oocytes in PFs, which is modulated by EGF (Jewgenow *et al.*, 1996). Isolated PFs also have been cryopreserved, showing that a small subpopulation of these follicles survive and are functionally intact after freezing with conventional cryoprotectants (Jewgenow *et al.*, 1998). There are no reports available on the production of embryos using oocytes retrieved from *in vitro* grown PFs in cat as well.

8. Horse and camel

Not much work has been carried out on equine and camel species on PF isolation and culture. Mare PFs are isolated from ovaries using collagenase treatment (Telfer and Watson 2000). Similarly the camel PFs are also successfully isolated (Saber *et al.*, 2009). No report on the successful PFs culture is available in these two species. The growth of mare ovarian follicle *in vivo* has been reviewed by Ginther *et al.*, 2004 and Donadeau and Pedersen, 2008. However, no report on *in vitro* follicle growth in mare has been reported. The growth of camel oocyte is reported to be associated with progressive increase in the number of mitochondria, endoplasmic reticulum, Golgi complexes and cytoplasmic vesicles as well as decrease in the number of lipid droplets and the nucleus migration from an eccentric in preantral to a peripheral location in antral follicles (Davoodian *et al.*, 2011). Ali and Abdel-Razek (2001) found that the average number of follicles/ovary is significantly higher in camel than cow and buffalo. The higher number of surface ovarian follicles in camels as compared to those reported in buffaloes and cows may be as a result of the high number of PFs presented in camel than buffalo and cow ovaries (EL-Harairy, 2007).

Conclusions

Apart from the benefits as source of oocytes for embryo production, *In vitro* culture of PFs can also be used to understand the factors controlling early ovarian folliculogenesis. In addition, follicular culture can also be used to evaluate *in vitro* effects of different substances that can affect ovarian function and fertility (*e.g.*, hormones, antibiotics and anti-inflammatory agents). Mammalian oocytes, especially of domestic animals, are in great demand because of increasing interest on cloning and transgenic studies. The oocytes are used as the recipient cells for transferring the karyoplast with a selected genome. Thus, a high oocyte yield from the animals utilizing the PFs as a source would fulfill the needs of transgenic and cloning works. Picton *et al.* (2008) opined that the follicle culture practitioners need to consider the direct effects of long-term culture and sub-optimal culture environments on the epigenetic information and methylation status of key imprinted genes in oocytes. Hence, further studies incorporating genomics are to be conducted for standardization of this technology in domestic animals. Formation of the theca cell layer is a key event that occurs during this transitional stage of preantral to early antral follicle. Granulosa cell factor(s) stimulates the recruitment of theca cells from cortical stromal cells, while oocyte-derived growth differentiation factor-9 (GDF-9) is involved in the differentiation of theca cells during this early stage of follicular development. It is a cystine knot-containing hormone of the transforming growth factor-beta superfamily produced by the oocyte. The GDF-9 promotes follicular survival and growth during transition from preantral stage to early antral stage by suppressing granulosa cell apoptosis and follicular atresia. The GDF-9 also enhances PF growth by up-regulating theca cell androgen production. Thecal factor(s) promotes granulosa cell proliferation and suppress granulosa cell apoptosis (Oriska *et al.*, 2009). Hence inclusion of GDF-9 in the *in vitro* culture medium of PFs of domestic animals may yield positive results. Technology to produce an offspring from domestic animal species from an embryo generated using oocytes from *in vitro* grown PFs may be made available in near future for the rapid multiplication of elite germplasm of livestock.

References

Ali A., Abdel-Razek A. (2001). Comparison of number and quality of oocytes in the Egyptian buffaloes (Bubalus bubalis), cows (Bos taurus) and camels (Camelus dromedarius). *Assiut Veterinary Medicine Journal* **45:** 317-325.

Amorim C.A., Rodrigues A.P.R., Lucci C.M., Figueiredo J.R., Gonçalves P.B.D. (2000). Effect of sectioning on the number of isolated ovine preantral follicles. *Small Ruminant Research* **37:** 269-277.

Araújo V.R., Chaves R.N., Duarte A.B.G., Celestino J.J.H., Silva G.M., Fernandes G.D., Matos M.H.T., Campello C.C., Figueiredo J.R. (2011). Effect of culture medium replacement protocol on the *in vitro* development of isolated caprine secondary follicles. *Small Ruminant Research* **95:** 139-143.

Arunakumari G., Shanmugasundaram N., Rao V.H. (2010). Development of morulae from the oocytes of cultured sheep preantral follicles. *Theriogenology* **74:** 884-894.

Arunakumari G., Vagdevi R., Rao B.S., Rajarajan K., Naidu K.S., Amarnath D., Vagedevi R., Rao V.H. (2007). Effect of hormones and growth factors on in vitro development of sheep preantral follicles. *Small Ruminant Research* **70:** 93-100.

Bharadwaz RL, Roy KS, 1999: Histomorophological study on the age related follicular atresia in the ovary of Indian buffaloes (Bubalus bubalis). *Buffalo Journal* **15:** 25-33.

Bolamba D., Borden-Russ K.D., Durrant B.S. (1998). In vitro maturation of domestic dog oocytes cultured in advanced preantral and early antral follicles. *Theriogenology* **49:** 933-942.

Bolamba D., Russ K.D., Olson M.A., Sandler J.L., Durrant B.S. (2002). In vitro maturation of bitch oocytes from advanced preantral follicles in synthetic oviduct fluid medium: serum is not essential. *Theriogenology* **58:** 1689-1703.

Cecconi S., Barboni B., Coccia M., Mattioli M. (1999). In vitro development of sheep preantral follicles. *Biology of Reproduction* **60:** 594-601.

Chelikani P.K., Amarnath D., Reddy K.K., Naidu K.S., Rao V.H. (1998). Isolation of preantral ovarian follicles in sheep and goats. *Theriogenology* **49:** 343 (Abstr.)

Choi M.H., Gong S.P., Lim J.M. (2008). Retrieval of porcine ovarian follicles by different methods. *Asian Australasian Journal of Animal Science* **21:** 353-357.

Danell B. (1987). Oestrus behaviour, ovarian morphology and cyclical variation in the follicular system and endocrine pattern in water buffalo heifers. *Ph. D Dissertation,* Sweedish University of Agricultural Sciences. Uppsala. Sweeden.

Davoodian N., Mesbah F., Kafi M. (2011). Oocyte ultrastructural characteristics in camel (Camelus dromedarius) primordial to large antral follicles. *Anatomia Histologia and Embryologia* **40:** 120-127.

Donadeau F.X., Pedersen H.G. (2008). Follicle development in mares. *Reproduction in Domestic Animals* **43:** 224-231.

Duarte A.B., Chaves R.N., Arau´jo V.R., Celestino J.J., Silva G.M., Lopes C.A., Tavares L.M., Campello C.C., Figueiredo J.R. (2010). Follicular interactions affect the *in vitro* development of isolated goat preantral follicles. *Zygote* DOI: 10.1017/S0967199410000237.

Durrant B.S., Pratt N.C., Russ K.D., Bolamba D. (1998). Isolation and characterization of canine advanced preantral and early antral follicles. *Theriogenology* **49:** 917-932.

EL-Harairy M.A., Shamiah S.M., Abdel-Khalek A.E., Khalil W.A. (2007). Effect of pregnancy status and harvesting technique on recovery rate and categories of dromedary camel oocytes. *Egyptian Journal of Basic and Applied Physiology* **6:** 255-268.

Eppig J.J., Schroeder A.C. (1989). Capacity of mouse oocytes from preantral follicles to undergo embryogenesis and development to live young after growth, maturation, and fertilization in vitro. *Biology of Reproduction* **41:** 268-276.

Figueiredo J.R., Hulshof S.C.J., Van den Hurk R., Ectors F.J., Fontes R.S., Nusgens B., Bevers M.M., Becker J.F. (1993). Development of a new mechanical and enzymatic method for the isolation of intact preantral follicles from fetal, calf and adult bovine ovaries. *Theriogenology* **40:** 789-799.

Figueiredo J.R., Hulshof S.C.J., Van den hurk R., Nusgens B., Bevers M.M., Ectors F.J., Beckers J.F., Van den hurk R. (1994). Preservation of oocyte and granulosa cell morphology in bovine preantral follicles cultured in vitro. *Theriogenology* **41:** 1333-1346.

Figueiredo J.R., Rodrigues A.P.R., Silva J.R.V., Santos R.R. (2011). Cryopreservation and *in vitro* culture of caprine preantral follicles. *Reproduction Fertility Development* **23:** 40-47.

Gigli I., Byrd D.D., Fortune J.E. (2006). Effects of oxygen tension and supplements to the culture medium on activation and development of bovine follicles *in vitro. Theriogenology* **66:** 344-353.

Ginther O.J., Beg M.A., Gastal M.O., Gastal E.L. (2004). Follicle dynamics and selection in mares. *Animal Reproduction* **1:** 45-63.

Gupta P.S.P., Nandi S., Ravindranatha B.M., Sarma P.V. (2001). Isolation of preantral follicles from buffalo ovaries. *Veterinary Record* **148:** 543-544.

Gupta P.S.P., Nandi S., Ravindranatha B.M., Sarma P.V. (2002a). In vitro culture of buffalo (Bubalus bubalis) preantral follicles. *Theriogenology* **57:** 1839-1854.

Gupta P.S.P., Nandi S., Ravindranatha B.M., Sarma P.V. (2002b). Trypan blue staining to differentiate live and dead buffalo oocytes and its effect on embryo development *in vitro. Buffalo Journal* **18:** 321-330.

Gupta P.S.P., Ramesh H.S., Nandi S., Ravindra J.P. (2007). Isolation of large preantral follicles from buffalo ovary: Effect of season and corpus luteum. *Animal Reproduction Science* **101:** 145-152.

Gupta P.S.P., Nandi S., (2010).Viability and growth of buffalo preantral follicles and their corresponding oocytes in vitro: Effect of growth factors and ß mercaptoethanol. *Reproduction in Domestic Animals* **45:** 147-154.

Gupta P.S.P., Ramesh H.S., Manjunatha B.M., Nandi S., Ravindra J.P. (2008). Production of buffalo embryos using oocytes from in vitro grown preantral follicles. *Zygote* **16:** 57-63.

Gutierrez C.G., Ralph J.H., Telfer E.E., Wilmut I., Webb R. (2000). Growth and antrum formation of bovine preantral follicles in long term culture *in vitro. Biology of Reproduction* **62:** 1322-1328.

Hemamalini N.C., Rao B.S., Tamilmani G., Amarnath D.,Vagdevi R., Naidu K.S., Reddy K.K., Rao V.H. (2003). Influence of transforming growth factor, insulin like growth factor,epidermal growth factor or follicle stimulating hormone on in vitro development of preantral follicles in sheep. *Small Ruminant Research* **50:** 11-22.

Huamin Z., Yong Z. (2000). *In vitro* development of caprine ovarian preantral follicles. *Theriogenology* **54:** 641-650.

Hulshof S.C.J., Figueiredo J.R., Beckers J.F., Bevers M.M., Vander donk J.A., Van den hurk R. (1995). Effects of fetal bovine serum, FSH and 17-Estradiol on the culture of bovine preantral follicles. *Theriogenology* **44:** 217-226.

Itoh T., Hoshi H. (2000). Efficient isolation and long-term viability of bovine small preantral follicles in vitro. *In vitro Cell Development and Biology* (Animal) **36:** 235-240.

Itoh T., Kacchi M., Abe H., Sendai Y., Hoshi H. (2002). Growth, antrum formation, and estradiol production of bovine preantral follicles cultured in a serum-free medium. *Biology of Reproduction* **67:** 1099-1105.

Jewgenov K., Penfold L.M., Meyer H.H.D., Wildt D.E. (1998). Viability of small preantral ovarian follicles from domestic cats after cryoprotectant exposure and cryopreservation. *Journal of Reproduction and Fertility* **112:** 39-47.

Jewgenow K. (1996). Impact of peptide growth factors on the culture of small preantral follicles of domestic cats. *Theriogenology* **45:** 889-895.

Jewgenow K., Göritz F. (1995). The recovery of preantral follicles from ovaries of domestic cats and their characterization before and after culture. *Animal Reproduction Science* **39:** 285-297.

Katska L., Alm H., Rynska B. (2000). Nuclear configuration of bovine oocytes derived from fresh and in vitro cultured preantral and early antral ovarian follicle. *Theriogenology* **54:** 247-260.

Katska L., Rynska B. (1998). The isolation and in vitro culture of bovine preantral and early antral follicles of different size classes. *Theriogenology* **50:** 213-222.

Lima G.L., Costa L.L., Cavalcanti D.M., Rodrigues C.M., Freire F.A., Fontenele-Neto J.D., Silva A.R. (2010). Short-term storage of canine preantral ovarian follicles using a powdered coconut water (ACP)-based medium. Theriogenology **74:** 146 – 152.

Lopes C.A.P., Santos R.R., Celestino J.J.H., Melo M.A.P., Chaves R.N., Campello C.C., Silva J.R.V., Báo S.N., Jewgenow K., Figueiredo J.R. (2009). Follicles (PAF). *Theriogenology* **51:** 308 (*Abstr.*).

Lucci C.M., Rodolfo R., Figuiredo J.R., Sonia N.B. (2002). Zebu (Bos indicus) ovarian preantral follicles: morphological characterization and development of an efficient isolation method. *Theriogenology* **57:** 1467-1483.

Magalhães D.M., Duarte A.B.G., Araújo V.R., Brito I.R., Soares T.G., Lima I.M.T., Lopes C.A.P., Campello C.C., Rodrigues A.P.R., Figueiredo J.R. (2011a). In vitro production of a caprine embryo from a preantral follicle cultured in media supplemented with growth hormone. *Theriogenology* **75:** 182-188.

Magalhães D.M., Fernandes D.D., Mororó M.B.S., Silva C.M.G., Rodrigues G.Q., Bruno J.B., Matos M.H.T., Campello C.C., Figueiredo J.R. (2011b). Effect of the medium replacement interval on the viability, growth and in vitro maturation of isolated caprine and ovine pre-antral follicles. *Reproduction in Domestic Animal* **46:** 134-140

Matos M.H.T., Van den Hurk R., Lima-Verde I.M., Luque M.C.A., Santos K.D.B., Martins F.S., Ba´o S.N., Lucci C.M., Figueiredo J.R. (2007). Effects of fibroblast growth factor-2 on the in vitro culture of caprine preantral follicles. *Cells Tissues and Organs* **186:** 112-120.

Metoki T., Iwata H., Itoh M., Kasai M., Takajyo A., Suzuki A., Kuwayama T., Monji Y. (2008). Effects of follicular fluids on the growth of porcine preantral follicle and oocyte. *Zygote* **16:** 239-247.

Mondadori R.G., Santin T.R., Fidelis A.A., Porfírio E.P., Báo S.N. (2010). Buffalo (*Bubalus bubalis*) pre-antral follicle population and ultrastructural characterization of antral follicle oocyte. *Reproduction in Domestic Animal* **45:** 33-37.

Morbeck D.E., Flowers W.L., Britt J.H. (1993). Response of porcine granulosa cells isolated from primary and secondary follicles to FSH, 8-bromo-cAMP and epidermal growth factor *in vitro. Journal of Reproduction and Fertility* **99:** 577-584.

Nandi S., Girish Kumar V., Manjunatha B.M., Ramesh H.S., Gupta P.S.P. (2009). Isolation and culture of ovine and bubaline small and large preantral follicles: effect of cyclicity and presence of a dominant follicle. *Reproduction in Domestic Animals* **44:** 74-79.

O'Brien M.J., Pendola J.K., Eppig J.J. (2003). A revised protocol for in vitro development of mouse oocyte from primordial follicles dramatically improves their development competence. *Biology of Reproduction* **68:** 1682-1686.

Orisaka M., Tajima K., Tsang B.K., Kotsuji F. (2009). Oocyte-granulosa-thecal cell interactions during preantral follicular development. *Journal of Ovarian Research* **2:** 9. DOI:10.1186/1757-2215-2-9.

Picton H.M., Harris S.E., Muruvi W., Chambers E.L. (2008). The in vitro growth and maturation of follicles. *Reproduction* **136:** 703-715.

Ping P.H., Xue F.G., Shun S.D. (2004). A method for isolation of buffalo preantral follicles. *Current Zoology* **50:** 291-296.

Rajarajan K., Rao B.S., Vagdevi R., Tamilmani G., Arunakumari G., Sreenu M., Amarnath D., Naik B.R., Rao V.H. (2006). Effect of various growth factors on the in vitro development of goat preantral follicles. *Small Ruminant Research* **63:** 204-212.

Ralph J.H., Wilmut I., Telfer E.E. (1996). The effect of FSH on bovine preantral to early antral ovarian follicle growth *in vitro. Biology of Reproduction (Suppl.1)* **54:** 5.

Ramesh H.S., Gupta P.S.P., Nandi S., Manjunatha B.M. (2010). In vitro development of buffalo preantral follicles in co-culture with cumulus cells and granulosa cells. *Veterinary Archives* **80:** 41-50.

Ramesh H.S., Gupta P.S.P., Nandi S., Manjunatha B.M., Girish Kumar V., Ravindra J.P. (2008). Co-culture of buffalo preantral follicles with different somatic cells. *Reprouction in Domestic Animals* **43:** 520-524.

Ramesh H.S., Ravindra J.P., Gupta P.S.P., Girishkumar V. (2007). Effect of individual or group culture on in vitro development of buffalo preantral follicles. *Indian Journal of Animal Science* **77:** 953-955.

Russ K.D., Harper S.A., Sandler J.L., Durrant B.S. (2006). Effects of epidermal growth factor and hormones on granulosa expansion and nuclear maturation of dog oocytes *in vitro. Theriogenology* **65:** 1037-1047.

Saber A.A. (2009). Effects of storing dromedary camel ovaries at 4 or 20°C for different periods of time on the morphology and viability of pre-antral follicles. *Medicina Veterinaria* DOI:10.2478/v10082-009-0007-4.

Saha S., Shimizu M., Geshi M., Izaike Y. (2002). Comparison of enzymatic and mechanical methods for the collection of bovine preantral follicles. *Animal Science* **74:** 155-161.

Saha S., Shimizu M., Izaike Y. (1999). In vitro culture and characterization of bovine preantral follicles. *Theriogenology* **51:** 308 (*Abstr.*)

Santos S.S.D., Biondi F.C., Cordeiro M.S., Miranda M.S., Dantas J.K., Igueiredo J.R., Ohashi O.M., (2006). Isolation, follicular density, and culture of preantral follicles of buffalo fetuses of different ages. *Animal Reproduction Science* **95:** 1-15.

Saraiva M.V.A., Rossetto R., Brito I.R., Celestino I.I.H., Silva C.M.G., Faustino L.R., Almeida A.P., Bruno I.B., Magalhaes D.M., Matos M.H.T., Campello C.C., Figuwiredo I.R.

(2010). Dynamic medium produces caprine embryo from preantral follicles grown *in vitro*. *Reproductive Science* **17:** 1135-1143.

Serafim M.K.B., Araújo V.R., Silva G.M., Duarte A.B.G., Almeida A.P., Chaves R.N., Campello C.C., Lopes C.A.P., Figueiredo J.R., Silva L.D.M. (2010). Canine preantral follicles cultured with various concentrations of follicle-stimulating hormone. *Theriogenology* **74:** 749-755.

Sharma G.T., Dubey P.K., Meur S.K. (2009). Survival and developmental competence of buffalo preantral follicles using three-dimensional collagen gel culture system. *Animal Reproduction Science* **114:** 115-124.

Sharma G.T., Dubey P.K., Kumar G.S. (2010). Localization of Follicle-stimulating hormonereceptor gene in buffalo (*Bubalus bubalis*) preantral follicles. *Reproduction in Domestic Animals* DOI:10.1111/j.1439-0531.2010.01604.

Short-term preservation of canine preantral follicles: Effects of temperature, medium and time. *Animal Reproduction Science* **115:** 201-214.

Shuttleworth G., Broughton pipkin F., Hunter M.G. (2002). *In vitro* development of pig preantral follicles cultured in a serum-free medium and the effect of angiotensin II. *Reproduction* **123:** 807-818.

Silva C.M.G., Matos M.H.T., Rodrigues G.Q., Faustino L.R., Pinto L.C., Chaves R.N., Araújo V.R., Campello C.C., Figueiredo J.R. (2010). *In vitro* survival and development of goat preantral follicles in two different oxygen tensions. *Animal Reproduction Science* **117:** 83-89.

Singh B., Chauhan M.S., Singla S.K., Gautam S.K., Verma V., Manik R.S., Singh A.K., Sodhi M., Mukesh M. (2008). Reproductive biotechniques in buffaloes (*Bubalus bubalis*): status, prospects and challenges. *Reproduction Fertility and Development* **21:** 499-510.

Sun F., Betzendahl I., Shen Y., Cortvrindt R., Smitz J., Eichenlaub-Ritter U. (2010). Preantral follicle culture as a novel in vitro assay in reproductive toxicology testing in mammalian oocytes. *Mutagenesis* **19:** 13-19.

Tamilmani G., Rao B.S., Vagdevi R., Amarnath D., Naik B.R., Mutharao M., Rao V.H. (2005) Nuclear maturation of ovine oocytes in cultured preantral follicles. *Small Ruminant Research* **60:** 295-305.

Telfer E.E. (2001). In vitro development of pig preantral follicles. *Reproduction (Suppl.)* **58:** 81-90.

Telfer E.E., Watson E.D. (2000). Method for isolating preantral follicles from mare ovaries. *Journal of Reproduction and Fertility (Suppl.)* **56:** 447-453.

Telfer E.E., Webb R., Moor R.M., Gosden R.G. (1999). New approaches to increase in oocyte yield from ruminants. *Journal of Animal Science* **68:** 285-298.

Thomas F.H., Campbell B.K., Armstrong D.G., Telfer E.E. (2007). Effects of IGF-I bioavailability on bovine preantral follicular development *in vitro*. *Reproduction* **133:** 1121-1128.

Van den Hurk R., Bevers M.M., Beckers J.F. (1997) *In-vivo* and *In-vitro* development of preantral follicles. *Theriogenology* **47:** 73-82.

Wandji S.A., Eppig J.J., Fortune J.E. (1996). FSH and growth factors affect the growth and endocrine function in vitro of granulosa cells of bovine preantral follicles. *Theriogenology* **45:** 817-832.

Wang X., Catt S., Pangestu M., Smith P.T. (2011). Successful in vitro culture of pre-antral follicles derived from vitrified murine ovarian tissue: oocyte maturation, fertilization, and live births. *Reproduction* **141:** 183-191.

Wu J., Benjamin R.E., Carrell D.T. (2001a). *In vitro* growth, maturation, fertilization, and embryonic development of oocytes from porcine preantral follicles. *Biology of Reproduction* **64:** 375-381.

Wu J., Carrell D.T., Wicox A.L. (2001b). Development of in vitro matured oocytes from porcine preantral follicles following intracytoplasmic sperm injection. *Biology of Reproduction* **65:** 1579-1585.

Wu J., Tian Q. (2007). Role of follicle stimulating hormone and epidermal growth factor in the development of porcine preantral follicle in vitro. *Zygote* **15:** 233-240.

Wu J., Xu B., Wang W. (2007). Effects of luteinizing hormone and follicle stimulating hormone on the developmental competence of porcine preantral follicle oocytes grown in vitro. *Journal of Assisted Reproduction and Genetics* **24:** 419-424.

□□□

Chapter 15

Embryo-Uterine Dialogue in Pregnancy Signalling

S. Mondal
National Institute of Animal Nutrition and Physiology, Adugodi, Bangalore-560 030, Karnataka, India

Summary

Early embryonic loss is a major cause of reproductive failure during preimplantation period when the embryo and uterus develop in a coordinated synchronous manner. Coordination of the synchrony of development depends on maternal hormones particularly ovarian steroids and the influence of embryo on uterine microenvironment. The survivality of embryo during early embryonic life is mostly dependent on the efficiency with which the maternal recognition of pregnancy (MRP) is established. Maternal recognition of pregnancy results from signalling between the trophoblast of conceptus and the maternal system. In ruminants, oxytocin (OT) triggers the pulsatile release of $PGF_{2\alpha}$ by the endometrium at the end of an infertile estrous cycle to induce luteolysis. Interferon-τ exerts its antiluteolytic action by suppressing the normal pattern of pulsatile $PGF_{2\alpha}$ release in late estrous cycle, possibly by a mechanism that involves down regulation of estrogen receptor in uterine epithelium which in turn prevents a rise in oxytocin receptor. Understanding the signal transduction pathway of OT-induced $PGF_{2\alpha}$ production will provide insight into the mechanisms underlying maternal recognition of pregnancy in ruminants. Several growth factors and cytokines secreted from the embryo, trophoblast, oviduct and endometrium during preimplantaion periods plays a crucial role in establishing the interaction between embryo and dam. Therefore the exploration of the complex interaction between the conceptus and maternal uterine environment will facilitate the development of optimal reproductive management strategies and paradigm to reduce early embryonic losses.

Early embryonic mortality is a major impediment hampering the reproductive efficiency of livestock. During early pregnancy, the growing embryo solely depends on uterine microenvironment for survival and growth as the uterine environment undergoes continual modifications to cope the needs of the embryo. If the embryo fails to signal its presence during this period (day 12 -18 of pregnancy), because of lack of synchrony between uterine environment and the embryo, premature expulsion of embryo occurs. The early embryonic development including implantation of foetus and maintenance of pregnancy are critically influenced by embryo-maternal crosstalk. The survivality of embryo during early embryonic life is mostly dependent on the efficiency with which the maternal recognition of pregnancy (MRP) is established. Maternal recognition of pregnancy results from dialogue between the trophoblast of conceptus and uterus. These signals ensure maintenance of structural and functional integrity of corpus luteum (CL). Establishment of pregnancy requires abrogation of luteolytic pulses of $PGF_{2\alpha}$ from uterus to maintain corpus luteum and progesterone production. The attenuation of pulsatile secretion of $PGF_{2\alpha}$ from the uterus is essential for prevention of luteolysis during pregnancy in ruminants. In early pregnancy, interferon-τ (IFN-τ), a protein secreted by trophoblast between days 15 and 24 of gestation acts as the embryogenic signal to inhibit the pulsatile secretory pattern of $PGF_{2\alpha}$ and corpus luteum regression. Progesterone from corpus luteum maintains endometrial functions that are permissive to early embryonic development, implantation, placentation and successful fetal/placental development.

1. Periimplantation embryo development

Embryogenesis, the period from fertilization to implantation, involves various morphological, cellular and biochemical changes related to activation of embryonic genome. These changes include several cleavage divisions of fertilized egg, compaction and blastocoel formation leading to the development of blastocyst. Before fertilization unfertilised oocytes occupy the entire space inside the zona pellucida. Soon after fertilization one cell embryo undergoes a series of cleavage division progressing through 2-cell, 4-cell, 8-cell, 16-cell stages and so on. The blastomeres (cells in cleavage stage embryo) form tight junctions with one another leading to formation of mulberry shaped mass of cells (morula). The change in shape of the embryo is called compaction and occurs around the 32 cell stage in both *in vitro* and *in vivo* embryos. Following activation of embryonic genome, the outer cells of morula begin to express various membrane transport molecules leading to accumulation of fluid inside the embryo which signals the formation of the blastocyst. The blastocyst continues to accumulate blastocoelic fluid (cavitation) and expands to form expanded blastocyst. Both compaction and cavitation are dependent on transcription of appropriate embryonic genes and their sequential activation. Transformation of morula to blastocyst stage gives rise to two different cell types: inner cell mass (ICM) and trophoblast cells (TC). The inner cell mass gives rise to the three germ layers of developing embryo (endoderm, mesoderm and ectoderm) whereas trophoblast cells develop the tissues of foetal placenta and associated extra-embryonic membrane. The zygote spends few days (up to 3 days) inside the oviduct and enters the uterine horn at the morula stage about 4-5 days after fertilization. The embryo then reached blastocyst stage at days 6-7 and day 6 in cow and sheep, respectively. At days 9-10 the zona pellucida ruptures and the blastocyst begins to elongate from about day 12-13. Bovine blastocysts are spherical on days 8-9, tubular on days 12-13 and then become filamentous by days 17-18 and by day 24 the conceptus occupies both uterine horns. Sheep blastocysts are spherical between days 4 and 10 and then elongate to the filamentous form by day 15. The pig blastocyst expands from about 0.5 to 1 mm diameter at hatching to 2-6 mm on days 10 before elongating rapidly to a filamentous form between days 11 and 14-16 of pregnancy (Bazer and First, 1983).

2. Molecular events of implantation

Implantation is a complex developmental process by which blastocyst comes in close contact with the uterine endometrium. It involves shedding of the zona pellucida, orientation, apposition, attachment and subsequent adhesion of the blastocyst to the endometrium. In ruminants and pigs, elongation of blastocyst takes place during the latter stages of implantation but this does not occur in rodents, horses, primates or humans (Guillomot *et al.*, 1993). During elongation of the blastocyst, the extra-embryonic endoderm originates from the inner cell mass and migrates under the trophoectoderm as the blastocoele expands. The mesoderm then originates from the inner cell mass and migrates between the endoderm and trophoectoderm. This interposed mesoderm then cavitates: the outer layer forms the chorion with the trophoectoderm whereas inner layer forms the yolk sac wall with endoderm. However, blastocyst implants rapidly before expansion and the extra-embryonic membranes are formed after implantation in rodents, primates and human. In sheep shedding of zona pellucida and blastocyst orientation occurs on day 8 and days 9-11, respectively. The antiadhesive mucin, MUC-1 present on the endometrial luminal epithelium (LE), prevents contact of the trophoblast with adhesive receptors (integrins). After day 12 the tubular blastocyst elongates to form a filamentous conceptus during which expression of MUC-1 declines on LE and exposes constitutively expressed integrins on the luminal epithelium and trophoblast. Apposition occurs between the trophoblast and endometrial LE and between trophoblasts papillae and germinal epithelium (GE) ducts. Finally adhesion of the trophoblast to the luminal epithelium occurs between days 15 and 16. Several molecules (Gly CAM-1, galectin-15 and osteopontin) have been found to interact with the receptors (integrins and glycoconjugates) on the apical surfaces of trophoblast and LE to fascilitate adhesion (Carson *et al.,* 2000). Recently several candidate adhesion molecules have been identified which mediate blastocyst implantation under the influence of progesterone. Progesterone plays a crucial role in establishment and maintenance of pregnancy. Progesterone receptors are expressed in the endometrial epithelium and stroma during early to mid-luteal phase and continuous exposure of the endometrium to progesterone down regulates the PR expression in the endometrial epithelium and expression of PR protein is undetectable in endometrial LE and GE in sheep after days 11 and 13 of pregnancy, respectively (Spencer and Bazer, 1995). The loss of PR in uterine epithelium immediately before implantation is coincident with onset of expression of genes of cell adhesion molecules such as MUC-1, glycosylated cell adhesion molecule (GlyCAM-1), galectin-15, integrins and osteopontin (Carson *et al.,* 2000). The MUC-1 is a large transmembrane glycoprotein with 120-220 kDa molecular mass and expression of MUC-1 by LE decrease at days 9-17 of early pregnancy in sheep which expose other glycoproteins involved in the adhesion between trophoblast and LE. The GlyCAM-1, a mucin family of glycoprotein mediates leukocytes-endometrial cell adhesion and expression increase on day 15 and abundant on days 17 and 19 of pregnancy. Galectin-15, a new galectin family member contains a conserved carbohydrate recognition domain (CRD) that binds b-galactosides and cell adhesion sequences (LDV and RGD) that mediate binding to integrins in ECM proteins. In endometrium of cyclic and pregnant ewes, expression of galectin-15 mRNA was undetectable by day 10, then appeared and increased 13 fold between days 10 and 14 but noticeably decreased between days 14 and 16 in sheep (Carson *et al.,* 2000). Integrins, a family of transmembrane glycoprotein receptors that bind ECM ligands to cause cytoskeletal reorganization, stabalize adhesion and mediate cell integration, proliferation and differentiation. Altered expression of integrin is associated with several causes of infertility and mutation of several integrins leads to periimplanbtation lethality. Osteopontin (OPN) is a member of the small integrins-binding ligand N-linked glyoprotein (SIBLING) family of ECM proteins. The OPN is a component of histotroph and its expression is detectable in some glands by day 13 and is present in all glands by day 19 in sheep. OPN binds integrin receptors and plays a crucial role in proliferation, migration, survival, adhesion, orientation and apposition, essential for implantation and placentation.

3. Uterine preparation for blastocyst implantation

Embryo implantation is a mutual interaction between blastocyst and uterus. Successful implantation is dependent on the cellular and molecular dialogue between embryo and receptive uterus. Uterine differentiation to support embryo development and implantation is coordinated by ovarian steroids. Ovarian progesterone and estrogens are crucial for preparation of progesterone primed uterus for implantation in mice and rats but progesterone alone is capable of initiating implantation in hamsters, guineapig, pig and rabbit. In mice and rats, the establishment of implantation window requires the presence of estrogens and progesterone. Estrogens stimulates proliferation of uterine epithelial cell whereas progesterone enhances stromal cell proliferation. In rodents uterine epithelial cells proliferate under the influence of preovulatory estrogens secretion during first two days of pregnancy. On third day progesterone from newly formed corpus luteum (CL) initiates stromal cell proliferation which is further potentiated by preimplantation estrogens secretion on day 4 of pregnancy. The preimplantation estrogens secretion is an absolute requirement for the establishment of uterine receptivity in rat and mouse. In cow, maternal recognition of pregnancy coincides with the formation of estradiol 17β by conceptus beginning on day 15 (Eley *et al.*, 1979) and with local increase in uterine blood flow. However, systemic administrations of high doses of estrogen are luteolytic in cow so that if estrogen is active, it acts as a short range rather than a systemic signal. However, uterine blood flow increased to the gravid horn during periimplantation period consistent with uterine vasodilation associated with local estrogen administration (Greiss and Miller, 1971). In contrast, considerable estrogen production by trophoblast has been found in pig and mare. Blastocyst estrogen production may prolong luteal function in early pregnancy by redirecting uterine PG secretion away from uterine venous blood towards the uterine lumen, thereby protecting CL from luteolytic effect of $PGF_{2\alpha}$ (Bazer and Thatcher, 1977). Further investigation is required to understand the molecular basis of differential role of estrogen and progeaterone in preparation of the receptive uterus and implantation among various species.

4. Molecular signalling during implantation

Current developments in molecular biology and biotechnology have lead to the discovery of numerous molecules involved in embryo-uterine crosstalk; however, the molecular signalling cascades have not been explored fully.

4.1 Steroid hormone signalling

Ovarian steroid, estrogen is prerequisite for differentiation of the uterus to the receptive stage and blastocyst implantation in progesterone primed uterus. The biological activity of steroid hormones (estrogen and progesterone) is manifested through high affinity receptors located in the nuclei of target cells. The presence of the receptor alone is sufficient to mediate the ability of cell to respond to hormone administration but the ultimate response of a cell to hormone is manifested by combination of receptor mediated genomic and nongenomic activities. For genomic action, the hormone activated receptor interacts directly with the regulatory region of a target gene and alters the rate of transcription (Beato *et al.*, 1995). Estrogen and progesterone receptors are a member of a superfamily of nuclear receptor. Members of the nuclear receptor family contain a highly conserved DNA binding domain, a moderately conserved C-terminal ligand binding domain and an N-terminal domain which is variable in length and sequence. The steroid hormone receptors reside in the nucleous of target cells in a latent form associated with a high molecular weight complex comprising of heat shock protein 90 (hsp90), 72 (hsp72) and 59 (hsp59) and possibly with other proteins. The role of hsp in steroid receptor action is unknown; however they are involved in assisting the folding of the nascent receptor peptide and in maintaining the receptor in a transcriptionally inactive state in absence of hormone. The estrogen-estrogen receptor complex form dimers that binds to steroid response element (SRE) in the regulatory regions of the target genes. Besides estrogen, many of the protein-protein interaction are mediated by ER. Cholera toxin and protein kinase C (PKC) has no ER binding capacity but mimic the mitogenic activation of estrogen in uterus. Xenoestrogens which induce implantation in progesterone primed rodents, have been found to interact with ER or other binding proteins that may not result in a similar kind of transactivation that normally occurs with the natural ligands. Increasing evidences suggest that rapid uterine effects of estrogenic compound do not involve classical genomic effects. Das *et al.* (1997; 2000) found that ER-α mutant female mice exhibited estrogenic responses to catecholestrogens or xenoestrogens via Wnt signaling, protein processing and calcium homeostasis. However, estrogen induces expression of many growth factors, their receptors and other secretory proteins to facilitate their transport to the membrane and/or secretion by activating membrane trafficking pathway via nuclear ER. Furthermore, gene targeting experiments in mice lacking ER or fail to initiate and support implantation due to failure of attachment. In contrast PR null mice (Lydon *et al.*, 1995) showed pleotropic reproductive effects including impaired ovulation, uterine hyperplasia and failure in decidualization. Although primary estrogen acts via uterine ER to prepare the uterus for implantation, catecholestrogens formed locally in the uterus play an important crucial role in blastocyst activation. Although nuclear ER-α present in both active and dormant blastocysts (Hou *et al.*, 1996), dormant blastocysts do not respond to estradiol and fail to gain implantation potency *in vitro.*

4.2 Signalling by growth factors

Among various growth factors, the EGF family of growth factors *viz.*, TGFβ, FGF, IGFs, HB-EGF (Heparin binding EGF like growth factor) platelet derived growth factors (PDGF), epiregulin and neuroregulin play a crucuial role in implantation. The earliest molecular marker is HB-EGF whose expression is found increased in luminal epithelium at the site of blastocyst apposition 6-7 h before initial attachment (Das *et al.,* 1994) and stimulates zona hatching, trophoblast outgrowth and ErbB1(Eukaryotic ribosome biogenesis protein 1) phosphorilation of murine blastocyst. This induction is followed by expression of betacellulin, epiregulin, neuroregulin and cyclooxygeanase – 2 (COX-2). However, amphiregulin is expressed throughout the uterine epithelium on day 4 of pregnancy during implantation of blastocyst but absent on day 5. The EGF-like growth factors interact with the receptor subtypes of the ErbB gene family comprising of four receptor tyrosine kinases ErbB1 (EGF R), ErbB2, ErbB3 and ErbB4. These receptors share common structural features but differ in their ligand specificity and tyrosine kinase activity. The initial dimerization between co-expressed receptors upon ligand binding initiates the classical mechanism of action of EGF-like ligands. Spatio-temporal expression patterns of EGF gene family members are ErbBs in the uterus during the periimplantation period suggest compartmentalized functions of EGF-like growth factors in implantation (Lim *et al.,* 1998). The HB-EGF is expressed as soluble and transmembrane forms in the uterine luminal epithelium at the site of blastocyst before attachment indicating paracrine and / or juxtacrine interaction. It has been observed that recombinant HB-EGF can promote blastocyst growth and differentiation but cells that express transmembrane form of HB-EGF can adhere to activate but not dormant blastocyst *in vitro*. HB-EGF mutant mice has been found to die early in postnatal life. Gene targeting experiment suggest that early events of implantation do not appear to be affected by blastocysts deficient in either ErbB1 or ErbB4.

Insulin-like growth factor family consisting of IGF-1, IGF-2, their receptors IGF-R1, IGF-R2, IGF binding proteins, plays a crucial role in embryo-maternal crosstalk. IGF-1 mediates the effects of estrogen on endometrial proliferation during the proliferative phase and IGF-2 mediates the effects of progesterone during the secretory phase of the endometrial cycle. IGF-1 and other related peptides such as insulin and IGF-2 stimulate preimplantation embryo development (Harvey and Kaye, 1988). Insulin in presence of amino acids, stimulates morphological development of the 8-cell embryo to the blastocyst stage and later, if the resulting blastocysts are replaced in a receptive uterus (Zhang and Armstrong, 1990). Multiple size transcripts of IGF-1 mRNA have been demonstrated in the uterus. Uterine IGF-1 mRNA levels increase during the preimplantation period in rats (Croze *et al.,* 1990), mice (Kapur *et al.,* 1992), pigs (Letcher *et al.,* 1989), sheep (Ko *et al.,* 1991) and cows (Geisert *et al.,* 1991). In pigs and sheep, the concentration of uterine luminal IGF-1 and its mRNA levels in the uterine tissues is higher during early pregnancy compared with its corresponding days in the estrous cycle (Ko *et al.,* 1991). IGF-1 mRNA levels in the uterine luminal fluids and IGF-1 mRNA in the uterus increase steadily throughout the preimplantation period followed by a rapid decline after the initiation of implantation in the pig (Letcher *et al.*, 1989). The IGFBPs are believed to play a central role in the uterine IGF system which is involved in regulating uterine growth and function. It has been hypothesized that IGF-2 stimulates implantation and invasion by promoting aggression, whereas IGFBP-1 counteract this effect by inhibiting IGF-2 action. Elevated level of IGFBP-1 has been found to cause implantation failure. The IGF/IGFBP system thus plays a role in establishing the implantation balance by stimulating and limiting inflammation.

4.3 Signaling by cytokines

Cytokines are not only involved in the establishment of the window of implantation but also embryo-uterine communication. The endometrium as well as embryo produces some of the cytokines in the various stages of development. Induction of inflammation can be seen as a form of aggregation by the embryo. All cytokines produced by the embryo are pro-inflammatory suggesting that implantation is a process of aggregation in which embryo induces or even forces the endometrium to accept it. Various cytokines are considered to be associated with various aspects of implantation. Among these cytokines IL-1, IL-6, TNFα and CSF-1 have been extensively studied. IL-6, a pro-inflammatory cytokine produced mostly by endometrial epithelial and stromal cells plays an important role in the implantation window. It has been found that low IL-6 production is associated with abortion due to decrease function of IL-6 in tissue remodelling, decidualization and placenta/ trophoblast development. IL-6 family comprises of numerous cytokines including LIF, IL-6, IL-11, neurotropic factor, oncostatin M and cardiotropin. The members of this class of cytokines shared intracellular signalling through gp130 suggesting that gp130 signalling is critically involved in implantation. A recent report shows that inactivation of gp130 by deleting all signal transducers and activators of transcription binding (STATs) sites result in implantation failure (Ernst *et al.*, 2001). Embryos lacking either LIF-R or gp130 develop to the blastocyst stage and implant normally; although disruption of these genes lead to embryonic and perinatal lethality (Yoshida *et al.*, 1996). IL-11 is another multifunctional cytokine with inflammatory properties produced by stromal and epithelial cells and stimulate decidulaization in humans (Dimitriadis *et al.*, 2005). It was observed that IL-11 Ra knockout mice were infertile due to disruption of decidualization and overinvassiveness of trophoblast. IL-1 system consists of two agonists IL-1a and IL-1b, two cell surface receptors, IL-1R1 and IL-1R2 which has inhibitory effect on IL-1 signalling is expressed at lower level around the window of implantation. IL-1 has been found to stimulate the production of LIF by endometrium and increases the expression of integrin β3 subunit which plays an important role in apposition, adhesion and decidualization.

LIF may control the proportion and amount of immune cells in the endometrium at the time of implantation. In uterus, LIF may mediate interaction between decidual leukocyte and invading trophoblast. In mouse knockout experiment it was found that LIF is necessary for successful implantation of the blastocyst but not for blastocyst viability suggesting its role in implantation (Stewart *et al.*, 1992). It has been observed that LIF R and gp130 are expressed at the blastocyst stage and administration of exogenous LIF improves embryo viability and hatching (Fry, 1992; Dunglison *et al.*, 1996; Nichols *et al.*, 1996). The LIF is transiently expressed in uterine gland on day 4 of pregnancy in mice and also expressed in stromal cells surrounding the blastocyst at the time of attachment reaction suggesting dual role of LIF – first in the preparation of uterus and later in the attachment reaction.

5. Luteolysis and early pregnancy – endocrine concept

Regulation of estrous cycle is a uterine dependent event in farm animals (Melampy and Anderson, 1968). Sheep, cattle and goats have oestrous cycles of about 17, 21 and 20 days respectively. Ovulation in ruminants occurs under the influence of ovalutory surge of luteinizing hormone (LH) around onset of oestrus. With the development of CL, concentrations of progesterone in peripheral circulation peak around mid to late diestrus phase and luteolysis is induced by pulsatile release of $PGF_{2\alpha}$ from endometrial epithelium on day 15 and/or 16. In ewes, $PGF_{2\alpha}$ is released from uterus into uterine vein in episodic surges lasting about 1 hr, beginning on days 12-13 and increasing in frequency to about 5-6 pulses/day during luteolysis on days 14-16 (McCracken *et al.*, 1984). The local $PGF_{2\alpha}$ passes from the uterine vein to ovarian artery via counter current exchange mechanism and acts in the ovary resulting in regression of CL. Uterine derived PGF binds to receptors on luteal cells and initiate intracellular events which terminate the production of progesterone and promote cell death. Endometrial production of luteolytic pulses of $PGF_{2\alpha}$ in ruminant is governed by the interplay of progesterone, estrogen and oxytocin on uterine epithelium. Oxytocin synthesised primarily from CL and secondarily from posterior pituitary stimulates the pulsatile secretion of $PGF_{2\alpha}$ from endometrial epithelium (Bazer, 1992). Oxytocin stimulate inositol phospholipid second messenger pathway by acting through receptors on endometrial epithelium which in turn release luteolytic pulses of $PGF_{2\alpha}$ (Flint and Sheldrick, 1986). In sheep (Flint and Sheldrick, 1986) and cows (Meyer *et al.*, 1986) endometrial receptors for oxytocin are present between estrus and about Day 4 of the cycle, low or undectable between Days 5 and 13 and increase rapidly between days 14 and 16 in sheep or Days 17 and 20 in cows. High levels of mRNA for oxytocin and its associated neurophysin are present in granulosa cells of the preovulatory follicle and corpus haemorragicum of cows, ewes and goats between days 0 and 7 after onset of estrus. Oxytocin and associated neurophysin are synthesized and stored in secretory granules of large luteal cells until their release into ovarian vasculature beginning on day 5 of estrous cycle or pregnancy.

Progesterone has a dual role in regulation of oxytocin receptor expression in uterus. During early luteal phase progesterone acts through endometrial progesterone receptors (PR) and inhibit estrogen receptor (ER) and oxytocin receptor (OTR) expression in endometrium for 10-12 days. This period is termed as progesterone block period. However, progesterone gradually down regulates PR expression in endometrial epithelium and losses its ability to suppress endometrial estrogen and oxytocin receptor expression. Estrogen then increases the formation of estrogen and oxytocin receptor. Endometrial ER and PR are highest during the first 10-12 days after onset of estrus in cows and then both decline to their lowest levels on about Day 13. The ER then increases between days 14 and 15, with OTR increasing rapidly between days 17 and 21. In sheep and goat, endometrial oxytocin receptor increase rapidly 48-72 h prior to estrus (Homeida and Khalafala, 1984; Wallace *et al.,* 1991). During luteolytic period the endometrium is characterized by low PR, increasing ER and increasing OTR. In cyclic ewes endometrial PR and PR mRNA decrease from Days 10-14 and then increase on Day 16 after increase between day 14 and estrus. This coincides with increasing ER, ER mRNA, OTR and OTR mRNA between day 14 and estrus. In pig, luteolysis occurs during late diestrus following stimulation of the uterine endometrium by progesterone for 10-12 days. Luteolysis occurs due to pulsatile release of uterine $PGF_{2\alpha}$ in the uterine venous drainage on about day 15 or 16 of the cycle (Bazer *et al.,* 1989). In contrast to ruminant CL, the CL of pigs contains only low levels of OT and vasopressin (Pitzel *et al.,* 1984) and OT mRNA is undetectable (Choy and Watkins, 1988). The uterine epithelium of mares release PGF which results in luteolysis but the pattern of PGF release did not require for luteolysis nor endocrine production of luteolytic PGF are established in this species (Irvine, 1995).

Prostaglandins (PGs) produced by the endometrium play a major role in dictating the course of pregnancy. Their release into uterine vein can cause luteolyis whereas their diffusion into myometrium stimulate uterine activity. Therefore, suppression of endometrial PG synthesis by the conceptus ensures the maintenance of a functional corpus luteum and inhibition of myometrial activity. The pulsatile release of $PGF_{2\alpha}$ which characterizes the luteal regression is not observed between days 12-16 of pregnancy and low concentration of $PGF_{2\alpha}$ in uterine venous plasma and PGFM in peripheral plasma throughout the pregnancy. The absence of a pulsatile pattern of $PGF_{2\alpha}$ release by the endometrium is due to inability of the endometrium to respond to oxytocin due to very low concentrations of oxytocin receptors in the endometrium of pregnant ewes during preimplantation period (Bazer, 1989). It has been postulated that since oxytocin receptors are under estrogenic control, the continued presence of progesterone during pregnancy would reduce the nuclear accumulation of estrogen receptor complex in endometrial cells and inhibit the synthesis of oxytocin receptors. Progesterone has been implicated in the maintenance of the corpus luteum during early pregnancy and acts by suppressing uterine prostaglandin synthesis. Expression of PR protein is not detectable in endometrial LE and GE in sheep after days 11 and 13 of pregnancy (Spencer and Bazer, 1995). In sheep continuous exposure of the uterus to progesterone induces expression of uterine milk protein (UTMP) and osteopontin (OPN). It has been observed that treatment of ovariectomized sheep with progesterone for 6 days induced very little UTMP mRNA and protein in the endometrium whereas treatment for 14 days or 30 days enhanced UTMP expression (Ing *et al.*, 1989). It is hypothesized that the loss of PR expression in GE is required for progesterone induction of UTMP and OPN gene expression.

6. Maternal recognition of pregnancy (MRP)

Maternal recognition of pregnancy occurs between days 16-19, 12-13 and around day 17 of pregnancy in cow, sheep and goat, respectively. The MRP in ruminants requires that the conceptus elongates from a spherical to a tubular and then filamentous form to produce IFNτ which is the pregnancy recognition signal. The IFNτ exerts a paracrine, antiluteolytic effect on the endometrium to inhibit endometrial production of luteolytic pulses of $PGF_{2\alpha}$. Antiluteolytic effect of IFNτ results in the maintenance of a functional CL and hence secretion of progesterone that is essential to maintain uterine environment, supports events critical to successful development of the conceptus to term. Ovine IFNτ (oIFNτ) is the first major protein secreted by trophoectoderm of periimplantation ruminant conceptus. Secretion of bovine IFNτ (bIFNτ) is maximal around days 16-19 of pregnancy; however, mRNA for bIFNτ can be detected as early as day 12. Secretion of bIFNτ increases during elongation of the conceptus and continues until at least day 38 of pregnancy. Potential mechanisms of action of this molecule includes (i) stabilization or upregulation of endometrial PR to extend progesterone block and prevent endometrial synthesis of OTR and/or ER (ii) direct inhibition of ER to attenuate pulsatile release of $PGF_{2\alpha}$ and (iii) direct inhibition of synthesis of endometrial ER and OTR. Available evidences indicate that endometrium of pregnant cows; ewes and goats have few or no receptors for oxytocin, progesterone and estradiol (Meyer *et al.*, 1986). The IFNτ does not act to stabilize PR expression in the endometrial epithelium during pregnancy; however, it acts in a paracrine fashion on endometrial LE and GE to suppress transcription of ERα and OTR genes (Spencer and Bazer, 1996). Interestingly, the increases in ERα and OTR gene expression detected in LE and GE on days 11-17 post-estrus in cyclic sheep do not occur in pregnant sheep or in cyclic sheep infused with IFNτ (Spencer and Bazer, 1995). The IFNτ prevents endometrial production of luteolytic pulses of $PGF_{2\alpha}$ by inhibiting increase in OTR expression. However, IFNτ does not inhibit basal production of $PGF_{2\alpha}$ which is higher in pregnant than cyclic ewes and the conceptus and IFNτ do not affect COX-2 expression in the pregnant sheep (Charpigny *et al.*, 1997). Thus the anti-luteolytic action of IFNτ are to prevent increase epithelial ERα, PR and OTR gene expression, which are all estrogen responsive, by directly inhibiting transcription of the ERα gene and maintaining secretion of progesterone by the CL.

Secretion of oIFNτ occurs between days 10 and 21 of pregnancy. Secretion of oIFNτ appears to be developmentally regulated beginning on about day 10 and increases as the conceptus change morphologically from spherical to tubular, and then to filamentous forms on days 12 to 30. Intrauterine infusions of either highly purified oIFNτ or recombinant oIFNτ from days 12 to 14 of the cycle extends the inter-estrous interval, life span of CL and reduce the number of OTR (Ott *et al.*, 1993). Intrauterine injection of recombinant oIFNτ between days 11-14 in cyclic ewes reduced ER and OTR gene expression and suppressed OT induced $PGF_{2\alpha}$ release (Spencer *et al.*, 1995). The ER mRNA was abundant in the LE and sGE of control ewes but absent in roIFNτ treated ewes. oIFNτ may inhibit synthesis of OTR directly or perhaps indirectly by down regulating endometrial ER and/or by stabilizing PR. Rapid replenishment of endometrial ER in ewes follows withdrawal of progesterone suggesting that failure of endometrial ER to increase during pregnancy is involved in either stabilization of PR or direct inhibition of ER synthesis by oIFNτ (Bazer, 1992). Prior to onset of luteolysis endometrium of cyclic ewes must be exposed to IFNτ. Once endometrial OTR numbers increase, IFNτ treatment will not block luteolysis. Endometrium of cyclic ewes must be exposed to IFNτ from days 11 or 12 to 14 (2-3 days before OTR increase in endometrium of cyclic ewes) to block expression of OTR and OT-induction of inositol phospholipid metabolism and luteolytic pulses of $PGF_{2\alpha}$. (Flint and Sheldrick, 1986). During early pregnancy, endometrial OTR are very low and OT cannot elicit pulsatile release of $PGF_{2\alpha}$. by the uterus. Available evidence suggests that IFNτ block transcription of ER and OTR genes in both LE and sGE. The IFNτ activates a signaling cascade in the endometrial epithelium which culminates in the production of a transcriptional repressor, such as IRF-2 which suppresses transcription of ER gene.

The IFNτ is a subclass of the 172 amino acids type I omega (ω) IFNs which competes with IFNα and β for binding of a common cell surface receptor. In cattle and sheep IFNτ s arise from multiple mRNAs approx 1 kb in length which arise from multiple genes. Like other type I interferon genes, IFNτ genes are intronless and consists of 585 bp ORF coding for a 195 amino acids pre-protein containing a 23 signal sequence which after cleavage yield a mature protein of 172 amino acids. Secreted forms of oIFNτ are not glycosylated. Bovine IFNτ transcripts contain potential N-glycosylation site at *Asn*78 and multiple glycosylation variants are present in the secreted proteins. Periimplantation goat conceptuses also express multiple isoforms of a caprine IFNτ which cross-react with the antisera to oIFNτ and bIFNτ. Both N-glycosylated and nonglycosylated forms of caprine IFNτ are secreted by goat conceptuses. Bovine, ovine and caprine IFNτ are more similar in sequence to each other than bIFNω. In the coding region, the nucleotide sequences exhibit approx. 90% identity and their inferred amino acid sequence about 80% identity (Roberts *et al.*, 1992). The predicted amino acid identity between bIFNτ and IFNα1 and IFN ω is 50% and 72%, respectively. Pontzer *et al.* (1990) demonstrated that a synthetic peptide corresponding to the carboxy-terminus (AA139-172) of oIFNτ blocked the antiviral activity of oIFNs and that of natural oIFNα, recombinant bIFNα and recombinant hIFNα but not of recombinant bIFNγ. A synthetic peptide corresponding to the amino terminus (AA1-39) of oIFNτ only blocked the antiviral activity of oIFNτ without affecting antiviral activity of IFNα s. These results suggest that the C-terminus may contain a receptor binding epitope common to type 1 IFNs whereas the amino terminus may mediate the biological activities of the IFNτ. IFNτ acts differently on the endometrial LE, GE and stroma to regulate expression of various IFN stimulated genes (ISGs) play crucial roles in endometrial differentiation and implantation of conceptus. The actions of IFNτ to signal pregnancy recognition (Ott *et al.*, 1992) and induce or increase expression of ISGs including ISG15 are dependent on the effects of progesterone. Type 1 IFN receptor subunits - IFNAR1 and IFNAR2 are expressed in all endometrial cell types with highest expression in endometrial LE. The majority of ISGs are induced or increased in response to the conceptus or IFNγ only in endometrial stroma and middle to deep GE of the ovine uterus (Choi *et al.*, 2001). In sheep IFNτ does not induce ISG in endometrial LE and sGE due to expression of potent repressor of gene transcription of IFN regulatory factor 2 (IRF 2). Bazer *et al.* (1997) proposed the mechanism of action of IFNτ on endometrial cells. oIFNτ binds to a dimeric IFN-R whose intracellular domain binds tyrosine kinases (Janus kinases, JAKs). After binding of IFNτ, JAKs *viz.*, JAK1 and Tyk2 are activated and subsequently phosphorylate tyrosine residues of signal transducers and activators of transcription (STATs: STAT1, STAT1A, STAT2). The STATs dimerize and bind DNA binding protein to form trimeric interferon simulated gene factor (ISGF) complex which then translocates to the nucleus where it binds an interferon stimulated regulatory element (ISRE) resulting in expression of the IRF-1 gene. The product of this gene in turn activates expression of negative acting transcription factor IRF2 which interact with other regulatory elements to control the expression of IFN-responsive genes including the OTR and ERs.

The theory of MRP in pigs has been proposed by Bazer (1992). The pig blastocysts expands and undergo morphological transition from about 0.5 to 1 mm diameter at hatching to 2-6 mm on day 10 before elongating rapidly to a filamentous form of 800-1000 mm between days 12 and 15 of the pregnancy. During the period of rapid elongation the trophoectoderm produces considerable amount of estrogens as well as interferon gamma (IFNγ) and delta (IFNδ). In pig, uterine endometrium secretes PGF and the conceptus produce estrogens from days 11 and 12 to day 15 of pregnancy that directs secretion of PGF away from uterine vasculature (endocrine secretion) to secretion into uterine lumen (exocrine secretion) and metabolized to prevent the luteolytic effects on the CL. Mean concentrations and amplitude of PGF in utero-ovarian vein are lower in pregnant and estrogen-induced pseudopregnant gilts than in cyclic gilts. However, significantly higher amount of PGF has been found in the uterine flushing from pseudopregnant and pregnant gilts than those from cyclic gilts.

Conclusions

Understanding the factors regulating conceptus development and exploration of the signal transduction systems would permit to understand the reciprocal regulation of trophoectoderm and adjacent endometrial cells. These in turn will facilitate the development of future strategies to ameliorate the early embryonic losses. Higher rates of early embryonic losses in bovines are a major cause of reproductive failure during preimplantation period. About 20% to 30% of fertilized ova are normally lost during early pregnancy with most losses happen in the first month when maternal recognition of pregnancy is occurring. If the embryo fails to signal its presence prior to Day 12 because of mortality or growth retardation and lack of synchrony between the uterine environment and the blastocyst, there is no extension of the lifespan of CL and the animal returns to service at the expected time. Maternal recognition of pregnancy is initiated at various times in the peri-implantation period by the embryological agent. Until we understand the paracrine signal transduction systems between embryonic trophoectoderm and endometrium, it is not possible to augment reproductive efficiency through amelioration of embryonic mortality in livestock.

References

Bazer F.W. (1989). Establishment of pregnancy in sheep and pigs. *Reproduction Fertility and Development* **1:** 237-242.

Bazer, F.W. (1992). Mediators of maternal recognition of pregnancy in mammals. *Proceeding of Society on Experimental Biology and Medicine* **93:** 373-384.

Bazer F.W. (1999). Effects of recombinant ovine interferon tau, placental lactogen, and growth hormone on the ovine uterus. *Biology of Reproduction* **61:** 1409-1418.

Bazer F.W. and First N.L. (1983). Pregnancy and parturition. *Journal of Animal Science (Suppl.)* **2:** 425-460.

Beato M., Herrlich P., Schutz G. (1995). Steroid hormone receptors: many actors in search of a plot. *Cell* **83:** 851-857.

Carson D.D., Bagchi I. Dey S.K., Enders A.C., Fazleabas A.T., Lessey B.A., Yoshinaga K. (2000). Embryo implantation. *Developmental Biology* **223:** 217-237.

Charpigny G.P., Reinaud J.P., Tamby C., Creminon J., Martal J., Maclouf M., Guillomot M. (1997b). Expression of cyclooxygenase-1 and -2 in ovine endometrium during the estrous cycle and early pregnancy. *Endocrinology* **138:** 2163-2171.

Choi Y., Johnson G.A., Burghardt R.C., Berghman L.R., Joyce M.M., Taylor K.M., Stewart M. D., Bazer F.W., Spencer T.E. (2001). Interferon regulatory factor-two restricts expression of interferon-stimulated genes to the endometrial stroma and glandular epithelium of the ovine uterus. *Biology of Reproduction* **65:** 1038-1049.

Choy V.J., Watkins W.B. (1988). Arginine vasopressin and oxytocin in the porcine corpus luteum. *Neuropeptides* **11:** 119-123.

Croze F., Kennedy T.J., Schroedter I.C., Freisen H.G., Murphy L.J. (1990). Expression of insulin like growth factor-1 and insulin like growth factor binding protein-1 in the rat uterus during decidualization. *Endocrinology* **71:** 1995-2000.

Das S.K., Wang X. N., Paria B. C., Damm D., Abraham J. A., Klagsbrun M., Andrews G. K., Dey S.K. (1994). Heparin-binding EGF-like growth factor gene is induced in the mouse uterus temporally by the blastocyst solely at the site of its apposition: a possible ligand for EGF-receptor in implantation. *Development* **120:** 1071-1083.

Das S.K., Taylor J.A., Korach K.S., Paria B.C., Dey S.K., Lubahn D.B. (1997). Estrogenic responses in estrogen receptor-deficient mice reveal a distinct estrogen signaling pathway. *Proceeding of National Academy of Science, USA* **94:** 12786-12791.

Das S.K., Tan J., Raja S., Halder J., Paria B.C., Dey S.K. (2000). Estrogen targets genes involved in protein processing, calcium homeostasis, and Wnt signaling in the mouse uterus independent of estrogen receptor α and β. *Journal of Biological Chemistry* **275:** 28834-28842.

Dimitriadis, E., White C.A., Jones R.L., Salamonsen L.A. (2005). Cytokines, chemokines and growth factors in endometrium related to implantation. *Human Reproduction Update* **11:** 613-630.

Dunglison G.F., Barlow D.H., Sargent I.L. (1996). Leukaemia inhibitory factor significantly enhances the blastocyst formation rates of human embryos cultured in serum-free medium. *Human Reproduction* **11:** 1911-1916.

Eley R.M., Thatcher W.W., Bazer F.W. (1979). Luteolytic effect of oesterone sulphate on cyclic beef heifers. *Journal of Reproduction and Fertility* **55:** 191-193.

Ernst M., Inglese M., Waring P., Campbell I. K., Bao S., Clay F.J., Alexander W.S., Wicks I.P., Tarlinton D.M., Novak U., Heath J.K., Dunn A.R. (2001). Defective gp130-mediated signal transducer and activator of transcription (STAT) signaling results in degenerative joint disease, gastrointestinal ulceration, and failure of uterine implantation. *Journal of Experimental Medicine* **194:** 189-203.

Flint A.P., Sheldrick E.L. (1986). Ovarian oxytocin and the maternal recognition of pregnancy. *Journal of Reproduction and Fertility* **76:** 831-839.

Fry R.C. (1992). The effect of leukaemia inhibitory factor (LIF) on embryogenesis. *Reproduction Fertility and Development* **4:** 449-458.

Geisert R.D., Lee C.Y., Simmen F.A., Zavy M.T., Fliss A.E., Bazer F.W., Simmen R.C.M. (1991). Expression of mRNAs encoding IGF-1, IGF-2 and insulin like growth factor binding protein -2 in the bovine endometrium during the estrous cycle and early pregnancy. *Biology of Reproduction* **45:** 975-983.

Guillomot M., Flechon J.E., Leroy F. (1993). Blastocyst development and implantation. In: Reproduction in Mammals and Man, (C. Thibault, M.C. Levasseur and R.H.F. Hunter, eds.), Ellipses, Paris, pp 387-411.

Greiss F.C., Miller H.B. (1971). Unilateral control of uterine blood flow in the ewe. *American Journal of Obstetrics and Gynaecology* **111:** 299-301.

Harvey M.B., Kaye P.L. (1988). Insulin stimulates protein synthesis in compacted mouse embryos. *Endocrinology* **122:** 1182-1184.

Homeida A.M., Khalafalla A.E. (1987). Effects of oxytocin antagonist injections on luteal regression in the goat. *British Journal of Pharmacology* **90:** 281-284.

Hou Q., Paria B.C., Mui C., Dey S.K., Gorski J. (1996). Immunolocalization of estrogen receptor protein in the mouse blastocyst during normal and delayed implantation. *Proceeding of National Academy of Science, USA* **93:** 2376-2381.

Ing, N.H., Francis H., McDonnell J.J., Amann J.F., Roberts R.M. (1989). Progesterone induction of the uterine milk proteins: major secretory proteins of sheep endometrium. *Biology of Reproduction* **41:** 643-654.

Irvine C.H.G. (1995). The nonpregnant mare: A review of some current research and of the last 25 years of endocrinology. In: Equine Reproduction IV, *Biology Reproduction Monograph* Series 1, (F.W. Bazer and D.C. Sharp, eds.), pp 343-360.

Kapur S., Tamada H., Dey S.K., Andrews G.K. (1992). Expression of growth factor-1 and its receptor in tthe periimplantation mouse uterua and cell specific regulation of IGF-1 gene expression by estradiol and progesterone. *Biology of Reproduction* **46:** 208-219.

Ko Y., Lee C.Y., Ott T. L., Davis M.A., Simmen R.C.M., Bazer F.W., Simmen F.A. (1991). Insulin like growth factors in sheep uterine fluids: concentrations and relationship to ovine trophoblast protein-1 production during early pregnancy. *Biology of Reproduction* **45:** 135-142.

Letcher R., Simmen R.C.M., Bazer F.W., Simmen F.A. (1989). Insulin like growth factor-1 expression during early conceptus development in the pig. *Biology of Reproduction* **41:** 1143-1151.

Lim H., Das S.K., Dey S.K. (1998). erbB genes in the mouse uterus: cell-specific signaling by epidermal growth factor (EGF) family of growth factors during implantation. *Developmental Biology* **204:** 97-110.

Lydon J.P., DeMayo F.J., Funk C.R., Mani S.K., Hughes A.R., Montgomery C.A., Shyamala G., Conneely O.M., O'Malley B.W. (1995). Mice lacking progesterone receptor exhibit pleiotropic reproductive abnormalities. *Genes Development* **9:** 2266-2278.

McCracken J.A., Scrhamm W., Okulicz W. (1984). Hormone receptor control of pulsatile secretion of $PGF_2\mu$ from the ovine uterus during luteolysis and abrogation in early pregnancy. *Animal Reproduction Science* **7:** 31-55.

Melampy R.M., Anderson A.L. (1968). Role of uterus in corpus luteum function. *Journal of Animal Science* **27** (Suppl.): 77-96.

Meyer H.H.D., Mittermeier T., Schams D. (1986). Dynamics of oxytocin, estrogen and progesterone receptors in the bovine endometrium during estrous cycle. *Acta Endocrinologica* **118:** 96-104.

Nichols, J., Davidson D., Taga T., Yoshida K., Chambers I., Smith A. (1996). Complementary tissue-specific expression of LIF and LIFreceptor mRNAs in early mouse embryogenesis. *Mechamisms of Development* **57:** 123-131.

Ott T.L., Zhou Y., Mirando M.A., Stevens C., Harney J.P., Ogle T.F., Bazer F.W. (1993).Changes in progesterone and oestrogen receptor messenger ribonucleic acid and protein during maternal recognition of pregnancy and luteolysis in ewes. *Journal of Molecular Endocrinology* **10:** 171-183.

Pitzel L., Welp K., Holtz W., Konig A. (1984). The content of oxytocin and vasopressin in the corpus luteum of the pig. *Acta Endocrinologica* (Suppl 264) **105:** 140-141.

Pontzer C.H., Ott T.L., Bazer F.W., Johnson H.M. (1990). Localization of an antiviral site on the pregnancy recognition hormone, ovine trophoblast protein 1. *Proceeding of National Academy of Science, USA* **87:** 5945-5949.

Roberts, R.M., Cross J.C., Leaman D.W. (1992). Interferons as hormones of pregnancy. *Endocrine Review* **13:** 432-452.

Spencer T.E., Gray A., Johnson G.A., Taylor K.M., Gertler A., Gootwine E., Ott and Bazer F.W., Johnson D.C., Sen M., Kogo H., Dey S.K. (1990) Initiation of embryo implantation and maintenance of early pregnancy in the rat by chlordecone (Kepone). *Proceeding of Society of Experimental Biology and Medicine* **195:** 44-50.

Spencer T.E., Bazer F.W. (1995). Temporal and spatial alterations in uterine estrogen receptor and progesterone receptor gene expression during the estrous cycle and early pregnancy in the ewe. *Biology of Reproduction* **53:** 1527-1543.

Spencer T.E., Ing N.H., Ott T.L., Mayes J.S., Backer W.C., Watson G.H., Mirando M.A., Bazer F.W. (1995). Intrauterine injections of ovine interferon-tau (oIFNô) alters oestrogen receptor and oxytocin receptor expression in the endometrium of cyclic ewes. *Journal of Molecular Endocrinology* **15:** 203-220.

Spencer T.E., Bazer F.W. (1996). Ovine interferon tau suppresses transcription of the estrogen receptor and oxytocin receptor genes in the ovine endometrium. *Endocrinology* **137:** 1144-1147.

Spencer T.E., Ott T.L., Bazer F.W. (1996). tau-Interferon: pregnancy recognition signal in ruminants. *Proceeding of Society of Experimental Biology and Medicine* **213:** 215-229.

Stewart C.L., Kaspar P., Brunet L.J., Bhatt H., Gadi I., Kontgen F., Abbondanzo S.J. (1992). Blastocyst implantation depends on maternal expression of leukemia inhibitory factor. *Nature* **359:** 76-79.

Wallace J.M., Helliwell R., Morgan P.J. (1991). Autoradiographical localization of oxytocin binding sites on ovine oviduct and uterus throughout estrous cycle. *Reproduction Fertility and Development* **3:** 127-135.

Wallace J.M., Helliwell R., Morgan P.J. (1991). Autoradiographical localization of oxytocin binding sites on ovine oviduct and uterus throughout estrous cycle. *Reproduction Fertility and Development* **3:** 127-135.

Yoshida K., Taga T., Saito M., Suematsu S., Kumanogoh A., Tanaka T., Fujiwara H., Hirata M., Yamagami T., Nakahata T., Hirabayashi T., Yoneda Y., Tanaka K., Wang W.Z., Mori C., Shiota K., Yoshida N., Kishimoto T. (1996). Targeted disruption of gp130, a common signal transducer for the interleukin 6 family of cytokines, leads to myocardial and hematological disorders. *Proceeding of National Academy of Science, USA* **93:** 407-411.

Zhang X., Armstrong D.T. (1990) presence of amino acids and insulin in a chemically defined medium improves development of 8 cell rat embryos *in vitro* and subsequent implantation *in vivo. Biology of Reproduction* **42:** 662-668.

❑❑❑

Chapter 16

Implantation Process, Associated Proteins and Applications in Assisted Reproductive Technologies in Ruminants

J. Ghosh, S.C. Roy, A. Dhali, K.S. Roy, S. Shree Vidhya, A. Mech.
National Institute of Animal Nutrition and Physiology, Adugodi, Bangalore 560 030, Karnataka, India

Summary

Establishment of physical communication between the conceptus and the maternal endometrium is late in ruminants. Therefore a continuous interaction between the developing conceptus and the maternal endometrium is noticed to have a successful conception in these species. The earliest reported conceptus released molecule which brings about a major change in the maternal system is interferone-τ. Based on the concept of antiluteolysis mechanism of this molecule the antiluteolytic package of practices came into being for enhancing the conception rate in large ruminants. Pregnancy associated glycoproteins are another group of glycoproteins found to be secreted in maternal circulation by the developing conceptus during early days of pregnancy. Detection of these molecules in maternal blood changed the whole concept of ruminant early pregnancy diagnosis. The concept, application, prospects and promises of both the aspects are discussed in detail.

The journey of life starts at the site of fertilization, the ampulla-isthmus junction of oviduct with the fusion of male and female pronuclei resulting in one cell zygote which subsequently divides by cleavage from 1 to 2, 2 to 4, 4 to 8 and so on. A successful development up to embryonic period, which is most important, proceed through sequential developmental events including genome activation, compaction, formation of blastocyst, hatching of eggs, elongation of trophoblast, secretion of pregnancy recognition molecule and development of inner cell mass into fetal organ and other system. These events are not only the developmental milestones but also the checkpoints that must be achieved for embryonic survival and all of these are established within a very short period of three weeks. By cellular multiplication, the developing embryo reaches a stage called morulla when it looks like the shape of mulberry around the day 3.5. The outer layer of cells gives rise to trophoblast, the earliest differentiated cells which cover the entire periphery of the developing embryo and ultimately form the fetal placenta. The cell division in the peripheral cells are more compared to the other cells and due to the increased permeability of the outer cells fluid starts accumulating in the embryo resulting a clump of cells remaining in one pole of the sphere called inner cell mass which later gives rise to the actual fetus and the structure is called blastocyst which is formed by 4-5 days in cattle and sheep. As the embryo develops, it continues to migrate towards the uterus, the actual organ of implantation with the help of oviduct cells and muscles. By the time it reaches the tip of uterine horn, it is 4-5 days old and still remains inside the oocyte covering called the zona pellucida. In sheep, the blastocyst looks spherical on day 8, measures 200 μm in diameter and contains approximately 300 cells. By day 10, it measures 400-900 μm in diameter and contains approximately 3000 cells (Spencer and Bazer, 2004). Zona escape/hatching of blastocyst by shedding egg shell can happen *in vitro* in rodents (Surani 1975), cow (Massip and Mulnard 1980), pig (Niemann and Elsaesser, 1987), rhesus monkey (Seshagiri and Hearn, 1993), and human (Lopata and Hay, 1989). In all the species, the fully expanded blastocysts exert a mechanical pressure due to accumulation of fluid, creating a nick in the zona and then the embryos actively extrude themselves through this hole, leaving the empty zona intact. There are reports proposing the involvement of protease-like hatching factor (s) of embryonic origin assisting in the rupture of zona *in vitro* (Sawada *et al.*, 1990; Vu *et al.*, 1997). Further, involvement of uterine zona lysin *in vivo* has been proposed in this process for mouse (Mintz, 1971), rat (Joshi and Murray, 1974), rabbit (Denker, 1977) and hamster (Gonzales and Bavister, 1995). In cattle, the hatching occurs at around day 9-11 and in mice by 4.5 days. In rodents (rat, mice) and primates (monkey and human) implantation occur soon after the blastocyst hatches out. However, in animals like horse, pig, sheep, goats, cattle and buffalo the conceptus remains free within the uterus for several days before implantation. The developing embryo remains protected and are not sensitive much to the uterine environment. As soon as the egg shell protection goes off, the embryos become vulnerable to the changes in uterine environment because they solely depend on the available secretion of the uterus and maximum number of conception failure occurs during this short period of hatching to implantation.

1. Molecules involved in maternal recognition of pregnancy

In primates and rodents there is a window of implantation which falls within the period of cycle and if hatched embryos are present at that time it will be implanted in the endometrium or they will perish. A similar event in animals like horse, pig, sheep, goats, cattle and buffalo which falls within the period of cycle is called the maternal recognition of pregnancy (MRP), wherein, the developing conceptus secretes some molecules to stop the luteolyis process of the uterine endometrium, so that the progesterone supply from the ovarian corpus luteum (CL) is maintained. The signal molecules essentially stop the initiation of these events locally in uterus. The developing conceptus sends a signal to the mother by releasing cytokines, called interferon tau (IFNτ) in cattle, sheep and other ruminant species or steroid (*e.g.*, estrogen) in pig for the continuing maternal support so that it can develop further (table 1).

Table 1 : Embryonic signal molecule in different farm animal species secreted in uterine environment during the different days of estrous cycle.

	Sow	Mare	Cow	Ewe	Doe
Embryonic Signal molecule	Estrogen	Unknown (Protein?)	Interferon τ	Interferon τ	Interferon τ
Days of estrous cycle	11 -13	14 - 16	15 - 17	14 -16	15 - 17

In this chapter, the IFNτ molecule will be discussed in detail since it is the important molecules for ruminant pregnancy establishment. In sheep, the mononuclear cells of the conceptus trophectoderm synthesize and secrete IFNτ between Days 10 and 21 to 25 with maximal production on Days 14 to 16 (Roberts *et al.*, 1999; Bazer, 1992). In terms of biological activity, a single sheep conceptus of Day 16 produces approximately 1×10^8 antiviral units of IFNτ in culture over 24 h (Ashworth and Bazer, 1989). The IFNτ is a member of the Type I IFN family cytokines, a small peptide by nature, secreted by conceptus membrane. It is involved in the cross talk between mother and the conceptus, considered to be the earliest important event which results in extensive changes of the maternal physiology. Considering its importance in sheep, goat, cattle and buffaloes this molecule has been the target of research for a long time. The molecule, its mechanism of action and other details are studied with more details in cattle and sheep. However, the concept of the results would equally be applicable in other ruminant species except the timing of occurrence of some of these events.

2. Antiluteolytic mechanism of Interferon-τ in uterus

Uterine endometrium contains two types of epithelial cells of which one lining the lumen is called the luminal epithelium (LE) and other is present in the uterine glands, which are coiled in endometrial stroma and are opened in the lumen, called glandular epithelium (GE). Interferon-tau (IFNτ) acts through type I-IFN receptor subunits, IFNAR1 and IFNAR2 and expresses a number of IFN-stimulated genes (ISGs) on the endometrial LE, GE and stromal cells that might play a role in endometrial differentiation and conceptus implantation (Kim *et al.,* 2003; Kerszberg and Wolpert, 1998). The IFNAR1 and IFNAR2 are expressed in all endometrial cell types, with the highest expression in endometrial LE (Rosenfeld *et al.,* 2002). The actions of IFNτ starting from signal of pregnancy recognition to induced or increased expression of ISGs, including ISG17 (Johnson *et al.,* 2000) and 2', 5'-oligoadenylate synthase (OAS) (Johnson *et al.,* 2001) are dependent on the effects of progesterone. However, the majority of ISGs increases in response to the conceptus or IFNτ are induced in the endometrial stroma and middle to deep glandular epithelium of the sheep uterus (Kim *et al.,* 2003, Johnson *et al.,* 2000, Johnson *et al.,* 2001). Interestingly, the inductions of many ISGs expression observed in the pig uterus during early pregnancy are limited only to the endometrial stroma (Cencic *et al.,* 2003). In the sheep uterus, the lack of ISG induction in the endometrial LE and other GE by IFNτ is apparently due to the expression of IFN regulatory factor-2 (IRF-2), a potent repressor of gene transcription that is constitutively expressed in the endometrial luminal epithelium LE and GE, and increased during early pregnancy (Choi *et al.,* 2001). In addition, IRF-2 appears to be involved in IFNτ inhibition of ERα gene transcription in the same endometrial epithelia (Fleming *et al.,* 2001).

Studies on sheep had shown that at estrus (Day 0), estrogens from Graafian follicles stimulate increased uterine estrogen receptor alpha (ERα), progesterone receptor (PR), and oxytocine receptor (OTR) expression (Wathes and Hamon, 1993; Spencer and Bazer, 1995) (Fig. 1). However, due to the absence of progesterone from CL the oxytocin would not be available to cause secretion of PGF2α and no luteolysis occurs. During early diestrus, progesterone from the newly formed CL stimulates the accumulation of phospholipids in LE and GE that liberates arachidonic acid for synthesis and secretion of PGF (Boshier and Holloway, 1973). During diestrus, progesterone level increases to block the expression of ERα and OTR via PR in the endometrial LE and GE (McCracken *et al.,* 1984), thus ERα and OTR expression is not detected between Days 5 and 11 of the cycle in sheep (Fig. 1). The precise molecular mechanism of progesterone dependant suppression of ERα gene transcription is unknown. However, it is speculated that the effects of progesterone on OTR gene expression may be indirect through suppression of ERα. This assumption is based on the evidence that the rat OTR gene contains palindromic ER response elements (EREs) that mediate the effects of estrogens (Bale and Dorsa, 1997), and the ovine OTR promoter DNA contains several Sp1 elements that appear to mediate responsiveness to ligand activated ERα (Spencer and Bazer, 2004).

In sheep, continuous exposure of uterus to progesterone for 8 to 10 days down-regulates expression of PR in endometrial LE and GE after Days 11 to 12 (Spencer *et al.,* 1995a). The long exposure of progesterone allows rapid increase in expression of ERα on Day 13 followed by OTR on Day 14 in LE and GE (Spencer *et al.,* 1995b). Oxytocin, secreted from Day 9 of the estrous cycle and pregnancy from the posterior pituitary and/or CL, then induces release of luteolytic PGF pulses from the endometrial LE and GE (Fig. 1) on Days 14 to 16 (Wathes and Lamming, 1995) causing regression of CL, allowing ewes to return to estrus at completion of the 17-day estrous cycle.

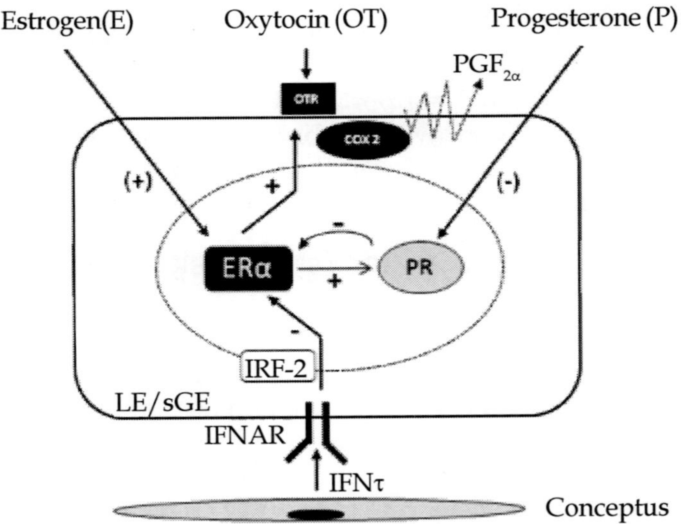

Fig. 1 : The proposed model of Spencer and Bazer (2004) describing the luteolytic mechanism and antiluteolytic effects of conceptus on sheep uterus wherein E: estrogen; ERα: estrogen receptor alpha; IFNô: interferon tau; IRF-2: interferon regulatory factor two; OT: oxytocin; OTR: oxytocin receptor; P: progesterone; PGF2α: prostaglandin F2 alpha; PR: progesterone receptor.

It has been observed that the IFNτ does not act to stabilize progesterone receptor expression in the endometrial epithelium rather, acts in a paracrine fashion on endometrial LE and GE to suppress transcription of estrogen receptor α (ERα) and oxytocin receptor (OTR) genes (Spencer and Bazer, 1996; Charpigny *et al.,* 1997), thereby nullify development of the endometrial luteolytic mechanism. This is inferred from the observation that increase in ERα and OTR gene expression occur only in LE and GE of days 11 to 17 post-estrus cyclic sheep but not in pregnant sheep (Spencer and Bazer, 1995) or in cyclic sheep infused with IFNτ (Spencer *et al.*, 1995). The IFNτ prevents increases in epithelial ERα and OTR gene expression, which are estrogen responsive by directly inhibiting transcription of the ERα gene and maintaining secretion of progesterone by the CL (Fleming *et al.*, 2001). It prevents endometrial production of luteolytic pulses of PGF2α by inhibiting increases in OTR expression. However, it does not inhibit basal production of PGF 2α, which is found higher in pregnant than cyclic ewes. Also, the conceptus and IFNτ of early pregnant sheep do not affect COX-2 expression in the endometrial epithelia (Charpigny *et al.*, 1997; Fig. 1) which is an intermediate important enzyme in the pathways of PGF2α synthesis.

3. Improving reproductive efficiency by antiluteolytic support system

The outcome of the discovery of antiluteolytic mechanism resulted in development of a whole practice of manipulating luteal support system for enhancement of reproductive efficiency in cattle (Table 2). These practices are essentially the maternal support to the developing embryo by uterine secretion so that the slow growing embryos can attain the expected growth size and are able to secrete the sufficient concentration of pregnancy recognition molecule enough for triggering the antiluteolytic mechanism.

4. Blastocyst elongation factor (s) and significance in maternal recognition of pregnancy

The most critical point for maternal recognition is that, the embryos must release enough amount of the pregnancy recognition molecules locally to initiate the anti-luteolytic mechanism by attaining a minimum size as in cattle and buffaloes (which bears only one conceptus) or by the presence of minimum number conceptus (as in litter bearing animals like pig). After day 10, elongation of the sheep blastocyst starts and it develops first into a tubular and then into a filamentous conceptus (Wintenberger-Torres and Flechon, 1974). Staring on day 11 the spherical or slightly tubular blastocyst begins to elongate until it reaches the length of 25cm or more by day 17 (Spencer *et al.*, 2004). In the initial phases of blastocyst development outer layers of cells grow faster than inner cell mass to ensure the earliest communication with the mother. In sheep by day 12, blastocysts elongate markedly, reaching a length of 10-22 mm and at day 14 when the filamentous conceptus is about 10cm long, the primitive streak appears and somites starts developing soon thereafter. The conceptus, first located in the uterine horn ipsilateral to the corpus luteum, elongates into the contralateral horn on day 13 and may fill more than half of its length on day 17 when only one ovulation has occurred (Rowson and Moor, 1966).

Table 2 : Different anti-luteolytic strategies adopted, procedure, mechanisms and the results obtained in different studies

Sl. No	Name of the Strategy	Procedure	Mechanism	Result
1	Increasing size of pre-ovulatory follicles	Administration of sub-luteal level progestagen during estrus	Allow follicle to grow more before ovulation and the size of the CL would be larger	Low conception rates because of altered oviduct environment (Binelli *et al.*, 1999) or early maturation of oocyte (Mihm, 1994) or both
2	Increasing rate of CL growth	GnRH agonist implant (Ambrose *et al.*, 1998) or administration	Produce LH surge of longer duration which support the CL growth and function to maintain the uterine support	Showed promise of use as
3	Increasing luteal phase progesterone	By adminis-tering GnRH, LH or hCG (Marques *et al.*, 2002)when preovulatory follicles are present at mid luteal phase	Allow formation of accessory CL which would secrete more progesterone	Administration of GnRH is promising but repeated administration of hCG or LH are limited due to development of antibodies
4	Decreasing effects of dominant follicles during critical period	Administration of GnRH to destroy the dominant follicle.	Stop supply of estrogen which initiates the process of luteolysis.	3.9 to 12% increase in conception rate reported in cattle (Peters, 1996)
5	Increasing antiluteolytic stimulus by conceptus unit	Administration of type I interferons (*eg.*, IFNτ; Meyer *et al.*, 1995)	Modulate the $PGF_{2\alpha}$ synthesis and secretion	Able to block luteolysis but, application is limited due to the side effect
6	Decreasing luteolytic response by maternal unit	i) By strategic feeding of essential fatty acids	Increases the ratio of linoleic to arachidonic acid in uterus cause alteration of PG synthesis resulting less $PGF_{2\alpha}$ release	15% improved conception (Wilkins *et al.*, 1996)
		ii) Adminis-tration of anti-inflammatory drugs (eg, Flunixin	Inhibits PG synthase	Able to control luteolysis (Odensvik *et al.*, 1998). Need further testing

The developing embryos have to achieve the targeted growth between hatching to the maternal recognition of pregnancy for continuing development and conception success. Many a times the conceptus fails to signal mother due to slower growth and is unable to reach the targeted size thereby not ensuring the availability of desired quantity of the maternal recognition molecule. It has been observed that elongation of blastocyst is critical for developmentally regulated production of interferon tau (Farin *et al.*, 1989, Guillomot *et al.*, 1990) that inhibits the development of the luteolytic mechanism. The cellular and molecular mechanisms regulating blastocyst elongation are not well understood, but are required for apposition and transient attachment of the trophoblast to the uterine luminal epithelium. Our current knowledge suggests that the uterine secretions are rich in nutrients which are essential for blastocyst elongation and subsequent development until the final attachment. Progesterone has a major influence on uterine secretion therefore supply of this hormone either from the ovarian corpus luteum or placenta is very critical during this period. This is evident from the fact that the microvillous epithelial cells of the uterine lumen present a high secretory activity during the luteal phase of the cycle and at the beginning of implantation (Guillomot *et al.*, 1981). Side by side the sheep trophoblast appears to be the site of intense pinocytotic activity that increases as the blastocyst develops (Wintenberger-Torres and Flechon, 1974) indicating the active involvement of trophoblast in assimilating the uterine secretions. It is interesting to note that the hatched blastocysts and trophoblastic vesicles are not able to elongate *in vitro* unless transferred into the uterus (Heyman *et al.*, 1984, Flechon *et al.*, 1986). This clearly reflects the role of uterine secretion in the elongation process. This notion is further strengthened from a series of studies conducted on uterine gland knockout (UGKO) ewes (Gray *et al.*, 2000, 2001, 2002), which were produced by continuous administration of a synthetic, nonmetabolizable progestin to neonatal ewes from birth to at least postnatal day 56. The exposure to progestin permanently ablates differentiation and development of the glandular epithelia from luminal epithelium in the endometrium without altering development of myometrium or other Mullerian duct-derived female reproductive tract structures or the hypothalamic–pituitary–ovarian axis. The UGKO ewes exhibit recurrent early pregnancy loss in which the blastocysts fail to elongate. Transfer of blastocysts from normal fertile ewes into the uteri of timed recipient UGKO ewes did not ameliorate this defect (Gray *et al.*, 2001). Morphologically normal blastocysts are present in uterine flushes of bred UGKO ewes on days 6 and 9 after mating, but not on day 14 (Gray *et al.*, 2002). On day 14, uterine flushes of mated UGKO ewes contain either no conceptus or a severely growth-retarded tubular conceptus. Therefore, histotrophic secretions from the endometrial epithelia are required for peri-implantation blastocyst survival and elongation in sheep. The exact molecule which is responsible for such action is yet to be characterized in uterine secretion. Available results indicated that the defects in blastocyst survival and elongation in UGKO ewes were not due to alterations in expression of steroid receptors, mucin glycoprotein 1 (MUC1) or adhesive integrins on the endometrial luminal epithelium, or to the responsiveness of the endometrium to the conceptus pregnancy recognition signal IFNô (Gray *et al.*, 2002). However, when uterine flushes of day 14 bred UGKO ewes were analyzed for the presence of adhesion proteins osteopontin (OPN) and glycosylated cell adhesion molecule 1 (GlyCAM-1), primarily secreted by glandular epithelium (Johnson *et al.*, 1999; Spencer *et al.*, 1999) were found very low compared to control day 14 pregnant ewes (Gray *et al.*, 2002). Therefore, the reduction or absence in adhesion proteins of endometrial epithelial origin is proposed as the cause of recurrent pregnancy loss in the UGKO ewe.

5. Process of implantation in ruminants

The implantation process enables the establishment of a physical communication with blastocyst and the maternal endometrium. The timing of implantation differs among species and not found related to the length of gestation (Guillomont *et al.*, 1993). However the completion of the attachment process might have relevance to the length of gestation as it is found finished early when gestation length is less and vice versa within the similar type of placentation process (Table 3).

Table 3 : Completion of placental attachment process in different farm animal species in relation to gestation length and placental type

	Cow	Ewe	Sow	Mare
Duration of placental attachments (days)	30 – 35	18 – 20	12 – 20	50 – 60
Gestation length (days)	281	148	114	337
Placental type	Cotyledonary	Cotyledonary	Diffuses	Diffused

The process of implantation starts with the shedding of zona pellucida/ hatching. Subsequently precontact with endometrium, orientation of blastocyst, apposition, adhesion and endometrial invasion occurs. True endometrial invasion does not happen in ruminants as it happens in rodents and primates. In these species, the blastocyst appears to be positioned and immobilized in the uterus after hatching although can easily be recovered from the uterus by lavage without causing structural damages.

5.1 The initial apposition

In sheep after day 14, the filamentous conceptus appears to be immobilized in the uterine lumen and maintains a close contact with the endometrial luminal epithelium. This is evident from the fact that a rounded shape of the endometrium is found imprinted on the trophectoderm in fixed specimens (Guillomot *et al.,* 1993). The apical membranes of both trophoblast and the uterine luminal epithelium cells remain in close association. However, the embryos can still be recovered easily at this stage too. A reduction of the apical microvilli covering the trophectoderm occurs between days 13 and 15 on the onset of apposition in sheep conceptus (Guillomot *et al.,* 1981, 1993). Similar modification of endometrial epithelium is found to occur in rodents (Enders and Schlafke, 1969), however, it does not appear to occur in sheep (Guillomot *et al.,* 1981, 1993). In this species the initial apposition is ensured by interdigitation of cytoplasmic projections of the trophectoderm cells and uterine epithelial microvilli which occur first near the inner cell mass then spread towards the extremities of the elongated conceptus (Guillomot *et al.,* 1981). Caruncular areas, the actual site of implantation in ruminants, are devoid of uterine glands which are available only in between areas called intercaruncular spaces. In histological sections the curuncular areas are found comprised of luminal epithelium, several types of stroma (stratum compactum and stratum spongiosum), blood vessels and immune cells. Interestingly, the uterine glands of the intercaruncular space also take part in this process of initial apposition in ruminants. The fingerlike villi or papillae developed from the trophoblast penetrate into the mouths of the superficial ducts of the uterine glands at days 15–18 (Guillomot *et al.,* 1981, Wooding *et al.,* 1982). These trophoblastic projections get vanished by day 20. The reason of this transient change is not known. However, trophoblastic differentiation for a short duration probably is required by the periattachment conceptus for a temporary anchor which helps in absorbing the histotrophic secretions from the uterine glands (Guillomot *et al.,* 1981). The trophoblast papillae may facilitate the formation of more robust adhesive interactions between the trophoblast and endometrial luminal epithelium (Wooding *et al.,* 1982). Similar features are described in the cow conceptus of day 15 pregnancy, but not seen in goat conceptus (Spencer *et al.,* 2004).

5.2 Caruncular folding

In sheep around day 14 the caruncles become edematous with a folded and depressed surface. These modifications are progressive and do not occur simultaneously on all caruncles. Caruncular folding is perhaps the first step in the formation of crypts that constitute the maternal side of the future placentomes, which are structures that form with placental cotyledons (Wimsatt, 1950). Dome-like cytoplasmic protrusions also appear on the caruncular epithelial cells, which have a convex apex. Similar protrusions, which are sites of endocytosis, termed pinopods have also been described on the uterine epithelium of mouse, rat, human and rabbit at the time of implantation (Guillomot *et al.,* 1981).

5.3 Formation of binucleate cells, syncytial plaque and planecntome

Mature sheep, goat, cattle and buffaloes placenta are called synepitheliochorial, being neither entirely syndesmochorial without uterine epithelium, nor completely epitheliochorial with two apposed cell layers whose only anatomic interaction is interdigitated microvilli, as in the pig. Formation of synepitheliochorial placentation involves the fusion of placental cotyledons with endometrial caruncles to form placentomes that serve a primary role in fetal–maternal gas exchange and derivation of nutrients by the placenta. In sheep on day 16, the trophoblast begins to adhere firmly to the endometrial luminal epithelium. The interdigitation of the trophectoderm and endometrial luminal epithelium occurs in both the caruncular and intercaruncular areas of the endometrium. Adhesion of the trophectoderm to the endometrial luminal epithelium progresses along the uterine horn and appears to be completed around day 22 in sheep (Guillomot *et al.,* 1981).

Binucleate trophoblast giant cells (BNC) are a characteristic feature of ruminant placenta (Wimsatt, 1951). The BNC develop from uninucleate trophoblast stem cells and become binucleate by acytokinetic mitosis (Wimsatt, 1951; Klisch *et al.,* 1999). In sheep, the trophoblast giant binucleate cells (BNC) differentiate from mononuclear trophoblast by day 16. Mature BNC migrate through the apical trophoblast tight junctions of the chorion towards the uterine epithelium and flatten as they fuse to the apical surface with the luminal epithelial cells resulting in formation of trinucleate feto maternal hybrid cells (Wooding, 1992) thereby assimilating and replacing the endometrial epithelium. Subsequently, the trinucleate cells enlarge by continued BNC migration and fusion to form syncytial plaques linked by tight junctions that appear to be limited in size about 20-25 nuclei in the ewes (Wooding 1984). Over time the syncytial plaques cover the caruncular surface and aid in formation of the placentome. Depending on the species the uterine luminal epithelium persists but with modification of varying degrees by the migration and fusion of the fetal BNC into a hybrid fetomaternal syncytium. The BNC of ruminant placenta may be analogous in many respects to the trophoblast giant cells of the syncytiotrophoblast in humans (Hoffman and Wooding, 1993). Interestingly, it has been noticed that the arrest of IFNτ gene expression occurs in regions of the mononuclear trophectoderm which have established cellular contacts with the luminal epithelium during the implantation process in sheep (Guillomot *et al.,* 1990).

6. Proteins of binucleate cells (BNC)

The BNC have at least two main functions: 1. to form a hybrid fetomaternal syncytium essential for successful implantation and subsequent placental growth; 2. to synthesize and secrete steroids (estrogen, progesterone) and placental lactogen that regulate maternal physiology including the other proteins of unknown function. During cell maturation, BNC become polyploid (Klisch *et al.,* 1999) and accumulate large amounts of dense core vesicles in their cytoplasm, which release their granules at the basal membrane of the uterine epithelium. Therefore, the BNC facilitate the transport of trophoblast-derived proteins across the otherwise protein-tight synepitheliochorial placental barrier (Wooding and Flint, 1994). The immune histochemical localization revealed that the granules of BNC bind some lectins (*Phaseolus vulgaris* leucoagglutinin, PHA-L; *Dolichos biflorus* agglutinin, DBA; *Vicia villosa* agglutinin, VVA) with high specificity (Klisch and Leiser, 2003). The lectins DBA, VVA recognize terminal N-acetylgalactosamine (Piller *et al.,* 1990) or an oligosaccharide motif in complex asparagine-linked glycans of the lactosamine-type (PHA-L; Kaneda *et al.,* 2002). These lectins bind to prolactin related protein I (PRP-I) and pregnancy associated glycoproteins in bovine BNC granules (Klisch and Leiser, 2003; Klisch *et al.,* 2005). Several different PRP-mRNAs have been identified in placenta (Ushizawa *et al.,* 2005) which belongs to a prolactin gene family which arose by gene duplication (Forsyth and Wallis, 2002). The PRP-I has been demonstrated on the protein level only and to date PRP-I has not been detected in the maternal circulation (Kessler and Schuler, 1997). Also the binding of PRP-I to prolactin or growth hormone receptors has not been observed (Kessler and Schuler, 1997), therefore the function and role of these molecules are still obscure.

7. Pregnancy associated glycoproteins and its biochemical characteristics

Another group of proteins known as pregnancy-associated glycoproteins (PAG), also called as pregnancy-specific protein B (Butler *et al.,*1982) constitute a large family of glycoproteins expressed in the outer epithelial cell layer (chorion/trophectoderm) of the placenta in several eutherian species like cattle (Butler *et al.,* 1982), sheep (Green *et al.,*2000), goat (Garbayo *et al.,* 1998) and pigs (Szafranska *et al.,* 2001). In cattle, 21 PAG mRNAs have been sequenced (Green *et al.,* 2000), but the number of PAG genes in the bovine and ovine genome has been estimated to be at least 100 (Xie *et al.,* 1997). They are members of the aspartic proteinase family, having high sequence homology with each other as well as with pepsin, pepsinogen, chymosin, cathepsin D, and cathepsin E (Xie *et al.,* 1991; Guruprasad *et al.,* 1996) but, to date no proteolytic activity of ruminant PAGs has been demonstrated. It has been indicated that although there are many PAG molecules, some of the PAG molecules are expressed during distinct stages of pregnancy in cattle and goats whereas others are not (Garbayo *et al.,* 2000; Green *et al.,* 2000).

These protein molecules (PSP-B) in cattle were originally thought to have a molecular weight of 47-53kDa (Butler *et al.,* 1982). However Zoli *et al.,* (1991) showed a larger molecular weight (67kDa) PAG in purified product of from fetal bovine cotyledonary tissues. The apparent molecular masses of the five N-terminal sequenced water buffalo PAG is reported to be 62 to 75 kDa as determined by SDS-PAGE (Barbato *et al.,* 2008). In all the species, the actual molecular weight of most PAG molecules exceeded the theoretical molecular weight 37 kDa, of the protein core (after removal of the signal sequence and the propeptide). The apparent large masses are partially attributable to the substantial posttranslational glycosylation in placenta tissues (Xie *et al.,* 1997; Garbayo *et al.,* 2000; Klisch *et al.,* 2006) as the PAG molecules undergo extensive posttranslational processing. Different numbers of N-glycosylation sites of asparagines (consensus sequence N-X-S/T, where X must not be P) have been observed in the PAG molecules isolated from the placentas of bovine (Xie *et al.,* 1991), ovine (Atkinson *et al.,* 1993), caprine (Garbayo *et al.,* 1998), and porcine origins (Szafranska *et al.,* 2004). In cattle for example, the dominant 67 kDa form of boPAG shows four potential glycosylation sites and 10% oligosaccharide content (Zoli *et al.,* 1991). Multiantennary oligosaccharides represent 17.83% of the relative molecular mass in ovine PAG/SBU3 and these large amounts of lateral-chain sugars are shown (Atkinson *et al.,* 1993) to be made up of N-acetyl glucosamine (5.26%), N-acetyl neuraminic acid (4.25%), N-acetyl galactosamine (3.62%), galactose (1.94%), and mannose (1.81%). A considerable scientific effort has been directed to elucidate the physiological role of PAG however the intricacies of the matter is still unraveled. As stated by Roberts *et al.* (1996), it is highly unlikely that PAGs are merely "inconsequential curiosities" but might perform some important function in the context of pregnancy. Whatever might be the reason its occurrence in blood circulation coincides with the time of firm trophoblast attachment with the uterine wall at the onset of placentation which provides the basis of a potential useful pregnancy test.

8. Assays for detection of pregnancy associated glycoproteins

The PAGs get transferred from the trophoblast to the maternal placental stroma and vasculature, to the maternal blood during pregnancy (Zoli *et al.,* 1992; Green *et al.,* 2005) and remained with detectable level in blood circulation around third week of pregnancy to term in cattle and other ruminant species (Zoli *et al.,* 1992; Zarauk *et al.,* 1998) including buffaloes (El-Battawy *et al.,* 2009). BioPrynTM (BioTracking, LLC, Moscow, ID, USA) is a commercially available enzyme-linked immunosorbent assay (ELISA) kit available in market designed to detect PSP-B based on the work of Butler and associates. Other groups have developed immunoassays for PAGs other than PSPB that are based on similar antigens. Whereas in one report the antigen was called pregnancy associated glycoprotein (Zoli *et al.*, 1992) and in the second it was named pregnancy serum protein-60 to denote its molecular weight (Mialon *et al.*, 1993). All are reported to have similar, if not identical, amino-terminal amino acid sequences (Xie *et al.*, 1991).

A lot of inter assay variations observed in bPAG-1 concentration measurement may be due to variations in the antiserum utilized. In two studies, one designed to determine factors affecting plasma bPAG-1 concentrations in pregnant high-producing dairy cows (Lopez-Gatius *et al.*, 2007) and the other to assess the predictive importance of maternal bPAG-1 concentrations in recipients carrying somatic clones to pregnancy outcome (Chavatte-Palmer *et al.*, 2006), bPAG-1 concentration varied with the assay and more specifically the primary antibody being used. It is likely that the different polyclonal antisera used in radioimmunoassay (RIA) systems to measure bPAG-1 recognize other PAG molecules and because more than 100 genes encode various PAG molecules in ruminant placenta (Xie *et al.*, 1997), the varying affinities would explain the inconsistent or varying inter-assay results. Assays utilizing heterologous bPAG-1 RIA systems may be more sensitive (Perenyi *et al.*, 2003) and demonstrate higher bPAG-1 concentrations, improving ability to detect early pregnancy. Sensitivity and specificity were improved when a monoclonal antibody raised against only a few bPAG-1 family members belonging to the binucleate trophoblasts cell-specific group was used to detect bPAG-1 (Green *et al.*, 2005) and permitted pregnancy to be detected in all animals by 28 days after AI.

9. Dynamic changes of PAG during pregnancy

In cattle, the mean bPAG-1 concentration begin to increase from days 15 to 35, however the variation in serum bPAG-1 concentrations among cows restricts their use as a reliable indicator of pregnancy until days 26–30 (Humbolt 2001; Zoli *et al.*, 1992).The dynamics of PAG in blood circulation varies between species. For example, in cattle the level of PAG continues to increase with the growth and development of placenta and reaches maximum around the time of parturition (Fig. 2; Zoli *et al.*, 1992). Whereas, in goats it reaches the maximum around the day 50 of gestation and remains high up to parturition (Fig. 3; Zarauk *et al.*, 1998). As the level of PAG reaches a maximum concentration in plasma at approximately the time of parturition in cattle, with their long half-life, they remain in circulation for 2–3 months after calving (Fig. 2 ; Zoli *et al.*, 1992). Therefore when using plasma bPAG-1 for pregnancy diagnosis, the concentrations expected at various times following conception and previous parturition must be taken into account (Zoli *et al.*, 1992; Szenci *et al.*, 1998). For example in cows < 2 months postpartum may have bPAG-1 concentrations above the pregnancy/open cut-off value, even if they had not been inseminated. Where as in goats, the level comes down very fast within 20 days postpartum (Fig 3; Zarauk *et al.*, 1998) therefore; similar precautions need not be taken.

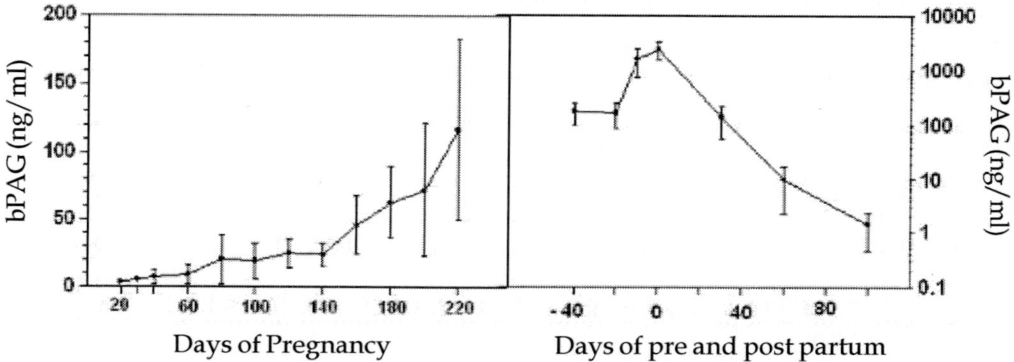

Fig. 2 : Profile of PAG (X axis; ng/mL) in cattle during different days of pregnancy (A), pre and post parturion (B). PAG level was determined using the homologous RIA. (Adopted from Zoli *et al.*, 1992)

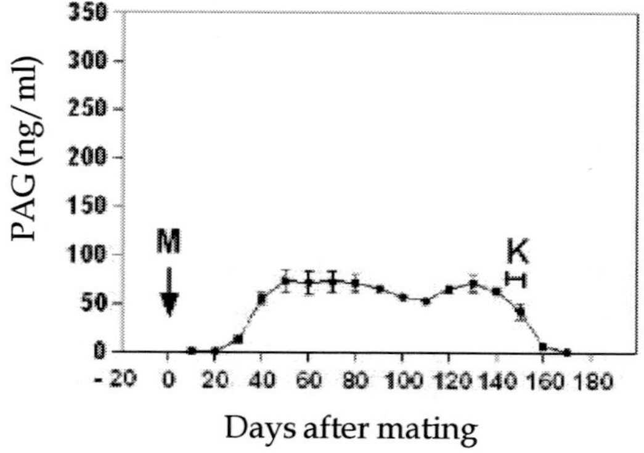

Fig. 3 : Profile of PAG concentrations (ng/mL) in goats (n=29) detected by heterologous assay system of bovine PAG during the whole gestation length (147±3 days). M indicates natural matting and K is the days of kidding, adopted from (Zarrauk *et al.*, 1999).

10. Ultrasonography vs PAG detection in pregnancy diagnosis

Transrectal ultrasonographic observation of embryonic and fetal heartbeat is the most attractive technique for the assessment of embryonic viability and pregnancy diagnosis. Studies for comparing the accuracy of pregnancy diagnosis in lactating dairy cows, by ultrasound and PAG1 detection method revealed that the pregnancy status after 27 days of timed AI as determined by plasma bPAG-1 ELISA (Green *et al.*, 2005) and transrectal ultrasonography, had a high level of agreement (kappa = 0.87–0.90; Silva *et al.*, 2007). This suggests that ultrasonography is no better than measurement of bPAG-1 at detecting day 27 pregnancy, however, when comparing the bPAG-1 ELISA to transrectal ultrasonography, the rate of false negative results was less than the rate of false positives. This is expected to happen because the half-life of bPAG-1 in maternal circulation can range from 4.3 to 7.0 days during the post-calving period and 2.7–7.0 days after induction of embryonic mortality (Semambo *et al.,* 1992; Szenci *et al.,* 2003). Thus the PAG1 levels would be shown as high in maternal circulation after embryonic death until it reaches to the value lower than the cut-off point of pregnancy and lead to false diagnosis. Thus the transrectal ultrasonography can be used as a supplementary test to visualize embryonic death and reduce the frequency of false positive results which is an advantage. In case the bPAG-1 concentrations decreased rapidly after embryonic death, the bPAG-1 ELISA might be used to detect losses earlier than transrectal palpation, due to the lag between embryonic death and expulsion of the conceptus (Kastelic *et al.,* 1991; Kastelic and Ginther, 1989).

11. Early embryonic and fetal loss, consequences and determination by PAG assay

Experiments in cattle (Hawk *et al.,* 1983) indicated that fertilization rates are usually high (85-95%), therefore the embryonic death is responsible for much of the reproductive wastage. In more recent studies fertilization rates have been shown lower averaging 75.0% in lactating (Breuel *et al.,* 1993) as compared to 98.6% in non-lactating beef cows (Maurer and Chenault, 1983). However, the fertilization rates were found similar between lactating and non-lactating dairy cows averaging 76.2 and 78.1%, respectively (Sartori *et al.,* 2002). These studies indicated that, although lactation may decrease fertilization in beef cattle, it is less important in dairy cows. In dairy cattle, within 5-6 days after insemination, only about 65% of fertilized oocytes resulted in viable embryos depending upon parity and lactation status. A study was conducted on the embryonic viability 5–6 days post-insemination as a percent of fertilization for dairy and beef cattle indicating that the embryonic viability in parous lactating, parous nonlactating and nulliparous cattle was 50.0, 57.9 and 71.9%, respectively (Santos *et al.,* 2004). The beef cows followed a similar pattern as in dairy cattle, except that rates were generally higher and comparable between parous nonlactating cows and nulliparous heifers (Santos *et al.,* 2004). Diskin and Sreenan (1980) reported that embryonic death prior to maternal recognition of pregnancy (14–19 days after fertilization) is 35–40% in the bovine. Loss of early embryos is of major concern for cattle, buffaloes and other animals which carry a singleton conceptus during the whole pregnancy period, since loss of a single conceptus results wastage of pregnancy and animal would repeat cycle. Such pregnancy loss can have a devastating effect on economic success in dairy and beef industry, where revenue is directly dependent upon reproduction efficiency and its associated effects on milk production. In dairy herds, the lost income as a result of reproductive waste or lost pregnancies is due to more days open, resulting in fewer days at peak milk production. A study in USA has estimated that each pregnancy loss in cattle results in an average of $US 640 lost income (Thurmond *et al.*,1990). Another report for dairy cattle of Pennsylvania State, USA, calculated the cost per day open beyond 60 days in milk would be as high as $3 (Groenendaal *et al.*, 2004). In beef herds on the other hand the pregnancy loss has a negative impact on economic returns, as herd income is heavily dependent on the number of calves sold. Retention of non-pregnant beef cows, which continue to consume feedstuff, is fiscally nonsensical (Whitlock and Maxwell, 2008). In economic term the monetary calculation cited above might be different in countries where feed and labor costs are cheaper than in USA and would vary with the current rates. However the fact remains that to make a dairy or beef farm profitable one has to know the pregnancy status at the earliest, at the same time there is a demand for a test which can determine the pregnancy loss too at the earliest.

Since blood sampling does not require the special equipment or skilled operators, detection of bPAG-1 in sequential samples could be a good alternative to identify late embryonic loss. Recently the profiles of bPAG-1 have been evaluated as a method of predicting embryonic and fetal loss in cattle (Zoli *et al.*, 1992). In diagnostics, receiver operator characteristic (ROC) curve is used to depict the true positive rate and the false positive rate when an increasing cut-off for the test is applied. When the test cut-off is set too low, the true positive rate becomes 100% (optimal) but the false positive rate also goes 100% (*e.g.*, all non pregnant are declared pregnant). Therefore, increasing the cut-off (moving to the left on the graph) will decrease the false positive rate. In the optimal scenario, the true positive rate will remain at 100% while the cut-off is increased and the false positive rate will progress toward 0%. If both the true positive rate and the false positive rate decrease when the cut-off is increased then the graph has a diagonal line through its center as shown in Fig. 4.

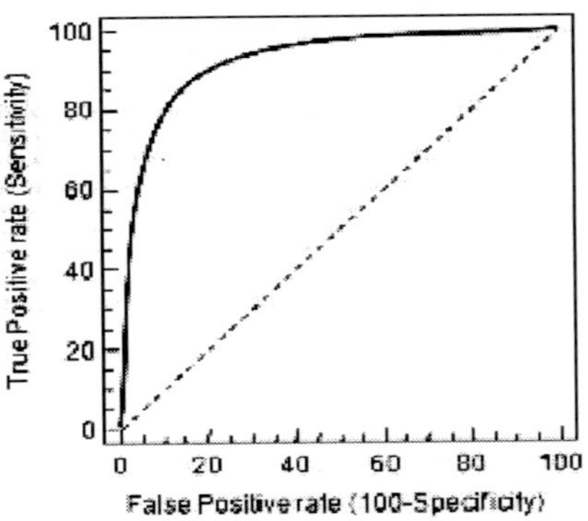

Fig. 4 : The receiver operator characteristic (ROC) curve showing when the test cut-off is set too low, the true positive rate becomes 100% (optimal) but the false positive rate also goes100% *i.e.*, all non pregnant are declared pregnant. Optimally, the true positive rate should remain at 100% while the cut-off is increased and the false positive rate is progress toward 0%.

Gabor *et al.* (2007) conducted a study in lactating dairy cows to develop a means of predicting embryonic loss at the time of early pregnancy detection by measuring both serum PSP-B and progesterone concentrations 30–36 days post-insemination. Over a 25-month interval they collected and analysed more than 8000 blood samples from three farms out of which 50.3% were classified as pregnant cows, according to the BioPrynTM assay. A total of 710 late embryonic losses (17.4%) were detected when cows were examined by transrectal palpation 60 days after AI. The authors have predicted late embryonic loss would occur when a sample's optical density (OD) reading in the BioPrynTM assay was between 0 and 30% above the cut-off OD for pregnancy. Using this criterion 31.8% of late embryonic losses were correctly predicted. However, when samples had both an OD value of 0–30% above cut-off OD for pregnancy, and serum progesterone concentrations were < 2ng/mL, 92% of late embryonic loss was accurately predicted. Although PSP-B concentrations alone did not accurately predict late embryonic loss, in combination with < 2ng/mL progesterone, PSP-B concentrations 0–30% above cut-off had high predictive value. In addition to accurately predicting early embryonic loss, only measuring progesterone in samples with an OD from 0 to 30% above pregnancy cut-off greatly reduced the number of progesterone determinations and thus assay cost. They concluded that a serial or single determination of bPAG-1 alone, or in combination with progesterone, may be superior to progesterone only, and provide an alternative to ultrasonography for detecting embryonic mortality in cattle.

12. Potential application of PAG detection for determination of multiple pregnancies

Determination of fetal numbers is desirable for better management of pregnant sheep, goat and other small ruminants which carry multiple pregnancies. It offers producers the opportunity to feed the groups of animals according to their precise needs in late gestation, which will prevent pregnancy toxemia, optimize the birth weights and increase the survivability of new born and mother. In addition the diagnosis helps decreasing the incidence of dystocia and the cost of feeding in animals carrying singletons (Robinson, 1983). The methods attempted to determine the number of fetuses in small ruminants includes recto-abdominal palpation, radiography, progesterone assay and ultrasonography techniques. Recto-abdominal technique has disadvantages of low accuracy for determination of multiples (57%) and hazardous with respect to rectal injury and abortion (Tyrrell and Plant, 1979). Radiography is accurate after Day 70 of pregnancy, however the cost of the portable X-ray, difficulty of using on farm and the health hazard to the operators and animals limit its use in the field. External Doppler ultrasonography gave accuracy rates of 83 and 93%, for the determination of singles and multiples, respectively at Days 80–95 of gestation (Fukui *et al.*, 1986). However, considerable expertise and relatively long (5 min/ewe) examination time is required. Real-time B-mode transabdominal ultrasonography (using a 3 or 3.5 MHz transducer) determined the fetal numbers in sheep with more than 90% accuracy between Days 50 and 100 of gestation (White *et al.*, 1984). However, pre-scanning shearing of wools of the ventral abdominal wall increases the cost of labor and needs a sophisticated system for rapid handling which is a major concern and limits its fast application. Several reports suggest that blood progesterone concentrations remains significantly higher in ewes carrying multiples than those carrying singles from week 4 until week 20 of pregnancy. The accuracy of a progesterone radioimmunoassay test to identify litter size reported in sheep ranged from 63 to 79% at Days 90–108 of gestation (Rawling *et al.*, 1983) which is far from ideal. A significant difference of PAG level had been shown in a homologous RIA for ovine PAG between ewes carrying singles and those carrying multiples during the early stage of pregnancy (Vandaele *et al.*, 2005). However, the accuracy of both progesterone and PAG tests for predicting the fetal numbers at present are still low to be used in the field.

13. Determination of placental function in abnormal offspring syndrome (AOS)

Somatic cell nuclear cloning in cattle, sheep and other species is associated with increased risk of fetal loss due to defects in formation or function of extra-embryonic membranes and developmental anomalies which may be manifested throughout pregnancy. The collective terms of these fetal and placental abnormalities is "abnormal offspring syndrome" (Farin *et al.*, 2006). It is difficult to identify recipients carrying clones that will develop the syndrome. In a study Chavatte-Palmer et al. (2006) utilized repeated ultrasonographic observations of the fetus and placenta and repeated measurement of maternal concentrations of bovine PAG-1 during the first 2 months of gestation in groups of pregnancies resulted from the embryos of SCNT and pregnancies without SCNT. Both the measurements they related to pregnancy outcome and occurrence of AOS. As measured by two different radio-immunoassays, concentrations of PAG were found significantly higher in cows carrying clone (SCNT) pregnancies which went to term than in vivo derived pregnancies that went to term. The two assays of bPAG-1 concentrations from days 34 to 50 also found significantly lower in clone recipient cows suffering an early pregnancy loss than those which maintained pregnancy to a later date. Thus measurement of bPAG-1 had shown a promise for practical non-invasive tool to follow pregnancy in clone recipients.

14. Future perspective

The conceptus while maintaining its growth and development brings changes in the maternal system by secreting a lot of biomolecules, some of which are characterized and some are yet to be discovered. Out of all the biomolecules, proteins always find a special place because they are the ultimate finish product of genes, effecter molecules and maintain the communication between and within the cells. Therefore the detection of these would reflect some of the important clues of physiological events and genetic defects.

The most important pregnancy related protein molecule which had found application earliest is pregnancy diagnosis in human by chorionic gonadotrophin (hCG). Maternal serum screening tests are all noninvasive biochemical methods developed for obtaining information about a fetus in human subject based on conceptus released molecules. The use of prenatal screening tests has expanded from identifying fetuses at risk for neural tube defects to those with fetal chromosome abnormalities and women at risk for third-trimester obstetrical complications. Maternal serum screening programs have shown the potential to decrease fetal morbidity and mortality by providing access to earlier diagnosis, by enabling families to make more informed reproductive decisions and by designing appropriate delivery strategies. Out of the three different markers *viz.*, alpha -fetoprotein (AFP), human chorionic gonadotropin (hCG), and unconjugated estriol used in maternal serum in screening programs, two are proteins. Other than confirming pregnancy the hCG has also been used and considered the most effective biochemical marker of Down syndrome screening (Bogart *et al.*, 1987).The association between the AFP value and fetal abnormalities is well known for detection of neural abnormality (Anderson and Brown, 2009). The identification of conceptus released protein interferon-tau finds its application in improvement of conception rate whereas the pregnancy associated glycoproteins has been used for diagnosis of early pregnancy in ruminant species. The nature, function and applications of the two very important protein molecules, *i.e.*, Interferon-τ and PAG, have been described in detail. The discovery of interferon-tau and the concept of luteal support system resulted in development of a whole set of managemental tools for reducing early pregnancy loss at the very critical period of maternal recognition of pregnancy. Similarly other than detection of early pregnancy, the PAG has shown its potential application in determination of abnormal offspring syndrome in pregnancies of the somatic nuclear transfer embryos. The use and applications of pregnancy associated proteins related to the detection of prenatal genetic defects has developed as a field of study in humans and is still obscure in animals since the animal breeding policies are more scientific which avoid genetic defects. There are considerable evidences to suggest that changes in concentration of PAGs in pregnant ruminants may have both diagnostic and predictive values for detection of pregnancy loss. However, practical application or translation of this technology to determine or predict abortion/pregnancy loss in cattle on farms is not yet realized. One of the main disadvantages of these molecules is that, in the maternal circulation, PAGs have an outstanding long half-life, which varies between different stages of pregnancy and also depends on the test systems applied. Persistence of bPAG-1 concentrations in the postpartum period or after pregnancy loss is another shortcoming of pregnancy determination based on bPAG-1. Therefore, one must be aware of the limitations of this testing technology. Another important consideration is that bPAG-1 detected by monoclonal antibodies have shown a relatively shorter half-life, averaging only 4.3 days during the post-calving period, and bPAG-1 detected with monoclonal antibodies were below pregnancy threshold concentrations by 8-week postpartum (Green *et al.*, 2005) and 2.7–7.0 days after induction of embryonic mortality (Semambo *et al.*,1992; Szenci *et al.*, 2003). Other than these two molecules there might still be many more awaiting discovery and application. Efforts are on and should be directed to identify those which can help in devising more and more managemental tools which can help in improvement of reproductive efficiency of the farm animals for the benefit of human being.

Conclusions

It has been demonstrated that some IFN-τ escape the uterus and can be detected in blood (Oliveira *et al.*, 2008; Bott *et al.*, 2010), however, the circulating concentrations of IFN-τ are extremely low thus precludes their use in a blood pregnancy test. An alternative strategy for pregnancy diagnosis has been proposed based on the measurement of the response proteins of circulatory leukocytes to IFN-τ. Leukocytes respond to IFN-τ by expressing interferon-stimulated genes (ISG). The utility of ISG for the purpose of pregnancy detection in dairy cattle has been demonstrated recently (Han *et al.*, 2006; Gifford *et al.*, 2007). Han *et al.* (2006) found that blood progesterone and ISG15 had acceptable results as a method of pregnancy diagnosis if samples were collected over a series of days. Gifford *et al.* (2007) demonstrated that ISG were up-regulated in peripheral blood leukocytes from pregnant cows on days 18 and 20 after AI compared with d 0 (day of AI). A test based on the gene expression status of Oas 1, an ISG of leukocyte, has been developed by Green *et al.*,(2010) which has shown an ideal cut-off for a day 18 pregnancy test, because the true positive rate reached 100% while the false positive rate was 0%. However there is a very narrow window that exists for its use as pregnancy diagnosis marker since pregnancy-associated glycoprotein (PAG) testing for bovine pregnancy is found highly effective after 26 days of AI (Green *et al.*, 2009). Such tools would find their way to future applications and benefit the use of assisted reproductive technologies.

References

Ambrose J.D., Pires M.F.A., Moreira F., Diaz T., Binelli M .,Thatcher W.W. (1998). Influence of Deslorelm (GnRH-agonist) implant on plasma progesterone, first wave dominant follicle and pregnancy in dairy cattle. *Theriogenology* **50:** 1157-1170.

Anderson ., Brown C.L. (2009). Fetal chromosomal abnormalities: Antenatal screening and diagnosis. *American Family Physician* **79:** 117-123.

Ashworth C.J., Bazer F.W. (1989). Changes in ovine conceptus and endometrial function following asynchronous embryo transfer or administration of progesterone. *Biology of Reproduction* **40:** 425-433.

Atkinson., Y. H., Gogolin-Evans K. J., Hounsell E. F., Davies M. J., Brandon M. R., Seamark R. F. (1993). Characterization of placentation-specific binucleate cell glycoproteins possessing a novel carbohydrate. Evidence for a new family of pregnancy-associated molecules. *Journal of Biological Chemistry* **268:** 26679-26685.

Bale T.L., Dorsa D.M. (1997). Cloning, novel promoter sequence and estrogen regulation of a rat oxytocin receptor gene. *Endocrinology* **138:** 1151-1158.

Barbato O., Sousa N.M., Klisch K., Clerget E., Debenedetti A., Barile VL., Malfatti A., Beckers J.F. (2008). Isolation of new pregnancy-associated glycoproteins from water buffalo *(Bubalus bubalis)* placenta by Vicia villosa affinity chromatography. *Research in Veterinary Science* **85:** 457-466.

Bazer F.W. (1992). Mediators of maternal recognition of pregnancy in mammals. *Proc Soc Exp. Biol. Med.* **199:** 373-384.

Binelli M., Hampton., Buhi W.C., Thatcher W.W. (1999). Persistent dominant follicle alters pattern of oviductal secretory proteins from cows at estrus. *Biology of Reproduction* **61:** 127-134.

Bogart M.H., Pandian M.R., Jones O.W. (1987). Abnormal maternal serum gonadotropin levels in pregnancies with fetal chromosome abnormalities. *Prenatal Diagnosis* **7:** 623-630.

Boshier D.P., Holloway H. (1973). Effects of ovarian steroid hormones on histochemically demonstrable lipids in the rat uterine epithelium. *Journal of Endocrinology* **56:** 59-67.

Bott R.C., Ashley R.L., Henkes L.E., Antoniazzi A.Q., Bruemmer J.E., Niswender G.D., Bazer F.W., Spencer T.E., Smirnova N.P., Anthony R.V., Hansen T.R. (2010). Uterine vein infusion interferon tau (IFNô) extends luteal life span in ewes. *Biology of Reproduction* **82:** 725-735.

Breuel K.F., Lewis P.E., Schrick F.N., Lishman A.W., Inskeep E.K., Butcher R.L. (1993). Factors affecting fertility in the postpartum cow: role of the oocyte and follicle in conception rate. *Biology of Reproduction* **48:** 655-661.

Brock D.J.H., Sutcliffe R.G. (1972). Alpha-fetoprotein in the antenatal diagnosis of anencephaly and spina bifida. *Lancet* **2:** 197-199.

Butler J.E., Hamilton W.C., Sasser R.G., Ruder C.A., Hass G.M., Williams R.J. (1982). Detection and partial characterization of two bovine pregnancy-specific proteins. *Biology of Reproduction* **26:** 925-33.

Cencic A., Guillomot M., Koren S., La Bonnardiere C. (2003). Trophoblastic interferons: do they modulate uterine cellular markers at the time of conceptus attachment in the pig? *Placenta* **24:** 862-869.

Charpigny G., Reinaud P., Tamby J.P., Creminon C., Martal J., Maclouf J., Guillomot M. (1997). Expression of cyclooxygenase 1 and 2 in ovine endometrium during the estrous cycle and early pregnancy. *Endocrinology* **138:** 2163-2171.

Chavatte-Palmer P., de Sousa N., Laigre P., Camous S., Ponter A.A., Beckers J.F. (2006). Ultrasound fetal measurements and pregnancy associated glycoprotein secretion in early pregnancy in cattle recipients carrying somatic clones. *Theriogenology* **66:** 829-840.

Choi Y., Johnson G.A., Burghardt R.C., Berghman L.R., Joyce M.M., Taylor K.M., Stewart M.D., Bazer F.W., Spencer T.E. (2001). Interferon regulatory factor-two restricts expression of interferon- stimulated genes to the endometrial stroma and glandular epithelium of the ovine uterus. *Biology of Reproduction* **65:** 1038-1049.

Denker H.W., Fritz H. (1979). Enzymatic characterization of rabbit blastocyst proteinase with synthetic substrates of trypsin-like enzymes. Hoppe-Seyler's Z. *Physiological Chemistry* **360:** 107-113.

Diskin M.G., Sreenan J.M. (1980). Fertilization and embryonic mortality rates in beef heifers after artificial insemination. *Journal of Reproduction and Fertility* **59:** 463-468.

El Amiri B., Remy B., Sousa N.M., Joris B., Ottiers N.G., Perenyi Z. (2003). Isolation and partial characterization of three pregnancy associated glycoproteins from the ewe placenta. *Molecular Reproduction and Development* **64:** 199-206.

El-Battawy K.A., Sousa N.M., Szenci O., Beckers J.F. (2009). Pregnancy-associated glycoprotein profile during the first trimester of pregnancy in Egyptian buffalo cows. *Reproduction in Domestic Animals* **44:** 161-166.

Farin C.E., Imakawa K., Roberts R.M. (1989). In situ localization of mRNA for the interferon, ovine trophoblast protein-1, during early embryonic development of the sheep. *Molecular Endocrinology* **3:** 1099-1107.

Farin P.W., Piedrahita J A., Farin C E. (2006). Errors in development of fetuses and placentas from in vitro-produced bovine embryos. *Theriogenology* **65:** 178-191.

Flechon J.E., Guillomot M., Charlier M., Flechon B., Martal J. (1986). Experimental studies on the elongation of the ewe blastocyst. *Reproduction Nutrition and Development* **26:** 1017-1024.

Fleming J.A., Choi Y., Johnson G.A., Spencer T.E., Bazer F.W. (2001). Cloning of the ovine estrogen receptor-alpha promoter and functional regulation by ovine interferon-tau. *Endocrinology* **142:** 2879-2887.

Forsyth I.A ., Wallis M. (2002). Growth hormone and prolactin–molecular and functional evolution. *Journal of Mammary Gland Biology and Neoplasia* **7:** 291-312.

Fukui Y., Kobayashi M., Tsubaki M., Tetsuka K., Shimoda K., Ono H. (1986). Comparison of two ultrasonic methods for multiple pregnancy diagnosis in sheep and indicators of multiple pregnant ewes in blood. *Animal Reproduction Science* **11:** 25-33.

Gabor G., Toth F., Ozsvari L., Abonyi-Toth Z., Sasser R.G. (2007). Early detection of pregnancy and embryonic loss in dairy cattle by ELISA tests. *Reproduction in Domestic Animals* **42:** 633-636.

Garbayo J.M., Green J.A., Manikkam M., Beckers J.F., Kiesling D.O., Ealy A.D., Roberts R.M. (2000). Caprine pregnancy-associated glycoproteins (PAG): their cloning, expression and evolutionary relationship to other PAG. *Molecular Reproduction and Development* **57:** 311-322.

Gifford C.A., Racicot K., Clark D.S., Austin K.J., Hansen T.R., Lucy M.C., Davies C.J, Ott T.L. (2007). Regulation of interferon-stimulated genes in peripheral blood leukocytes in pregnant and bred, non-pregnant dairy cows. *Journal of Dairy Science* **90:** 274-280.

Gonzales D.S., Bavister B.D. (1995) Zona pellucida escape by hamster blastocysts in vitro is delayed and morphologically different compared with zona escape in vivo. *Biology of Reproduction* **52:** 470-480.

Gray C., Bartol F.F., Taylor K.M., Wiley A.A., Ramsey W.S., Ott T.L., Bazer F.W., Spencer T.E. (2000). Ovine uterine gland knock-out model:effects of gland ablation on the estrous cycle. *Biology of Reproduction* **62:** 448-456.

Gray C.A., Burghardt R.C., Johnson G.A., Bazer F.W., Spencer T.E. (2002). Evidence that absence of endometrial gland secretions in uterine gland knockout ewes compromises conceptus survival and elongation. *Reproduction* **124:** 289-300.

Gray C.A., Taylor K.M., Ramsey W.S., Hill J.R., Bazer F.W., Bartol F.F., Spencer T.E. (2001). Endometrial glands are required for preimplantation conceptus elongation and survival. *Biology of Reproduction* **64:** 1608-1613.

Green J.A., Xie S., Quan X., Bao B., Gan X., Mathialogan N., Beckers J.F., Roberts R.M. (2000). Pregnancy-associated bovine and ovine glycoproteins exhibit spatially and temporally distinct expression patterns during pregnancy. *Biology of Reproduction* **62:** 1624-1631.

Green J.A., Parks T.E., Avalle M.P., Telugu B.P., McLain A.L., Peterson A.J., McMillan W., Mathialagan N., Hook R.R., Xie .S., Roberts R.M. (2005). The establishment of an ELISA for the detection of pregnancy-associated glycoproteins (PAGs) in the serum of pregnant cows and heifers. *Theriogenology* **63:** 1481-1503.

Green J.A., Parks T.E., Avalle M.P., Telugu B.P., McLain A.L., Peterson A.J. (2005).The establishment of an ELISA for the detection of pregnancy-associated glycoproteins (PAGs) in the serum of pregnant cows and heifers. *Theriogenology* **63:** 1481-1503.

Green J.C., Okamura C.S., Poock S.E., Lucy M.C. (2010). Measurement of interferon-tau (IFN-τ) stimulated gene expression in blood leukocytes for pregnancy diagnosis within 18–20 d after insemination in dairy cattle. *Animal Reproduction Science* **121:** 24-33.

Green J.C., Volkmann D.H., Poock S.E., McGrath M.F., Ehrhardt M., Moseley A.E., Lucy M.C. (2009). Technical note: a rapid enzyme-linked immunosorbent assay blood test for pregnancy in dairy and beef cattle. *Journal of Dairy Science* **92:** 3819-3824.

Groenendaal H., Galligan D.T., Mulder H.A. (2004). An economic spreadsheet model to determine optimal breeding and replacement decisions for dairy cattle. *Journal of Dairy Science* **87:** 2146-2157.

Guillomot M., Flechon J.E., Leroy F. (1993). Blastocyst development and implantation. In Reproduction in Mammals and Man, Eds. C Thibault, MC Levasseur and RHF Hunter. Paris: Ellipses pp 387-411.

Guillomot M., Flechon J.E., Wintenberger-Torres S. (1981). Conceptus attachment in the ewe: an ultrastructural study. *Placenta* **2:** 169-182.

Guillomot M., Michel C., Gaye P., Charlier N., Trojan J., Martal J. (1990). Cellular localization of an embryonic interferon, ovine trophoblastin and its mRNA in sheep embryos during early pregnancy. *Biology of the Cell* **68:** 205-211.

Guruprasad K., Blundell T.L., Xie S., Green J., Szafranska B., Nagel R.J., McDowell K., Baker C.B., Roberts R.M. (1996). Comparative modeling and analysis of amino acid substitutions suggests that the family of pregnancy-associated glycoproteins includes both active and inactive aspartic proteinases. *Protein Engineering* **9:** 849-856.

Han H., Austin K.J., Rempel L.A., Hansen T.R. (2006). Low blood Isg15 mRNA and progesterone levels are predictive of non-pregnant dairy cows. *Journal of Endocrinology* **191:** 505-512.

Hawk H.W. (1983). Sperm survival and transport in the female reproductive tract. *Journal of Dairy Science* **66:** 2645-2660.

Heyman Y., Camous S., Fevre J., Meziou W., Martal J. (1984). Maintenance of the corpus luteum after uterine transfer of trophoblastic vesicles to cyclic cows and ewes. *Journal of Reproduction and Fertility* **70:** 533-540.

Hoffman L.H., Wooding F.B. (1993). Giant and binucleate trophoblast cells of mammals. *Journal of Experimental Zoology* **266:** 559-577.

Humblot P. (2001). Use of pregnancy specific proteins and progesterone assays to monitor pregnancy and determine the timing, frequencies and sources of embryonic mortality in ruminants. *Theriogenology* **56:** 1417-1433.

Johnson G.A., Burghardt R.C., Spencer T.E., Newton G.R., Ott T.L., Bazer F.W. (1999). Ovine osteopontin. II. Osteopontin and alpha(v)-beta(3) integrin expression in the uterus and conceptus during the periimplantation period. *Biology of Reproduction* **61:** 892-899.

Johnson G.A., Spencer T.E., Burghardt R.C., Joyce M.M., Bazer F.W. (2000). Interferon-tau and progesterone regulate ubiquitin cross-reactive protein expression in the ovine uterus. *Biology of Reproduction* **62:** 622-627.

Johnson G.A., Stewart M.D., Gray C.A., Choi Y., Burghardt R.C., Yu-Lee L.Y., Bazer F.W., Spencer T.E. (2001) Effects of the estrous cycle, pregnancy, and interferon tau on 2',5'- oligoadenylate synthetase expression in the ovine uterus. *Biology of Reproduction* **64:** 1392-1399.

Jones C.J., Koob B., Stoddart R.W., Hoffmann B., Leiser R. (1994). Lectin histochemical analysis of glycans in ovine and bovine near-term placental binucleate cells. *Cell and Tissue Research* **278:** 601-610.

Joshi M.S., Murray I.M. (1974). Immunological studies of the rat uterine fluid peptidase. *Journal of Reproduction and Fertility* **37:** 361-365.

Kaneda Y., Whittier R.F., Yamanaka H., Carredano E., Gotoh M., Sota H., Hasegawa Y., Shinohara Y. (2002). The high specificities of Phaseolus vulgaris erythro- and leukoagglutinating lectins for bisecting GlcNAc or beta 1-6-linked branch structures, respectively, are attributable to loop B. *Journal of Biological Chemistry* **277:** 16928-16935.

Kastelic J.P., Ginther O.J. (1989). Fate of conceptus and corpus luteum after induced embryonic loss in heifers. *Journal of American Veterinary Medical Association* **194:** 922-928.

Kastelic J.P., Northey D.L., Ginther O.J. (1991). Spontaneous embryonic death on days 20 to 40 in heifers. *Theriogenology* **35:** 351-363.

Kerszberg M., Wolpert L. (1998). Mechanisms for positional signaling by morphogen transport: a theoretical study. *Journal of Theoritical Biology* **191:** 103-114.

Kessler M.A., Schuler L.A. (1997). Purification and properties of placental prolactin-related protein-I. *Placenta* **18:** 29-36.

Kim S., Choi Y., Bazer F.W., Spencer T.E. (2003). Identification of genes in the ovine endometrium regulated by interferon tau independent of signal transducer and activator of transcription 1. *Endocrinology* **144:** 5203-5214.

Klisch K., Leiser R. (2003). In bovine binucleate trophoblast giant cells,pregnancy-associated glycoproteins and placental prolactin-related protein-I are conjugated to asparagine-linked N-acetylgalactosaminyl glycans. *Histochemistry and Cell Biology* **119:** 211-217.

Klisch K., Pfarrer C., Schuler G., Hoffmann B., Leiser R. (1999). Tripolar acytokinetic mitosis and formation of feto-maternal syncytia in the bovine placentome: different modes of the generation of multinuclear cells. *Anatomy and Embryology* **200:** 229-237.

Klisch K., Boos A., Friedrich M., Herzog K., Feldmann M., Sousa N., Beckers J., Leiser R., Schuler G .(2006). The glycosylation of pregnancy-associated glycoproteins and prolactin-related protein-I in bovine binucleate trophoblast giant cells changes before parturition. *Reproduction* **132:** 791-798.

Klisch K., De Sousa N.M., Beckers J.F., Leiser R., Pich A. (2005). Pregnancy-associated glycoprotein-1, -6, -7 and -17 are major products of bovine binucleate trophoblast giant cells at midpregnancy. *Molecular Reproduction and Development* **71:** 453-460.

Lopata A., Hay D.L .(1989). The potential of early human embryos to form blastocysts, hatch from their zona and secrete HCG in culture. *Human Reproduction* **4:** 87-94.

Lopez-Gatius F., Garbayo J.M., Santolaria P., Yaniz J., Ayad A., de Sousa N.M. (2007). Milk production correlates negatively with plasma levels of pregnancy-associated glycoprotein (PAG) during the early fetal period in high producing dairy cows with live fetuses. *Domestic Animal Endocrinology* **32:** 29-42.

Marques M.O., Madureira E.H., Oliveira C.A., Bo G.A., Baruselli P.S. (2002). Ovarian ultrasonography and plasma progesterone concentration in Bos taurus x Bos indicus heifers administered different treatments on Day 7 of the estrous cycle. *Theriogenology* **57:** 548.

Massip A ., Mulnard J. (1980). Time-lapse cinematographic analysis of hatching of normal and frozen-thawed cow blastocysts. *Journal of Reproduction and Fertility* **58:** 475-478.

Maurer R.R ., Chenault J.R. (1983). Fertilization failure and embryonic mortality in parous and nonparous beef cattle. *Journal of Animal Sciences* **56:** 1186-1190.

McCracken J., Schramm W., Okulicz W.C. (1984): Hormone Receptor control of pulsatile secretion of $PGF_{2\alpha}$ from the ovine uterus during luteolysis and its abrogation in early pregnancy. *Animal Reproduction Sciences* **7:** 31-55.

Meyer M.D., Hansen P.J., Thatcher W.W., Drost M., Badinga L., Roberts R.M., Li J., Ott T.L., Bazer F.W. (1995). Extension of corpus luteum life span and reduction of uterine secretion of prostaglandin F2α of cows in response to recombinant interferon-tau. *Journal of Dairy Science* **78:** 1921-1931.

Mialon M.M., Camous S., Renand G., Martal J., Menissier F. (1993). Peripheral concentrations of a 60-kDa pregnancy serum protein during gestation and after calving and in relationship to embryonic mortality in cattle. *Reproduction Nutrition and Development* **33:** 269-282.

Mihm M., Currant N., Hytell P., Boland M.P., Roche J.F. (1994). Resumption of meiosis in cattle oocytes from pre-ovulatory follicles with a short and long duration of dominance. *Journal of Reproduction and Fertility*. Abstr Ser 1994: 13-14.

Mintz B (1971). Control of embryo implantation and survival. *Advances in Biosciences* **6:** 317-341.

Munson L., Kao J.J., Schlafer D.H. (1989). Characterization of glycoconjugates in the bovine endometrium and chorion by lectin histochemistry. *Journal of Reproduction and Fertility* **87:** 509-517.

Niemann H., Elsaesser F. (1987). Steroid hormones in early pig embryo development. In Bavister, B.D. (ed.) The Mammalian Preimplantation Embryo. Plenum Press, New York, USA, pp. 117-132.

Odensvik K., Gustafsson H., Kindahl H. (1998). The effect on luteolysis by intensive oral administration of flunixin granules in heifers. *Animal Reproduction Science* **50:** 35-44.

Oliveira J.F., Henkes L.E., Ashley R.L., Purcell S.H., Smirnova N.P., Veeramachaneni D.N., Anthony R.V., Hansen T.R. (2008). Expression of interferon (IFN)-stimulated genes in extrauterine tissues during early pregnancy in sheep is the consequence of endocrine IFN-tau release from the uterine vein. *Endocrinology* **149:** 1252-1259.

Perenyi Z.S., Szenci O., Sulon J., Drion P.V., Beckers J.F. (2002). Comparison of the ability of three radioimmunoassay to detect pregnancy-associated glycoproteins in bovine plasma. *Reproduction in Domestic Animals* **37:** 100-104.

Peters A.R. (1996). Embryo mortality in the cow. *Animal Breeding Abstract* **64:** 587-598.

Piller V., Piller F., Cartron J.P. (1990). Comparison of the carbohydrate binding specificities of seven N-acetyl-D-galactosamine-recognizing lectins. *European Journal of Biochemistry* **191:** 461-466.

Rawlings N.C., Jeffcoate I.A., Savage N.C., Steuart D.M.K., Steuart L.H.M. (1983). Pregnancy diagnosis and assessment of fetal numbers in the ewe in a commercial setting. *Theriogenology* **19:** 655-663.

Roberts R.M., Ealy A.D., Alexenko A.P., Han C.S., Ezashi T.(1999). Trophoblast interferons. *Placenta* **20:** 259-264.

Roberts R.M., Xie S., Mathialagan N. (1996). Maternal recognition of pregnancy. *Biology of Reproduction* **54:** 294-302.

Robinson J.J. (1983) .Nutrition of pregnant ewes. In: HaresignW, editor. Sheep production. London: Butterworth p. 111.

Rose N.C., Mennuti M.T. (1993). Maternal serum screening for neural tube defects and fetal chromosome abnormalities, In: Fetal Medicine [Special Issue]. *The Western Journal of Medicine* **159:** 312-317.

Rosenfeld C.S., Han C.S., Alexenko A.P., Spencer T.E., Roberts R.M. (2002). Expression of interferon receptor subunits, IFNAR1 and IFNAR2, in the ovine uterus. *Biology of Reproduction* **67:** 847-853.

Rowson L.E., Moor R.M. (1966). Development of the sheep conceptus during the first fourteen days. *Journal of Anatomy* **100:** 777-785.

Santos J.E., Thatcher W.W., Chebel R.C., Cerri R.L., Galvao K.N. (2004). The effect of embryonic death rates in cattle on the efficacy of estrus synchronization programs. *Animal Reproduction Science* **82/83:** 513-535.

Sartori R., Sartor-Bergfelt R., Mertens S.A., Guenther J.N., Parrish J.J., Wiltbank M.C. (2002). Fertilization and early embryonic development in heifers and lactating cows in summer, lactating and dry cows in winter. *Journal of Dairy Sciences* **85:** 2803-2812.

Sawada H., Yamazaki K., Hoshi M. (1990). Trypsin-like hatching protease from mouse embryos: evidence for the presence in culture medium and its enzymatic properties. *Journal of Experimental Zoology* **254:** 83-87.

Semambo D.K., Eckersall P.D., Sasser R.G., Ayliffe T.R. (1992). Pregnancyspecific protein B and progesterone in monitoring viability of the embryo in early pregnancy in the cow after experimental infection with Actinomyces pyogenes. *Theriogenology* **37:** 741-748.

Seshagiri P.B., Hearn J.P. (1993). In-vitro development of in-vivo produced rhesus monkey morulae and blastocysts to hatched, attached, and post-attached blastocyst stages: morphology and early secretion of chorionic gonadotrophin. *Human Reproduction* **8:** 279-287.

Silva E., Sterry R.A., Kolb D., Mathialagan N., McGrath M.F., Ballam J.M. (2007). Accuracy of a pregnancy-associated glycoprotein ELISA to determine pregnancy status of lactating dairy cows twenty-seven days after timed artificial insemination. *Journal of Dairy Science* **90:** 4612-4622.

Spencer T.E., Bartol F.F., Bazer F.W., Johnson G.A., Joyce M.M. (1999).Identification and characterization of glycosylation-dependent cell adhesion molecule 1-like protein expression in the ovine uterus. *Biology of Reproduction* **60:** 241-250.

Spencer T.E., Bazer F.W. (1995). Temporal and spatial alterations in uterine estrogen receptor and progesterone receptor gene expression during the estrous cycle and early pregnancy in the ewe. *Biology of Reproduction* **53:** 1527-1543.

Spencer T.E., Bazer F.W. (1996). Ovine interferon tau suppresses transcription of the estrogen receptor and oxytocin receptor genes in the ovine endometrium. *Endocrinology* **137:** 1144-1147.

Spencer T.E., Becker W.C., George P., Mirando M.A., Ogle T.F., Bazer F.W. (1995). Ovine interferon-tau regulates expression of endometrial receptors for estrogen and oxytocin but not progesterone. *Biology of Reproduction* **53:** 732-745.

Spencer T.E., Ing N.H., Ott T.L., Mayes J.S., Becker W.C., Watson G.H., Mirando M.A., Brazer F.W. (1995b). Intrauterine injection of ovine interferon-tau alters oestrogen receptor and oxytocin receptor expression in the endometrium of cyclic ewes. *Journal of Molecular Endocrinology* **15:** 203-220.

Spencer T.E., Johnson G.A., Burghardt R.C., Bazer F.W. (2004). Progesterone and placental hormone actions on the uterus: insights from domestic animals. *Biology of Reproduction* **71:** 2-720.

Spencer T.E., Johnson G.A., Bazer F.W., Burghardt R.C. (2004). Implantation mechanisms: insights from the *Reproduction* **128:** 657-668.

Surani MAH.(1975). Zona pellucida denudation, blastocyst proliferation and attachment in rats. *Journal of Embryology and Experimental Morphology* **33:** 343-353.

Szafranska B., Majewska M., Panasiewicz G. (2004). N-glycodiversity of the pregnancy-associated glycoprotein family (PAG) produced *in vitro* by trophoblast and trophectoderm explants during implantation, placentation and advanced pregnancy in pig. *Biology of Reproduction* **4:** 67-89.

Szafranska B., Panasiewicz G., Waclawik A. (2001). Length polymorphism of PCR-amplified genomic fragments of the pregnancy-associated glycoprotein (PAG) gene family in the pig and some other domestic and wild mammals. *Journal of Applied Genetics* **42:** 335-349.

Szenci O., Beckers J.F., Humblot P., Sulon J., Sasser G., Taverne MA. (1998). Comparison of ultrasonography, bovine pregnancy-specific protein B, and bovine pregnancy-associated glycoprotein 1 tests for pregnancy detection in dairy cows. *Theriogenology* **50:** 77-88.

Szenci O., Beckers J.F., Sulon J., Bevers M.M., Borzsonyi L., Fodor L. (2003). Effect of induction of late embryonic mortality on plasma profiles of pregnancy associated glycoprotein 1 in heifers. *The Veterinary Journal* **165:** 307-313.

Thurmond M.C., Picanso J.P., Jameson C.M. (1990). Considerations for use of descriptive epidemiology to investigate fetal loss in dairy cows. *Journal of American Veterinary and Medical Association* **197:** 1305-1312.

Tyrrell R.N., Plant J.W. (1979). Rectal damage in ewes following pregnancy diagnosis by rectal-abdominal palpation. *Journal of Animal Science* **48:** 348-350.

Ushizawa K., Takahashi T., Hosoe M., Kaneyama K., Hashizume K. (2005). Cloning and expression of two new prolactin-related proteins, prolactin-related protein-VIII and -IX, in bovine placenta. *Reproductive Biology and Endocrinology* **3:** 68.

Vandaele L., Verberckmoes S., El-Amiri J., Sulon J., Duchateau L., Van Soom A. (2005). Use of homologous radioimmunoassay (RIA) to evaluate the effect of maternal and fetal parameters on pregnancy associated glycoprotein (PAG) concentrations in sheep. *Theriogenology* **63:** 1914-1924.

Vu T.K.H., Liu R.W., Haaksma C.J.(1997). Identification and cloning of the membrane-associated serine protease, hepsin, from mouse preimplantation embryos. *Journal of Biological Chemistry* **272:** 31315-31320.

Wathes D.C., Hamon M. (1993). Localization of oestradiol, progesterone and oxytocin receptors in the uterus during the oestrous cycle and early pregnancy of the ewe. *Journal of Endocrinology* **138:** 479-492.

Wathes D.C., Lamming G.E. (1995): The oxytocin receptor, luteolysis and the maintenance of pregnancy. *Journal of Reproduction and Fertility.(Supplement)* **49:** 53-67.

White I.R., Russel A.J.F., Fowler D.G. (1984). Real-time ultrasonic scanning in the diagnosis of pregnancy and the determination of fetal numbers in sheep. *Veterinary Record.* **115:** 140-143.

Whitlock B.K., Maxwell H.S. (2008). Pregnancy-associated glycoproteins and pregnancy wastage in cattle. *Theriogenology* **70:** 550-559.

Wilkins J.F., Hoffman W.D., Larsson S.K., Hamilton B.A., Hemressy D.W., Hillard M.A. (1996). Protected lipid/protein supplement improves synchrony of estrous and conception rate in beef cows. 13th Intern Congr Anim Reprod, Sydney, Australia **3:** 19-29.

Wimsatt W.A. (1950). New histological observations on the placenta of the sheep. *American Journal of Anatomy* **87:** 391-436.

Wimsatt W.A. (1951). Observations of the morphogenesis, cytochemistry and significance of the binucleate giant cells of the placenta of ruminants. *Journal of Anatomy* **89:** 233-282.

Wintenberger-Torres S., Flechon J.E. (1974). Ultrastructural evolution of the trophoblast cells of the pre-implantation sheep blastocyst from day 8 to day 18. *Journal of Anatomy* **118:** 143-153.

Wooding F.B. (1984) Role of binucleate cells in fetomaternal cell fusion at implantation in the sheep. *American Journal of Anatomy* **170:** 233-250.

Wooding F.B. (1992). Current topic: the synepitheliochorial placenta of ruminants: binucleate cell fusions and hormone production. *Placenta* **13:** 101-113.

Wooding F.B., Staples L.D., Peacock M.A. (1982). Structure of trophoblast papillae on the sheep conceptus at implantation. *Journal of Anatomy* **134:** 507-516.

Wooding F.B.P., Flint A.P.F. (1994). Placentation. In: Marshall's Physiologyof Reproduction, edn 4 Ed. GE Lamming. London:Chapman & Hall., pp 233-460.

Xie S., Green J., Bixby J.B., Szafranska B., DeMartini J.C., Hecht S.(1997).The diversity and evolutionary relationships of the pregnancy- associated glycoproteins, an aspartic proteinase subfamily consisting of many trophoblast-expressed genes. *Proceedings of National Academy of Science*, USA. **94:** 12809-12816.

Xie S., Low B.G., Nagel R.J., Kramer K.K., Anthony R.V., Zoli A.P., Beckers J.F., Roberts R.M. (1991). Identification of the major pregnancy-specific antigens of cattle and sheep as inactive members of the aspartic proteinase family. *Proceedings of the National Academy of Sciences* of USA. **88:** 10247-10251.

Zarrouk A., Engeland I., Sulon J., Beckers J.F. (1999). Determination of pregnancy-associated glycoprotein concentrations in goats *(Capra hircus)* with unsuccessful pregnancies: A retrospective study. *Theriogenology* **51:** 1321-1331.

Zoli A.P., Guilbault L.A., Delahaut P., Ortiz W.B., Beckers J.F. (1992). Radioimmunoassay of a bovine pregnancy-associated glycoprotein in serum: its application for pregnancy diagnosis. *Biology of Reproduction* **46:** 83-92.

Zoli A.P., Beckers J.F., Wouters-Ballman P., Closset J., Falmagne P., Ectors F. (1991). Purification and characterization of a bovine pregnancy-associated glycoprotein. *Biology of Reproduction* **45:** 1-10.

□□□

Chapter 17

Reactive Oxygen Species, Oxidative Stress and Antioxidant Mechanisms in Utero-Ovarian Microenvironment of Livestock

S.C. Roy, J. Ghosh, K.S. Roy, A. Dhali, A. Mech
National Institute of Animal Nutrition and Physiology, Adugodi, Bangalore-560 030, Karnataka, India

Summary

In mammalian tissues, reactive oxygen species (ROS) are generated as by-products of aerobic respiration and metabolism. Low or physiological concentrations of ROS are required to cater diverse physiological functions including cellular signaling involved in cell proliferation and differentiation. However, an excess production of ROS beyond the scavenging capacity of cellular and extracellular antioxidants leads to oxidative stress (OS). This in turn leads to several OS-associated pathologies including disorders of the mammalian reproductive processes. Lipids, proteins and DNA, three vital components of cellular architecture, are the major targets of ROS attack. To maintain the physiological level as well as to scavenge excess production of ROS and as a part of adaptation mechanism, the mammalian tissue produces and secretes an array of enzymatic and non-enzymatic antioxidant molecules. Thus, in healthy animals, there exists a fine balance between the pro-oxidants and the antioxidants to maintain the reduction and oxidation (redox) status of cellular microenvironment. In undernourished animals and certain pathological or inflammatory conditions such as endometritis, the antioxidant defense arsenal of endometrium or uterine microenvironment becomes weak and causes OS-associated early pregnancy loss (EPL) in livestock. Possible ways to treat the above problem could be either potentiating endometrial antioxidant defenses through administration of vital micronutrients or enhancing the antioxidant gene expression by factors that remain to be explored and identified.

Reactive oxygen species (ROS) are highly reactive oxidizing agents belonging to the class of free-radicals. A free radical is any compound (not necessarily derived from oxygen) which contains one or more unpaired electrons in its outermost orbital. They initiate chain reactions by removal of an electron from another molecule to complete its own orbital. The most common ROS that have potential implications in reproductive biology includes superoxide anion (O_2·-), hydrogen peroxide (H_2O_2), hydroxyl radical (OH) and nitric oxide (NO•). Sometimes, NO• is classified under reactive nitrogen species (RNS). Out of these, OH·reacts rapidly with almost every molecule, whereas O_2·-, H_2O_2 and NO• only react quickly with a few molecules.

In mammalian tissues, ROS are generated as by-products of aerobic respiration and metabolism. Low or physiological concentrations of ROS are required to cater diverse physiological functions including cellular signaling involved in cell proliferation and differentiation. Any excess production of these ROS is controlled or scavenged by an array of antioxidants that are produced by mammalian cells. Excess production of ROS beyond the capacity of antioxidants induces oxidative stress (OS) in cellular microenvironment that damage lipids, proteins and DNA of cells.

The ROS and antioxidants have been implicated in the regulation of various reproductive processes in mammals such as cyclic endometrial and luteal changes, follicular development, ovulation, fertilization, embryogenesis, embryonic implantation, placental differentiation and growth. In contrast, imbalances between ROS production and their scavenging by antioxidant systems induce oxidative stress that negatively affects the reproductive processes. High levels of ROS production during embryonic, fetal and placental development is a feature of pregnancy due to dynamic remodeling of the endometrium/developing embryo and associated angiogenesis. To maintain the physiological level as well as to scavenge excess production of ROS, the endometrium must produce and release an array of enzymatic and non-enzymatic antioxidant biomolecules in to the uterine luminal fluid (ULF). In case of any pathology, if this antioxidant defense arsenal is breached then it leads to oxidative stress and has been suggested as a cause of mammalian pregnancy related disorders such as recurrent early pregnancy loss (EPL), intrauterine growth restriction and fetal death. Among the ruminants; the incidence of EPL has been observed more in buffaloes as compared to cattle based on the several *in vivo* and *in vitro* studies.

1. Sources and nature of ROS

Under physiological conditions, majority of ROS are produced as by-products of oxidative phosphorylation (OXYPHOS) at electron transport chain (ETC) of mitochondria as it is the site of cellular respiration to convert molecular oxygen (O_2) to water (H_2O) (Boveris *et al.*, 1975). During the electron transfer, O_2·- are generated at complexes I and III. The formation of O_2·-, by single electron donation to molecular oxygen (O_2), is a very reactive unpaired electron state which is the initial step in the formation of ROS. The half-life of $O_2^{\cdot -}$ in cellular environment is approximately 10^{-6}s (Pryor, 1986). The $O_2^{\cdot -}$ spontaneously dismutates to H_2O_2 by intracellular enzyme superoxide dismutase (SOD) (McCord and Fridovich, 1969) which in turn may be reduced to H_2O and O_2. For the reason, in any system producing $O_2^{\cdot -}$, substantial amounts of H_2O_2 are also produced. Unlike $O_2^{\cdot -}$, H_2O_2 is very stable and can cross the cell membrane. The toxicity of H_2O_2 is mostly due to the formation of hydroxyl radicals (OH·) through the well established Fenton (Fenton and Jackson, 1899) and Haber-Weiss (Haber and Weiss, 1934) reactions in the presence of transient metal ions such as iron (Fe^{3+}). The OH· is the most toxic free radical of all ROS and responsible for majority of oxidative damages in mammals. The half-life of OH· at 37°C is 10^{-9} s (Pryor, 1986). It does not survive for more than a few collisions after its formation and its reaction with other molecules are site-specific.

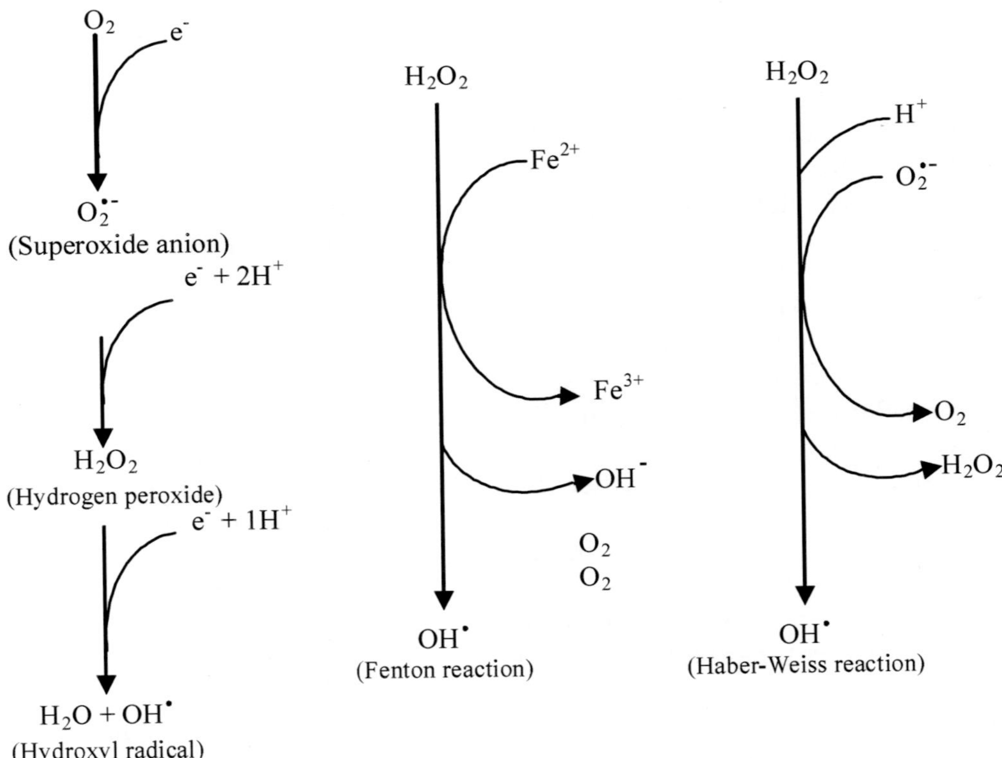

Fig. 1 : Genesis of various ROS in mitochondria and cytosol.

2. Extra-mitochondrial sources of ROS production

ROS are also generated via other extra-mitochondrial sources that include enzymatic pathways such as NADPH oxidase, xanthine oxidase, cyclooxygenases, lipoxygenases, monooxygenases, and cytochrome P450 systems. Polymorphonuclear leukocytes (PMNs) and phagocytes possess membrane bound NADPH-oxidase that generate $O_2^{\cdot-}$ for killing invading pathogens. A huge amount of $O_2^{\cdot-}$ is produced during respiratory burst of neutrophils for microbicidal action.

Nitric oxide (NO•), another free radical is produced from L-arginine substrate by nitric oxide synthases (NOSs) using NADPH as electron donor (Bredt, 1999). In mammals, NOS enzyme is of three different types that includes neuronal NOS (nNOS or NOS I), inducible NOS (iNOS or NOS II) and endothelial NOS (eNOS or NOS III). Neuronal NOS and endothelial NOS are constitutive NOSs and responsible for basal release of NO•. Inducible NOS is generally present in mononuclear phagocytes and produces a large amount of NO• for killing of bacteria. This is expressed in response to pro-inflammatory cytokines and lipopolysaccharides (LPS). The expression of iNOS is highly induced under pathological conditions of the female reproductive tract. The endothelial NOS (eNOS) is involved in vascular relaxation. The eNOS is expressed in theca cells, granulosa cells, and the surface of oocyte during the follicular development and involved in oocyte maturation and the ovulatory processes (Rosselli et al., 1998). In most organs, inducible NOS is expressed only in response to immunological stimuli. The pathological effect of NO• is often due to the formation of reactive nitrogen intermediates such as peroxynitrite ($ONOO^-$) rather than NO• itself. NO• reacts with $O_2^{\cdot-}$ to form $ONOO^-$. The $ONOO^-$ ion can diffuse freely within and out of the cell and react with lipids, proteins and DNA leading to lipid peroxidation, DNA damage and apoptosis. When cellular NO• production is higher than 1μM then it reacts with $O_2^{\cdot-}$ to form highly reactive $ONOO^-$ (Beckman and Koppenol, 1996). Peroxynitrite is a potent oxidant and has been shown to react with virtually all classes of biomolecules. Peroxynitrite can induce nitrosylation of several tyrosine residues that regulate enzyme function as well as lipid peroxidation.

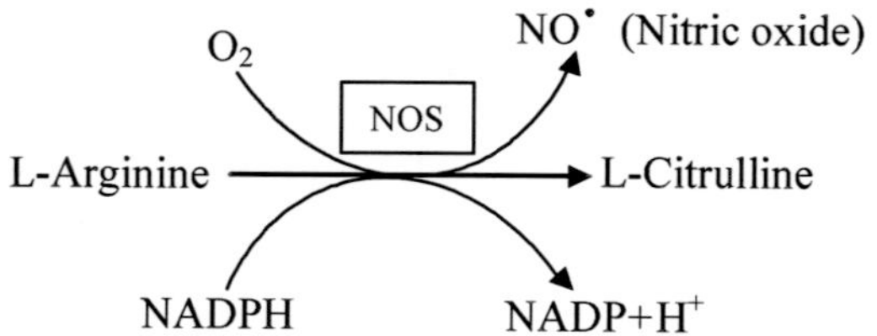

Fig. 2 : Production of nitric oxide by nitric oxide synthase

3. Physiological effect of ROS on reproductive processes

Earlier it was thought that ROS production is always harmful for body. But, now it has been established that these ROS at their physiological concentrations are highly essential to drive several physiological processes of body that includes follicular growth, corpus luteum (CL) formation, endometrial differentiation, growth of placental vessels, angiogenesis and apoptosis.

The ROS have been recognized as key molecules, which can selectively modify proteins and therefore regulate cellular signaling including apoptosis. Apoptosis or programmed cell death is a fundamental physiological process of mammalian systems which helps eliminating cells during early embryonic development (Pierce *et al.*, 1989) and plays an important role during tissue remodeling of the uterine endometrium and embryo implantation (Zhang and Paria, 2006). Mitochondria-generated ROS promotes apoptosis through activation of an intrinsic pathway. It is clear that ROS are involved in normal physiology and important in fighting infections.

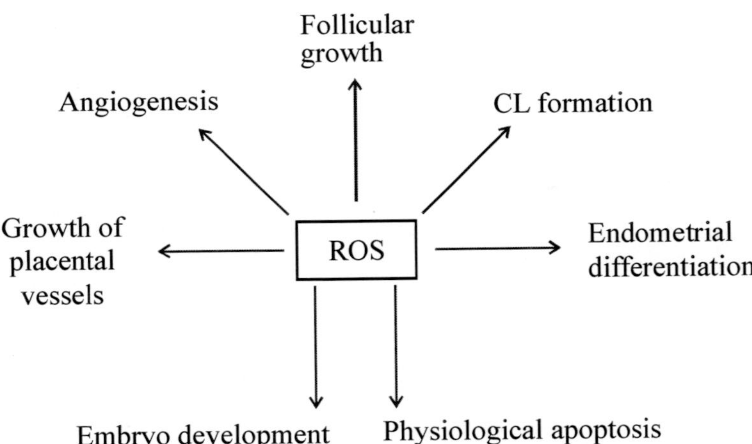

Fig. 3 : Reactive oxygen species drives diverse physiological functions of the body system.

4. Toxic effect of ROS

In a normal situation, there exists a fine balance between the ROS production and their scavenging to cater diverse physiological processes of mammals. However, in several diseases or infections (*e.g.*, endometritis, rheumatoid arthritis, inflammatory bowel disease) and environmental stress (*e.g.*, UV or heat exposure) the local production of ROS increases dramatically. An increased production of ROS by any cell beyond the capacity of the cellular antioxidant defenses leads to oxidative stress (OS), which ultimately cause significant cell damage through irreversible modification of vital cellular structures such as lipids, proteins and nucleic acids (Halliwell and Gutteridge, 1989).

4.1. Damage to DNA (DNA fragmentation)

The direct effect of high concentrations of H_2O_2 and O_2·- cause DNA damage which can be seen in the form of a base damage (depurination or depyrimidination), single strand breaks and double strand breaks.

4.2. Damage to lipid membranes (Lipid peroxidation)

Lipid peroxidation (LPO) is a process by which lipid hydroperoxides (ROOH) are formed from polyunsaturated fatty acids (PUFA) of cell membranes in a chain reaction providing continuous supply of free radicals that initiate further lipid peroxidation (Fig 4). In the process, malondialdehyde (MDA), a product of LPO, is formed, which can be measured by spectrophotometric technique. Lipid peroxidation alters functional properties of membranes and delivery of lipid to tissues (Halliwell and Gutteridege, 1999).

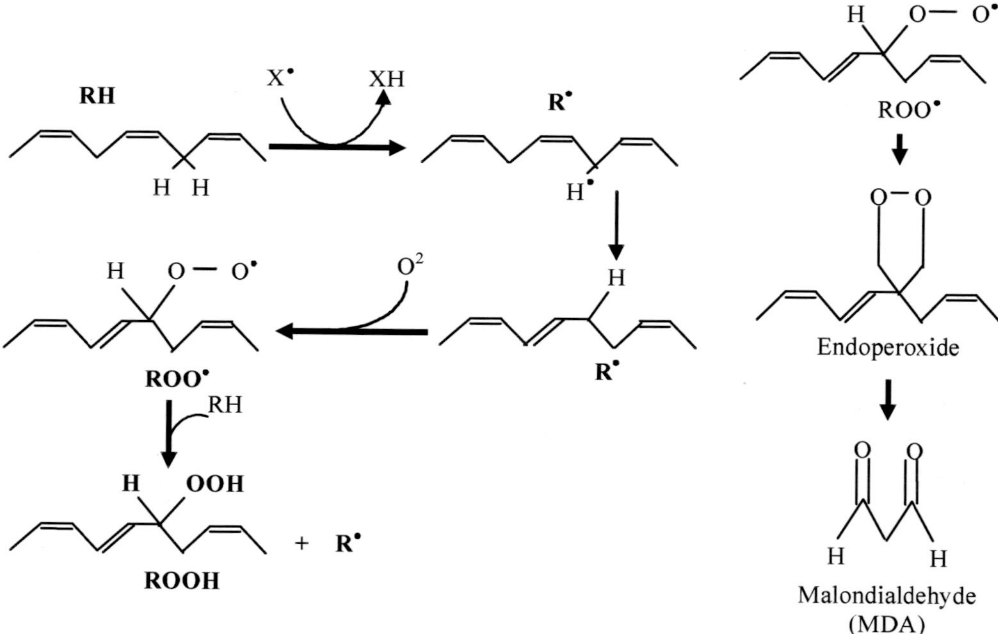

Fig. 4 : The process of lipid peroxidation: Membrane polyunsaturated fatty acid RH is attacked by a free radical (X·) producing alkyl (R·) and alkoxyl radicals (ROO·) in a chain reaction. The end product formed is malondialdehyde, the quantification of which serves as an indicator of degree of lipid peroxidation.

4.3 Damages to proteins

Excess ROS production causes oxidation of critical side chains of proteins including sulfhydril (-SH) groups leading to enzyme, receptor and carrier protein dysfunction. Proline, histidine, arginine, cysteine and methionine are prone to attack by ROS with subsequent fragmentation of proteins and cross-linking leading to inactivation.

5. Antioxidants

Maintaining a physiological equilibrium between intracellular levels of antioxidants and the production of ROS is crucial for the survival of the developing conceptus (embryo and its associated membranes). Tightly controlled ROS generation appears to be one of the central elements in the mechanisms involved in cell function, growth, differentiation and death (Valko *et al.,* 2007). Intracellular ROS production and propagation are controlled by highly complex and integrated antioxidant systems. The antioxidant defense system of mammals is comprised of two subsystems *viz.,* i) enzymatic antioxidant systems and the low molecular mass ii) non-enzymatic antioxidant systems that enable to cope with the oxidative stress environments (Table 1). Both the systems act coordinately to protect tissues and body fluids from damage by ROS whether produced physiologically or as a response to inflammation, infection or disease.

Table 1 : List of antioxidant defense molecules of mammals

Major enzymatic antioxidants	Major non-enzymatic antioxidants
1. Superoxide dismutases (SOD)	1. Vitamin E (α-tocopherols)
2. Catalase (CAT)	2. Vitamin C (Ascorbic acid)
3. Glutathione peroxidases (GPx)	3. Vitamin A (β-Carotene)
4. Glutathione reductase (GR)	4. Glutathione (GSH)
5. Peroxiredoxins (PRX)	5. Uric acid
6. Thioredoxins (TRX)	6. Pyruvate
	7. Lipoic acid
	8. Bilirubin
	9. Albumin
	10. Metal binding proteins *viz.,* Transferin, ceruloplasmin, lactoferrin
	11. Micronutrients (Cu, Zn, Se, Mn)

5.1 Enzymatic antioxidants

Mammalian cells have been bestowed with an array of antioxidant enzymes (Table 2) that include superoxide dismutases (SODs), catalases (CATs), glutathione peroxidases (GPxs), glutathione reductases (GSR), peroxiredoxins and thioredoxins to defend them against ROS damage.

5.1.1 Superoxide dismutases (SODs)

Superoxide dismutases are a class of closely related metalloenzymes that catalyze the dismutation of $O_2^{\bullet-}$ into H_2O_2 (Fig. 5). The SOD enzymes are present in almost all aerobic cells and in extracellular fluids. Thus, they constitute the first line of defense against the cellular production of $O_2^{\bullet-}$.

$$2O_2^{\bullet-} + 2H^+ \xrightarrow{\boxed{\textbf{SOD}}} H_2O_2 + O_2$$

Fig. 5 : Reaction catalyzed by super oxide dismutase (SOD) enzymes

Three distinct isoforms of SOD have been identified in mammals. The SOD1 or Cu,Zn-SOD contains Cu and Zn as metal cofactors and is present in the cytosol, while, SOD2 or manganese superoxide dismutase (Mn-SOD), is present in the mitochondrion and contains Mn as the metal cofactor. The SOD3 or extracellular form SOD (EC-SOD), is structurally similar to Cu,Zn-SOD, and also contains Cu and Zn as metal cofactors and present in high levels in the extracellular fluid of epididymis as well as the lung (Mruk *et al.,* 2002). The Cu,Zn-SOD consists of two subunits of identical molecular weight joined by a disulfide bond. There are two Cu and two Zn atoms per molecule (Bannister *et al.,* 1971) at its active site (Fridovich and Freeman, 1986). Copper is essential for the enzyme's catalytic activity, and zinc imparts stability to the protein structure (Fridovich, 1975, 1995).

In a gene knockout experiment, mice lacking SOD2 or Mn-SOD gene died within 10 days with cardiac abnormalities, fat accumulation in liver and skeletal muscle and metabolic acidosis (Melov *et al.,* 1998). Mn-SOD deficient mice also succumb to variety of pathologies including severe neurodegeneration and anaemia (Lebovitz *et al.,* 1996). The lethal nature of Mn-SOD knockout shows how biologically important is this enzyme in removing $O_2^{\bullet-}$. In contrast, the mice lacking Cu,Zn-SOD are viable but have numerous pathologies and a reduced lifespan, while mice without the extracellular SOD have minimal defects (Ho *et al.,* 1998). The importance of removal of $O_2^{\bullet-}$ is highlighted by the presence of three different forms of SODs in different cell compartments.

5.1.2 Catalases

The catalase is heme-containing enzyme that exclusively detoxifies H_2O_2 and converts it to water and oxygen (Fig. 6) using either an iron (Fe) or manganese (Mn) cofactor (Zamocky and Koller, 1999; Chelikani *et al.,* 2004). This protein is found in highest concentrations in peroxisomes of most eukaryotic cells and in lesser concentration in mitochondria and cytosol (del Rio *et al.,* 1992). Despite its apparent importance in H_2O_2 removal, humans with genetic deficiency of catalase or mice genetically engineered to lack catalase completely, suffer few ill effects (Muller *et al.*, 1997). It plays its specific role in liver.

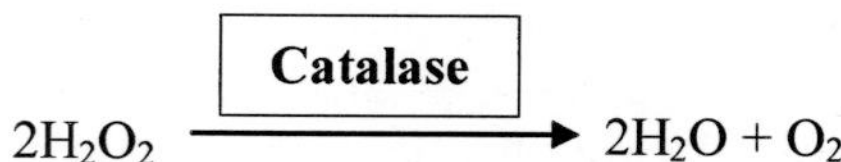

Fig. 6 : Reaction catalyzed by catalase enzyme

5.1.3 Glutathione peroxidases (GPXs)

Glutathione peroxidases (GPXs) are located within the mitochondrial matrix and cytoplasm and constitute the secondary antioxidant defense mechanisms that catalyze the conversion of lipid hydroperoxides (ROOH) and H_2O_2 to H_2O. Conventional GPX contains seleno-cysteine (SeC) at its active center and uses sulfhydril group (-SH) of glutathione (GSH) as an electron donor forming oxidized disulfide form of glutathione (GSSG) and play pivotal role in detoxification of these peroxides.

There are several isozymes of GPX encoded by different genes, which vary in cellular location and substrate specificity. So far, eight different isoforms of glutathione peroxidase (GPX1-8) genes have been identified in humans. Of these, GPX1, GPX2, GPX3, and GPX4 have been shown to be selenium-containing enzymes. The gene sequences of other three GPX (GPX 6, -7, and -8) have been deduced from whole genome sequence of bovine (Zimin *et al.*, 2009) but the proteins still remain uncharacterized.

Glutathione peroxidase 1(GPX1) or Cellular GPX is the most abundant version, found in the cytoplasm of nearly all mammalian tissues (intracellular erythrocytes, liver and kidney) whose preferred substrate is H_2O_2. Surprisingly, GPX1 is dispensable, as mice lacking this enzyme have normal lifespans, (Ho *et al.*, 1997) but they are hypersensitive to induced oxidative stress (de Haan *et al.*, 1998). GPX-1 is a tetrameric glycoprotein, requires selenium (Se) as a co-factor and contains a seleno-cysteine amino acid residue in the active site of each monomer that participates in the actual reaction mechanism of this enzyme. As the integrity of cellular and sub-cellular membranes depends heavily on GPX, the antioxidative protective system of GPX itself depends heavily on the presence of Se. The bovine cellular GPX-1 enzyme monomer has a molecular mass of 22.5 kDa.

Glutathione peroxidase 2 (GPX2) or gastrointestinal GPX is an intestinal and extracellular enzyme, is a selenium-dependent glutathione peroxidase responsible for the majority of the glutathione-dependent hydrogen peroxide-reducing activity in the epithelium of the gastrointestinal tract. Studies in knockout mice indicate that mRNA expression levels respond to luminal microflora, suggesting a role of the glutathione peroxidases in preventing inflammation in the GI tract.

Glutathione peroxidase 3 (GPX3) or plasma GPX is the principal extracellular form has been found in blood plasma (Martin *et al.*, 1993), breast milk and fluid lavaged from alveolar lungs and also present in amniotic and exo-coelomic fluid surrounding the embryonic tissue. It is a ~100 kDa homotetramer consisting of four identical 23 kDa subunits, each containing a seleno-cysteine residue at the active site.

Glutathione peroxidase 4 (GPX4) or phospholipid hydroperoxide GPX (PHGPX) catalyzes the reduction of hydrogen peroxide, organic hydroperoxides, and lipid peroxides at the expense of reduced glutathione and functions in the protection of cells against oxidative stress. The oxidized form of glutathione (GSSG)), which is generated during the reduction of hydroperoxides by GPX4 is recycled by glutathione reductase (GR) and NADPH/H^+. GPX4 differs from the other GPX family members in terms of its monomeric structure, a less restricted dependence on glutathione as reducing substrate, and the ability to reduce lipid-hydroperoxides (ROOH) inside biological membranes. GPX4 encodes an isoform that specifically detoxifies phospholipid hydroperoxides and is referred as PHGPX, and is expressed at high levels in the testes.

Glutathione peroxidase 5 (GPX-5) or epididymal androgen related GPX is mostly expressed in epididymis. Its activity is not dependant on Se.

5.1.4 Glutathione reductase and the glutathione-redox system

The glutathione-redox system includes glutathione (GSH), glutathione reductase (GR), glutathione peroxidases (GPXs) and glutathione *S*-transferases (Meister and Anderson, 1983). Glutathione is a tripeptidyl (γ-glutamyl-cysteinyl-glycine) molecule and is present in either the reduced (GSH) or the oxidized (GSSG) state by forming a disulfide bond between two molecules. It has pleiotropic roles, which include the maintenance of cells in a reduced state and the formation of conjugates with some harmful endogenous and xenobiotic compounds (Meister, 1995). In addition, GSH serves as an electron donor for GPX that reduces hydroperoxides to the corresponding alcohols. The GSH levels are maintained by de novo synthesis that is catalyzed by two

$$\begin{matrix} H_2O_2 \\ ROOH \end{matrix} + 2GSH \xrightarrow{\boxed{GPX}} GSSG + O_2 + \begin{matrix} 2H_2O \\ R\text{-}OH \end{matrix}$$

$$GSSG + NADPH + H^+ \xrightarrow{\boxed{GR}} 2GSH + NADP^+$$

R

Fig. 7 : Reaction catalyzed by glutathione peroxidases (GPX) and glutathione reductase (GR) enzymes

enzymes, γ-glutamylcysteine synthetase (γ-GCS) and glutathione synthetase (GS). Glutathione reductase converts the disulfide form of glutathione *i.e.,* GSSG back the sulfhydril form using NADPH produced in the pentose phosphate pathway (Fig. 6).

Table 2 : Gene and protein character of bovine (*Bos taurus*) antioxidant enzymes/protiens

Gene Name	Name of the enzyme	mRNA accession no.	mRNA nucleotides (bp)	Protein accession no.	Protein length (aa)	Protein mass (in Dalton)
SOD1	Cu,Zn-SOD	NM_174615	867	NP_777040	152	15551
SOD2	Mn-SOD	NM_201527	1438	NP_963285	222	22096
SOD3	Extracellular SOD	NM_001082610	1143	NP_001076079	241	24500
Catalase	Catalase	NM_001035386	2291	NP_001030463	527	59784
GPX1	Cellular GPX	NM_174076	926	NP_776501	205	22528
GPX2	Gastrointestinal GPX	NM_001163139	927	NP_001156611	190	21890
GPX3	Plasma GPX	NM_174077	1585	NP_776502	226	23586
GPX4	Phospholipid hydroperoxide GPX	NM_174770	913	NP_777195	197	19625
GPX5	Epididymal androgen related GPX	NM_001025335	1652	NP_001020506	219	22694
GPX6	Olfactory GPX	NM_001163142	1412	NP_001156614	221	23045
GPX7	GPX7	NM_001101113	1234	NP_001094583	186	19182
GPX8	GPX8	NM_001046088	1120	NP_001039553	209	23852
GSR	Mitochondrial glutathione reductase	NM_001114190	2366	NP_001107662	519	56231
PRDX1	Peroxiredoxin 1	NM_174431	883	NP_776856	199	22034
TXNRD1	Thioredoxin reductase 1	NM_174625	3532	NP_777050	499	54640

[Source: http://www.ncbi.nlm.nih.gov. The details of authors/ references of each of the gene or protein can be found in the website by searching the particular accession number]

5.1.5 Peroxiredoxins (PRDX)

Peroxiredoxins are peroxidases that catalyze the reduction of H_2O_2, organic hydroperoxides, as well as peroxynitrite (Rhee *et al.,* 2005). All PRDX enzymes contain a conserved Cys residue that undergoes a cycle of peroxide-dependent oxidation and thiol-dependent reduction during catalysis. Mammalian cells express six isoforms of PRDX (I to VI), which are classified into three subgroups (2-Cys, atypical 2-Cys, and 1-Cys) based on the number and position of Cys residues that participate in catalysis (Wood *et al.,* 2003). These enzymes share the same basic catalytic mechanism, in which a redox-active cysteine (the peroxidatic cysteine) in the active site is oxidized to a sulfenic acid by the peroxide substrate (Claiborne *et al.,* 1999). Over-oxidation of this cysteine residue in peroxiredoxins inactivates these enzymes, but this can be reversed by the action of sulfiredoxin (Jönsson and Lowther, 2007). Peroxiredoxins seem to be important in antioxidant metabolism, as mice lacking peroxiredoxin 1 or 2 have shortened lifespan and suffer from hemolytic anaemia (Neumann *et al.,* 2003; Lee *et al.,* 2003).

5.1.6 Thioredoxins (TRX)

The thioredoxin system is comprised of thioredoxin (TRX), thioredoxin reductase (TXNRD) and NADPH. This is one of the best representative systems for its protective function against oxidative stress in various cells. There are three isoforms of mammalian TRX, i.e. cytosolic TRX-1 (Holmgren, 1985), mitochondrial TRX-2 (Spyrou *et al.,* 1997), and spermatid specific TRX (Jimenez *et al.,* 2004). Similarly, there are three isoenzymes of TRXR in mammalian cells, that is, cytosolic TRXR-1, mitochondrial TRXR-2 and testis-specific TRXR. The active site of all of these TRXs and TRXRs consists of two neighboring cysteines, as part of a highly conserved CXXXXC or CXXC motif that can cycle between an active dithiol form (reduced) and an oxidized disulfide forms. In its active state, thioredoxin acts as an efficient reducing agent, scavenging ROS and maintaining other proteins in their reduced state (Arner and Holmgren, 2000). The thioredoxin system contains the 12-kDa protein thioredoxin and its companion thioredoxin reductase (Nordberg and Arner, 2001). After being oxidized, the active thioredoxin is regenerated by the action of thioredoxin reductase, using NADPH as an electron donor (Mustacich and Powis, 2000).

5.2 Non-enzymatic antioxidants

The non-enzymatic antioxidants include glutathione (GSH), vitamin C (ascorbic acid), vitamin E (α-tocopherol), vitamin A (β-carotene), trace elements (Cu, Zn, Se, Mn), uric acid, polyphenols *etc.* Antioxidant micronutrients are the major dietary antioxidants that directly scavenge ROS, providing a major source of protection against the damaging effects of ROS (Asworth and Antipatis, 2001; Johnson *et al.,* 2003,). The primary antioxidant capacity of serum is derived from non-enzymatic antioxidants such as glutathione, α-tocopherol, β-carotene and uric acid (Halliwell and Gutteridge, 1989). Similarly, recently discovered polyphenol antioxidants such as epigallocatechin-3-gallate (a green tea polyphenol), curcumin (an active principle of turmeric powder) assist in preventing ROS damage by scavenging free radicals (Sharma, 1975; Ruby *et al.*, 1995; Frei and Higdon, 2003).

Dietary antioxidants play important roles in protecting cells from ROS damage. Both dietary and enzymatic antioxidants interact each other to control ROS production. Trace minerals may modulate cellular antioxidant capacities because many micronutrients form part of the active site necessary for the antioxidant function or act as cofactors in the regulation of antioxidant enzymes. Mitigation of oxidative stress-induced effect on cells may be mediated by modulation of gene expression of key antioxidant enzymes through feeding of vital antioxidant micronutrients.

6. Roles of oxidative stress and antioxidant defenses in pregnancy of livestock

In primates, oxidative stress affects a variety of reproductive functions such as oocyte maturation, ovarian steroidogenesis, ovulation, implantation, formation of blastocyst, luteolysis and luteal maintenance in pregnancy in mammals (Agarwal *et al.*, 2005). The pathological effect of OS on female reproduction is associated with lipid peroxidation, inhibition of protein synthesis, and depletion of ATP. Oxidative stress has been found to be related with several pregnancy-related disorders, most notably preeclamsia and intra-uterine growth retardation of primates leading to pregnancy loss (Gupta *et al.*, 2007). In preeclampsia, the placentation process is affected in the first trimester of pregnancy by abnormal decidualization and trophoblast invasion (Founds *et al.*, 2009). Endometriosis, polycystic ovary syndrome and recurrent abortions have been associated with inflammatory cytokines and an increased level of ROS (Iborra *et al.*, 2005). Cytokines and antioxidant defense system forms a network to promote the dialogue between the conceptus and maternal paracrine system that are associated with apposition, attachment and invasion leading to establishment of pregnancy. During an insult of OS, the above network is disrupted leading to pregnancy failure. However, the biological system has evolved several mechanisms to offset the potential deleterious effects of ROS. Mammalian pre-implantation embryos could vary in the capacity to reduce these deleterious effects of exposure to ROS, and this may contribute in part to their differential capacities to sustain development *in vitro*. Though, the effect of OS in livestock reproduction has not been fully elucidated, it appears that it affects livestock reproduction at various levels. In the dairy cow, oxidative stress has been associated with several pathological conditions, such as retained placenta, udder edema, mastitis, which in turn may impair reproductive performances leading to embryonic mortality (Hansen *et al.*, 2004, Ahmed *et al.*, 2009). Nitric oxide (NO•) has been shown to affect to an array of reproductive processes including tubal and uterine muscle contractility, smooth muscle relaxation and thus absence of this free radical may impair tubal motility and uterine contractility (Rosselii *et al.*, 1998; Norman *et al.*, 1999). Nitric oxide generating system has been detected in human and bovine oviduct (Roselli *et al.*, 1996). Uterine tract infections associated increase in NO• production may be toxic to the incoming sperm, as sperm viability and motility is found affected by excess local concentration of NO• (Roselli *et al.*, 1995).

In corpus luteum, ROS are integrally involved in luteolysis and apoptosis. $O_2^{\bullet}$-, OH• and H_2O_2 are the primary ROS generated in steroidogenic cells. An appreciable amount of OS experienced during luteolysis is possibly produced by macrophages within the regressing corpus luteum. The potentially toxic effects of these substances are attenuated by antioxidant enzymes such as catalase, superoxide dismutase and glutathione peroxidase (Rueda *et al.*, 1995, Sugino, 2006). Low expression level of catalase was found in the mouse corpus luteum during luteolysis. Catalase activities increased 6-8 folds on day 6-16 of the estrous cycle and then decreased during the luteal regression at different development stage of bovine corpus luteum (Rapoport *et al.*, 1998).

Transcripts encoding catalase was detectable in all stages of *in vivo* pre-implantation mouse embryos (from 1-cell to blastocyst stages) and there was decreased abundance at the second cell stage, which was probably due to degradation of maternal mRNA. In early embryos, transcripts for catalase were expressed in all pre-implantation embryo stages (Harvey *et al.*, 1995).

In bovines, an increased catalase activity was seen in oviductal fluid during the estrous cycle, to reach maximal activity just before ovulation (day's 18-20, Lapointe *et al.*, 1998). In cow, the oviductal fluid catalase activity increased by 2-fold from day 1 to day 20 during the cycle. Catalase levels increase during the estrous cycle, specifically in ampulla section of the oviduct (Lapointe and Bilodeau, 2003).

In bovine oviduct, the dynamic expression of the classical cytosolic GPX-1, the gastrointestinal GPX-2, and the extracellular GPX-3 emphasizes the importance of the control of H_2O_2 and lipid hydroperoxides (ROOH) in the female reproductive tract (Lapointe *et al.*, 2005). However, without the help of a phospholipase, these enzymes are unable to reduce membrane-bound lipid hydroperoxides. Thus, GPX-1, -2, and -3 alone cannot counteract the numerous effects generated by the peroxidation of membrane lipids. The phospholipid hydroperoxide glutathione peroxidase (PHGPx) is the only known intracellular enzymatic antioxidant that can directly reduce both phospholipid and cholesterol hydroperoxides located in cell membranes (Thomas *et al.*, 1990; Ursini *et al.*, 1985). Recently, the relationship between sex steroid hormones and the cellular antioxidant enzyme system has also been investigated. The expression of antioxidant enzymes in cow oviduct are differentially modulated during estrous cycle (Lapointe and Bilodeau, 2003).

In uterine endometrium, estrous cycle-dependent changes in superoxide radical and the superoxide dismutase levels were reported in rats (Laloraya *et al.*, 1991). It was suggested that superoxide radicals are involved in regulating the edema and cell proliferation of the uterus. Significantly higher activity of Cu,Zn-SOD was observed in early pregnant endometrium of human compared to non-pregnant endometrium (Sugino *et al.*, 1996). A decreased Cu,Zn-SOD expression and an increased concentrations of lipid peroxide and $PGF_{2\alpha}$ in human deciduas was associated with spontaneous abortion (Sugino *et al.*, 2000). This suggests that Cu,Zn-SOD contributes to the maintenance of pregnancy by preventing the accumulation of superoxide radicals that causes $PGF_{2\alpha}$ synthesis. The decrease in Cu,Zn-SOD activity after ovarian steroid withdrawal may be involved in endometrial breakdown (Sugino *et al.*, 2002). The activities of Cu,Zn-SOD was significantly increased in late luteal and early pregnant buffalo uterine luminal fluid (Roy *et al.*, 2008). The activities of key antioxidant enzymes have also been reported to change in sheep placentomes during early placental development (Garrel *et al.*, 2010). The progesterone has very less or no effect on the antioxidant enzyme system whereas the treatment with estrogen, either alone or in combination with progesterone, decreased SOD1 ($P < 0.01$), CAT ($P < 0.01$) and GPX ($P < 0.05$) activities in endometrial tissues (Al-Gubory *et al.*, 2008). In human, early pregnancy loss was associated with reduced activities of Cu,Zn-SOD, peroxiredoxin3 (PRX3) and thioredoxin-like 1 proteins (TXNL1) in placental villous tissue (Liu *et al.*, 2006). All of these proteins are part of the cellular defense mechanism against ROS under biological or pathological status during pregnancy (Sawicki *et al.*, 2003; Shibata *et al.*, 2003; Vorum *et al.*, 2004).

Glutathione (GSH), a tripeptide antioxidant, has been implicated in maintaining the meiotic spindle morphology of the oocyte. After fertilization, this thiol plays an active role in the formation of the male pronucleus, and has a beneficial effect on early embryogenesis to the blastocyst stage. GSH concentrations change within the oocytes during meiotic maturation and its synthesis is regulated by gonadotropins. Cumulus cells surrounding oocytes are structurally and metabolically linked with the gametes and involved in the process of glutathione synthesis (Luberda, 2005). It has been shown that the cumulus cells play an important role in the intracellular GSH synthesis in the oocytes of cow (de Matos *et al.*, 1997). Earlier studies have demonstrated that GSH concentration decreases about 90% (from 7 mM to 0.7 mM) from the unfertilized oocyte to the blastocyst stage (Gardiner *et al.*, 1994), while the total mass of the embryo remains constant. It was also demonstrated that the mouse embryo has substantial GPX and GPR activity throughout pre-implantation development. However, the pre-implantation mouse embryo does not have the capacity for *de novo* synthesis of GSH until the blastocyst stage, and further development *in vitro* is adversely affected by low levels of GSH-depleting or -oxidizing chemicals (Gardiner and Reed, 1994; 1995).

Blocking GSH synthesis during oocyte maturation prevents sperm nuclear decondensation after fertilization. Inhibition of GSH synthesis for two days preceding ovulation reduces ovum GSH content below 0.20 pmol and results in abnormal development of zygotes due to lack of transformation of the sperm nucleus (Calvin *et al.*,1986). Supplementation of culture medium with cysteine increases the GSH content of pig oocytes matured *in vitro* and subsequent male pronucleus formation (Yoshida *et al.*, 1993). Chemically induced oxidation of oocyte GSH content disrupts normal microtubule function and fertilization of hamster oocytes (Zuelke *et al.*, 1997). In oocytes, GSH levels change rapidly during progression of meiosis and early embryonic development, and high oocyte glutathione at the time of fertilization is required for male pronucleus formation and for embryonic development to the blastocyst stage (for review see Devine *et al.*, 2011). These studies demonstrate that GSH has an important role during fertilization of the oocyte and early embryo development.

Several studies have reported that there is an improvement in pregnancy outcome in animals through feeding of feed supplements rich antioxidant principles. The reproductive performance of sow was enhanced by administration of b-carotene or vitamin A (Coffey and Britt, 1993). Combined treatment of vitamin E and vitamin C decreased oxidative stress and improved fetal outcome in experimental diabetic pregnancy (Cederberg *et al.*, 2001). Administration of b-carotene associated to a-tocopherol improved embryo quality in superovulated Holstein cows (Sales *et al.*, 2008). Thus, pre-conception nutrition plays a major role in programming the offspring susceptibility to disease, which may be mediated by macro- and micronutrient deficiencies and oxidative stress (Chavatte-Palmer *et al.*, 2008).

Micronutrients *viz.*, Cu, Zn, Mn, and Se deficiencies impair cellular antioxidant capacities as they are essential constituents of enzymatic antioxidants *viz.*, Cu,Zn-SOD (SOD1), Mn-SOD (SOD2) and Se-GPX. In human, deficiencies of trace minerals such as Cu and Zn during pregnancy have been associated various pregnancy related disorders (Pathak and Kapil, 2004). Dietary Cu deficiency may impact the activity of SOD1 (Chung *et al.*, 1988), which has anti-oxidative function during fetal development (Jankowski *et al.*, 1993). Rat embryos cultured in Cu-deficient medium develop abnormally and have impaired antioxidant system (Hawk *et al.,* 1998). Maternal Cu deficiency was associated with multiple fetal development defects (Keen *et al.,* 2003). Increased ROS levels in the Cu-deficient embryo may cause oxidative damage and contribute to the occurrence of developmental defects (Hawk *et al.,* 2003). Embryos recovered from mice fed a zinc-deficient diet had fewer cells and delayed blastocyst development (Peters *et al.,* 1991). Zinc deficiency induces apoptosis of embryonic cells in rats (Jankowski-Hennig *et al.,* 2000). Supplementation of trace minerals in the form of mineral mixture to breedable cows yielded better estrous cycle pattern and conception rates (Selvaraju *et al.,* 2009). Cetin *et al.,* (2010) indicated that micronutrients may affect fertility, embryogenesis and placentation and prophylactic use of some micronutrients may be useful in preventing adverse pregnancy outcomes. Retention of placenta (RP) in Egyptian buffaloes was shown to be associated with oxidative stress as there was increase of blood OS markers such as malondialdehyde (MDA) and nitric oxide (NO) and decreases of catalase, superoxide dismutase, ascorbic acid, glutathione reduced (R-GSH) and total antioxidant capacity (TAC) values along with low zinc, copper, iron and selenium (Se) concentrations (Ahmed *et al.,* 2009).

7. Assessment of extent of OS in animals

Various methods have been developed and described to assess the extent of OS in animals in general and reproductive tissues/fluid in particular. Qualitative and quantitative assays of various OS biomarkers have been developed for the purpose. Superoxide dismutase (SOD) has been assayed using either the principle of autoxidation of pyrogallol (Marklund and Marklund, 1974) or reduction of acetylated ferricytochrome C using xanthine + xanthine oxidase system (McCord and Fridovich, 1969 as modified by Holand *et al.,* 1982). Catalase is assayed using the method of Aebi 1984. The GPX activities can be assayed using the method of Paglia and Valentine (1967). Glutathione and glutathione disulfied are assayed using method of Anderson (1985). The mRNA levels of SOD, Catalse and GPx enzyme genes in any tissues can be quantified by quantitative-PCR assay. Extent of lipid peroxidation can be assayed by the method of Ohkawa *et al.,* (1979) using the thiobarbituric acid reactive substances (TBARS). The assay of TAC relies on the ability of combined antioxidants (vitamin, protein, lipids, glutathione, uric acid, etc.) present in the cell lysate or tissue to inhibit the oxidation of 2, 2-azino-di-(3-ethylbenzthiazoline sulfonate) (ABTS) by metmyoglobin (Miller *et al.,* 1993; Benzie and Strain 1996; Benzie and Szeto, 1999). Various other methods are also available to assess the extent of DNA damage or apoptosis. Specific enzyme/protein products in tissues/fluids can be detected by Western blot technique.

8. Possible strategies to mitigate OS-induced pregnancy loss in animals

Thus, the current evidence suggests that OS can have significant negative impacts on female fertility and gamete health. Domestic ruminants especially cow and buffaloes may be under severe oxidative stress during peri-parturient period without showing any clinical symptoms. Studies have shown that the antioxidant defense system of these species is highly compromised. Hence, supplements in the form of dietary antioxidants may prove to be effective strategies to protect female fertility and recurrent pregnancy failure. Cetin *et al.* (2010) indicated that micronutrients may affect fertility, embryogenesis and placentation and prophylactic use of some micronutrients may be useful in preventing adverse pregnancy outcomes. Discovery of OS-responsive genes and proteins and their regulation by any modulators may be an interesting area of research for development of newer strategies for mitigating of OS-induced recurrent pregnancy loss in livestock.

Conclusions

In vivo, antioxidant enzymes operate in co-ordination to prevent excess production of ROS. The ROS and antioxidants have been implicated in the regulation of various reproductive processes including endometrial remodeling, fertilization, embryonic implantation, placentation and fetal growth. A fine balance exists between the ROS production and their control by antioxidant systems. The mechanism of oxidative stress-associated early pregnancy loss is not clear and could not be adequately investigated in large animal species because of ethical reasons. Also there is a lack of fundamental insights regarding cellular, biochemical and molecular regulation of these antioxidant enzymes' adaptive responses to an oxidant environment under both physiological and disease states which needs an urgent study on these aspects. There is also an urgent need to elucidate the mechanisms whereby conceptus development and survival are enhanced by essential trace minerals and vitamins. This in turn may lead to development of specific feeding programs to increase the reproductive efficiency of livestock.

References

Aebi H. (1984). Catalase in vitro. *Methods in Enzymology* **105:** 121-126.

Agarwal A., Gupta S., Sharma R.K. (2005). Role of oxidative stress in female reproduction. *Reprodive Biology and Endocrinology* **3:** 28.

Ahmed W.M., El Hameed A.R.A., ElKhadrawy H.H., Hanafi E.M. (2009). Investigations on retained placenta in Egyptian buffaloes. *Global Veterinaria* **3:** 120-124.

Anderson M.E. (1985). Determination of glutathione and glutathione disulfide in biological samples. *Methods in Enzymology* **113:** 548-555.

Arner E.,Holmgren A. (2000).Physiological functions of thioredoxin and thioredoxin reductase. *European Journal of Biochemistry* **267:** 6102-6109.

Al-Gubory K.H.,Bolifraud P., Garrel C. (2008).Regulation of key antioxidant enzymatic systems in the sheep endometrium by ovarian steroids. *Endocrinology* **149:** 4428-4434.

Asworth C.J., Antipatis C. (2001). Micronutrient programming of development through gestation. *Reproduction* **122:** 527-535.

Bannister J., Bannister W., Wood E. (1971). Bovine erythrocyte cupro-zinc protein. I. Isolation and general characterization. *European Journal of Biochemistry* **18:** 178.

Beckman J.S., Koppenol W.H. (1996). Nitric oxide, superoxide, and peroxynitrite-the good, the bad, and the ugly. *American Journal of Physiology* **271:** C1424-C1437 .

Benzie I.F.F., Strain J.J. (1996). The ferric reducing ability of plasma (FRAP) as a measure of "antioxidant power": the frap assay. *Analytical Biochemistry* **239:** 70-76.

Benzie I.F.F.,Szeto Y.T.(1999). Total antioxidant capacity of teas by the ferric reducing/ antioxidant power assay. *Journal of Agricultural and Food Chemistry* **47:** 633-636.

Boveris A.,Cadenas E.(1975). Mitochondrial production of superoxide anions and its relationship to the antimycin-insensitive respiration. *FEBS Letters.* **54:** 311-314.

Bredt D.S.(1999). Endogenous nitric oxide synthesis: biological functions and pathophysiology. *Free Radical Research* **31:** 577-596.

Calvin H.I., Grosshans K., Blake E.J. (1986). Estimation and manipulation of glutathione levels in prepuberal mouse ovaries and ova: relevance to sperm nucleus transformation in the fertilized egg. *Gamete Research* **14:** 265-275.

Cederberg J., Simán C.M., Eriksson U.J. (2001). Combined treatment with vitamin E and vita- min C decreases oxidative stress and improves fetal outcome in experimental diabetic pregnancy. *Pediatric Research* **49:** 755-762.

Cetin I., Berti C., Calabrese S. (2010). Role of micronutrients in the periconceptional period. *Human Reproduction Update* **16:** 80-95.

Chavatte-Palmer P., Al-Gubory K.H., Picone O., Heyman Y. (2008). Maternal nutrition: effects of offspring fertility and importance of the periconceptional period on long-term development. *Gynecologie Obstetrique & Fertilite* **36:** 920-929.

Chelikani P., Fita I., Loewen P. (2004). Diversity of structures and properties among catalases. *Cellular and Molecular Life Sciences* **61:** 192-208.

Chung K., Romero N., Tinker D., Keen C.L., Ameniya K., Rucker R.(1988). Role of copper in the regulation and accumulation of superoxide dismutase and metallothionein in rat liver. *Journal of Nutrition* **118:** 859-864.

Claiborne A., Yeh J., Mallett T., Luba J., Crane E., Charrier V., Parsonage D.(1999). Protein-sulfenic acids: diverse roles for an unlikely player in enzyme catalysis and redox regulation. *Biochemistry* **38:** 15407-15416.

Coffey M.T., Britt J.H. (1993). Enhancement of sow reproductive performance by B-carotene or vitamin A. *Journal of Animal Science* **71:** 1198-202.

de Haan J., Bladier C., Griffiths P., Kelner M., O'Shea R., Cheung N., Bronson R., Silvestro M., Wild S., Zheng S., Beart P., Hertzog P., Kola I.(1998). Mice with a homozygous null mutation for the most abundant glutathione peroxidase, Gpx1, show increased susceptibility to the oxidative stress-inducing agents paraquat and hydrogen peroxide. *Journal of Biological Chemistry* **273:** 22528-22536.

de Matos D.G., Furnus C.C., Moses D.F. (1997). Glutathione synthesis during in vitro maturation of bovine oocytes: Role of cumulus cells. *Biol. Reprod.* **57:** 1420-1425

Devine P.J., Perreault S.D., Luderer U. (2011). Roles of reactive oxygen species and antioxidants in ovarian toxicity. *Biology of Reproduction* (In press) DOI:10.1095/ biolreprod. 111.095224.

del Río L., Sandalio L., Palma J., Bueno P., Corpas F.(1992). Metabolism of oxygen radicals in peroxisomes and cellular implications. *Free Radical Biology and Medicine* **13:** 557-580.

Fenton H.J.H., Jackson H. (1899). The oxidation of polyhydric alcohols in the presence of iron. *Journal of the Chemical Society, Farday Transactions* **75:** 1-11.

Founds S.A., Conley Y.P., Lyons-Weiler J.F., Jeyabalan A., Hogge W.A., Conrad KP. (2009). Altered global gene expression in first trimester placentas of women destined to develop pre-eclampsia. *Placenta* **30:** 15-24.

Fridovich I. (1975). Superoxide dismutases. *Annual Review of Biochemistry* **44:** 147-159.

Fridovich I., Freeman B. (1986). Antioxidant defenses in the lung. *Annual Review of Physiology* **48:** 693-702.

Fridovich I. (1995). Superoxide radical and superoxide dismutases. *Annual Review of Biochemistry* **64:** 97-112.

Frei B., Higdon J.V. (2003). Antioxidant activity of tea polyphenols *in vivo*: evidence from animal studies. *Journal of Nutrition* **133:** 3275S-3284S.

Gardiner C.S., Reed D.J.(1994). Status of glutathione during oxidant-induced oxidative stress in the preimplantation mouse embryo. *Biology of Reproduction* **51:** 1307-1314.

Gardiner C.S., Reed D.J.(1995). Glutathione redox cycle driven recovery of reduced glutathione after oxidation by tertiary-butyl hydroperoxide in preimplantation mouse embryos. *Archives of Biochemistry and Biophysics* **321:** 6-12.

Garrel C., Fowler P.A., Al-Gubory K.H. (2010). Developmental changes in antioxidant enzymatic defences against oxidative stress in sheep placentomes. *Journal of Endocrinology* **205:** 107-116.

Gupta S., Agarwal A., Banerjee J., Alvarez J. (2007). The role of oxidative stress in spontaneous abortion and recurrent pregnancy loss: a systematic review. *Obstetrical & Gynecological Survey* **62:** 335-347.

Haber F., Weiss J. (1934). The catalytic decomposition of hydrogen peroxide by iron salts. *Proceedings of the Royal Society* **147:** 332-351.

Halliwell B., Gutteridge J.M.C. (1989). Protection against oxidants in biological systems: the superoxide theory of oxygen toxicity. *Free Radical in Biology and Medicine, Oxford: Clarendron Press*, pp 86-123.

Halliwell B, Gutteridge J.M.C. (1999). Free Radical Biology and Medicine, 3rd Edition. *Oxford: Oxford University Press.*

Hansen., P.J., Soto., P.Natzke., R.P. (2004). Mastitis and fertility in cattle - possible involvement of inflammation or immune activation in embryonic mortality. *Americal Journal of Reproductive Immunology* **51:** 294-301.

Harvey M.B., Arcellana P.M.Y., Zhang X. (1995). Expression of gene encoding antioxidant enzymes in preimplantation mouse and cow embryos and primary bovine oviduct cultures employed for embryo coculture. *Biology of Reproduction* **13:** 532-540.

Hawk S.N., Uriu-Hare J.Y., Daston G.P., Jankowski M.A., Kwik-Uribe C., Rucker R.B, Keen C.L. (1998). Rat embryos cultured under copper-deficient conditions develop abnormally and are characterized by an impaired oxidant defense system. *Teratology* **57:** 310-320.

Hawk S.N., Lanoue L., Keen C.L., Kwik-Uribe C.L., Rucker R.B., Uriu-Adams J.Y. (2003). Copper-deficient rat embryos are characterized by low superoxide dismutase activity and elevated superoxide anions. *Biology of Reproduction* **68:** 896-903.

Ho Y., Magnenat J., Bronson R., Cao J., Gargano M., Sugawara M., Funk C. (1997). Mice deficient in cellular glutathione peroxidase develop normally and show no increased sensitivity to hyperoxia. *Journal of Biological Chemistry* **272:** 16644-16651.

Ho Y.S., Magnenat J.L., Gargano M., Cao J. (1998). The nature of antioxidant defense mechanisms: a lesson from transgenic studies. *Environmental Health Perspectives* **106** (Suppl 5): 1219-1228.

Holand M.K., Alvarez J.G., Storey B.T. (1982). Production of superoxide and activity of superoxide dismutase in rabbit epididymal spermatozoa. *Biology of Reproduction* **27:** 1109-1118.

Holmgren,A. (1985). Thioredoxin. *Annual Review of Biochemistry* **54:** 237-271.

Iborra A., Palacio J.R., Martinez P. (2005). Oxidative stress and autoimmune response in the infertile woman. *Chemical Immunology and Allergy* **88:** 150-162.

Jankowski M.A., Uriu-Hare J.Y., Rucker R.B., Keen C.L.(1993). Effect of maternal diabetes and dietary copper on fetal development in rats. *Reproductive Toxicology* **7:** 589-598.

Jankowski-Hennig M.A., Clkegg M.S., Daston G.P., Rogers J.M., Keen C. (2000). Zinc-deficient rat embryos have increased capase 3-like activity and apoptosis. *Biochemical Biophysical Research Communications* **271:** 250-256.

Jimenez A., Zu., Rawe V.Y., Pelto-Huikko M., Flickinger C.J., Sutovsky P., Gustafsson J.A., Oko R., Miranda-Vizuete A. (2004). Spermatocyte/spermatid-specific thioredoxin-3, a novel Golgi apparatus-associated thioredoxin, is a specific marker of aberrant spermatogenesis. *Journal of Biological Chemistry* **279:** 34971-34982.

Johnson L.J., Meacham S.L., Kruskall L.J. (2003). The antioxidants-vitamin C, vitamin E, selenium and carotenoids. *Journal of Agromedicine.* **9:** 65-82.

Jönsson T.J., Lowther W.T. (2007). The peroxiredoxin repair proteins. *Sub-Cellular Biochemistry* **44:** 115-141.

Keen C.L., Clegg M.S., Hanna L.A., Lanoue L., Rogers J.M., Daston G.P. (2003). The plausibility of micronutrient deficiencies being a significant contributing factor to the occurrence of pregnancy complications. *Journal of Nutrition* **133:** 1597S-1605S.

Laloraya M., Kumar G.P., Laloraya M.M. (1991). Changes in the superoxide radical and superoxide dismutase levels in the uterus of *Rattus norvegicus* during the estrous cycle and a possible role for superoxide radical in uterine oedema and cell proliferation at proestrous. *Biochemistry and Cell Biology* **69:** 313-316.

Lapointe J., Bilodeau J. (2003). Antioxidant defenses are modulated in the cow oviduct during the estrous cycle. *Biology of Reproduction* **68:** 1157-1164.

Lapointe J., Kimmins S., MacLaren L.A., Bilodeau J. (2005). Estrogen selectively upregulates the phospholipid hydroperoxide glutathione peroxide in the oviducts. *Endocrinology* **146:** 2583-2592.

Lapointe S., Sullivan R., Sirad M.A. (1998). Binding of a bovine oviductal fluid catalase to maintain spermatozoa. *Biology of Reproduction* **58:** 747-753.

Lebovitz R.M., Zhang H., Vogel H, Cartwright J.Jr. Dionne L., Lu N., Hang S., Matzuk M.M. (1996). Neurodegeneration, myocardial injury and perinatal death in mitochondrial superoxide dismutase-deficient mice. *Proceedings of the National Academy of Sciences of the USA* **93:** 9782-9787.

Lee T., Kim S., Yu S., Kim S., Park D., Moon H., Dho S., Kwon K., Kwon H., Han Y., Jeong S., Kang S., Shin H., Lee K., Rhee S., Yu D. (2003). Peroxiredoxin II is essential for sustaining life span of erythrocytes in mice. *Blood* **101:** 5033-5038.

Liu A.X., Jin F., Zhang W.W., Zhou T.H., Zhou C.Y., Yao W.M. (2006). Proteomic analysis on the alteration of protein expression in the placental villous tissue of early pregnancy loss. *Reproductive Biology* **75:** 414-420.

Luberda Z.(2005). The role of glutathione in mammalian gametes. *Reproductive Biology* **5:** 5-16.

Marklund, S., Marklund. G. (1974). Involvement of superoxide anion radical in the autoxidation of pyrogallol and a convenient assay for superoxide dismutase. *European Journal of Biochemistry* **47:** 469-474.

Martin A.J.M., Ghosh. S., Coco-prados. M.(1993). Cloning of the bovine plasma selenium-dependent GPx (GP) cDNA from the ocular ciliary epithelium: expression of the plasma and cellular forms within the mammalian eye. *Journal of Biochemistry* **114:** 284-292.

McCord.I., Fridovich J.M. (1969). Superoxide dismutase. An enzyme function for erythrocuprein. *Journal of Biological Chemistry* **244:** 6049-6055.

Meister A., Anderson M. (1983). Glutathione. *Annual Review of Biochemistry.* **52:** 711-760.

Meister A. (1995). Glutathione biosynthesis and its inhibition. *Methods in Enzymology* **252:** 26-30.

Melov S., Schneider J.A., Day B.J., Hinerfeld D., Coskun P., Mirra S.S., Crapo J.D., Wallace D.C.(1998). A novel neurological phenotype in mice lacking mitochondrial manganese superoxide dismutase. *Nature Genetics* **18:** 159-163.

Miller N.J., Rice-Evans C., Davies M.J. (1993). A novel method for measuring antioxidant capacity and its application to monitoring the antioxidant status in premature neonates. *Clinical Science* **84:** 407-412.

Mruk D.D., Silvestrini B., Mo M.Y., Cheng C.Y. (2002). Antioxidant superoxide dismutase- a review: its function, regulation in the testes, and role in male fertility. *Contraception.* **65:** 305-311.

Mueller S., Riedel H., Stremmel W. (1997). Direct evidence for catalase as the predominant H_2O_2 -removing enzyme in human erythrocytes. *Blood* **90:** 4973-4978.

Mustacich D., Powis G. (2000). Thioredoxin reductase. *Biochemical Journal* **346:** 1-8.

Neumann C., Krause D., Carman C., Das S., Dubey D., Abraham J., Bronson R., Fujiwara Y., Orkin S., Van Etten R. (2003). Essential role for the peroxiredoxin (Prdx1) in erythrocyte antioxidant defence and tumour suppression. *Nature* **424:** 561-565.

Nordberg J., Arner E.S. (2001). Reactive oxygen species, antioxidants, and the mammalian thioredoxin system. *Free Radical Biology and Medicine* **31:** 1287-1312.

Norman J.E.,Thomson A.J., Telfer J.F.(1999). Myometrial constitutive nitric oxide synthase expression is increased during human pregnancy. *Molecular Human Reproduction* **5:** 175-181.

Ohkawa H., Ohishi N., Yagi .K. (1979). Assay for lipid peroxidation in animal tissues by thiobarbituric acid reaction. *Analytical Biochemistry* **95:** 351-358.

Paglia D.E.,Valentine W.N. (1967). Studies on the quantitative and qualitative characterization of erythrocyte glutathione peroxidase. *Journal of Laboratory and Clinical Medicine* **70:** 158-168.

Pathak P., Kapil U. (2004). Role of trace elements zinc, copper and magnesium during pregnancy and its outcome. *Indian Journal of Pediatrics* **71:** 1003-1005.

Peters J.M., Wiley L.M., Zidenburg-Cherr.S., Keen C.L. (1991). Influence of short-term maternal zinc deficiency on the in vitro development of preimplantation mouse embryos. *Proceedngs of the Society of Experimental Biology and Medicine* **198:** 561-568.

Pierce G.B., Lewellyn A.L., Parchment R.E. (1989). Mechanism of programmed cell death in the blastocyst. *Proceedings of the National Academy of Sciences of the USA* **86:** 3654-3658.

Pryor W.A. (1986). Oxy-radicals and related species: Their formation, lifetimes, and reactions. *Annual Review of Physiology* **48:** 657-667.

Rapoport R., Sklan D., Wolfenson D., Shanam A.A., Hanukoglu I. (1998). Antioxidant capacity is correlated with steroidogenic status of the corpus luteum during the bovine estrous cycle. *Biochemical Pharmacologoy* **1380:** 133-140.

Rhee S., Chae H., Kim K. (2005). Peroxiredoxins: a historical overview and speculative preview of novel mechanisms and emerging concepts in cell signaling. *Free Radical Biology and Medicine* **38:** 1543-1452.

Rosselli M., Dubey R., Imthurn B. (1995). Effects of nitric oxide on human spermatozoa: evidence that nitric oxide decreases sperm motility and induces sperm toxicity. *Human Reproduction* **10:** 1786-1790.

Rosselli M., Dubey R.K., Rosselli M.A., Macas E. (1996). Identification of nitric oxide synthase in human and bovine oviduct. *Molecular Human Reproduction* **2:** 607-612.

Rosselli M., Keller P.J .,ubey R.K. (1998). Role of nitric oxide in the biology, physiology and pathophysiology of reproduction. *Human Reproduction Update.* **4:** 3-24.

Roy S.C., Ghosh J., Roy K.S. (2008). Estrouc cycle and pregnancy-dependent modulation of antioxidant enzymes in buffalo (*Bubalus bubalis*) uterine secretions. In*: Compendium of 2nd International Conference on Trends in Cellular and Molecular Biology held at School of Life Sciences, Jawaharlal Nehru University, New Delhi from January 5-7, 2008. (Abstr. 40).*

Ruby A.J., Kuttan G., Babu K.D., Rajasekharan K.N., Kuttan R. (1995). Antitumor and antioxidant activity of natural curcuminoids. *Cancer Letters* **94:** 79-83.

Rueda B.R., Tilly K.I., Hansen T.R., Hoyer P.B., Tilly J.L. (1995). Expression of superoxide dismutase, catalase and glutathione peroxidase in the bovine corpus luteum: evidence supporting a role for oxidative stress in luteolysis. *Endocrine* **3:** 227-232.

Sales J.N.S., Dias L.M.K., Viveiros A.T.M., Pereira M.N., Souza J.C. (2008). Embryo production and quality of Holstein heifers and cows supplemented with b-carotene and tocopherol. *Animal Reproduction Science* **106:** 77-89.

Sawicki G., Dakour J., Morrish D.W. (2003). Functional proteomics of neurokinin B in the placenta indicates a novel role in regulating cytotrophoblast antioxidant defenses. *Proteomics.* **3:** 2044-2051.

Selvaraju S., Reddy I.J., Gowda N.K.S., Prasad C.S., Ananthram K., Sampath K.T.(2009). Effect of supplementation of area specific mineral mixture in improving reproductive efficiency in crossbred dairy cattle-a field study. *Indian Journal of Animal Science* **79:** 599-601.

Sharma O.P. (1975). Antioxidant activity of curcumin and related compounds. *Biochemical Pharmacology* **25:** 1811-1812.

Shibata E., Nanri H., Ejima K., Araki M., Fukuda J., Yoshimura K., Toki N., Ikeda M., Kashimura M. (2003). Enhancement of mitochondrial oxidative stress and up-regulation of antioxidant protein peroxiredoxin III/SP-22 in the mitochondria of human pre-eclamptic placentae. *Placenta.***24:** 698-705.

Spyrou G., Enmark E., Miranda-Vizuete A., Gustafsson J. (1997). Cloning and expression of a novel mammalian thioredoxin. *Journal of Biological Chemistry* **272:** 2936-2941.

Sugino N., Karube-Harada A., Sakata A., Takiguchi S., Kato H.(2002). Different mechanisms for the induction of copper-zinc superoxide dismutase and manganese superoxide dismutase by progesterone in human endometrial stromal cells. *Human Reproduction* **17:** 1709-1714.

Sugino N., Nakata M., Kashida S., Karube A., Takiguchi S., Kato H. (2000). Decreased superoxide dismutase expression and increased concentration of lipid peroxide and prostaglandin F (2alpha) in the decidua of failed pregnancy. *Molecular Human Reproduction* **6:** 642-647.

Sugino N., Shimamura K., Takiguchi S., Tamura H., Ono M., Nakata M., Nakamura Y., Ogino K., Uda T., Kato H.(1996). Changes in the activity of superoxide dismutase in the human endometrium throughout the menstrual cycle and in early pregnancy. *Human Reproduction* **11:** 1073-1078.

Sugino N. (2006). Roles of reactive oxygen species in the corpus luteum. *Animal Science Journal* **77:** 556-565.

Thomas J.P., Maiorino M., Ursini F., Girotti A.W. (1990). Protective action of phospholipid hydroperoxide glutathione peroxidase against membrane-damaginglipid peroxidation. In situ reduction of phospholipid and cholesterol hydroperoxides. *Journal of Biological Chemistry* **265:** 454-461.

Ursini F., Maiorino M., Gregolin C. (1985). The selenoenzyme phospholipid hydroperoxide glutathione peroxidase. *Biochimical Biophysical Acta.* **839:** 62-70.

Valko M., Leiter D., Moncol J., Cronin M.T.D., Mazur M., Telser J. (2007). Free radicals and antioxidants in normal physiological functions and human disease. *International Journal of Biochemistry and Cell Biology* **39:** 44-84.

Vorum H., Ostergaard M., Hensechke P., Enghild J.J., Riazati M., Rice G.E. (2004). Proteomic analysis of hyperoxia-induced responses in the human choriocarcinoma cell line JEG-3. *Proteomics* **4:** 861-867.

Wood Z., Schröder E., Robin Harris J., Poole L. (2003). Structure, mechanism and regulation of peroxiredoxins. *Trends in Biochemical Science* **28:** 32-40.

Yoshida M., Ishigaki K., Nagai T., Chikyu M., Pursel V.G. (1993). Glutathione concentration during maturation and after fertilization in pig oocytes: relevance to the ability of oocytes to form male pronucleus. *Biology of Reproduction* **49:** 89-94.

Zámocký M., Koller F. (1999). Understanding the structure and function of catalases: clues from molecular evolution and in vitro mutagenesis. *Progress in Biophysics and Molecular Biology* **72:** 19-66.

Zhang Q., Paria B.C. (2006). Importance of uterine cell death, renewal, and their hormonal regulation in hamsters that show progesterone-dependent implantation. *Endocrinology* **147:** 2215-2227.

Zimin A.V., Delcher A.L., Florea L., Kelley D.R., Schatz M.C., Puiu D., Hanrahan F., Pertea G., Van Tassell C.P. (2009). A whole genome assembly of the domestic cow, *Bos Taurus*. *Genome Biology* **10:** R42.

Zuelke K.A., Jones D.P., Perreault S.D. (1997). Glutathione oxidation is associated with altered microtubule function and disrupted fertilization in mature hamster oocytes. *Biology of Reproduction* **57:** 1413-1419.

❏❏❏

Chapter 18

Concepts and Advances in Prediction of Semen Quality and Fertility in Ruminants

S. Selvaraju, A. Arangasamy, J.P. Ravindra
National Institute of Animal Nutrition and Physiology, Adugodi, Bangalore-560 030, Karnataka, India

Summary

Selection of fertile bull and semen evaluation are main components of artificial insemination (AI) program. It has been estimated that up to 40% bulls maintained in the semen banks are inferior quality in terms of achieving pregnancy after artificial insemination. Hence selection of bulls plays an important role. Even today most of the semen banks select semen for freezing based on concentration, mass activity, progressive motility and total abnormalities. After freezing, the semen is evaluated based on post thaw progressive forward motility. Variations in conception rate between and within animals (between ejaculates) warrants inclusion of various parameters ranging from simple functional tests to molecular tests for efficient and accurate analysis of semen quality. An accurate laboratory test(s) that would give immediate results of fertility status would be very valuable. In this chapter, both the conventional as well as the recent methods of semen evaluation are discussed.

Reproductive biotechnologies continue to be developed for genetic improvement of mammals. In dairy sector, improving reproductive efficiency is 5 to 10 times economically more important than any other production parameters. The first biotechnology applied to improve reproduction and genetic gain in farm animals is AI. It has an enormous impact worldwide in many species, particularly in dairy cattle. Though AI using frozen semen emerged 50 years back, fertility rate with AI is less and unpredictable (Larson and Rodriquez-Martinez, 2000). Fertility is a multifaceted phenomenon influenced by various factors like male, female and the managemental including the technique and the time of insemination, *etc.*

Selection of fertile bull is very important to improve reproductive efficiency in dairy animals. The problem is also compounded due to the variation in fertility rate among bulls. In the dairy industry it has been reported that 20-40% of the bulls are sub-fertile. It is relatively easy to identify infertile bulls because their spermatozoa usually are considerably less motile or have abnormal shapes. However, identifying sub-fertile bulls with below average fertility or individual sub-fertile semen collections is typically more difficult because the defects are not always obvious. Sperm from sub-fertile bulls may appear normal, but insemination with this semen may produce conception rates 25 to 30 percent lower than the most fertile bulls. Since a single bull is used to inseminate hundreds of cows, the use of sub-fertile or infertile semen can have devastating consequences in the breeding industry. Identification of sub-fertile bulls prior to being used for AI would increase reproductive efficiency. More accurate and sensitive methods of fertility estimation are needed to identify these sub-fertile bulls.

The major problem in AI appears to be an inaccurate semen analysis before freezing and as well as after freezing/post-thaw. Hence, efficient semen evaluation methods are needed to predict fertility potential of a bull with high productivity trait.

1. Conventional semen evaluation

Conventional semen evaluation procedure includes macroscopic and microscopic methods. Using these techniques, semen fertility is being estimated to date. Though these techniques are employed with a minimum cutoff values in all the bulls, the fertility varies between bulls, suggesting that these techniques of semen evaluation are not sufficient to detect fertility of a semen sample.

1.1 General examination

The general examination consists of directly observing and examining the ejaculate in the tube to rule out any defect due to volume, color, odor or presence of dust particles (Table 1).

1.2 Mass activity

Mass activity is determined by placing a drop of semen on a slide, and observing it under a bright field microscope with maximum of 10X magnification (Fig. 1). The mass activity is estimated based on the presence and intensity of waves and eddies.

Table 1 : General examination of bull semen

Parameters	Normal sample	Remarks
Volume	6 ml (range, 1-8ml)	
Color	Milky or creamy white colour.	Watered milk: low concentration. Yellow: contaminated with urine Pink: presence of blood.
Odor	Similar to fresh milk	Smell of urine: presence of urine Unpleasant: disease in the testicles or in the reproductive tract.
Appearance	Opaque	Transparent: low concentration
pH	6.4-6.9	Above 6.9 are indicative of low semen quality

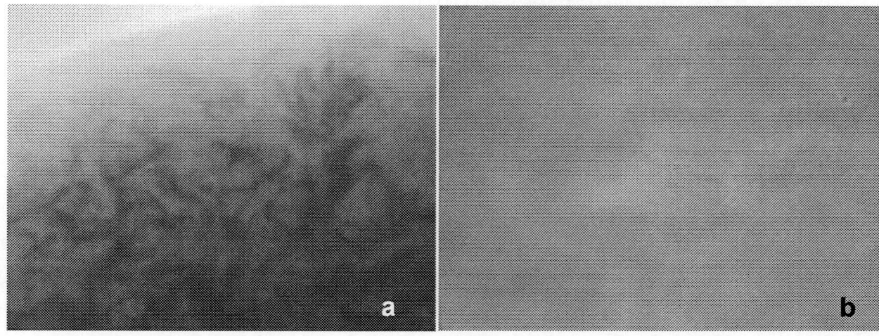

Fig. 1 : Semen mass activity: The good quality semen with extremely rapid waves and eddies (a, grade 5+) can be used for further processing and a poor quality semen with no motion waves and eddies mostly oscillatory (b, grade 2+) is discarded.

The rating of microscopic appearance

0 No swirl – immotile sperm
1 No swirl - stationary bunting (weak rotatory movements),
2 Oscillatory movements with no wave motions or eddies,
3 Motions with slowly moving waves and eddies
4 Rapid waves and eddies
5 Extremely rapid waves and eddies

1.3 Sperm concentration

Accurate and precise determination of sperm concentration in an ejaculate is important for AI stations in order to determine the number of insemination doses with an adequate number of sperm. The hemocytometer has often been referred to as the "gold standard" for assessing sperm numbers (Fig. 2). The use of a spectro-photometer is probably the most frequent method used by AI stations for assessment of sperm concentration. Electronic particle counters allow rapid determination of sperm concentration but tend to include any debris in the size range of sperm (Evenson *et al.,* 1993). Fluorometric measurement of the amount of DNA, using DNA-specific fluorochromes has been investigated (Fenton *et al.,* 1990; Hansen *et al.,* 2002), but this method requires stoichiometric staining of all DNA and minimal nonspecific fluorescence from the extender. Presently, photometers are commonly used in all AI centers. Photometric evaluation of sperm concentration reduces human error and the time consumption. The concentration of the spermatozoa in the ejaculate of the fertile bull varies from 3×10^5 to 2×10^6 per ml, with an average of 8×10^5 (Roberts, 1971).

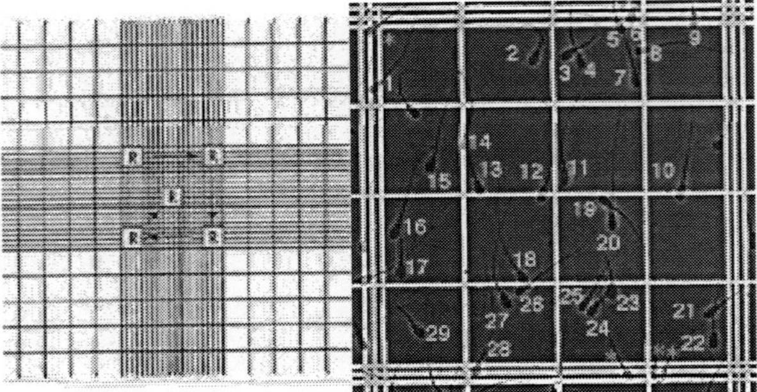

Fig. 2 : Assessment of sperm concentration using hemocytometer

1.4 Sperm motility

Motility of spermatozoa at the time of collection has been used commonly as a measure of the fertilizing ability of the sperm (Roberts, 1971; Bhosrekar, 1990). In addition to being a measure of spermatozoon viability, motility provides an indication that spermatozoa are able to navigate the barrier in the female reproductive tract that must be overcome to reach the oocyte. Although sperm motility does not correlate well with bull fertility, it can reflect the physiological status of bull spermatozoa after semen collection or cryopreservation. Spermatozoa have been found to lose their fertilizing capacity before they lose motility. Hence motility estimation not necessarily indicating the fertilizing capacity of the sperm (Hafez, 1993). Even under physiological conditions, expression of motility is not an entirely reliable parameter of sperm integrity and the poor motility does not always indicate cellular damage (Harrison and Vickers, 1990).

Normally 40-80% of bull sperm has been found motile (Hafez, 1993; Bearden and Fuquay, 2000), however, spermatozoa motility below 50% (Roberts, 1971, Bearden and Fuquay, 2000) has been known to be associated with low conception rate or poor fertility. The easiest and simple method of estimation of motility is a visual appraisal of the percentage of motile spermatozoa and the quality of the motility of individual spermatozoa under microscope (Hafez, 1993).

1.5 Sperm abnormalities

Sperm abnormalities are evaluated with an eosin-nigrosin stain (background stain) to highlight the cells. Abnormalities are classified as primary and secondary. Primary abnormalities are thought to arise in the testes, whereas secondary abnormalities arise in the epididymis or ejaculate. Some of the primary abnormalities include, head (micro and macro) defect, knobbed acrosomal defect, mid piece abnormalities, dag defect etc. Some of the secondary abnormalities include detached head, bent tail, protoplasmic droplets, *etc*. Some abnormalities are compensable, some are non-compensable. A non-compensable abnormality gives the animal a poor prognosis for any recovery.

Criteria for selection of semen sample for freezing should be mass activity 3+; progressive forward motility, >60%; spermatozoa concentration >500million /ml; total abnormalities - not to exceed 20%. In the post thaw semen samples, the progressive forward motility should be more than 40%.

2. Recent advances

2.1 Progressive forward motility by computer assisted semen analysis

Spermatozoa progressive forward motility along with certain velocity parameters are essential for the spermatozoa to achieve fertilization. Spermatozoa kinematic variables such as progressive forward motility, straight-line velocity (VSL), curvilinear velocity (VCL), lateral head displacement (ALH) and linearity (LIN) were correlated with bull fertility (Farrel *et al.*, 1996; Perumal *et al.*, 2011). The VSL (μm/s) is the average path velocity of the spermatozoa head along a straight line from its first to last position). The VCL (μm/s) is the average path velocity of the spermatozoa head along its actual trajectory. The percentage of LIN is the ratio between VSL and VCL. The ALH (μm/s) is the average value of the extreme side-to-side movement of the spermatozoa head in each beat cycle. A significantly higher VCL and ALH of the spermatozoa indicate major bending of the mid piece and large amplitude of lateral head displacement. This signifies the hyper-activation of the spermatozoa. Hyper-activation in turn implies high energy state of the spermatozoa, which is essential for sperm penetration through cervical mucus and fuse with the oocytes (Aitken *et al.*, 1985). Spermatozoa motility and velocity reflect their mitochondrial function indirectly. In bovine, specific motion parameters have been reported to be related to fertility (Budworth *et al.*, 1988; Kjaestad *et al.*, 1993; Farrell *et al.*, 1996). But the threshold levels for these motion characteristics have not yet been established to meet a general consensus. Such motion parameters can be measured using computer assisted semen analyzer (Fig. 3).

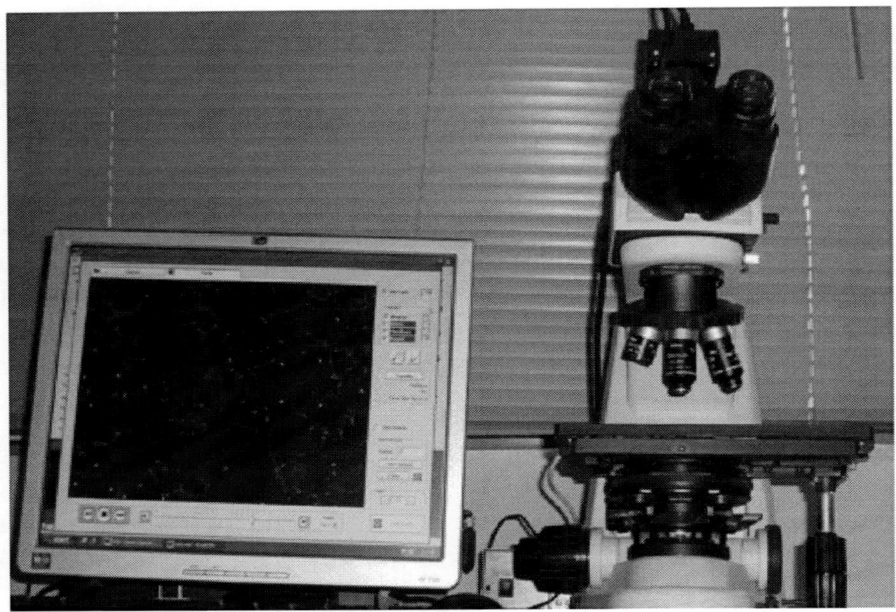

Fig. 3 : Computer assisted semen analyzer: Assessment of computer assisted semen analyzer has been used to assess semen motility as well as velocity parameters

2.2 Assessment of plasma membrane integrity

Assessment of plasmalemma characteristics is useful for predicting the fertilizing ability of sperm. Sperm plasmalemma integrity is essential for sperm metabolism, capacitation, ova binding and acrosome reaction. Various tests are being done to evaluate sperm plasmalemma include, permeability to stains and biochemical function. Sperm stains such as eosin/nigrosin, have been used to evaluate whether the plasmalemma is physically damaged or not. Sperm membrane functional status is essential since an intact and functionally active membrane is required for metabolism, capacitation and acrosome reaction, attachment and penetration of the oocyte (Jeyendran *et al.*, 1984).

A correlation was observed among spermatozoa positive for hypoosmotic swelling test (HOST), motility, viability and intact acrosome. Jeyendran *et al.* (1984) showed a good correlation between the percentage of spermatozoa undergoing swelling and the percentage of denuded hamster oocytes penetrated by capacitated spermatozoa of the same sample. The HOST is simple and inexpensive and has proved useful in predicting the spermatozon's ability to fertilize. After incubation in a hypoosmotic medioum (e.g. 100-150mOSm), the hairpin bend occurs in the principal piece of the spermatozoa tail as compared to iososmotic(300mOsm) solution, in which no tail bend occur (Fig. 4).

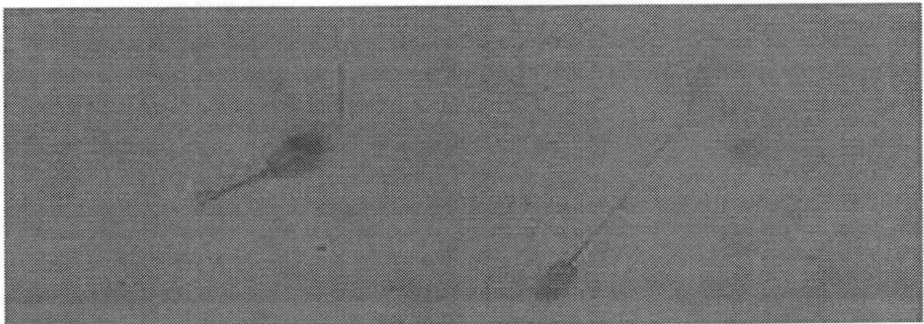

Fig. 4 : Evaluation of spermatozoa after hypoosmotic swelling reaction test Hairpin bend in the principal tail piece is considered as positive for HOST (a) as compared to other forms of tail bend (b) or no tail bend.

It has been reported that loss of the sperm plasma membrane integrity is frequently associated with infertility in males, despite normal semen parameters. Spermatozoa membrane integrity is measured using various tests like: plasmalemma integrity using dye-exclusion principle (eosin-nigrosin staining, carboxy fluorescein di-acetate-propidium iodide, *etc.*), functional membrane integrity using HOST, acrosomal integrity using Giemsa staining, *etc.* The HOS test to evaluate the functional sperm membrane integrity appears to give high repeatability and accuracy. This test was suggested to be a useful addition to the standard semen analysis. It is clear that measures of single sperm traits, or the results of single functional tests, are poorly correlated with fertility.

Evaluation of acrosomal status is very important because it is directly correlated with the fertilizing capacity (Henkel *et al.*, 1993). The use of morphological stains to characterize acrosomal status along with vital stains to differentiate live vs. dead sperm cells has been reported for cattle (Didone and graves, 1986), buffalo (Selvaraju *et al.*, 2008b). Using a stain that will differentiate acrosomal status as well as living from nonliving cells makes it possible to distinguish true acrosome reacted sperm (Fig. 5). Although maximum limit for acrosome alterations is not fixed, it is reported that the samples should not contain more than 40% of spermatozoa with acrosomal alterations.

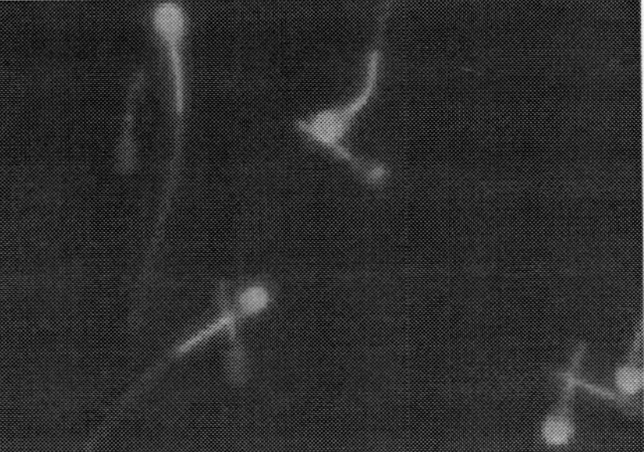

Fig. 5 : Assessment of acrosomal integrity in spermatozoa using fluorogenic stain (Carboxy fluorescin diacetate and propidium iodide). Note: Acrosome is present even in the moribund (head is read), which won't take part in fertilization. Hence mere assessment of only acrosome may not be helpful to analyse semen fertility.

2.3 Simultaneous assessment of functional membrane integrity (Hypo-osmotic swelling test) and acrosomal integrity

The independence of different regions plasma membrane surrounding the spermatozoa has been reported. As a result, the emphasis now is focused on analyses that incorporate multiple variables to examine how different sperm parameters interact to determine fertility. In this direction, sperm functional membrane integrity and acrosomal integrities are estimated in spermatozoa using hypo-osmotic swelling-Giemsa (HOS-G; Fig. 6) test (Selvaraju *et al.,* 2008b). This test is found have good correlation with *in vitro* (r = 0.9). If a sperm is positive for both these attribute suggest that the sperm can reach the site of fertilization (due to functional membrane integrity positivity) and penetrate through zona pellucida (due to acrosomal integrity positivity). This can be used to assess sperm fertility at the field levels (Selvaraju *et al.,* 2008b).

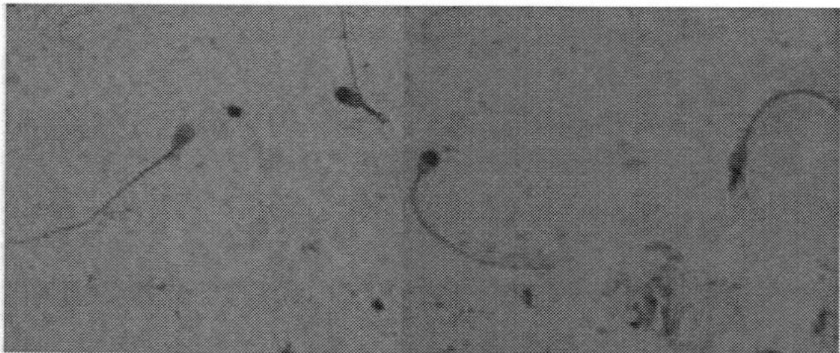

Fig. 6 : Hypo-osmotic swelling-Giemsa (HOS-G) test: A combination test evaluates functional membrane integrity and acrosomal integrities in spermatozoa

2.4 Mitochondrial membrane potential

Assessment of mitochondrial membrane potential can be considered as the most sensitive semen evaluation test. Mitochodrial membrane potential was assessed by using JC-1 (5,5′, 6,6′-tetrachloro-1, 1′, 3,3′-tetra-ethylbenzimidazolyl-carbocyanine iodide). The spermatozoa with yellowish to orange fluorescence (aggregates) in the mid piece were considered as cells positive for mitochondrial membrane potential (Fig. 7). The mitochondrial membrane potential varies significantly between animals and

Fig. 7 : Assessment of mitochondrial membrane potential. Note: Mitochondrial membrane potential varies between live spermatozoa) in spermatozoa. Spermatozoa with yellowish to orange color indicate spermatozoa with maximum membrane potential.

between groups and has a significant correlation with cleavage rate (Kasai *et al.*, 2002; Selvaraju *et al.*, 2009a). The reduction in mitochondrial membrane potential defines an early stage of apoptosis preceding DNA fragmentation, reactive oxygen species production and the late increase in membrane permeability (Garner *et al.*, 1997; Marchetti *et al.*, 2002). Hence, determination of mitochondrial membrane potential may be considered as an important parameter in buffalo semen analysis. The mitochondrial membrane potential found have good correlation with *in vitro* (r = 0.9; Selvaraju *et al.*, 2008b) as well as field fertility (r = 0.8, Perumal *et al.*, 2011).

2.5 DNA integrity and distribution

Existence of subtle sperm abnormalities that are unrecognized by conventional semen analysis may explain reduced fertility in assisted reproductive technologies in males. Therefore a greater understanding of the molecular basis of male fertility is essential for sperm egg interaction and embryo development. Sperm with abnormal DNA distribution has been associated with improper zygotic, embryonic and or fetal development (Saacke, 1998). Most of the sperm evaluation methods concern primarily the viability and functional status of spermatozoa, which influence the fertilizing ability of the gamete. However, vital factors essential for the sperm to produce a healthy and viable offspring primarily depends on the genetic material content. Since sperm DNA is uniquely condensed and organized, any abnormality associated with DNA, chromatin packing, or the sperm nuclear matrix should be reflected by a change in sperm nuclear shape (Fig. 8). The evaluation of sperm DNA distribution could be useful for assessing male fertility (Selvaraju *et al.*, 2008a).

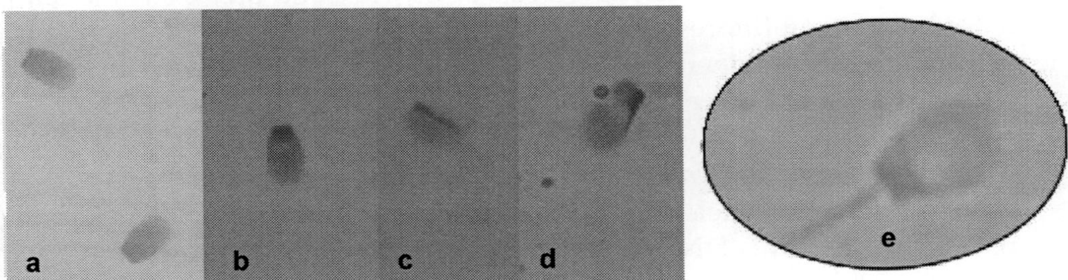

Fig. 8 : Sperm DNA distribution using Feulgen's straining: the spermatozoa DNA is evenly distributed in the spermatozoa without patches (a), Spermatozoa abnormalities include, abnormal distribution (b), folded DNA (c), vacuole (d), etc. The spermatozoa DNA abnormalities can also be seen under phase contrast microscope (e).

One of the most important parameters of spermatozoa fertilizing potential and to produce viable young one is sperm chromatin integrity. Sperm chromatin integrity has direct positive correlation with *in vitro* fertilization rate, embryo quality, pregnancy and successful delivery rate. The sperm DNA chromatin integrity provides better diagnostic and prognostic approaches than standard semen parameters. Over the last decade, rapid advances in reproductive molecular biology have resulted in numerous techniques to assess sperm DNA integrity. The ability of these techniques to accurately estimate sperm DNA damage depends on many technical and biological aspects. Various methods to assess spermatozoa chromatin integrity include, aniline blue staining, Feulgen's staining, FISH (fluorescence *in situ* hybridization) techniques, *in-situ* nick translation, acridine orange staining sperm chromatin structure assay (SCSA), spermatozoa chromatin dispersion (SCD) test, comet assay, terminal deoxynucleotidyl transferase-mediated deoxyuridine triphosphate-nick end labeling (TUNEL), *etc.* The each method to evaluate sperm chromatin integrity needs to be studied for routine use in diagnostic andrology lab. Among all these methods, SCD is easy to perform, fast reliable and does not need to detect the color or fluorescence intensity. SCSA is highly constant over a long period of time as compared to the standard semen analysis tests and may be applied successfully in the field of andrology.

2.5.1 Single-cell gel electrophoresis (SCGE), or comet assay

Comet assay is a simple, rapid, visual and sensitive method for detecting primary DNA damage at the individual cell level. The comet assay measures DNA damage by quantifying the single- and double-stranded breaks associated with DNA damage. One of the principles of the comet assay is that nicked double-stranded DNA tends to remain in the comet head, whereas short fragments of nicked double- and single-stranded DNA migrate into the tail area. Thus, spermatozoa with high levels of DNA strand breaks would show increased comet tail fluorescent intensity (Hughes *et al.,* 1996) and comet tail length (Singh and Stephens, 1998; Selvaraju *et al.,* 2009a). However, useful thresholds have not been established for the comet assay.

2.5.2 Sperm nuclear protein

The spermatozoa nuclear proteins have a role in fertilization. For example, transcription factors, DNA-binding proteins and proteins involved in chromatin metabolism have been identified in cells that are transcriptionally inactive and have most of its DNA tightly packaged with protamine. The presence of some of these proteins represent leftovers from spermiogenesis. Identification of these proteins could be useful as they could represent a 'window' to the later stages of spermatogenesis with potential clinical implications. Recent reports indicate the presence of a complex chromatin organization of the genes in sperm, with an appreciable fraction containing both nucleohistone and nucleoprotamine domains that is suggested to be of potential relevance for embryo development. Whether these nuclear proteins are marking some regions of the male genome and may have an epigenetic function is not clear. In addition to the DNA sequence, the existence of imprints determined by the DNA methylation status is also important for a proper embryonic development, and that infertile patients have an aberrant DNA methylation at specific loci.

2.6 Sperm acrosomal enzyme quality and acrosomal reaction test

Maintaining the molecular features of the sperm acrosme during the process of preservation, thawing, and transport in the female reproductive tract are essential for successful fertilization. Sperm penetration into zona pellucida is aided by hydrolytic enzymes in the sperm acrosome. In mammals, acrosin proteolytic activity is related to the fertilizing capacity of the spermatozoa (Mohsenian *et al.,* 1982). Gelatin substrate film assay can be used to assess the acrosin proteolytic activity (APA) of the sperm (Selvaraju *et al.,* 2010).

For successful fertilization, sperm should undergo capacitation and acrosomal reaction. Without this essential facet of fertilization, the sperm cannot be fertile. Various studies reported positive correlation between sperm undergoing acrosomal reaction in vitro and fertilization outcome either *in vitro* (Selvaraju *et al.,* 2010) or *in vivo* (Grippo *et al.,* 1995).

2.7 Seminal plasma proteins

Sub-optimal fertility in males is a concern in humans and animals. In sub-fertile males, the factors contributing to their sub-fertility are largely unknown. In these situation analyzing fertility regulating protein, if any is considered to be helpful to improve fertility.

The presence or absence of the critical concentration of proteins in seminal plasma could potentially responsible for the effects of seminal plasma on sperm fertility (Killian *et al.,* 1993). Low fertility seminal plasma contains anti-fertility factors that have a greater negative effect on high fertility spermatozoa than on low fertility spermatozoa (Henault and Killian, 1996). In bulls, heparin-binding proteins in seminal plasma have been correlated with fertility (Kandell *et al.,* 1992). Studies indicate that identification and manipulation of such fertility regulating proteins are highly important in cattle industry.

2.8 Sperm membrane protein

The fertilization is a complex event, every single steps leading to fertilization represents a critical point which could alter semen fertility (Thacker *et al.,* 2011). Depending on the steps involved in the process of fertilization, many sperm components such as lipids, proteins, ions and nucleic acids have been proposed to vary in quantity or quality according to the male fertility status in many mammalian species. Soluble and structural proteins have an important role in the spermatozoal metabolism and bull's fertility (Killian *et al.*, 1993). Since the proteins present on the sperm membrane take part during zona binding and penetration, the spermatozoa protein profiles are investigated (Peddinti *et al.*, 2008). Analysis of sperm membrane protein revealed proteins with a molecular weight ranging from 19 kDa to 137 kDa (Author's unpublished observation). The semen preservation process causes alterations in some protein molecules that may influence the fertility characteristics of the ejaculate. A 30-kDa heparin-binding protein named fertility-associated antigen was identified in sperm membranes of beef bulls with greater fertility potential (Bellin *et al.*, 1998; D'Armours *et al.*, 2010). Levels of P25b, a bovine sperm membrane antigen, are lower in semen from sub-fertile bulls than in the semen from high fertile bulls (Parent *et al.*, 1999). These studies also suggested that the effects of these antigens can carry over to the next generation.

2.9 Sperm transcripts profile

The application and use of spermatozoa transcripts as markers of male factor fertility status continues to evolve. Some spermatozoal transcripts were associated with non-return rate, a field fertility index (Bissonnette *et al.*, 2009; Arangasamy *et al.*, 2011). The spermatozoa mRNA reflect spermatogenesis gene expression, and/or a prognosis value for fertilization. The process of spermatogenesis would naturally lead to a well conserved set of spermatozoal transcripts in the healthy fertile male. Since these RNAs are delivered to oocytes, analysing mRNA profiles in spermatozoa could be helpful as a diagnostic tool to evaluate male fertility. Studies on the role of spermatozoa mRNA on sperm function and early embryonic development will be useful for diagnosis of bull fertility.

2.10 *In vitro* fertilization tests

To assess male fertility by mating or AI is expensive and time consuming, and only allows a limited number of males to be tested. Hence, interest has lately been focused on methods related to *in vitro* fertilization. Assays based on the number of sperm bound to zona (Fig. 10a,b) and penetrated through zona (Fig. 10c) have been studied as diagnostic tests to predict the fertility of the bull in the field (Zhang *et al.*, 1998; Selvaraju *et al.*, 2009b). However, cleavage rate after *in vitro* fertilization is the best available end point for expressing bull fertility (Fig. 11) since, early embryonic development as measured by the cleavage varies between different bulls, and these differences are used to discriminate between bulls of high and low bull field fertility (Totey *et al.*, 1993).

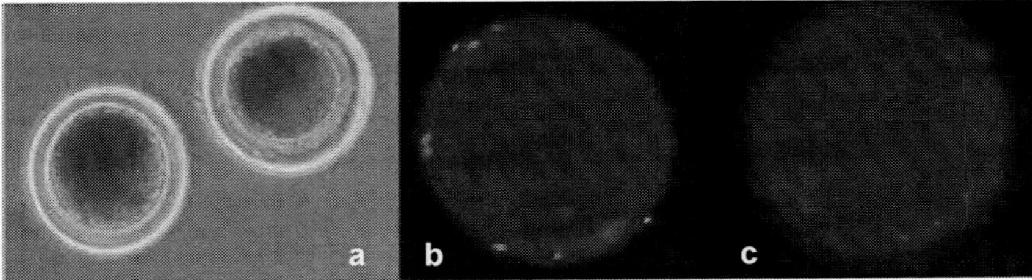

Fig. 9 : Assays based on the number of sperm bound to zona, phase contrast (a), fluorescent staining (b) and penetration through zona (c) have been used as diagnostic tests to predict the fertility of the semen (Adapted from Selvaraju *et al.*, 2009b).

3. Routine analysis versus recent concept

Knowledge of fertility in bulls is of great importance for the production of bovine semen, which is achieved by good analysis of the semen, among other assessments. The routine semen analysis relies on assessing a number of parameters such as sperm concentration, motility and morphology for the prediction of fertility in the male (Correa *et al.*, 1996). These tests provide the information about the status of spermatogenesis and cannot be used as reliable predictors of sperm fertilizing ability (Amann, 1989).

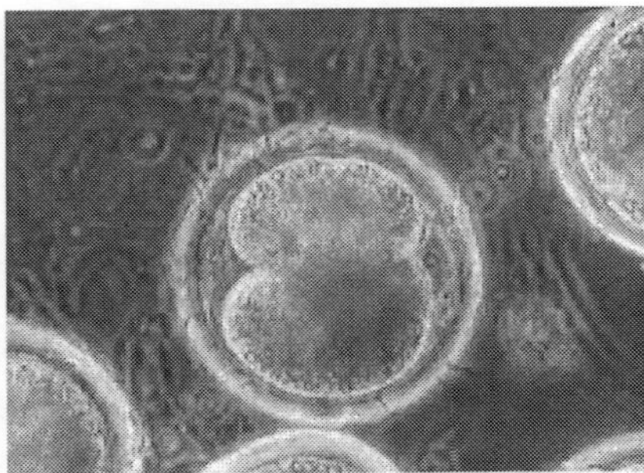

Fig. 10 : Cleavage rate could be used as one of the best end points to assess *in vitro* spermatozoa fertility.

The ability to predict the fertility of semen with laboratory tests is limited due to the complexity of the spermatozoon and the fertilization process. Many laboratory assays that examine spermatozoon's single cellular attribute. Testing a single attribute is unlikely to measure fertility since the spermatozoa must meet many requirements for successful fertilization. Right combination of laboratory assays should test not only the ability to reach the site of fertilization, but also the ability of the spermatozoa to fertilize the oocyte and activate successful embryonic development. The most reliable approach is to use a combination of tests to evaluate different sperm attributes, thereby increasing the accuracy of the estimate (Amann and Hammerstedt, 1993).

4. Possibilities of predicting bull fertility accurately

Since fertilization is a complex process and involves many interrelated factors, developing a test using a single attribute may not predict fertility accurately. Some of the important sperm assessment techniques involving array of tests such as sperm motility, sperm membrane integrity, sperm membrane proteins, sperm chromatin quality and transcripts profile may predict fertility potential of a bull to a significant extent.

5. Improving semen fertility

Preserving good quality semen after cryopreservation is imperative in order to obtain acceptable non-return and/or conception rates. Sperm cryopreservation induces cryoinjury to (formation of intracellular ice crystals as well as solution effect) to the spermatozoa that causes damage mainly to cytoplasm, cytoskeleton or genome related structures. During freezing, reactive oxygen species are generated that affect sperm membrane integrity. Incorporating antioxidants into freezing extenders is a way to overcome this cascade. A variety of antioxidants have been tested to either scavenge ROS directly or to counter ROS toxicity in semen of a variety of mammalian and avian species. The addition of various substances like prostaglandin and oxytocin (Arangasamy and Singh, 2002), oviductal proteins (Kumaresan *et al.,* 2006), IGF-I (Selvaraju *et al.,* 2010), glutathione (Perumal *et al.,* 2011), *etc.,*before freezing may improve semen quality. Ram seminal plasma, in TRIS-egg yolk extender consistently increased pregnancy rates after cervical AI of ewes with ram semen stored at 5 °C for 24 h (López-Pérez and Pérez-Clariget, 2012). The action of seminal plasma in improving semen fertility is not clear (Henault and Killian, 1996; Maxwell *et al.,* 2007). The seminal plasma proteins tightly adhere to the spermatozoa and the attachment is very strong; even after extensive washing it may not be possible to separate them from the spermatozoa. Few studies suggested that the addition of seminal plasma increased spermatozoa viability and fertility in ram (Maxwell *et al.,* 1997; Maxwell *et al.,* 1999). The positive effect of ram seminal plasma on fertility may be due to a decrease in the number of capacitated sperm (López-Pérez and Pérez-Clariget, 2012).

The ultimate way to improve semen quality is modulating spermatogenesis in the testicular compartment itself. In this regard nutraceuticals may play an important role in improving semen quality (Wathes *et al.,* 2007; Adeel *et al.,* 2011). Modulating growth factor levels especially IGF-I in the testis play an important role in testicular function (Sauerwein *et al.,* 2000). In the testis, IGF-I is secreted from the Sertoli cells and Leydig cells under the control of FSH and LH, respectively. The IGF-I receptor has been reported in spermatogonia, spermatocytes, spermatids and spermatozoa (Henricks *et al.,* 1998; Vannelli *et al.,* 1988). It has been suggested that IGF-I is an important factor for the germ cell development, maturation and motility of the spermatozoa (Henricks *et al.,* 1998; Vickers *et al.,* 1999). An association of seminal plasma IGF-I concentration with spermatozoa motility and morphology has been reported in equines (Macpherson *et al.,* 2002). The

IGF-I concentrations in the seminal plasma of healthy breeding bulls were found positively correlated with pregnancy rates (Sauerwein *et al.,* 2000). Modulating seminal plasma IGF-I levels either by changing the level of dietary energy or different energy source (mainly polyunsaturated fatty acids) may improve semen quality in rams (Selvaraju *et al.,* 2011; Selvaraju *et al.,* 2012).

Conclusion

The semen analysis and predicting semen fertility is very difficult for many reasons, including the use of subjective techniques. Since fertilization is a complex phenomenon, use of any single parameter may not suffice to predict semen quality. Studies in author's lab and elsewhere suggest that some of the microscopic evaluation parameters such as progressive forward motility, functional membrane integrity, mitochondrial membrane potential and DNA integrity measurements (sperm nuclear morphology, DNA distribution, DNA fragmentation tests) may constitute valuable markers for the assessment of male fertility. In future, spermatozoa membrane protein and transcripts profiles will be valuable and indispensable components in semen evaluation for selection of fertile bulls. The recent research on semen constituents and modulation of spermatogenesis through nutraceuticals may improve semen quality and fertility in male animals.

References

Adeel M., Ijaz A., Aleem M., Rehman H., Yousaf M.S., Jabbar M.A. (2009). ?Improvement of liquid and frozen-thawed semen quality of Nili-Ravi buffalo bulls (*Bubalus bubalis*) through supplementation of fat. *Theriogenology* **71:** 1220-1225.

Aitken R.J., Sutton M., Warner P., Richardson D.W. (1985). Relationship between the movement characteristics of human spermatozoa and their ability to penetrate cervical mucus and zona-free hamster oocytes. *Journal of Reproduction and Fertility* **73:** 441-449.

Amann R.P. (1989). Can the fertility potential of a seminal sample be predicted accurately?. *Journal of Andrology*. **10:** 89-98.

Amann R.P. Hammerstedt R.H. (1993). *In vitro* evaluation of sperm quality: an opinion. *Journal of Andrology* **14:** 397-406.

Arangasamy A., Kasimanickam V.R., DeJarnette J.M. (2011). Association of CRISP2, CCT8, PEBP1 mRNA abundance in sperm and sire conception rate in Holstein bulls. *Theriogenology* **76:** 570-577.

Arangasamy A., Singh L.P. (2002). In vitro assessment of fertilizing potential of post-thaw crossbred bull (HFxH) spermatozoa with added prostaglandin $F_{2\alpha}$, oxytocin and BHT. *Indian Journal of Animal Sciences* **72:** 61-63.

Bearden J.H., Fuquay J.W. (2000). In: *Applied Animal Reproduction*. (H.J. Bearden, J.W. Fuquay, S. T. Willard. Eds). 5th Edn. Prentice-Hall, Englewood Cliffs, NJ, USA.

Bellin M.E., Oyarzo J.N., Hawkins H.E., Zhang H., Smith R.G., Forrest D.W., Sprott L.R., Ax R.L. (1998). Fertility-associated antigen on bull sperm indicates fertility potential. *Journal of Animal Science* **76:** 2032-2039.

Bhosrekar M.R. (1990). Semen production and artificial insemination, (1st ed). BAIF Development Research Foundation, India.

Bissonnette N., Lévesque-Sergerie J.P., Thibault C., Boissonneault G. (2009). Spermatozoal transcriptome profiling for bull sperm motility: a potential tool to evaluate semen quality. *Reproduction* **138:** 65-80.

Budworth P.R., Amann R.P., Chapman P.L. (1988). Relationships between computerized measurements of motion of frozen thawed bull spermatozoa and fertility. *Journal of Andrology* **9:** 41-54.

Correa J.R., Rodriguez M.C., Patterson D.J., Zavos P.M. (1996). Thawing and processing of Cryopreserved bovine spermatozoa at various temperatures and their subsequent effects on sperm viability, osmotic shake and sperm membrane functional integrity. *Theriogenology* **46:** 413-420.

D'Amours O., Frenette G., Fortier M., Leclerc P., Sullivan R. (2010). Proteomic comparison of detergent-extracted sperm proteins from bulls with different fertility indexes. *Reproduction* **139:** 545-556.

Didione B.A., Graves C.N. (1986). In vivo capacitation and acrosome reaction of bovine sperm in estrous and diestrous cows. *Journal of Animal Science* **62:** 1029-1033.

Evenson D.P., Parks J.E., Kaproth M.T., Jos L.K. (1993). Rapid determination of sperm cell concentration in bovine semen by flow cytometry. *Journal of Dairy Science* **76:** 86-94.

Farrell P.B., Presicce G.A., Brockett C.C., Foote R.H. (1998). Quantification of bull sperm characteristics measured by computer assisted sperm analysis (CASA) and their relationship to fertility. *Theriogenology* **49:** 871-879.

Fenton S.E., Ax R.L., Cowan C.M., Coyle T., Gilbert G.R., Lenz R.W. (1990). Validation and application of an assay for deoxyribonucleic acid to estimate concentrations of bull sperm. *Journal of Dairy Science* **73:** 3118-3125.

Garner D.L., Thomas C.A., Joerg H.W., DeJarnette J.M., Marshall C.E. (1997). Fluorometric assessments of mitochondrial function and viability in cryopreserved bovine spermatozoa. *Biology of Reproduction* **57:** 1401-1406.

Grippo A.A., Way A.L., Killian G.J. (1995). Effect of bovine ampullary and isthmic oviductal fluid on motility, acrosome reaction and fertility of bull spermatozoa. *Journal of Reproduction and Fertility* **105:** 57-64.

Hafez E.S.E. (1993). In: *Reproduction in Farm Animals.* (B. Hafez, ESE Hafez, Eds). 6th Edn. Philadelphia: Lea and Febiger, 405-439.

Hansen C., Christensen P., Stryhn H., Hedeboe A.M., Rode M., Boe-Hansen G. (2002). Validation of the FACS Count AF system for determination of sperm concentration in boar semen. *Reproduction in Domestic Animals* **37:** 330-334.

Harrison R.A.P., Vickers Sally E. (1990). Use of fluorescent probes to assess membrane integrity in mammalian spermatozoa. *Journal of Reproduction and Fertility* **88:** 343-352.

Henault M.A., Killian G.J. (1996). Effect of homologous and heterologous seminal plasma on the fertilizing ability of ejaculated bull spermatozoa assessed by penetration of zona-free bovine oocytes. *Journal of Reproduction and Fertility* **108:** 199-204.

Henkel R., Muller C., Miska W., Gips H., Schill W.B. (1993). Determination of the acrosome reaction in human spermatozoa is predictive of fertilization in vitro. *Human Reproduction* **8:** 2128-2132.

Henricks D.M., Kouba A.J., Lackey B.R., Boone W.R., Gray S.L. (1998). Identification of insulin-like growth factor I in bovine seminal plasma and its receptor on spermatozoa: influence on sperm motility. *Biology of Reproduction* **59:** 330-337.

Hughes C.M., Lewis S.E., McKelvey-Martin V.J., Thompson W. (1996). A comparison of baseline and induced DNA damage in human spermatozoa from fertile and infertile men, using a modified comet assay. *Molecular Human Reproduction* **2:** 613-619.

Jeyendran R.S., Van der Ven H.H., Perez-Pelaez M., Crabo B.G., Zaneveld L.J.D. (1984). Development of an assay to assess the functional integrity of the human sperm membrane and its relationship to other semen characteristics. *Journal of Reproduction and Fertility* **70:** 210-229.

Kandell R.L., Bellin M.E., Hawkins H.E., Ax R.L. (1992). Bull fertility was related to distributions of heparin binding proteins in sperm membranes and seminal plasma. *Journal Andrology (Suppl.)* **1:** 13-30.

Kasai T., Ogawa K., Mizuno K., Nagai S., Uchida Y., Ohta S., Fujie M., Suzuki K., Hirata S., Hoshi K. (2002). Relationship between sperm mitochondrial membrane potential, sperm motility, and fertility potential. *Asian Journal of Andrology* **4:** 97-103.

Killian G.J., Chapman D.A., Rogowski L.A. (1993). Fertility associated proteins in Holstein bull seminal plasma. *Biology of Reproduction* **49:** 1202-1207.

Kjaestad H., Ropstad E., Berg K.A. (1993). Evaluation of spermatological parameters used to predict the fertility of frozen bull semen. *Acta Veterinaria Scandinavica* **34:** 299-303.

Kumaresan A., Ansari M.R., Garg A., Kataria M. (2006). Effect of oviductal proteins on sperm functions and lipid peroxidation levels during cryopreservation in buffaloes. *Animal Reproduction Science* **93:** 246-257.

Larson B., Rodriquez-Martinez H. (2000). Can we use in vitro fertilization tests to predict semen fertility. *Animal Reproduction Science* **60-61:** 327-336.

López-Pérez A., Pérez-Clariget R. (2012). Ram seminal plasma improves pregnancy rates in ewes cervically inseminated with ram semen stored at 5°C for 24 hours. *Theriogenology* **77:** 395-399.

Macpherson M.L., Simmen R.C.M., Simmen F.A., Hernandez J., Sheerin B.R., Varner D.D., Loomis P., Cadario M.E., Miller C.D., Brinsko S.P., Rigby S., Blanchard T.L. (2002).

Insulin-like growth factor-I and insulin-like growth factor binding protein-2 and -5 in equine seminal plasma: association with sperm characteristics and fertility. *Biology of Reproduction* **67:** 648-654.

Marchetti C., Obert G., Deffosez A., Formstecher P., Marchetti P. (2002). Study of mitochondrial membrane potential, reactive oxygen species, DNA fragmentation and cell viability by flow cytometry in human sperm. *Human Reproduction* **17:** 1257-1265.

Maxwell W. M., de Graaf S. P., Ghaoui Rel H., Evans G. (2007). Seminal plasma effects on sperm handling and female fertility. *The Society for Reproduction and Fertility (Suppl.)* **64:** 13-38.

Maxwell W.M.C., Evans G., Mortimer S.T., Gillan L., Gellatly E.S., McPhie C.A. (1999). Normal fertility after cervical insemination with frozen-thawed spermatozoa supplemented with seminal plasma. *Reproduction Fertility and Development* **11:** 123-126.

Maxwell W.M.C., Welch G.R., Johnson L.A. (1997). Viability and membrane integrity of spermatozoa after dilution and flow cytometric sorting in the presence or absence of seminal plasma. *Reproduction Fertility and Development* **8:** 1165-1178.

Mohsenian M., Syner F.N., Moghissi K.S. (1982). A study of sperm acrosin in patients with unexplained infertility. *Fertility and Sterility* **37:** 223-229.

Parent S., Lefievre L., Brindley Y., Sullivan R. (1999). Bull subfertility is associated with low level of a sperm membrane antigen. *Molecular Reproduction and Development* **52:** 57-65.

Peddinti D., Nanduri B., Kaya A., Feugang J.M., Burgess S.C., Memli E. (2008). Comprehensive proteomic analysis of bovine spermatozoa of varying fertility rates and identificationof biomarkers associated with fertility. *BMC System Biology* **2:** 1-13.

Perumal P., Selvaraju S., Barik A.K., Mohanty D.N., Das S., Mishra P.C. (2011). Role of reduced glutathione in improving post-thaw seminal parameters in poor freezable Jersey crossbred bull semen. *Indian Journal of Animal Sciences* **81:** 807-810

Perumal P., Selvaraju S., Selvakumar S., Barik A.K., Mohanty D.N., Das S., Das R.K., Mishra P.C. (2011). Effect of pre-freeze addition of cysteine hydrochloride and reduced glutathione in semen of crossbred Jersey bulls on sperm parameters and conception rates. *Reproduction in Domestic Animals* **46:** 636-641.

Roberts S. J. (1971): In: *Veterinary Obstetrics and Genital Disease*, (S.J. Roberts, Ed). 2nd Edn. CBS Publishers and Distributors, India.

Saacke R.G., Dejarnette J.M., Barne J.H., Karabinus D.S., Whitman S.S. (1998). can spermatozoa with abnormal heads gain access to the ovum in artificially inseminated super- and single-ovulating cattle?. *Theriogenology* **50:** 117-128.

Sauerwein H., Breier B.H., Gallaher B.W., Götz C., Küfner G., Montag T., Vickers M., Schallenberger E. (2000). Growth hormone treatment of breeding bulls used for artificial insemination improves fertilization rates. *Domestic Animal Endocrinology* **18:** 145-158.

Selvaraju S., Ghosh J., David C.G., Reddy I.J., Ravindra J.P. (2008a). Sperm nuclear morphology in relation to sperm functional tests in assessing buffalo semen. *Indian Veterinary Journal* **85:** 505-507.

Selvaraju S., Ravindra J.P., Ghosh J., Gupta P.S.P., Suresh K.P. (2008b). Evaluation of sperm functional attributes in relation to in vitro sperm-zona pellucida binding ability and cleavage rate in assessing frozen thawed buffalo (*Bubalus bubalis*) semen quality. *Animal Reproduction Science* **106:** 311-321.

Selvaraju S., Reddy I.J., Nandi S., Rao S.B.N., Ravindra J.P. (2009a). Influence of IGF-I on buffalo (*Bubalus bubalis*) spermatozoa motility, membrane integrity, lipid peroxidation and fructose uptake in vitro. *Animal Reproduction Science* **113:** 60-70.

Selvaraju S, Ghosh J, Ravindra JP. (2009b). Prognostic value of various spermatological attributes as predictors of zona binding and zona penetration of buffalo (*Bubalus bubalis*) semen. *Reproduction in Domestic Animals* **44:** 6-11.

Selvaraju S., Nandi S., Subramani T.S., Raghavendra B.S., Rao S.B., Ravindra J.P. (2010). Improvement in buffalo (*Bubalus bubalis*) spermatozoa functional parameters and fertility *in vitro*: Effect of insulin-like growth factor-I. *Theriogenology* **73:** 1-10.

Selvaraju S., Priyadarshini R., Rao S.B.N., Raghavendra S., Nandi S., Dineshkumar D., Allen Thayakumar., Parthipan S., Ravindra J.P. (2011). Evaluation of maize grain and polyunsaturated fatty acid (PUFA) as energy sources for breeding rams based on hormonal, sperm functional parameters and fertility. *Reproduction Fertility and Development* http://dx.doi.org/10.1071/RD11229.

Selvaraju S., Sivasubramani T., Raghavendra B.S., Raju P., Rao S.B.N., Dinesh Kumar D., Ravindra J.P. (2012). Effect of dietary energy on seminal plasma insulin-like growth factor-I (IGF-I), serum IGF-I and testosterone levels, semen quality and fertility in adult rams. *Theriogenology*. doi 10.1016/j. theriogenology. 2012.03.010.

Singh N.P., Stephens R.E. (1998). X-ray induced DNA double-strand breaks in human sperm. *Mutagenesis* **13:** 75-79.

Thacker S., Yadav S.P., Sharma R.K., Kashou A., Willard B., Zhang D., Agarwal A. (2011). Evaluation of sperm proteins in infertile men: a proteomic approach. *Fertility and Sterility* **95:** 2745-2748.

Totey S.M., Pawshe C.H., Singh G.P. (1993). Effects of bull and heparin and sperm concentrations on in vitro fertilization of buffalo (*Bubalus bubalis*) oocytes matured *in vitro*. *Theriogenology* **39:** 887-898.

Vannelli B.G., Barni T., Orlando C., Natali A., Serio M., Balboni G.C. (1988). Insulin-like growth factor-I (IGF-I) and IGF-I receptor in human testis: an immunohistochemical study. *Fertility and Sterility* **49:** 666-669.

Vickers M.H., Casey P.J., Champion Z.J., Gravance C.G., Breier B.H. (1999). IGFI treatment increases motility and improves morphology of immature spermatozoa in the GH-deficient dwarf (dw/dw) rat. *Growth Hormone and IGF Research* **9:** 236-240.

Wathes D.C., Abayasekara D.R., Aitken R.J. (2007). Polyunsaturated fatty acids in male and female reproduction. *Biology of Reproduction* **77:** 190-201.

Zhang B.R., Larsson B., Lundeheim N., Rodriguez-Martinez H. (1998). Sperm characteristics and zona pellucida binding in relation to field fertility of frozen-thawed semen from dairy AI bulls. *International Journal of Andrology* **21:** 207-216.

❑❑❑

Chapter 19

Role of Paternal Transcripts on Sperm Function and Fertility

A. Arangasamy, S. Selvaraju, J. P. Ravindra
National Institute of Animal Nutrition and Physiology, Adugodi, Bangalore-560 030, Karnataka, India

Summary

Initially it was thought that RNA present in semen relates to contamination from somatic cells and/or immature sperm both containing substantially higher amounts of RNA than the fertilizing sperm. However, recent molecular techniques confirmed the presence of mRNA in mature sperm cells. During fertilization along with sperm DNA, some of its RNA is also introduced into the oocyte. The spermatozoa RNA are stable until the activation of the embryonic genome. The possible role of spermatozoa RNA on sperm motility, capacitation, acrosome reaction, sperm-egg fusion, fertilization and early embryo development has been explored. This chapter summarizes key aspects of some spermatozoal messenger RNA expression; its function, role in the male reproductive tract and possible key events of fertilization and bull fertility.

Fertility is one of the most important critical factors controlling biological and financial performance of animal production systems and genetic improvement of lines (Feugang *et al.*, 2009). Sperm morphology and motility, number of sperm per insemination, percentage of acrosome reacted sperms and *in vivo* and *in vitro* fertilization have been extensively evaluated as an indication of sperms ability to fertilize an egg. Many proteins in sperm are adsorbed/modified during the processes of fertilization (Naz and Rajendran, 2006). Recent studies show that, there are mRNAs for several proteins present in mature sperm, probably left over after spermatogenesis/spermiogenesis. Some laboratories reported the presence of mRNAs in mature sperm nearly two decades ago (Kumar *et al.*, 1993; Pessot *et al.*, 1989). Since then, several labs have confirmed the presence of mRNAs in spermatozoa (Ostermeier *et al.*, 2002; Wang *et al.*, 2004; Rui Pires Martins *et al.*, 2005; Dadoune *et al.*, 2005). It is evident that there is a residual mRNA present in sperm cell for the receptors, which were synthesized during sperm development/maturation in testis/epididymis. Apart from DNA, the sperm provides the egg with paternal centrioles, proteins, and RNAs (Miller *et al.*, 2005). Though functional significance of mRNA in mature spermatozoa remains unexplored (Lalancette *et al.*, 2008), it is understood that mRNA is necessary from the embryo cleavages until the activation of the embryonic genome (Ostermeier *et al.*, 2004) and thus mRNA can affect phenotypic traits of embryos (Meseguer *et al.*, 2006) and offspring (Miller and Ostermeier, 2006a and 2006b).

Reverse transcription-polymerase chain reaction (RT-PCR), *in situ* hybridization (ISH), testicular microarray and/or serial analysis of gene expression (SAGE) experiments revealed that the ejaculated bovine (Gilbert *et al.*, 2007) and human (Wykes *et al.*, 1997; Miller *et al.*, 1999; Zhao *et al.*, 2006) spermatozoa evidently retain a complex yet specific population of transcripts. These transcripts might play an important roles in spermatozoal development, chromatin repackaging, genomic imprinting, early zygotic development, male-derived factors that underlie idiopathic infertility in males, and possibly provide the key to more successful animal cloning using somatic-cell nuclear transfer (Ostermeier *et al.*, 2004; Martins and Krawetz, 2005). Some of the spermatozoal mRNA transcripts might not have effect on the embryogenesis and degraded rapidly in embryos at late 1-cell stage (Hayashi *et al.*, 2003). However, some of these spermatozoal mRNA transcripts were found to survive upto 4-cell stage. Therefore, the spermatozoa deliver not only the genetic materials but also spermatozoal RNAs into the oocyte during the process of fertilization. Because of its origins and the peculiarities of spermatogenesis, spermatozoal RNA can be regarded not only as remnants that escape cytoplasmic extrusion during the last steps of spermiogenesis, but also as a fingerprint of spermatogenesis quality and fertility outcome. The various mRNA transcripts expression is associated with sire conception rate deviation (SCRD) scores in Holstein bulls (Arangasamy *et al.*, 2011).

1. Sperm RNA

At the end of spermatogenesis, highly differentiated haploid spermatozoa are produced. Spermatozoa are transcriptionally inactive specialized cell containing minimal cytoplasm and compact nucleus. In the spermatozoa RNA levels are substantially lower than in the oocyte. An amount of 100fg RNA per sperm was first reported (Pessot *et al.*, 1989) but recently Krawetz (2005) observed a lower 10–20fg RNA per human spermatozoa. It should be realized that this small amount of paternal RNA is brought to a multitude of maternal RNA present in mammalian oocytes 0.5–1.5ng per oocyte (Fig. 1) depending on the mammalian species tested (Olszanska and Borgul, 1990). Sperm mRNA appears to be fully processed, in that they contain 30-poly-A-tails and lack intron sequences (Ostermeier *et al.*, 2002; Concha *et al.*, 1993; Miller, 1997).

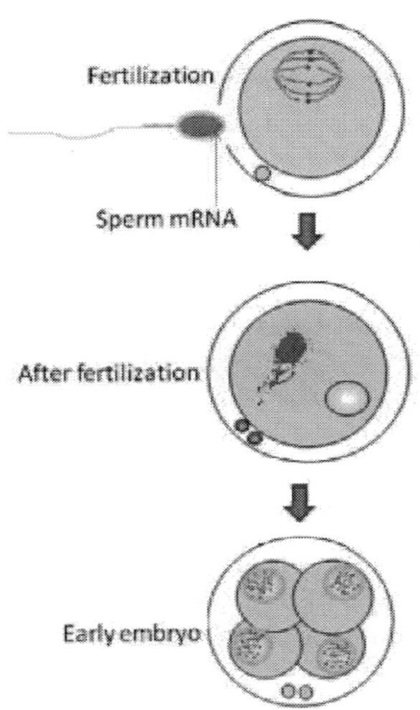

Fig. 1 : Delivering of spermatozoa RNA to early embryo

2. Analysis of sperm transcriptome

Transcriptome profiling is a technique that can be used to identify messengers that are potential markers of fertility on the basis of their presence/absence in mature spermatozoa. Approximately 3,000–5,000 mRNA transcripts have been reported to be present in human spermatozoa (Wykes *et al.*, 1997; Krawetz *et al.*, 2005). This method permits the identification of novel genes by enriching transcripts that are differentially expressed. The RNA content of a spermatozoon could be used as a pattern for the genomic analysis of semen quality, in terms of both spermatogenesis and fertility potential. The various transcripts that are present in spermatozoa affecting different metabolic pathways or functions raise many questions about the complexity of spermatogenesis and the significance of the transcripts that are generated. The mammalian ejaculated spermatozoa are highly differentiated terminal cells with an extremely compacted nucleus of haploid genome. Accumulated evidences from the use of recent high throughput techniques in fields of molecular andrology, convincingly suggesting that human ejaculated spermatozoa retain a complex yet specific population of RNAs (Lambard *et al.*, 2004; Miller *et al.*, 2005). The existence of transcriptional and translational activities in human sperm during capacitation and acrosome reaction has been suggested, which could also explain the presence of mRNA in mature sperm (Naz, 1998). Under certain conditions, at least some cytoplasmic mRNAs can apparently be translated *de novo*, possibly on mitochondrial polysomes. The mature spermatozoa are indeed metabolically active with respect to transcription but restricted to the mitochondrion. Protein phosphorylation, transcription and translation steps have been observed in human sperm. Indeed, the histone-to-protamine exchange process seems to be incomplete in human spermatids, which suggest a putative transcription and/or translation in sperm (Gatewood *et al.*, 1987). Also, accumulation of a certain mRNA may indicate that translation has not occurred; suggesting that protein content for that specific gene may be lower. The association between a lower gene-to-protein turnover and infertility may assist in establishing potential targets for therapeutic intervention.

3. Sperm mRNAs as fertility markers

The application and use of spermatozoa transcripts as markers of male fertility status continues to evolve. This arose from the initial hypothesis that the spermatogenesis is well orchestrated process and would naturally lead to a well conserved set of spermatozoal transcripts in the healthy fertile male. Microarray studies revealed a series of very promising clinical markers of spermiogenic dysgenesis. Analyzing mRNA profiles in spermatozoa could be helpful either as a diagnostic tool to evaluate male fertility, since they reflect spermatogenesis gene expression, and/or a prognosis value for fertilization, since these RNAs are delivered to oocytes. Some studies witnessing the emergence of a myriad of diverse transcripts identified using different transcript profiling platforms for humans, cattle, boar and recently reported in stallion sperm (Gilbert *et al.*, 2007; Lalancette *et al.*, 2008; Olivier D'Amours *et al* ., 2010; Goodrich *et al.*, 2007; Yang *et al.*, 2009; Das *et al.*, 2010). Transcripts encoding a serine/threonine testis-specific protein kinase (TSSK6) and a metalloproteinase non-coding RNA (ADAM5P) is associated with high-motility status (Bissonnette *et al.*, 2009). These results demonstrate that some transcripts previously identified in association with field fertility are also found in association with *in vitro* motility. It is therefore pertinent to discuss some of the specific transcripts which are reported to be associated with the sperm function and/or fertility.

4. Specific transcripts associated with sperm function and fertility

4.1 Adenylate kinase isoenzyme 1 (AK1)

The presence of AK1 in bovine and murine sperm flagella has been reported, strongly suggesting a function in motility (Schoff *et al.*, 1989; Cao *et al.*, 2006). This provide a mechanism to buffer the adenylate energy charge for sperm motility, which was found to be more abundant on sperm from high fertile bull group and contributing to the energy homeostasis of the cell by catalysing the reaction: 2ADP $\rightarrow$ ATP+cAMP (Atkinson, 1968). The fluctuation of nucleotide concentrations in normal and metabolically stimulated sperm suggests that AK1 is mostly active when the cell is highly motile (Schoff *et al.*, 1989). The ATP is required by the dynein ATPase in the axoneme to produce the deep flagellar bends characteristic to hyperactivation. Hyperactivation may be critical to the success of fertilization, because it enhances the ability of sperm to detach from oviductal epithelium and to penetrate the ZP (Suarez and Ho, 2003). Relationship of AK1 with male fertility could be to sustain energy needs during hyperactivated motility of spermatozoa. This enzyme is acquired during the epididymal transit with functions in sperm motility (Schoff *et al.*, 1989; Cao *et al.*, 2006). The AK1 mRNA was first seen in condensing spermatids associated with the outer microtubular doublets and outer dense fibers of sperm. The level of AK1 mRNA expression and its positive association to sire conception rate deviation (SCRD) score were reported in Holstein bulls (Kasimanickam *et al.*, personal communication).

4.2 Phosphatidylethanolamine-binding protein 1 (PEBP1)

The roles of PEBP1 in sperm remain to be established. The PEBP1 was found in higher abundance in sperm from high fertile bulls. It acts either as a decapacitation factor that is released during capacitation (Nixon *et al.*, 2006) or as a membrane bound, glycophosphatidylinositol (GPI) anchored receptor for a decapacitation factor (Gibbons *et al.*, 2005). This anti-capacitation effect is further supported by the observation that sperm from PEBP1K-/K-mice are precociously capacitated compared with their wild-type counterparts (Moffit *et al.*, 2007). Although PEBP1K-/K-male mice remain fertile, data from mating experiments indicate significant decreased reproduction rates between crosses with either heterozygous or PEBP1K+/K-females, but interestingly, not with wild-type females. The level of mRNA expression and its association to sire conception rate deviation (SCRD) score were reported in Holstein bulls (Arangasamy *et al.*, 2011).

4.3 Subunit 8 of the T-complex protein 1 (CCT 8)

The subunits 8 of the T-complex protein 1 (CCT 8), a member of the class II chaperonins, were found in higher concentration in the low fertile bull sperm samples. Chaperonins are involved in the proper folding of other proteins, with actin and tubulin being the major substrates for CCT (Sternlicht *et al.*, 1993). In rat spermatids, cytoplasmic CCT is localized in centrosomes and microtubules of the manchette during spermatogenesis and would be discarded in residual bodies at spermiation and subpopulation remains in mature cells (Soue's *et al.*, 2003). The presence of three CCT subunits, including CCT5, has been reported in ejaculated sperm from fertile men (de Mateo *et al.*, 2007). Since CCT is supposed to be discarded at spermiation, high levels of CCT subunits in sperm samples from low fertile bulls may reflect incomplete processes involving these proteins during spermatogenesis. The CCT8 mRNA expression and its association to sire conception rate deviation (SCRD) score were reported in Holstein bulls (Arangasamy *et al.*, 2011).

4.4 Cystine rich secretary proteins

This protein is produced by testicular germ cells and becomes localized to the sperm tail and to the acrosome (Mizuki *et al.*, 1992; Foster *et al.*, 1996; Bryan *et al.*, 2001). The CRISP2 also known as testis-specific protein 1 (Tpx1), expressed exclusively in the testis (Foster *et al.*, 1996; Giese *et al.*, 2002; Kasahara *et al.*, 1989; Kratzschmar *et al.*, 1996). This is an intra-acrosomal protein of testicular origin, antibodies against which caused the accumulation of perivitelline spermatozoa during *in vitro* fertilization in mouse (Busso *et al.*, 2007). In a zona-free fertilization assay, CRISP2 seemed to compete with CRISP1 for the oolemma binding sites, suggesting that the two proteins bind to complementary/overlapping sites. Murine CRISP1 has been shown to inhibit sperm-egg fusion and to block capacitation in rat sperm (Ellerman *et al.*, 2006; Roberts *et al.*, 2003; Cohen *et al.*, 2000). More recently, rat CRISP2 has also been shown to inhibit sperm-egg fusion, suggesting that CRISP2 has a molecular activity in common with CRISP1 (Busso *et al.*, 2007). The molecular mechanism for both of these activities remains unknown. Given that rat CRISP1 and CRISP2 share a similar activity in sperm egg fusion, and CRISP2 may also have some efficacy in inhibiting sperm capacitation. The results of this experiment revealed just the opposite; including rpCRISP2 (recombinant porcine CRISP2) in the *in vitro* capacitation incubation resulted in an increased number of sperm undergoing an acrosomalreaction (AR) and concluded that rpCRISP2 can induce an AR with the same efficiency as calcium ionophore (Da *et al.*, 2007). The level of CRISP2 mRNA expression and its positive association to sire conception rate deviation (SCRD) score were reported in Holstein bulls (Arangasamy *et al.*, 2011).

4.5 Nerve growth factors (NGF)

Expression of NGF and its receptor tyrosine kinase (TrkA) was detected in animal testes (Robinson *et al.*, 2003) and found to have role on Leydig cell steroid production (Müller *et al.*, 2006). The NGF affects leptin secretions, viability and apoptosis of ejaculated bovine sperm. These observations provided growing evidence that NGF played important roles in animal reproduction (Li *et al.*, 2010). The mRNA of NGF has been localized on sperm and early spermatids of adult mice suggesting that it may be involved in sperm maturation (Mutter *et al.*, 1999). Treatment of sperm with NGF increases motility and acrosome reaction in time and dose dependant manner in golden hamster sperm (WanZho *et al.*, 2010). Higher sperm NGF mRNA abundances in positive SCR bulls suggests an association between NGF and fertility in bulls (Kasimanickam *et al.*, personal communication).

4.6 Doppel

Doppel was initially identified as a prion-like protein due to its structural and biochemical similarities to prion protein (PrPC). Recent report claimed that the doppel protein is mainly expressed in the reproductive system, more specifically in sertoli cells and spermatozoa (Peoc'h *et al.*, 2002; Li *et al.*, 2000). The exact biological function is still unclear, but its deregulation causes male sterility (Behrens *et al.*, 2002). A possible association between PRND (prion protein 2 doublets) gene polymorphisms and ram semen traits/freezability and fertility was recently suggested (Pereira *et al.*, 2009). The presence of significantly higher Doppel mRNA in bulls with high SCR indicates its positive role in sperm acrosome reaction and higher fertilization rates (Kasimanickam *et al.*, personal communication).

4.7 Tissue inhibitor of metalloproteinases type-2 (TIMP-2)

Tissue inhibitor of metalloproteinases type-2 (TIMP-2) is a member of the TIMP gene family. It has been described that TIMP-2 extracted from bovine seminal plasma binding to sperm. Influence of TIMP2 on bull fertility was postulated by McCauley *et al.* (2001). The TIMP-2 is found associates with bovine and human sperm membranes (McCauley *et al.*, 2001; Bechman-Shaked *et al.*, 2002). The expression of TIMP-2 mRNA was detected in bovine bulbo-urethral gland, prostate, and seminal vesicles. This protein is involved in interaction and remodeling of the extracellular matrix at the time of sperm interaction with cumulus cells, zona pellucida and oocyte membrane. Metalloproteinases released from the sperm during acrosome reaction facilitate sperm-egg fusion in hamsters (D´ýaz-Perez and Meizel, 1992). Presence of those proteins detected in bull's ejaculate corresponded to a 13-19% increase in fertility (Bellin *et al.*, 1994, 1996, 1998). The observation of higher mRNA abundance of TIMP-2 in positive SCR-score in Holstein bulls, evidence the role of TIMP-2 in semen quality and fertility (Kasimanickam *et al.*, Personal communication).

4.8 Leptin

Presence of leptin mRNA in the bull spermatozoa suggests that leptin might be involved in the physiological processes of bovine spermatozoa (Abbas *et al.*, 2010). Potential actions of leptin and its receptors (Ob-R) in bovine spermatozoa have not been studied properly, however its existence (Ob-R mRNA and leptin) indicate involvement of leptin in metabolism, capacitation and survival of bovine sperm (Nikbakht *et al.*, 2010).

Recently few more mRNA genes like integrin β (IB) 5, lactate dehydrogenase C (LDHC) 1, small nuclear ribonucleoprotein polypeptide N

(SNRPN) 2, outer dense fiber of sperm tails (ODF) 2, phospholipase C zeta (PLCz)1 were investigated in Holstein bulls and their correlation to sire conception rate deviation scores were established (Kasimanickam *et al.*, personal communication).

Conclusions

The mRNA genes are involved with sperm motility, capacitation, acrosome reaction, sperm-egg fusion, fertilization induction and early embryo development. Therefore, there is need to study the important spermatozoa RNA in elaborate and their possible correlation with *in vivo* and *in vitro* fertility. This will lead to the road for developing the sperm bio-marker for predicting the desired quality bulls in future.

References

Abbas A., Ali B., Parviz S., Hesam D. (2011). Leptin mRNA in bovine spermatozoa. *Research Veterinary Science* **90:** 439-442.

Arangasamy A., Kasimanickam V., DeJarnette M., Kasimanickam R. (2011). Association of CRISP2, CCT8, PEBP1 mRNA abundance in spermatozoa and sire Conception rate in Holstein Bulls. *Theriogenology* **76:** 570-577.

Atkinson D.E. (1968). The energy charge of the adenylate pool as a regulatory parameter. Interaction with feedback modifiers. *Biochemistry* **7:** 4030-4034.

Bechman-Shaked O., Kraiem Z., Gonen Y., Goldman S. (2002). Presence of metalloproteinases and tissue inhibitor of metalloproteinases in human sperm. *Journal of Andrology* **23:** 702-708.

Behrens A., Genoud N., Naumann H., Rülicke T., Janett F., Heppner F.L., Ledermann B. Aguzzi A. (2002). Absence of the prion protein homologue Doppel causes male sterility. *EMBO Journal of Animal Science* **21:** 3652-3658.

Bellin M.E., Hawkins H.E., Ax R.L. (1994). Fertility of range beef bulls grouped according to presence or absence of heparin-binding proteins in sperm membranes and seminal fluid. *Journal of Animal Science* **72:** 2441-2448.

Bellin M.E., Hawkins H.E., Oyarzo J.N., Vanderboom R.J., Ax R.L. (1996). Monoclonal antibody detection of heparin-binding proteins on sperm corresponds to increased fertility of bulls. *Journal of Animal Science* **74:** 173-182.

Bellin M.E., Oyarzo J.N., Hawkins H.E., Zhang H.M., Smith R.G., Forrest D.W., Sprott L.R., Ax R.L. (1998). Fertility associated antigen on bull sperm indicates fertility potential. *Journal of Animal Science* **76:** 2032-2039.

Bissonnette N., Sergerie J.P.L., Thibault C., Boissonneault G. (2009). Spermatozoal transcriptome profiling for bull sperm motility: a potential tool to evaluate semen quality. *Reproduction* **138:** 65-80.

Busso D., Nadia M.. Goldweic H.M., Kasahara M., Cuasnicu P.S. (2007). Evidence for the involvement of testicular protein CRISP2 in mouse sperm-egg fusion. *Biology of Reproduction* **76:** 701-708.

Cao W., Gerton G.L., Moss S.B. (2006). Proteomic profiling of accessory structures from the mouse sperm flagellum. *Molecular Cell Proteomics.* **5:** 801-810.

Cohen D.J., Ellerman D.A., Cuasnicu P.S. (2000). Mammalian sperm-egg fusion: evidence that epididymal protein DE plays a role in mouse gamete fusion. *Biology of Reproduction* **63:** 462-468.

Concha I.I., Urzua U., Yanez A., Schroeder R., Pessot C., Burzio L.O. (1993). U1 and U2 snRNA are localized in the sperm nucleus. *Experimental Cell Research* **204:** 378-381.

D´ýaz-Perez, E., Meizel S. (1992). Importance of mammalian endoprotease activity during the acrosome reaction to subsequent sperm-egg fusion: inhibitor studies with human sperm and zona-free hamster eggs. *Molecular Reproduction Devevelopment* **31:** 122-130.

D'Amours O., Frenette G., Fortier M., Leclerc P., Sullivan R. (2010). Proteomic comparison of detergent-extracted sperm proteins from bulls with different fertility indexes. *Reproduction* **139:** 545-556.

Da Ros V., Busso D., Cohen D.J., Maldera J., Goldweic N., Cuasnicu P.S. (2007). Molecular mechanisms involved in gamete interaction: evidence for the participation of cysteine-rich secretory proteins (CRISP) in sperm-egg fusion. *Society of Reproduction Fertility (Suppl.)*, **65:** 353-356.

Dadoune J.P, Pawalak A, Alfonsi M.F and Siffroi J.P. (2005). Identification of transcripts by macroarrys, RT-PCR and in situ hybridization in human ejaculate spermatozoa. *Human Reproduction* **11:** 133-140.

Das P.J., Paria N., Gustafson-Seabury A., Monika V., Sankar P.C., Charles C.L., Dickson D.V., Chowdhary B.P., Terje R. (2010). Total RNA isolation from stallion sperm and testis biopsies. *Animal Reproduction Science* **74:** 1099-1106.

de Mateo S., Martý´nez-Heredia J., Estanyol J.M., Domý´nguez-Fandos D., Vidal-Taboada J.M., Ballesca' J.L., Oliva R. (2007). Marked correlations in protein expression identified by proteomic analysis of human spermatozoa. *Proteomics* **7:** 4264-4277.

Ellerman D.A., Cohen D.J., Da Ros V.G., Morgenfeld M.M., Busso D, Cuasnicu P.S. (2006). Sperm protein "DE" mediates gamete fusion through an evolutionarily conserved site of the CRISP family. *Development Biology* **297:** 228-237.

Feugang F.M., Abdullah K., Grier P.P., Chen L., Mehta T., Hirani K., Lynne N., Einko T., Gibbs R., Memili E. (2009). Two-stage genome-wide association study identifies integrin beta 5 as having potential role in bull fertility. *BMC Genomics* **10:** 176-185

Foster J.A., Gerton G.L. (1996). Autoantigen 1 of the guinea pig sperm acrosome is the homologue of mouse Tpx-1 and human TPX1 and is a member of the cysteine-rich secretory protein (CRISP) family. *Molecular Reproduction and Development* **44:** 221-229.

Gatewood J.M., Cook G.R., Balhorn R., Bradbury E.M., Schmid C. (1987). Sequence-specific packaging of DNA in human sperm chromatin. *Science* **236:** 962-964.

Gibbons R., Adeoya-Osiguwa S.A., Fraser L.R. (2005). A mouse sperm decapacitation factor receptor is phosphatidylethanolamine-binding protein 1. *Reproduction* **130:** 497-508.

Giese A., Jude R., Kuiper H., Raudsepp T., Piumi F., Schambony A., Guerin G., Chowdhary B.P., Distl O., Topfer-Petersen E., Leeb T. (2002). Molecular characterization of the equine testis-specific protein 1 (TPX1) and acidic epididymal glycoprotein 2 (AEG2) genes encoding members of the cysteine-rich secretory protein (CRISP) family. *Gene* **299:** 101-109.

Gilbert I., Bissonnette N., Boissonneault G., Vallee M., Robert C. (2007). A molecular analysis of the population of mRNA in bovine spermatozoa. *Reproduction* **133:** 1073-1086.

Goodrich R., Johnson G., Krawetz S.A. (2007). The preparation of human spermatozoal RNA for clinical analysis. *Archives of Andrology* **53:** 161-167.

Hayashi S., Yang J., Christenson L., Yanagimachi R., Hecht N.B. (2003) Mouse preimplantation embryos developed from oocytes injected with round spermatids or spermatozoa have similar but distinct patterns of early messenger RNA expression. *Biology of Reproduction* **69:** 1170-1176.

Kasahara M., Gutknecht J., Brew K., Spurr N., Goodfellow P.N. (1989). Cloning and mapping of a testis-specific gene with sequence similarity to a spermcoating glycoprotein gene. *Genomics* **5:** 527-534.

Kratzschmar J., Haendler B., Eberspaecher U., Roosterman D., Donner P., Schleuning W.D. (1996). The human cysteine-rich secretory protein (CRISP) family. Primary structure and tissue distribution of CRISP-1, CRISP-2 and CRISP-3. *European Journal of Biochemistry* **236:** 827-836.

Krawetz S.A. (2005). Paternal contribution: new insights and future challenges. *Nature Reviews Genetics* **6:** 633-642.

Kumar G., Patel D., Rajesh K. (1993). c-MYC mRNA is present in human sperm cells. *Cell. Molecular Biology Research* **39:** 111-117.

Lalancette C., Miller D., Li Y., Krawetz S.A. (2008). Paternal contributions: new functional insights for spermatozoa RNA. *Journal of Cell Biochemistry* **104:** 1570-1579.

Lambard S., Galeraud-Denis I., Martin G., Levy R., Chocat A., Carreau S. (2004). Analysis and significance of mRNA in human ejaculated sperm from normozoospermic donors: relationship to sperm motility and capacitation. *Molecular Human Reproduction* **10:** 535-541.

Li A., Sakaguchi S., Shigematsu K., Atarashi R., Roy B.C., Nakaoke R., Arima K., Okimura N., Kopacek J., Katamine S. (2000). Physiological expression of the gene for PrP-like protein, PrPLP/Dpl, by brain endothelial cells and its ectopic expression in neurons of PrP-deficient mice ataxic due to Purkinje cell degeneration. *American Journal of Pathology* **157:** 1447-1452.

Li C., Sun Y., Yi K., Ma Y., Sun Y., Zhang W.X. (2010). Detection of nerve growth factor (NGF) and its specific receptor (TrkA) in ejaculated bovine sperm, and the effects of NGF on sperm function. *Theriogenology* **74:** 1615-1622.

Martins R.P., Krawetz S.A. (2005). RNA in human sperm. *Asian Journal of Andrology* **7:** 1-4.

McCauley T.C., Zhang H.M., Bellin M.E., Ax R.L. (2001). Identification of a heparin-binding protein in bovine seminal fluid as tissue inhibitor of metalloproteinases-2. *Molecular Reproduction and Development* **58:** 336-341.

Meseguer M., de los Santos M.J., Simon C., Pellicer A., Remohi J., Garrido N. (2006). Effect of sperm glutathione peroxidases 1 and 4 on embryo asymmetry and blastocyst quality in oocyte donation cycles. *Fertility and Sterility* **86:** 1376-1385.

Miller D. (1997). RNA in the ejaculate spermatozoon: a window into molecular events in spermatogenesis and a record of the unusual requirements of haploid gene expression and post-meiotic equilibration. *Molecular Human Reproduction* **3:** 669-676.

Miller D., Ostermeier G.C. (2006a). Towards a better understanding of RNA carriage by ejaculate spermatozoa. *Human Reproduction Update* **12:** 757–767.

Miller D., Ostermeier G.C. (2006b). Spermatozoal RNA. Why is it there and what does it do? *Gynecology Obstetrics and Fertility* **34:** 840-846.

Miller D., Briggs D., Snowden H., Hamlington J., Rollinson S., Lilford R., Krawetz S.A. (1999). A complex population of RNAs exists in human ejaculate spermatozoa: implications for understanding molecular aspects of spermiogenesis. *Gene* **237:** 385-392.

Miller D., Ostermeier G.C., Krawetz S.A. (2005). The controversy, potential and roles of spermatozoal RNA. *Trends in Molecular Medicine* **11:** 156-163.

Mizuki N., Sarapata D.E., Garcia-Sanz J.A., Kasahara M. (1992). The mouse male germ cell-specific gene Tpx-1: molecular structure, mode of expression in spermatogenesis, and sequence similarity to two non-mammalian genes. *Mammalian Genome* **3:** 274-280.

Moffit J.S., Boekelheide K., Sedivy J.M. and Klysik J. (2007). Mice lacking Raf kinase inhibitor protein-1 (RKIP-1) have altered sperm capacitation and reduced reproduction rates with a normal response to testicular injury. *Journal of Andrology* **28:** 883-890.

Müller D., Davidoff M.S., Bargheer O., Paust H.J., Pusch W., Koeva Y., Jezek D., Holstein A.F., Middendorff R. (2006). The expression of neurotrophins and their receptors in the prenatal and adult human testis: evidence for functions in Leydig cells. *Histochemistry and Cell Biology* **126:** 199-211.

Mutter D., Middendorff R., Davidoff M.S. (1999). Neurotrophic factors in the testis. *Biomedical Reviews* **10:** 25-30.

Naz R.K., Rajendran S. (2006). Receptors in Spermatozoa: Are They Real? *Journal of Andrology* **27:** 627-636.

Naz R.K. (1998). Effect of actinomycine D and cycloheximide on human sperm function. *Archiews of Andrology* **41:** 135-142.

Nikbakht G., Ali M., Baghbanzadeh M.R., Tajik A.P., Tamanini C., Emam M. (2010). Leptin receptor mRNA in bull ejaculated spermatozoa. *Reproduction in Domestic Animals* **45:** 237-242.

Nixon B., MacIntyre D.A., Mitchell L.A., Gibbs G.M., O'Bryan M., Aitken R.J. (2006). The identification of mouse sperm-surface-associated proteins and characterization of their ability to act as decapacitation factors. *Biology of Reproduction* **74:** 275-287.

O'Bryan M.K., Sebire K., Meinhardt A., Edgar K., Keah H.H., Hearn M.T., De Kretser D.M. (2001). Tpx-1 is a component of the outer dense fibers and acrosome of rat spermatozoa. *Molecular Reproduction and Development* **58:** 116-125.

Olszanska B., Borgul A. (1990). Quantitation of nanogram amounts of nucleic acids in the presence of proteins by the ethidium bromide staining technique. *Acta Biochimea Polomica* **37:** 59-63.

Ostermeier G.C., Dix D.J., Miller D., Khatri P., Krawetz S.A. (2002). Spermatozoal RNA profiles of normal fertile men. *Lancet* **360:** 772–777.

Ostermeier G.C., Miller D., Huntriss J.D., Diamond M.P., Krawetz S.A. (2004). Reproductive biology: delivering spermatozoan RNA to the oocyte. *Nature* **429:** 154.

Peoc'h K., Serres C., Frobert Y., Martin C., Lehmann S., Chasseigneaux S., Sazdovitch V., Grassi J., Jouannet P., Launay J.M., Laplanche J.L. (2002). The human "prion-like" protein Doppel is expressed in both Sertoli cells and spermatozoa. *Journal of Biological Chemistry* **277:** 43071-43078.

Pereira R.M., Mesquita P., Batista M., Baptista M.C., Barbas J.P., Pimenta J., Santos I.C., Marques M.R., Vasques M.I., Silva Pereira M., Santos Silva F., Oliveira Sousa M.C., Fontes C.M., Horta A.E., Prates J.A, Marques C.C. (2009). Doppel gene polymorphisms in Portuguese sheep breeds: insight on ram fertility. *Animal Reproduction Science* **114:** 157-166.

Pessot C.A., Brito M., Figueroa J., Concha I.I., Yanez A., Burzio L.O. (1989). Presence of RNA in the sperm nucleus. *Biochemistry, Biophysics, Research Communications* **158:** 272-278.

Roberts K.P., Wamstad J.A., Ensrud K.M., Hamilton D.W. (2003). Inhibition of capacitation-associated tyrosine phosphorylation signaling in rat sperm by epididymal protein Crisp-1. *Biology Reproduction* **69:** 572-581.

Robinson L.L., Townsend J., Anderson R.A. (2003). The human fetal testis is a site of expression of neurotrophins and their receptors: regulation of the germ cell and peritubular cell population. *Journal of Clinical Endocrinology and Metabolism* **88:** 3943-3951.

Rui Pires Martins R.P., Krawetz S. A. (2005). RNA in human sperm. *Asian Journal of Andrology* **7:** 115-120.

Schoff P.K., Cheetham J., Lardy H.A. (1989). Adenylate kinase activity in ejaculated bovine sperm flagella. *Journal of Biological Chemistry* **264:** 6086-6091.

Souès S., Kann M.L., Fouquet J.P., Melki R. (2003). The cytosolic chaperonin CCT associates to cytoplasmic microtubular structures during mammalian spermiogenesis and to heterochromatin in germline and somatic cells. *Experimental Cell Research* **288:** 363-373.

Sternlicht H., Farr G.W., Sternlicht M.L., Driscoll J.K., Willison K., Yaffe M.B. (1993). The T-complex polypeptide 1 complex is a chaperonin for tubulin and actin *in vivo*. *Proceeding National Academy of Science, USA*. **90:** 9422-9426.

Suarez S.S., Ho H.C. (2003). Hyperactivated motility in sperm. *Reproduction in Domestic Animals* **38:** 119-124.

Wang H., Zhou Z., Xu M., Li J., Xiao J., Xu Z.Y., Sha J. (2004). A spermatogenesis-related gene expression profile in human spermatozoa and its potential clinical applications. *Journal of Molecular Medicine* **82:** 317-324.

WanZho J.,Tanaka A., Watanabe G., Matsuda H., Taya K. (2010). Effect of NGF on the motility and acrosome reaction of Golden hamster spermatozoa *in vitro*. *Journal of Reproduction and Development* **56:** 437-443.

Wykes, S. M., Visscher D.W., Krawetz S.A. (1997). Haploid transcripts persist in mature human spermatozoa. *Molecular Human Reproduction* **3:** 15-19.

Yang C.C., Lin Y.S., Hsu C.C., Wu S.C., Lin E.C., Cheng W.T. (2009). Identification and sequencing of remnant messenger RNAs found in domestic swine (*Sus scrofa*) fresh ejaculated spermatozoa. *Animal Reproduction Science* **113:** 143-155.

Zhao Y., Li Q., Yao C., Wang Z., Zhou Y.,Wang Y., Liu L.,Wang L., Qiao Z. (2006). Characterization and quantification of mRNA transcripts in ejaculated spermatozoa of fertile men by serial analysis of gene expression. *Human Reproduction* **21:** 1583-1590.

❑❑❑

Chapter 20

Sexing of Spermatozoa and Embryos in Farm Animals: Achievements and Challenges

S. Selvaraju, A. Arangasamy, J.P. Ravindra
National Institute of Animal Nutrition and Physiology, Adugodi, Bangalore-560 030, Karnataka, India

Summary

Since ages, human beings have been interested in controlling the sex of their own offspring and of the animals. Predetermination of sex in the animals is in great demand since they provide food for the ever increasing human population. Gender pre-selection has been focused prior to or after coitus, at insemination and also manipulation of sperm and embryo. Various theories of sexing such as females developed on the left side and males on the right of the uterus originated with the Greek philosophers but without scientific explanation. Even in eighteenth century it was believed that sperm from the right testes produced more male while sperm from the left produced more females. The scientific break through that the differences in DNA content between X and Y sperm led to the conclusion that sex control could be accomplished. The flowcytometric method of XY separation has been validated on the basis of live births. Promising various other approaches like immunological sexing and manipulation of maternal environment are simultaneously focused to select sex of the offspring. In addition varying methods f embryo sexing is also discussed.

The main objectives of using reproductive biotechnologies in livestock are to increase production, efficiency of reproduction and rates of genetic gain. Over the years, many options have become available for managing the reproduction of the major large and small ruminants. Artificial insemination (AI) and cryopreservation of semen and embryos are the main technologies that are used extensively. Both of these technologies enable preservation of superior paternal/maternal genetic resources and facilitate international trade in germplasm.

In India, livestock sector is an important source of livelihood to a large proportion of landless labourers and small and marginal farmers. The birth of a male calf in a dairy farm leads to the loss of future female animal for breeding. Further this also makes the farmer to wait with uncertainty for at least one more year to get a female calf. This is not in the interest of the farmer's economy. Juxtaposed to this, in country like India, there is a ban on cow slaughter; a selective production of male calves becomes imminent to meet the protein requirement of the growing population and also to enhance beef export. Under these circumstances, production of calves of desired sex using sex selected semen will be helpful to improve farm productivity and economy of the farmer. This also improves export oriented meat industry by assuring the birth of a sex selected calf. As well, it could enhance the effect of livestock genetic research in general by increasing the rate at which animals of the required sex would be available for breeding.

Despite high costs and complex procedures, sexing of spermatozoa, usually followed by cryopreservation, is being used commercially for cattle and horse production in several countries. In India there is a lack of extensive research on this area even for the cattle and buffalo, which are the two important animals for milk and meat production.

1. Importance of sexing

Biotechnological means can greatly help in accelerating the speed of introducing the desirable characteristics such as better growth rates, or increased milk production into animals. Sexing of spermatozoa is one such technique which helps in increasing the rate of genetic improvement and reduces the cost of livestock production. For feeding ever increasing human population with the pressure to improve productivity with limited resources, it is essential to produce desired type of calf such as female for dairy industry in cattle and male for export oriented meat industry in buffalo. Further, sex selection will conserve the desired germplasm of endangered species like zebu cattle. In equine breeding industry, producing fillies for more genetically advanced brood mares including racing purpose, results in high economic return.

Implementation of systems for *in vitro* embryo production (IVEP) in bovine has been limited by costs, inefficiencies, and compromised conception rates. The IVEP program with sex sorted sperm would allow these technologies to be combined effectively in modern breeding programs. The efficiency of IVEP programs could be enhanced dramatically by skewing the sex ratio in favor of females.

In future, the requirement for sex sorted semen for IVEP, transgenesis and cloning will be more. As such the success rate of transgenic animal production is very low (0.7-0.9%) because of limitations of the available technologies. Success rate would be lower by half for the genes which are expressed only in a particular sex if a mixed XY population of spermatozoa is used for breeding the animals. Use of sexed semen will greatly improve the success rate in such a scenario. For example, if the idea is to produce a transgenic animal wherein the gene of interest is only expressed in milk, production of embryos using female sexed sperm is desirable.

2. Research in sex selection

Major breakthrough in sexing of spermatozoa happened in the year 1968, when Gardner and Edward sexed the rabbit blastocyst based on the presence or absence of the Barr body. The presence of a Barr body (formed from the inactive X-chromosome) in female cells is not a reliable indicator of sex in the domestic farm animal species. Then in the year, 1973, Dane and Rowson (cited by Polge and Rowson, 1973) sexed the sheep embryos based on karyotyping. The first successful gender pre-selected calf was produced during the year 1975. The differences in DNA content between X and Y chromosome bearing spermatozoa is being used since 1980's. Latter on Larry Johnson in the year 1989 introduced the method of sexing by flow cytometry using the differential DNA content between X and Y chromosome bearing spermatozoa.

3. Spermatozoa sexing

Manipulation of sperm has attracted the greatest interest among the end users and the scientific community since sex determination in mammals is based on the chromosome content of the fertilizing sperm. Successful separation of X and Y chromosome bearing spermatozoa is dependent on the existence of some fundamental differences between the two types of cells (Table 1).

Swimming of sperm through sperm albumin gradient has been used for many years in an effort to distort sex ratio. However, it has not been fully effective in animal studies. Separating sperm by using physical characters remains a subject of controversy. Hence researchers are focusing the difference in DNA content between X and Y chromosome bearing spermatozoa to preselect sex of the offspring (Table 2).

Table 1 : Proposed phenotypic differences between X and Y chromosome bearing sperm

	Phenotypic characters	Reference
1.	Plasma membrane surface charge (Relatively negative on X-sperm)	Kaneko *et al.*, 1984
2.	Differences in density	Harvey, 1946
3.	Morphological differences in nucleus and head of spermatozoa	Shelters, 1961
4.	Unique lactate dehydrogenase isozyme in Y sperm	Stambaugh and Buckley, 1971
5.	H-Y antigen present on Y-bearing sperm	Goldberg *et al.*, 1971
6.	Swimming velocity	Ericsson *et al.*, 1973
7.	Motility characteristics	Sarkar *et al.*, 1984.
8.	DNA content	Moruzzi, 1979.

Table 2 : Differences in DNA content (percent) between X and Y containing spermatozoa in different species

Species	Percent difference
Human	2.9
Swine	3.6
Cattle	3.8
Dog	3.9
Horse	4.1
Sheep	4.2

4. Flow cytometric sorting of sexed spermatozoa

Isolation of X-bearing sperm, in particular, could have important consequences with respect to the availability and affordability of replacement of dairy heifers. It is speculated that farmers could achieve financial benefits even if the cost of sex-sorted semen was twice that of unsorted semen from a comparable sire. At present, the only proven method for sexing sperm is the fluorescence-activated cell sorting approach, commonly known as the "Beltsville sperm sexing technology,"

Sorting of semen, one sperm at a time, into males and females, using staining procedure and detecting by laser beam with the help of standard flow cytometry equipment is the brief procedure behind the flow cytometric sorting of spermatozoa (Johnson and Welch, 1999). Thus, sperms with an X or Y chromosome could be used to produce male or female embryos/animals. Offsprings have been produced via artificial insemination with spermatozoa sexed by flow cytometry and cell sorting. The pregnancy rate after sorting and cryopreservation is reported to be lower, regardless of species, following AI (Seidel Jr., *et al.*, 1999; Hollinshead *et al.*, 2002). The differential expression of developmentally important mRNA transcripts in bovine blastocysts derived from sex-sorted and non-sorted sperm may partially explain the reasons for reduction in embryo production efficiency (Morton *et al.*, 2007). Refinement in the sorting process such as reduced sorting pressure and use of pulse lasers reduces damage to sperm and increases fertility (Schenk *et al.*, 2009; Sharpe and Evans, 2009). Further, modification in semen preservation protocols during and after sorting may result in pregnancy rates near those of unsorted semen (Rath *et al.*, 2009). Similarly, *in vitro* sperm characteristics, including motility, viability, mitochondrial activity, and acrosome integrity, are no longer reduced after modified flow cytometry (de Graaf *et al.*, 2006). The advancement is sexing of spermatozoa in one species may not be equally applicable to all domestic animals. For example, despite sheep and cattle being closely related species, ovine embryos were more tolerant or adaptive to changing culture conditions, as quantified through morphology, cryotolerance, and relative mRNA abundance (Rizos *et al.*, 2004). Hence, the embryo production and pregnancy rate after sorting may be more efficient in ovine as compared to bovine.

4.1 Constraints and probable solutions of flow cytometry based sperm sexing

Offsprings from sexed spermatozoa appear to have no abnormalities both genotypically and phenotypically. However the accuracy of spermatozoa sexing is found to be 85–95% in most species. About a quarter of the spermatozoa processed are sexed and the rest are discarded in the process or lost due to logistical constraints. The resulting loss reduces the number of available spermatozoa for routine artificial insemination use. Spermatozoa also undergo some damage during sorting. When similar numbers of spermatozoa per dose have been used, pregnancy rates with sexed spermatozoa usually have been 60–80% of unsexed control spermatozoa. This is due to the amount of damage to DNA and mortality of spermatozoa (for review see Garner and Seidel Jr., 2003).

During routine practice for cattle, 20×10^6 sperm/ dose is used to inseminate. Since sexing technology drastically reduces the available spermatozoa numbers, low dose insemination seem a viable option with sexing of spermatozoa for wide spread use of this technique. However, insemination with low concentration of sexed sperm per dose resulted in low conception rate in heifers (Seidel *et al.*, 1999). Fertility may be increased by improving sexing technology and animal management. The efficient methods which may improve fertility are intra uterine insemination and deep cornual insemination ipsilateral to ovary having mature follicle (Hunter, 2001).

Since the duration of sexing of sperm is longer and seminal plasma is absent in the sexed semen, various factors influence the spermatozoa viability and membrane integrity during and after sexing. Development of freezing and thawing methods that improve fertility and survival of cryopreserved sexed spermatozoa is also important.

Although the technique is expensive and the applications are limited for routine use, sexed spermatozoa has tremendous application in biomedical research. For example changes in membrane protein patterns from sorted X- and Y- chromosome bearing spermatozoa will be helpful to understand the molecular factors involved during sexed semen processing.

5. Immunological method of sperm sexing

Surface antigenic differences between male and female sperm cells can be exploited to sex the spermatozoa. The antibody raised against unwanted sex may cause the sperm to clump. Various immunological approaches to sex the spermatozoa of mammals have been tested without repeatable success.

An immunological approach, however, would be highly desirable because inexpensive batch processing could be used to enrich for either X- or Y-chromosome-bearing spermatozoa. The conventional approach to immunological sexing, utilization of a surface protein has shown little promise of being successful to date. In a recent study, rabbit antisera was purified against X- or Y- bovine sperm were used to immunoprecipitate sex-specific proteins (SSPs) in bovine sperm proteins. The antibody of 30 kDa protein specifically was captured by the rabbit antisera against X-sperm. This 30 kDa protein might be a sex-specific protein in bovine X-sperm, which has the potential to be used in immunological procedures for sexing sperm (Sang *et al.,* 2011). A viable immunological sperm sexing procedure can be developed using a more rigorous method to isolate SSPs (Blecher *et al.,* 1999; Sang *et al.,* 2011). However, to date there are no reports of producing sex-selected offspring with this procedure despite considerable improvement in scientific knowledge (Ellis *et al.,* 2011).

6. Embryo sexing

Determination of the sex of the preimplantation embryos is important for the management and breeding of livestock as well as for the prenatal diagnosis of genetic disorders. Generally embryos have been sexed either by invasive (biopsy) or non-invasive (without biopsy of embryonic tissues) method.

6.1 Invasive method

6.1.1 Karyotyping

Identification of one Y or two X chromosome in the cultured biopsied cells from embryos.

6.1.2 Y- specific chromosomal DNA probes

In this method, cells from biopsies are spread on a slide treated with proteinase to expose the DNA and then hybridized with radioactively labeled Y chromosome specific probe. This technique is reliable and required only a few non-dividing cells, so the viability of embryos is not affected. This technique is quite complicated, expensive, time consuming and requires the cryopreservation of embryo biopsy (Thomson *et al.*, 1991).

6.1.3 PCR method

This method shortened the time of the sexing assay to less than 6 h and has minimized the number of cells required (1-3 cells). The sex of the buffalo embryos could be able to predict with 100% accuracy, using three different sets of bovine Y-chromosome specific primers (Appa Rao *et al.*, 1993). In spite of the speed and accuracy, there are risks of contamination and requirement of micromanipulator to invade zona pellucida. Under farm conditions sexing could be more rapid (within 1-2 h) possibly by replacing enzymatic lysis of the biopsies with chemical lysis and reducing the number of cycles in the PCR (Bredbacka *et al.*, 1994).

6.2 Non-invasive Method

6.2.1 Quantitative comparison of the X-linked enzymes between male and female embryos

Two enzymes *viz.*, glucose-6-phosphate dehydrogenase (Williams, 1986) or hypoxanthine phosphoribosyl transferase (Monk and Handyside, 1988) activities are proposed to be measured between the embryos. This method is based on the hypothesis that the ratio of X-linked enzyme activity to autosomal enzyme activity is higher in female than in male embryos. The activity of the enzyme is scored as high or low, based on whether embryos stain a light or dark color, respectively in the presence of the indicator dye. However, early inactivation of some of the female embryos and the toxicity of the dye to the embryos make this technique ineffective for sex determination.

6.2.2 Detection of male specific H-Y antigen

H-Y antigen is controlled by Y chromosome. Bovine 4-cell embryos to blastocyst have been used for this purpose. The H-Y antigen is identified by cytotoxicity or through immuno fluorescence assays. Success rate of sex determination is 84% (White *et al.*, 1987).

6.2.3 Differences in developmental rates between male and female embryos

Sexual dimorphism might occur from the time of fertilization, because much younger male and female embryo differences can be shown on day 8 of *in vitro* cultured cattle embryos. A lower average meiotic index is seen in male than in female embryos in cattle (Xu *et al.*, 1992).

7. Sperm sexing vs embryo sexing

Manipulation of sperm has attracted the greatest interest since sex determination in mammals is based on the chromosome content of the fertilizing sperm. Sperm sexing is simple and abnormalities in offspring are not common than with embryo sexing. In embryo sexing only 50% of the embryos are of desired sex, whereas in sperm sexing more than 85% embryos are of desired sex. Hence, sex determination at conception is more economical than embryo sexing. It is reasonable to believe that sexing of spermatozoa will replace sexing of embryos. With sexed spermatozoa additional technologies such as AI, *in vitro* fertilization and embryo transfer technology, cloning and transgenics can also be effectively used to get desired offspring and end product like milk and meat (animal pharming).

8. Economic benefits of sexed semen

Sex selection is also essential for various production purposes. Male calves are highly essential for open nucleus breeding scheme, bull mother farm and production of genetically advanced breeding bull. In a beef industry, where the sex ratio is skewed toward males, the value is in the difference between the weaning weight of the steers' vs heifers plus the higher selling price for steers.

Female calves are highly essential for progeny testing programs and for breeding heifers, in which the female calves leads to less dystocia and obstetrical complications. In a dairy industry, to propagate and exploit high quality maternal characteristics, sex selection is highly essential.

The cost of a unit of sexed semen would probably range from 1.5 to 2.25 times the present value of semen depending upon the genetic worth of the bull. Based upon these costs there will be situations where the value of sexed semen will be economically justified, however, every operation will have a different set of factors that will need to be considered. Commercial application of this technology depends on type of separation and its efficiency (cost), and resulting pregnancy rates. This application has the potential to revolutionize cattle breeding strategies in both beef and dairy sectors.

9. Skewing of sex ratio in farm animals

9.1 Effect of synchronization

PGF_2 alpha treatment favors male calf probably by reducing progesterone levels (James, 1989). Whereas, combination of PGF_2 alpha+GnRH treatment favors female calf probably by elevating gonadotrophin levels (Ostrowsji, 1988). If this is the case, progesterone synchronization may favor female calves in cattle (Xu and Burton, 1999).

9.2 Timing of mating relative to ovulation

Earlier in cattle it was suggested that, early breeding at estrus resulted in more female calves, however, such findings could not be confirmed (Foote, 1977). Recent studies with more precise technological control of the reproductive cycle demonstrate that a small degree of distortion of sex ratio may be possible by timing of insemination (Rorie, 1999). Though it has been advocated for years, it simply has not been repeatable because precise prediction of timing of ovulation has not been possible as yet.

Different rates of development between male and female embryos under *in vitro* condition provide a plausible mechanism for sex selection (Rorie, 1999).

9.3 Cryopreservation and AI results in sex selection

It is reported that frozen semen resulted in 1.24– 1.66% more male calves than fresh AI semen. And the difference may be due to the effect of freezing on the survival and function of the X or Y-bearing sperm or on the subsequent effect on the survival of the embryos after fertilization. A 1% increase in the probability of a male calf being born following artificial insemination has been reported (Berry and Cromie, 2007).

9.4 Nutraceuticals- a way to alter sex ratio

The young dams (mice) fed high-fat diet and bred within 40 weeks of age had a sex ratio of 0.67:0.33 (male/female). The mature dams fed the low fat-high carbohydrate diet had more females as compared to male (0.39:0.61 male/female). Explanations for these observations have been proposed (Rivers and Crawford, 1974), but not scientifically tested. Finding that the females in better body condition would produce more male than female progeny with some exception has been observed in domestic ruminants and monogastric species, (for review, Rosenfeld and Roberts, 2003). The cows, that have problems in becoming pregnant by artificial insemination, also tend to produce more males (King *et al.*, 1985). If sex-ratio skewing due to diet could occur in dairy cows, how long the feeding period would be needed to effect the change has to be tested. Clearly, any technique, nutritional or otherwise, that would yield more female calves would be of great benefit to the dairy industry.

Altering, follicular fluid, uterine and vaginal environment is also proposed to skew sex ratio towards a particular gender. The offsprings sex ratios in female mammals are significantly related to maternal dominance (Clutton-Brock *et al.,* 1984). It was hypothesized that the higher levels of follicular testosterone was associated with a greater likelihood of conceiving a male. Bovine ova that developed in follicular fluid with high concentrations of testosterone *in vivo* were significantly more likely to be fertilized by Y chromosome-bearing spermatozoa (Grant *et al.,* 2008). But a recent study could not relate the testosterone concentration in the follicular fluid with that of the offspring's sex (García-Herreros *et al.,* 2010). Uni and divalent cationic elements in seminal and female reproductive tract fluids influence the allosteric properties of enzymatic systems and chemotactic properties within and around the unfertilized eggs. High sodium and potassium ions around the egg leads to male, whereas calcium and magnesium ions around the egg leads to female offspring.

Altering vaginal environment is also proposed to skew sex ratio. X-sperm have a survival advantage in acidic secretions, while Y-sperm have a motility advantage in more alkaline secretions. The viscoelastic properties of the mucopeptides secreted within the cervical mucus are highly dependent upon both the pH of the fluid and on the electrolyte content.

Conclusions

Sex pre-selection has generated great interest and controversy over the years. Medical and commercial benefits outweigh the ethical issues. Despite the costs and complexities involved in sexing of spermatozoa, the method of sexing could be commercially viable for niche applications in several species. Much simpler equipment as compared to flowcytometric sorting designed specifically for sperm sexing probably will reduce the cost of sexed semen. As efficiencies improve and costs decline, sperm sexing will be applied more widely. Maternal diet, possibly its caloric content, can play a directive role in skewing offspring sex ratio. Sexed sperm combined with AI makes it possible to pre-determine the sex of offspring and may make revolution in the field of research/dairy industry. Sexed semen could markedly increase genetic improvement rates and have major implications for end-product commercial production. It is likely that no method will be capable of being 100% accurate in selection because of the large number of spermatozoa produced in each ejaculate, and the fact that only one spermatozoa results in fertilization. Therefore, once a selection technique becomes available it will probably skew the sex ratio of calves born by some percentage rather than being 100% predictable. With all of the above factors considered, it is reasonable to assume that the sexing of semen will decrease the production potential of a bull by greater than one-half.

"I formerly thought that when a tendency to produce the two sexes in equal numbers was advantageous to the species, it would follow from natural selection, but I now see that the whole problem is so intricate that it is safer to leave its solution for the future."- Charles Darwin. In: *Descent of Man*, 1874.

References

Appa Rao K.B.C., Pawshe C.H., Totey S.M. (1993). Ex determination of in vitro developed buffalo (*Bubalus bubalis*) embryos by DNA amplification. *Molecular Reproduction and Development* **36:** 291-296.

Berry D.P., Cromie A.R. (2007). Artificial insemination increases the probability of a male calf in dairy and beef cattle. *Theriogenology* **67:** 346-352.

Blecher S.R., Howie R., Li S., Detmar J., Blahut L.M. (1999). A new approach to the immunological sexing of sperm. *Theriogenology* **52:** 1309-1321.

Bodmer M., Janett F., Hässig M., den Daas N., Reichert P., Thun R. (2005). Fertility in heifers and cows after low dose insemination with sex-sorted and non-sorted sperm under field conditions. *Theriogenology* **64:** 1457-1474.

Bredbacka P., Velmala R., Peippo J., Bredbacka K. (1994). Survival of biopsied and sexed bovine demi embryos. *Theriogenology* **41:** 1023-1031.

Clutton-Brock T.H., Albon S.D., Guinness F.E. (1984). Maternal dominance, breeding success and birth sex ratios in red deer. *Nature* **308:** 358-360.

de Graaf S.P., Evans G., Maxwell W.M., O'Brien J.K. (2006). In vitro characteristics of fresh and frozen-thawed ram spermatozoa after sex sorting and re-freezing. *Reproduction Fertility and Development* **18:** 867-874.

Ellis P.J.I., Yu Y., Zhang S. (2011). Transcriptional dynamics of the sex chromosomes and the search for offspring sex-specific antigens in sperm. *Reproduction* **142:** 609-619.

Ericsson R.J., Langevin C.N., Nishino M. (1973). Isolation of fractions rich in human Y sperm. *Nature* **246:** 421-424.

Foote R. (1997). Sex ratios in dairy cattle under various conditions. *Theriogenology* **8:** 349-357.

García-Herreros M., Bermejo-Alvarez P., Rizos D., Gutiérrez-Adán A., Fahey A.G., Lonergan P. (2010). Intrafollicular testosterone concentration and sex ratio individually cultured bovine embryos. *Reproduction Fertility and Development* **22:** 533-538.

Gardner R.L., Edwards R.G. (1968). Control of the sex ratio at full term in the rabbit by transferring sexed blastocysts. *Nature* **218:** 346-348.

Garner D.L., Seidel Jr, G.E. (2003). Past, present and future perspectives on sexing sperm. *Canadian Journal of Animal Science* **83:** 375-384.

Goldberg E.H., Boyse E.A., Bennet D., Scheid M., Carswell E.A. (1971). Serological demonstration of H-Y (male) antigen on mouse sperm. *Nature* **232:** 478-480.

Grant V.J., Irwin R.J., Standley N.T., Shelling A.N., Chamley L.W. (2008). Sex of bovine embryos may be related to mothers' preovulatory follicular testosterone. *Biology of Reproduction* **78:** 812-815.

Harvey E.N. (1946). Can the sex of mammalian offspring be controlled? *Journal of Heredity* **37:** 71-73.

Hollinshead F.K., O'Brien J.K., Maxwell W.M.C., Evans G. (2002). Production of lambs of predetermined sex after the insemination of ewes with low numbers of frozen-thawed sorted X- or Y-chromosome-bearing spermatozoa. *Reproduction Fertility and Development* **14:** 503-508.

Hunter R.H.F. (2001). New breeding opportunities with deep cornual insemination: exploiting modern sperm technologies in cattle. *Reproduction in Domestic Animals* **36:** 217-222

James WH. (1989). The sex ratio of offspring of estrus-synchronised heifers. *Dtsch Tierarztl Wochenschr* **96:** 424-425.

Johnson L.A., Flook J.P., Hawk H.W. (1989). Sex preselection in rabbits: Live births from Xand Y sperm separated by DNA and cell sorting. *Biology of Reproduction* **4:** 199-203.

Johnson L.A., Welch G.R. (1999). Sex preselection: High speed flow cytometirc sorting of X and Y sperm for maximum efficiency. *Theriogenology* **52:** 1323-1342.

Kaneko S., Oshio S., Kobiashi T. (1984). Human X and Y bearing sperm differ in cell surface sialic acid content. *Biochemical and Biophysical Research Communications* **124:** 950-955.

King Jr K.K., Seidel G.E., Elsden R.P. (1985). Bovine embryo transfer pregnancies. I. Abortion rates and characteristics of calves. *Journal of Animal Science* **61:** 747-757.

Monk M., Handyside A.H. (1988). Sexing of preimplantation mouse embryos by measurement of X-linked gene dosage in a single blastomere. *Journal of Reproduction and Fertility* **82:** 365-368.

Morton K.M., Herrmann D., Sieg B., Struckmann C., Maxwell W.M., Rath D., Evans G., Lucas-Hahn A., Niemann H., Wrenzycki C. (2007). Altered mRNA expression patterns in bovine blastocysts after fertilisation in vitro using flow-cytometrically sex-sorted sperm. *Molecular Reproduction and Development* **74:** 931-940.

Moruzzi J.F. (1979). Selecting a mammalian species for the separation of X and Y chromosome bearing spermatozoa. *Journal of Reproduction and Fertility* **57:** 319-323.

Ostrowsji J.E.B. (1988). Pasture breeding of oestrus-synchronized beef heifers and its apparent effect on sex-ratio of offspring. *Dtsch Tierarztl Wochenschr* **95:** 365-368.

Polge C., Rowson L.E.A. (1973). Recent progress in techniques for increasing reproductive potential in farm animals. In: *Proceedings of the Third World Conference on Animal Production* (R.L. Reid, Ed.), Melbourne. Sydney University Press, Sydney, pp 633-643.

Rath D., Moench-Tegeder G., Taylor U., Johnson. L.A. (2009). Improved quality of sex-sorted sperm: A prerequisite for wider commercial application. *Theriogenology* **71:** 22-29.

Rivers J., Crawford M. (1974). Maternal nutrition and the sex ratio at birth. *Nature* **252:** 297-298.

Rizos D., Gutierrez-Adan A., Moreira P., O'Meara C., Fair T., Evans A.C.O., Boland M.P., Lonergan P. (2004). Species-related differences in blastocyst quality are associated with differences in relative mRNA transcription. *Molecular Reproduction and Development* **69:** 381-386.

Rorie R.W. (1999). Effect of timing of artificial insemination on sex ratio. *Theriogenology* **52:** 1273-1280.

Rorie R.W., Lester T.D., Lindsey B.R., McNew R.W. (1999). Effect of timing of artificial insemination on gender ratio in beef cattle. *Theriogenology* **52:** 1035-1041.

Rosenfeld C.S., Roberts R.M. (2004). Maternal diet and other factors affecting offspring sex ratio: A review. *Biology of Reproduction* **71:** 1063-1070.

Sang L., Yang W.C., Han L., Liang A.X., Hua G.H., Xiong J.J., Huo L.J., Yang L.G. (2011). An immunological method to screen sex-specific proteins of bovine sperm. *Journal of Dairy Science* **94:** 2060-2070.

Sarkar S., Jolly D. J., Friedmann T., Jones O.W. (1984). Swimming behaviour of X and Y human sperm. *Differentiation* **27:** 120-125.

Schenk J.L., Cran D.G., Everett R.W., Seidel Jr G.E. (2009). Pregnancy rates in heifers and cows with cryopreserved sexed sperm: Effects of sperm numbers per inseminate, sorting pressure and sperm storage before sorting. *Theriogenology* **71:** 717-728.

Seidel Jr G.E., Schenk J.L., Herickhoff L.A., Doyle S.P., Brink Z., Green R.D., Cran D.G. (1999). Insemination of heifers with sexed sperm. *Theriogenology* **52:** 1407-1420.

Sharpe J.C., Evans K.M. (2009). Advances in flow cytometry for sperm sexing. *Theriogenology* **71:** 4-10.

Shelters L.B. (1961). Human spermatozoa shape in relation to sex ratio. *Fertility and Sterility* **12:** 502-508.

Stambaugh R., Buckley J. (1971). Association of the lactic dehydrogenase X4 isozyme with male producing rabbit spermatozoa. *Jornal of Reproduction and Fertility* **25:** 275-278.

Thomson P.D., Schwerin M., Poulsen P.H., Avery B. (1991). Sex determination of bovine embryo biopsies using in situ hybridization. *Reproduction in Domestic Animals* **26:** 66-69.

White K.L., Anderson G.B., Bondurant R.H. (1987). Expression of a male–specific factor on various stages of preimplantation bovine embryos. *Biology of Reproduction* **37:** 867-873.

Williams T. J. (1986). A technique for sexing mouse embryos by a visual colorimetric assay of the X-linked enzyme, glucose-6-phosphate dehydrogenase. *Theriogenology* **25:** 733-739.

Xu K.P., Yadav B.R., Kines W.A., Betteridge K.J. (1992). Sex related differences in developmental rates of bovine embryos produced and cultured in vitro. *Molecular Reproduction and Development* **31:** 249-252.

Xu Z.Z., Burton L.J. (1999). Reproductive performance of dairy heifers after estrus synchronization and fixed-time artificial insemination. *Journal of Dairy Science* **82:** 910-917.

□□□

Section - 3

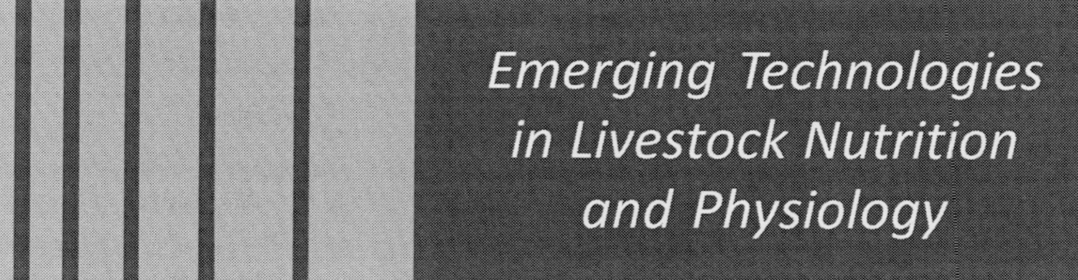
Emerging Technologies
in Livestock Nutrition
and Physiology

Chapter 21

Stem Cell Technologies: Present Status and Prospects in Farm Animal Research

J. Ghosh, S. Shree Vidhya
National Institute of Animal Nutrition and Physiology, Adugodi, Bangalore 560 030, Karnataka, India

Summary

Stem cell technologies are developing in a rapid pace for its potential application in human therapeutics. The present state of knowledge, development and areas of applications are highlighted in this chapter especially for embryonic and induced pluripotent stem cells. Spermatogonial stem cells are also described which have long been the interests of the entire reproductive biologist's community and the best understood *in vivo* system available in mammals for adult stem cell studies. Some avenues of research are described such as: 1) *in vitro* model for genetic studies, specifically for those genes whose homozygous mutants cause embryonic lethality; 2) *in vitro* differentiation of male or female germ cells from the pluripotent or unipotent stem cells which gives an opportunity to treat the infertile couples; and 3) differentiation of embryonic stem cells to trophoblast cells for studying the *in vitro* development of placenta from the beginning which were not possible in earlier days. In this whole endeavor, animals have been looked at as models for testing the efficiency of tissue or organ transplants because of their long life compared to rodent. The potential attractive applications of stem cell technologies on which animal scientists should reap the benefit are improvement of breeds and biopharming by genetic manipulation of stem cells followed by production of chimera or somatic cell nuclear transfer clones.

Stem cells are unspecialized cells which have the capacity to develop into many different specialized cell types of the body during early life and growth. In early life they are available in the inner cell mass and in adults they are present in different tissues where they serve as an internal repair system, which divide without limit to replenish other cells as long as the person or animal is alive. Stem cells after cell division either remain as stem cells or become differentiated to another type of cell with a more specialized function. For example, if the cells are of the embryonic stem cell type, after division some cells remain as pluripotent stem cells whereas others differentiate to become muscle cells, beating cells of heart, blood cells, or brain cells (Fig. 1).

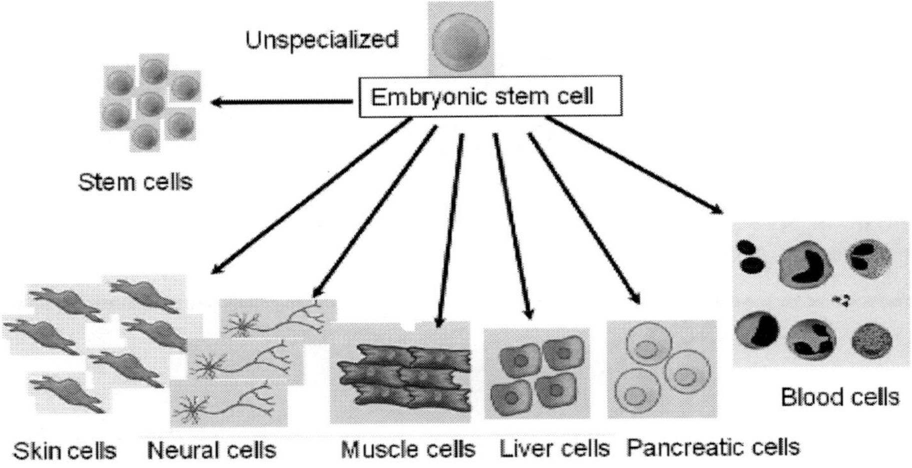

Fig. 1 : Fate of embryonic stem cells after cell division. They either remain unspecialized after cell division or become varying specialized cells of the body system after differentiation.

The excitement surrounding stem cells is enormous because of its potential in human regenerative medicine, the controversies related to therapeutics and the ethical issues involved in such technologies. In animal science this technology has huge potential applications which need to be explored by careful considerations. In animals these cells may provide a powerful tool for gene targeting, as disease model, cloning and can also facilitate development of efficient methods for somatic cell nuclear transfer (SCNT), transgenesis and gene regulation.

1. Types of stem cells and sources

Stem cells are named after the source from which they are derived such as embryonic stem cells, germ stem cells, fetal stem cells and adult stem cells. Embryonic stem (ES) cells are available in the inner cell mass of the early developing embryos. The germ line stem cells are available in the gonads.

Of the existence of two germ line stem cells, spermatogonial stem cells are known, however, female germ line stem cells in the ovary are not yet proved with certainty. The varying sources of fetal stem cells are the fetal tissues (tissue specific), blood circulation (mesenchymal stem cells, haemopoetic stem cells), placenta ectoplacental cone (EPC), mesenchymal stem cells, amniotic and allantoic fluids (ES cell like mesenchymal stem cells, haemopoetic stem cells) and umbilical cord. The adult stem cells are found in different types of tissue and organs (*e.g.,* bone marrow, endometrium, prostate and skin).

Stem cells are also classified as uni, bi, multi and pluripotent types based on the differentiation potential to one, two or more than two specific lineage types. The germ line stem cells are unipotent which can generate either male or female germ cells. Fetal stem cells are of pluripotent to multipotent types whereas, the adult stem cells are either unipotent, bipotent or multipotent. The mesenchymal and haemopoteic stem cells are examples of multipotent cells as they can generate cells of only a specific lineage such as red blood cells, white blood cells and platelets. Embryonic stem cells are pluripotent since they have the potential to generate all the tissues types of three germ cell lineages (*viz.,* ectoderm, mesoderm and endoderm) present in the embryo and adult.

2. Fundamental properties of stem cells

Stem cells have three fundamental properties:

1. Ability to self renewal without differentiation.
2. Capability to generate one or more lineage of specialized cells (ectoderm, mesoderm and endoderm)
3. Indefinite proliferative potential.

The pluripotent cells possess some more properties (Wobus, 2001) such as :

4. High alkaline phosphatases activity.
5. Expression of stage specific embryonic antigens (SSEA) such as SSEA-1 in mouse *etc.*
6. Expression of the germ-line transcription factor Oct-4, Nanog and Sox-2 form the core regulatory network that ensures the suppression of genes that lead to differentiation and the maintenance of pluripotency (Boyer *et al.,* 2005).
7. Cells with high nucleo-cytoplasm ratio.
8. High telomerase activity; and
9. Regulation of self renewal by IL6 family cytokines such as leukemia inhibiting factor (LIF) and other membrane bound factors.

The emerging evidences indicate that a complex reciprocal regulatory circuit involving the Nanog, Oct-4 and Sox-2 pluripotency transcription factors, polycomb repressive complexes (PRC) and microRNAs regulate stem cell pluripotency and differentiation (Kashyap *et al.*, 2009). These factors cooperate in the transcriptional and epigenetic regulation of key stem cell genes.

3. Culture and derivation of pluripotent embryonic stem cells

Standard protocols are available for mouse, rat, monkey and human ES cell derivation, culture and propagation which are routinely used in various laboratories all over the world. The pluripotent stem cells in mouse and other successful species are cultured in knockout Dulbeco's modified eagle's medium (DMEM) with specific batch of serum or knockout serum replacer. These cells normally grow in co-culture system with feeder cell support. Fibroblast cells arrested for further mitosis are used as feeder cells for *in vitro* culture of mouse embryonic stem cells in presence of leukemia inhibiting factor (LIF) and other known and unknown growth factors. The LIF belongs to the interleukin-6 cytokine family that binds to the heterodimeric receptor consisting of LIF receptor and gp130 and maintains ESC in proliferative and undifferentiated state (Suda *et al.*, 1987). The binding of LIF to the receptors results in activation of canonical JAK/STAT (Janus kinase-signal transduction and activation of transcription) pathways in mouse however human ESC do not require gp130 signaling (Humphrey *et al.*, 2004). Embryonic stem cells are classified into two categories across the species '*naïve/authentic*' which are LIF dependant and '*primed*' which are LIF independent.

4. '*Naïve*' vs '*primed*' pluripotent stem cells

Established '*naïve/authentic*' embryonic stem cells (ESC) for example in mouse are characterized by:

1. Their dependency on the LIF/STAT3 signaling pathways for maintenance of pluripotency (Hall *et al.*, 2009).
2. The positive effects of bone morphogenic protein 4 (BMP-4) for self renewal and resistance to differentiation (Ying *et al.*, 2003); and
3. Tendency to differentiate in response to activation of fibroblast growth factor 2 (FGF2) and Activin/transforing growth factor-β (TGF-β) signal transduction pathways (Li *et al.*, 2009).
4. *Naïve* cells are tolerant to passaging as single cells; show no signs of aging over extended culture doubling or X chromosome inactivation in female cell lines. *Naïve* ES cells derivation in some mouse is successful but not in all strains.

Mouse and human ESC are not morphologically similar despite being derived from inner cell mass (ICM). Human embryonic stem cells (ESC) colony appears flattened and are dependent on FGF2 and TGFβ/Activin/Nodal signaling rather than on LIF/STAT3 for maintenance of their pluripotency (Dvorak *et al.,* 2005; Xu *et al.,* 2005). Human ESC rapidly differentiate when exposed to BMP 4 (Das *et al.,* 2007; Xu *et al.,* 2002) and at least a partial inactivation of one of the X chromosomes occurs in female cell lines even when they are cultured under conditions that maintain an undifferentiated state (Silva *et al.,* 2008). The primate ESC undergoes apoptosis if they are dissociated into single cells for routine sub culture. The human ESCs are much more prone to undergo spontaneous differentiation than mouse and they divide more slowly (Ezashi *et al.,* 2005; Westfall *et al.,* 2008). Also both the human and mouse ESC differ in the display of cell surface antigens. For example carbohydrate antigen SSEA1 is expressed in mouse ESC where as a series of complex carbohydrate entities including SSEA 3 and 4 are displayed on the human cells (Henderson *et al.,* 2002). Thus mouse and primate ESC in many respects are distinct despite exhibiting the pluripotency character. Interestingly, the ESC derived from the egg cylinder of gastrulation stage mouse embryo share striking similarities with the human ESC interms of their flattened morphology, lack of dependence on LIF for maintenance and susceptibility of differentiation to trophoblast and germ cells upon BMP4 treatment. Such stem cells are called *"primed"* ESC and are considered as more advanced differentiated state than the earlier one possibly because of perturbation of ground state as a result of ERK1 pathways block (Nichols and Smith, 2009) while derivation. Such *'primed'* ESC can be altered to the *naïve* type by genetic manipulation (Hanna *et al.,* 2010) or even by changing the culture condition (Bao *et al.,* 2009; Xu *et al.,* 2010). This rose the question whether the ESC derived from human ICM are in a more differentiated state than their mouse counterpart? However the present evidences suggest that there are existences of two ESC types, the first one is *'naïve'* whose pluripotent state is dependent on LIF/STAT3 and BMP4. The other one is *'primed'* whose pluripotency is dependent on FGF2 and Activin/Nodal signaling.

5. Derivation of embryonic stem cells

Derivation of embryonic stem cell culture is major breakthrough in the recent past. Mouse ESC have been derived first from blastocyst/epiblast stage preimplantation embryos (Evans and Kaufman, 1981; Martin, 1981). Subsequently the derivation protocol for human (Thomson *et al.,* 1998) and monkey (Thomson *et al.,* 1996) ESC have been standardized after 16-18 years. Attempts to standardize derivation protocol and culture methods in farm animals mostly remained unsuccessful probably because the culture systems applicable in rodents and humans does not fit to be applied in these species.

Appreciation of biochemical network maintaining the pluripotent state and application of pharmacological agents, especially the inhibitors of intracellular signaling pathways has resulted in successful development of *naïve* stem cell lines from the previously known '*difficult*' species such as rat (Buehr *et al.*, 2008), human (Li *et al.*, 2008) and non permissive mouse strains such as *non obese diabetic* (NOD) mouse (Hanna *et al.*, 2009). '*Naïve*' mouse embryonic stem cells are normally derived by mechanical dissociation of the inner cell mass and culture on the feeder cells in presence of a protein kinase inhibitor PD0325901 (PD), a compound which blocks the mitogen activated protein kinase (ERK) pathways. However in rat in addition to PD, a second compound CHIR99021, an inhibitor of glycogen synthase kinase 3β (GSK-3β) is added in the culture system (Buehr *et al.*, 2008). Addition of two inhibitors for derivation made this system popular as 2i system. Success in derivation of 'difficult to derive' species such as rats also raises the possibility of deriving ESC from the different livestock species.

Maintaining the embryonic stem cells in a pluripotent state over multiple passages remained a challenge and most of the attempts failed to generate cell lines which survive for a prolonged period. In some instances porcine ESC lines have shown some degrees of stemness such as the ability to be maintained in culture for a prolonged period (Evans *et al.*, 1990) to form teratomas, and in one instance the chimeras (Chen *et al.*, 1999). In recent time, porcine cell lines have been generated from the embryonic discs of day 10.5 - 12 pig conceptuses that were dependent on Activin/Nodal signaling but not on LIF, and differentiated into trophoblast and germ cells upon BMP4 treatment and could give rise to teratomas (Alberio *et al.*, 2010). These cell lines are similar to the primed/human ESC cell line class. Attempts have been made to derive the ES cell lines from other farm animal species such as cattle (Evans *et al.*, 1990; Wang *et al.*, 2005), buffalo (Verma *et al.*, 2007; Anand *et al.*, 2011), horse (Saito *et al.*, 2002), sheep (Notarianni *et al.*, 1991) and goats (Tillmann and Meinecke, 1996), however, most of the cases the cells did not conform the classical properties of *naïve or primed* ESC therefore, are termed as "*ES like*" cells. The success to generate *naïve* ESC remained elusive in most of the farm animal species. The ungulate ESCs are more similar to primate colony cell morphology. These cells, in most of the cases failed to undergo continuous self renewal, clear description of morphology, expression of cell specific pluripotency markers. Also the ungulate ESC barring a few reported cell lines in pig fail to form teratomas, the common proof of pluripotency in primate and mouse ESC, when transplanted in immuno compromised mice.

6. Pluripotency markers in embryonic stem cells

The morphological criteria of ESC sometimes are not linked to the parameter of pluripotency and self renewal therefore; cellular and molecular markers are used to define the state of cell lines derived from a particular species. Two categories of genetic markers are used to identify the stem cells of which some are expressed on the cell surface and others are intracellular:

6.1 Cell surface markers

Under this category there are two class of proteins- alkaline phosphatases (AP) and stage specific embryonic antigen (SSEA). There are species specific differences exist in expressions of SSEA but not with AP. Alkaline phosphatases were first demonstrated as a reliable cell surface marker of ESC in pig and sheep by Talbot *et al* (1993). The SSEA1 and 4 genes are found expressed in both ICM and trophoectoderm of caprine embryo (He *et al.*, 2006). In equine, ESC like cells express AP, SSEA-1, 3 and 4 in addition to TRA 1-60 and TRA 1-81 (Guest and Allen, 2007). Similarly in buffaloes AP, SSEA 1, 3 and 4 are used as markers to identify pluripotent cells (Verma *et al.*, 2007; Huang *et al.*, 2007). Both the proteins have multiple isoforms, are considered ES cell characteristic markers but not the definite markers of pluripotency.

6.2 Intracellular markers

There are three transcription factors under this category *viz.*, the Oct4 also known as Pou5F1, Nanog and Sox2. Since these genes are expressed after embryonic genome activation, they are considered definite markers of pluripotency for mouse, human and pig. The Oct3/4 is found expressed in ICM and trophoectoderm cells of pig, cattle and goat embryos (van Eijk *et al.*, 1999; Kirchhof *et al.*, 2000, He *et al.*, 2004; Yadav *et al.*, 2005). In cattle, since Oct4 is not restricted to be expressed in ICM of blastocyst therefore may not be the ideal marker for pluripotency (Kurosaka *et al.*, 2004). The Nanog is detected in bovine and caprine embryos and are considered as the specific pluripotency marker in these species. The expression of Nanog mRNA is found strongly down regulated in the trophoectoderm of caprine blastocyst (He *et al.*, 2005, 2006). The pig pluripotent cells express all the three markers *viz.*,Oct4, Nanog and Sox2 but there are quantitative variations in the expression of such genes for *in vitro* and *in vivo* produced embryos. The Nanog expression in pig is not only restricted to pluripotent cells but also detected in somatic adult tissues such as ovary, heart and muscles cells (Brevini *et al.*, 2005).

7. Induced pluripotent stem cells (iPSC) from reprogrammed somatic cells

With the latest development the pluripotent stem cells can be derived from cells isolated from the inner cell mass of early stage blastocysts which are called ESC (Fig. 2A) and by epigenetic reprogramming of differentiated adult cell types employing Yamanaka or Thomson factors called as induced pluripotent stem cells (iPSC, Fig 2B). The innovation of iPSC in the year 2006 has given stem cell research a new impetus because it allows the creation of normal and disease specific stem cells.

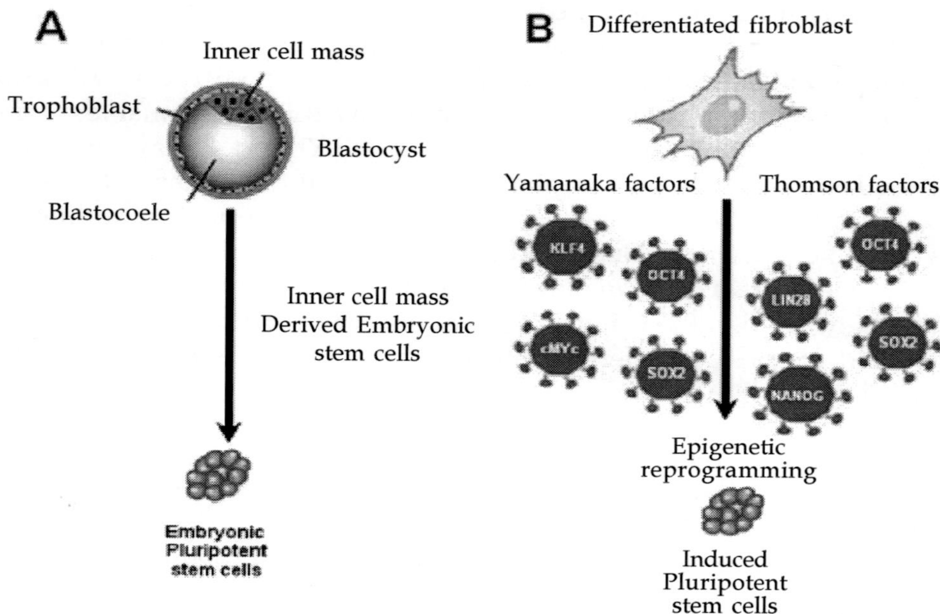

Fig. 2 : Derivation of pluripotent embryonic stem cells from the inner cell mass of developing embryos (panel A) and induced pluripotent stem cells from the adult cells (panel B) by epigenetic reprogramming introducing different transcription factors (concept from Kashyap *et al.*, 2009).

7.1 Induction of iPSC by transcription factors

In mouse iPSC is reprogrammed from fibroblast by retroviral delivery of four transcription factors Oct3/4, Sox2, Klf4 and cMyc (Takahashi and Yamanaka, 2006). This path breaking discovery was followed by generation of human iPSC in the similar manner by several groups (Takahashi *et al.*, 2007, Yu *et al.*, 2007; Park *et al.*, 2008). Since then a large number of reports have described reprogramming many somatic cells types using different number of transcription factors and various methods of introducing the transcription factors genes or proteins into the somatic cells (Yamanaka, 2009). It was proved that mature tissue cells can be induced to pluripotent state with the introduction of four transcription factors (Takahashi and Yamanaka, 2006; Takahashi *et al.*, 2007). Subsequently it has been shown that the greatest reprogramming efficiency is achieved when combinations of 4 factors, *Oct4, Sox2,* cMyc, and Klf4, or Oct4, Sox2, Nanog, and Lin28 genes are introduced into the differentiated cell (Fig. 2B). However, Oct4 and Sox2 appear critically required to induce pluripotency (Kashyap *et al.,* 2009). Viral vector delivery system of transcription factor genes is efficient however the major concern of using this method is integrations of the vector in random location of the chromosomes which may disturb the vital gene functions (Varas *et al.,* 2009). The solution to this problem can be sorted out by determining the viral integration sites by reverse PCR and then exclude the colonies which show dangerous integration. However, the introduction of reprogramming factors by integrated viral delivery system compromise the integrity of the target cell genome, thus generating the mutant iPSC. Another possible obstacle in iPSC technology is the reactivation of transgene. It has been observed that retroviral carried cMyc gets reactivated in the ~ 50% chimeric mice resulting tumor formation (Okita *et al.,* 2007). The iPSC can be generated without cMyc (Nagakawa *et al.,* 2008) but reactivation of any of the transcription factor might lead to tumor formation. Further, sustained expression of transgene might suppress the differentiation potential of iPSC resulting higher propensities to produce teratoma when transplanted into the patient for regenerative therapy (Yamanaka, 2009).

Several alternate methods have been tried to address these issues which includes use of lentiviral vector with limited insertion sites (Sommer *et al.,* 2009), non integrating vector such as plasmid (Okita *et al.,* 2008), adenoviral (Stadtfeld *et al.,* 2008), OriP/Epstein-Barr nuclear antigen-1 (EBNA1)-based episomal vectors (Yu *et al.,* 2009), piggy Bac vector for insertion into transposons (Woltjen *et al.,* 2007) and bacteriphage integrase which favors integration in the intergenic regions (Ye *et al.,* 2010) even by direct delivery of proteins. Although all of these approaches improved the technology it did not completely bypass the preclinical road block as each approach has a relatively minor but specific limitation in respect to the efficiency of reprogramming. Even when the inserted transgenes were removed using the Cre-LoxP system, as attempted in mouse, permanent modifications were left in the host genome (Kaji *et al.,* 2009) and resulted in creating the mutant iPSCs again. A new innovative approach is described by Warren *et al.* (2010) which relies on delivery of cocktail of *in vitro* generated engineered mRNA that encodes the reprogramming factors (Klf4, cMyc, Oct 4, Sox 2 and Lin 28). The assumption made was that these mRNAs are translated in the cytoplasm and their transfection into the cells does not cause permanent genetic change. This approach shows promise because it does not pose danger related to safety issues of transgenes.

7.2 Somatic cells for iPSC induction

Induced pluripotent stem cells in mouse have been generated varying from fibroblast, hepatocytes, gastric epithelial cells, bone marrow, pancreatic cells, neural stem cells to B lymphocytes whereas, in humans such iPSC are generated from skin fibroblast, keratinocyte and blood progenitor cells (Yamanaka, 2009). In fact any somatic cells can be chosen for generation of iPSC if collections of donor cells are easy and safe. The derived iPSC in human and other species is found more similar to '*primed*' pluripotent cells than '*naïve*' type. However, in pig recently it has been shown that induction of *naïve* iPSC is possible from fibroblast cells by adding two inhibitors (2i) of rats ESC derivation system with addition of DNA methyl transferase inhibitor, 5-azacytidine to prevent *de novo* DNA methylation (Telugu *et al.*, 2010).

An important consideration for iPSC generation is that different tissue sources of somatic cells might show different differentiation potential and pluripotent character. Certain cells might be the better candidate for complete reprogramming with a reduced risk of teratoma formation whereas others are not. Thus, endodermal origin gastric epithelial cells might be the better somatic cells to start with for generation of pancreatic β cells or hepatocytes. Notably, iPSC generated from hepatocytes (Aoi *et al.*, 2008; Aasen *et al.*, 2008) have fewer retroviral integration sites than do iPSC generated from fibroblast cells therefore, can be better cells for iPSC generation (Yamanaka, 2009).

Induced pluripotent cells provide a new dimension in the biomedical research and tissue therapies but we still are in the process of understanding the mechanism of proliferation and trans-differentiation of these cells. The iPSC derivation from adult cells have a high developmental potential, however might have several limitations:

1. They may not have the same development and proliferation capacity as the embryonic or fetal cells.
2. Adult somatic cells may contain DNA abnormalities caused by environmental factors which would be propagated when stem cells are generated either by somatic cell nuclear transfer or by iPSC technologies.
3. Somatic cells of some individuals might contain genetic defect and if not selected properly might be the source of spreading genetic defects in the cells or in the established transgene lines.

8. Bottle neck of using ESC and iPSC for transplantation therapies

The derivation of ESC opened up a new area of research in regenerative medicine and yielded an unimaginable progress in identifying functions of many genes within the mammalian genome. Similarly the induction of iPSC from somatic cells is also considered as a major step forward in stem cell research as they ensure an endless supply of compatible cells for regenerative medicine. However, before the ESC or iPSC are used for human cell or tissue therapy following prerequisites need to be fulfilled:

1. Methods for directed differentiation and selective isolation of pure defined cell populations.
2. The somatic donor cells from which pluripotent cells would be derived are not tumorogenic.
3. Transplanted cells must show the tissue specific function and get integrated with the existing cells of the tissues.
4. The transplanted cells must be immunologically compatible.

The last problem is addressed in the newer strategies of generating ESC or iPSC from the patients themselves, but the other three obstacles remain, which still prevent the use of this technology in human transplantation therapies.

9. Opportunities of ESC, iPSC and other stem cell

9.1 Toxicological screening of drugs

The most suitable short term application of this technology remaining is toxicological screening of drugs for pharmacological research. One such hypothetical example is that liver cells generated from the iPSC of individuals with different cytochrome P450 enzyme would be suitable to predict the liver toxicity of the new drugs. The iPSC has tremendous potential to create a model for *in vitro* drug screening of disease which are caused by mutation. One such example is long QT syndrome in humans. This diesase is characterized by mutation of the gene involved in generation of action potential in heart causing lethal cardiac arrhythmia. Induced pluripotent cells can be generated from such patients, which can be differentiated to cardiomyocytes and be used for screening candidate drugs for desirable effects (Yamanaka, 2009). Both ESC and iPSC are helping to unravel the mysteries of early embryonic development and differentiation *in vitro*, including test and development of therapeutic products, analyze the effect of xenobiotics or teratogenic drugs, screen embryo toxicity and finally generation of novel *in vitro* models for human diseases in other species.

9.2 Pluripotent stem cells in testing function of lethal genes

The stem cells can be used to analyze the effect of over expressed genes (gain-of-function; Rohwedel *et al.*, 1995) or testing the phenotypic effects of homozygous mutants (loss-of-function) by *in vitro* cell differentiation model. The *in vitro* differentiation model is most suited for those genes whose loss-of-function (homozygous mutants) result in early embryonic death (Fassler *et al.*, 1996; Rohwedel *et al.*, 1998) *in vivo*. The *in vitro* technology allows the differentiation of wild-type cells, mutant cells by 'loss-of-function' and 'gain-of-function' and are useful for the analyzing the effects of exogenous differentiation factors. The figure given below (Fig 3) describes the concept of how gain-of-function or loss-of-function effects of $\beta_1$intergin gene can be studied in *in vitro* differentiation of embryoid body and three germ cell layer formation model. The effects of different exogenous factors such as retinoic acid (RA), signaling molecules, BMP-4, extracellular matrix proteins (ECM) or embryotoxic/teratogenic compounds including some physical factors can be studied. The differentiated cells show the phenotype *in vitro* whereas, embryos showing homozygous deficiency (loss-of-function) of β_{1-}intergin gene do not survive *in vivo*.

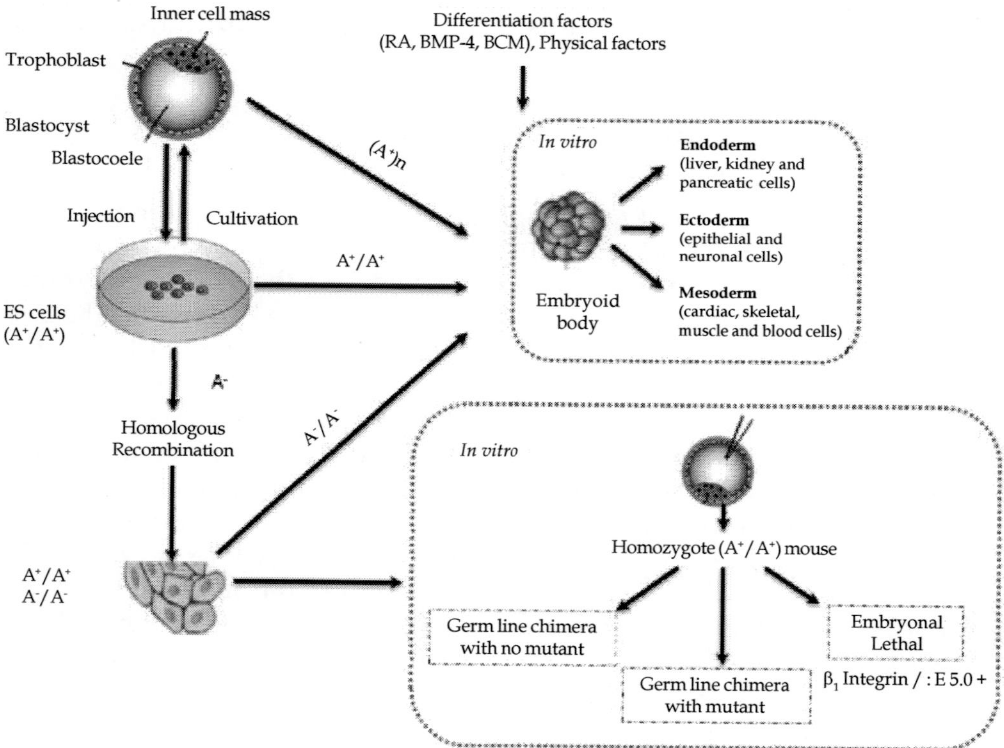

Fig. 3 : *In vivo* genetic studies showing homozygous deficient β_1 integrin gene results in death of embryo shortly after implantation at day 5. However, the homozygous deficiency of the same gene *i.e.*, phenotypic effects of the mutation can easily be analysed by *in vitro* ES cells differentiation model. Examples of different exogenous factors whose effects can be assessed in such models are shown (concept taken from Wobus, 2001).

9.3 Animal origin pluripotent stem cells as human model for transplantation therapies

The iPSC technology has a tremendous application in human therapeutics because it generates patient specific stem cells that bypass the ethical questions surrounding ESC derivation and somatic cell nuclear transfer- a state of the art model for studying genetic disease *in vitro.* Many questions related to the mechanism although remain unanswered in humans; the current focus of research may bring iPSC to clinical application sooner or later. The safety of such extraordinary endeavor must be checked in an animal model close enough to human. Mice and rats are easiest animal model to learn the reprogramming machinery and to improve methodology, but their size, physiology and reduced life span remain the major handicaps for making any serious assumptions on safety for humans. Monkey is theoretically the best suited model for human application because of phylogenetic similarities but the ethical concerns remain and these animals are very difficult to breed. Swine is a much cheaper and publicly acceptable alternative to primate model (Brevini *et al.,* 2007, Hall 2008, Roberts *et al.,* 2009, Vackova *et al.,* 2007) which provides an unprecedented opportunity for creating a genetic model for human disease. There are number of reasons in its favour :

1. Pig farming has been adopted since ages as a regular source of food for human therefore, are easily available, easy to breed and obtain a large number of litters.
2. Its physiology is remarkably similar to humans, have similar body size, organ physiology and morphology (Telugu *et al,* 2009).
3. The relatively long lifespan make this species ideal for investigating the long term effects of transplantation therapies.

   The other reasons include:

4. Porcine origin insulin is widely used for treating the human diabetes.
5. Pig origin heart valve and skin have been transplanted and used in burn victims for decades (Hall, 2008).
6. Transgenic pig devoid of α (1-3) galactosyl transferase gene, the major xenoantigen involved in acute rejection hold promise of use in xenogenous transplantation of organs in humans (Kobler–Simond *et al.,* 2004).

The engineered animals can be made for transplantation therapies, to improve production traits, disease resistance and biopharming. The transgenic animal models for a specific human disease can be produced by engineering iPSC or ESC which would result in an offspring of desired genetic makeup. These goals are achievable by chimera production, which is well established in producing the genetically modified mice (Capecchi, 1989) or through improving the efficiency of somatic cell nuclear transfer (Campbell *et al.,* 1996; Lai *et al.,* 2002). These applications are not only limited to porcine species but most of the farm animal species. Keefer *et al.*, (2007) rightly pointed out that animal ESC have tremendous prospect of application for improving production traits and products, producing disease resistant animal and pharmacological proteins for human diseases (biopharming).

9.4 Trophoblast cells differentiation from pluripotent stem cells and opportunities

Differentiation of trophoblastic cells from embryonic stem cells provides opportunity to study placental morphogenesis and interactions with other cells. Overall placental growth and villous morphogenesis are widely recognized as crucial for pregnancy success in animals and human being. Therefore, understanding early trophoblast differentiation, villous morphogenesis and placenta formation, and extra villous trophoblast differentiation and process of invasion, non invasion or formation of syncytium are fundamental before considering the therapeutic approaches for preventing or treating suboptimal implantation and pregnancy complications related to placental development. Possibility of obtaining a static histological sample poses a limitation for designing such studies; therefore these processes are not traceable at the time of implantation in many species. The differentiation of ESC to trophoblast was first noticed by Thomson *et al.* (1998) who reported the first derivation of hESCs. They noticed differentiation of ESC to trophoblasts in the colonies undergoing spontaneous differentiation, and judged by the secretion of human chorionic gonadotropin (hCG), the commonly used trophoblast marker. At that time they thought the secretion of hCG was as a result of the activation of the component of gene expression program during differentiation to the trophoectoderm and interpreted as the indication that these ESCs could serve as a surrogate for blastocyst-stage embryos at least from the perspective of trophectoderm/trophoblast formation. Later on it was proved indeed ESC can generate the extra-embryonic lineage cells since the yolk sac specific marker alpha feto protein is found expressed in the rhesus monkey (Thomson *et al.*, 1995) and human (Reubinoff *et al.*, 2000) ESC. The formation of these extra-embryonic lineages from ESC is exciting since it allowed the study of placenta formation, not from tissues which had already undergone morphogenesis and differentiation to villous and extravillous lineages (i.e. first trimester placental tissues, or term delivered placentas), but from the 'blank slate' represented by ESCs.

9.5 Male and female gametes differentiation for assisted reproduction

Differentiation of gametes from embryonic stem cells has the potential for use in assisted reproductive technology. The potential to produce gametes as derivatives of mouse and human embryonic stem cells (Hubner *et al.*, 2003; Clark *et al.*, 2004) has generated much excitement over the utility of these cells as tools for basic developmental research and in more practical applications as an alternative source of gametes for fertility treatments. It has been proved that mouse ES cells are capable of differentiating into oocytes (Hubner *et al.,* 2003). Future experiments will reveal whether the oocytes generated in culture from ES cells can be fertilized or not, whether they have undergone a gender-specific resetting of the epigenetic marks (imprinting), and also whether they can be used as starting material to derive ES cell lines after nuclear transfer.

9.6 Spermatogonial stem cells as a study model

Adult stem cells have now been characterized in most of the tissues and organ of the body system. The best characterized are those cells which are found in organs and undergo rapid cellular turnover such as haemopoetic tissues of the bone marrow, lining of the gut, epidermis of skin, mammary gland and uterine endometrium. Adult stem cells are derived from varying sources and culture methods are standardized, however, hurdles in derivation process limit its applicability and potential. Other than haemopoetic/ mesenchymal stem cells in bone marrow, fetal cord blood stem cells also found application in human regenerative medicines. Similarly spermatogonial stem cells as an area of research has long been the interest of the entire reproductive biologists' community since the time they became known and till date it is the best understood *in vivo* system available in mammals. These cells are integral constituents of the male germ line and are required for the maintenance of a pool of diploid germ cells, which enter spermatogenesis and guarantee a constant high sperm output. In contrast to other adult stem cells, spermatogonial stem cells inherit several unique features:

1. These cells are theoretically immortal. In mouse, it has been observed that spermatogonia have a very long lifespan, since serial transplantations lead to enormous expansion of the spermatogonial stem cell pool and induction of spermatogenesis for several generations (Kanatsu-Shinohara *et al.,* 2003, Ogawa *et al.,* 2003). This indicates that the aging mechanisms in spermatogonia might be different from other adult stem cells.

2. Spermatogonial cells maintain a high degree of DNA integrity throughout the fertile life of a male which is important from the evolutionary point of view. Since the male genome in spermatogonia relies on almost error-free proliferation leading to production of excellent quality male gametes. Thus, spermatogonial stem cells hold a key position in driving a balanced evolutionary modification of the genome. This is a demanding task, as spermatogonial stem cells are reserve cells, which can recolonize the seminiferous epithelium following DNA damage. It is striking that recovery of spermatogenesis from radiodepletion leads to healthy

gametes after a transient period of poor DNA integrity, indicating a highly efficient repair or cell selection mechanisms in spermatogonial stem cells (Stahl *et al.*, 2004).

3. These stem cells generate differentiating progeny with sperm as the only type of final differentiated phenotype therefore are the only stem cells in the adult organism which give rise to cells undergoing meiosis.
4. Spermatogonial stem cells provide a unique mammalian system where the entire process of stem cell self-renewal, progenitor formation and all stages of differentiation can be followed in a single organ, *in situ*.

This system has been instrumental in development of present understanding on the principles of spermatogonial stem cell biology and helped in defining the role of these stem cell niches in regulating stem cell function. Researches in many laboratories across the world are directed to understand several unanswered questions of this system. The understanding on species-specific kinetics and mechanisms of spermatogonial stem cell expansion in different mammalian species remained unexplored that needs study in greater details which otherwise would pose dangers of extrapolating assumptions across the species. The main purposes of culturing these cells are *in vitro* production of sperm from azospermic human males for *in vitro* fertilization in treatment of infertility. However, such developments have limited application in animals because males with azospemia are normally culled and are not allowed to propagate. Certainly these cells would help understanding the basic mechanism of sperm cell differentiation and species specific kinetic studies which still are not well understood in all the animal species.

Conclusions and future perspectives

Stem cell research is on the cutting edge of biological science research today however, it is still in its infancy. Embryonic, induced pluripotent or adult stem cells are mainly studied aiming at advancing the scientific and therapeutic potential most efficiently in human. Research has mainly been focused on directing the differentiation of embryonic stem cells into desired cell types for the study of developmental processes that otherwise cannot be studied in early development. The major questions still remain about the importance of genetic or environmental factors during various stages of cell differentiation in the body that control the fate of ESCs or iPSCs. It has been proved that these unique tools would help in conducting basic research critical for the foundation of human regenerative therapies. It has been possible, to create a lineage of mouse ESCs that generate neural cell precursors (Li *et al.*, 1998). Similarly there are other studies which reports generation of precursors of different other cell lineages as well.

Due to the tremendous interest and development in this area, several other avenues of research have opened up. A better understanding on the genetic controls of tissue differentiation (Duncan *et al.,* 1998) came into existence due to the studies related to the genes which get turned on and off as the ESCs begin to differentiate. Stem cell studies also have provided the opportunity to explore the role of biochemicals which are produced in the normal cellular environment that induce stem cells to differentiate, to migrate to a site needing repair, and to assimilate into tissues (Schuldiner *et al.,* 2000). Outcome of all these efforts resulted in development of protocols for deriving cells of somatic lineages, cardiomyocytes, pancreatic, neuronal, and hematopoietic lineages, hepatocytes, and germ lines. Both ESC and iPSC offers unprecedented opportunities for developing therapies for debilitating human diseases having no cures. However, two identifiable risks associated with this approach are: tumor formation and immune rejection. If human ESCs are injected into mice, they produce benign tumors made up of diverse tissues popularly known as teratoma. This response is related to the multipotency of the undifferentiated cells in an *in vivo* environment. However, a small number of short-term studies in mice and human had shown that when the ESCs were allowed to begin differentiation before transplantation they did not result in significant tumor formation (Odorico *et al.,* 2001). This is a critical problem to understand and control. It is too early to consider using human ESCs or iPSCs directly as regenerative medicine. A great deal of research must be conducted to understand how body controls differentiation of the stem cells and how these can reliably be reproduced *in vitro*. The behavior of ESC or iPSCs implanted in a specific organ has not been studied well and need a thorough investigation.

Among the adult stem cells bone marrow cells have so far been provided most of the examples of successful therapies for replacement of diseased or destroyed cells. Despite the enthusiasm generated by recent reports, the potential of adult stem cells to differentiate fully into other cell types such as brain, nerve, pancreatic cells is still poorly understood and remains to be clarified. Embryonic or induced pluripotent stem cells either in human or mice have shown that these cells have potential to differentiate into multiple tissue types and exhibit long-term self-renewal in culture. These features are not demonstrated in many adult stem cells. Nevertheless adult stem cells are identified as the potential target cells for inducing pluripotent stem cells since these cells are less specialized and have the indefinite proliferation potential.

Another dimension of research that stem cell technologies presented is to explore the fundamental questions of biology, such as determining the basic mechanisms of tissue development and specialization, which are required for the development of therapies. While those possibilities in human are still under experimental investigations, application of stem cell technology in animal science is finding its way. Any proof of the concept needs doing experiment in mice and other animals because of ease, quickness and best alternative available in place of human. However, it should be kept in mind that substantial biological differences exist between the animal and human development and stem cell characteristics. It is important to understand the full range of similarities and differences between the species by thorough study in each of them. Until now, the derivation and culture system is developed and successful in mouse, rat, monkey, human and pigs but not in other species which still remain a challenge. The directed differentiation is successful only for some of the tissues and cell types but not for all tissues or cells of the entire body system. Transdifferention of iPSC is another challenge which needs to be sorted out soon to make use of these cells for human therapeutics. With the efforts of so many people it might happen someday that ES cell is transplanted only by adding some growth factors to stimulate the production of a particular cell type or multiple cell types. There are possibilities to co-transplant inducer tissues that interact with stem cells to achieve a similar result. Potential applications of these technologies in farm animal species are beginning with their application as a model for genetic studies and human tissue transplantation. The need of the hour is to cater to the advantages of such a cutting edge technology for the benefit of human and animal species.

References

Aasen T., Raya A., Barrero M.J., Garreta E., Consiglio A., Gonzalez F., Vassena R., Biliæ J., Pekarik V., Tiscornia G., Edel M., Boué S., Izpisúa Belmonte J.C. (2008). Efficient and rapid generation of induced pluripotent stem cells from human keratinocytes. *Nature Biotechnology* **26:** 1276-1284.

Alberio R., Croxall N., Allegrucci C. (2010). Pig epiblast stem cells depend on activin/nodal signaling for pluripotency and self-renewal. *Stem Cells Development* **19:** 1627-1636.

Anand T., Kumar D., Singh M.K., Shah R.A., Chauhan M.S., Manik R.S., Singla S.K., Palta P. (2011). Buffalo (Bubalus bubalis) embryonic stem cell-like cells and preimplantation embryos exhibit comparable expression of pluripotency-related antigens. *Reproduction in Domestic Animal* **46:** 50-58.

Aoi T., Yae K., Nakagawa M., Ichisaka T., Okita K., Takahashi K., Chiba T., Yamanaka S. (2008). Generation of pluripotent stem cells from adult mouse liver and stomach cells. *Science* **321:** 699-702.

Bao S., Tang F., Li X., Hayashi K., Gillich A., Lao K., Surani M.A. (2009). Epigenetic reversion of post-implantation epiblast to pluripotent embryonic stem cells. *Nature* **461:** 1292-1295.

Boyer L.A., Lee T.I., Cole M.F., Johnstone S.E., Levine S.S., Zucker J.P., Guenther M.G., Kumar R.M., Murray H.L., Jenner R.G., Gifford D.K., Melton D.A., Jaenisch

R., Young R.A. (2005). Core transcriptional regulatory circuitry in human embryonic stem cells. *Cell* **122:** 947-956.

Brevini T.A., Antonini S., Cillo F., Crestan M., Gandolfi F. (2007). Porcine embryonic stem cells: Facts, challenges and hopes. *Theriogenology* **68** (*Suppl.1*): S206-S213.

Brevini T.A.L., Cillo F., Antonini S., Gandolfi F. (2005). Expression pattern of Nanog gene in porcine tissue and parthenogenetic embryos. *Reproduction in Domestic Animals* **40:** 384.

Brevini T.A.L., Tosetti V., Crestan M., Antonini S., Gandolfi F. (2007). Derivation and characterization of pluripotent cell lines from pig embryos of different origins. *Theriogenology* **67:** 54-63.

Buehr M., Meek S., Blair K., Yang J., Ure J., Silva J., McLay R., Hall J., Ying QL, Smith A. (2008). Capture of authentic embryonic stem cells from rat blastocysts. *Cell* **135:** 1287-1298.

Campbell K.H., McWhir J., Ritchie W.A., Wilmut I. (1996). Sheep cloned by nuclear transfer from a cultured cell line. *Nature* **380:** 64-66.

Capecchi M.R. (1989). Altering the genome by homologous recombination. *Science* **244:** 1288-1292.

Clark A.T., Bodnar M.S., Fox M., Rodriquez R.T., Abeyta M.J., Firpo M.T., Pera R.A. (2004). Spontaneous differentiation of germ cells from human embryonic cells *in vitro*. *Human Molecular Genetics* **13:** 727-739.

Duncan S.A., Navas M.A., Dufor D., Rossant J., Stoffel M. (1998). Regulation of a transcription factor network required for differentiation and metabolism. *Science* **281:** 692-695.

Dvorak P., Dvorakova D., Koskova S., Vodinska M., Najvirtova M., Krekac D., Hampl A. (2005). Expression and potential role of fibroblast growth factor 2 and its receptors in human embryonic stem cells. *Stem Cells* **23:** 1200-1211.

Das P., Ezashi T., Schulz L.C., Westfall S.D., Livingston K.A., Roberts R.M. (2007). Effects of fgf2 and oxygen in the bmp4-driven differentiation of trophoblast from human embryonic stem cells. *Stem Cell Research* **1:** 61-74.

Chen L.R., Shiue Y.L., Bertolini L., Medrano J.F., BonDurant R.H., Anderson G.B. (1999). Establishment of pluripotent cell lines from porcine preimplantation embryos. *Theriogenology* **52:** 195-212.

Evans M.J. and Kaufman M.H. (1981). Establishment in culture of pluripotential cells from mouse embryo. *Nature* **292:** 154-156.

Evans M.J., Notarianni E. Laurie S., Moor R.M. (1990). Derivation and preliminary characterization of pluripotent cell lines from porcine and bovine blastocysts. *Theriogenology* **33:** 125-128.

Ezashi T., Das P., Roberts R.M. (2005). Low O2 tensions and the prevention of differentiation of hES cells. *Proceedings of National Academy of Sciences*, USA **102:** 4783-4788.

Fässler R., Rohwedel J., Maltsev V., Bloch W., Lentini S., Guan K., Gullberg D., Hescheler J., Addicks K., Wobus A.M. (1996). Differentiation and integrity of cardiac muscle cells are impaired in the absence of β_1 integrin. *Journal of Cell Science* **109:** 2989-2999.

Guest D.J., Allen W.R. (2007). Expression of cell-surface antigens and embryonic stem cell pluripotency genes in equine blastocysts. *Stem Cells Development* **16:** 789-796.

Hall J., Guo G., Wray J., Eyres I., Nichols J., Grotewold L., Morfopoulou S., Humphreys P., Mansfield W., Walker R., Tomlinson S., Smith A. (2009). Oct4 and LIF/Stat3 additively induce Krüppel factors to sustain embryonic stem cell self-renewal. *Cell Stem Cell* **5:** 597-609.

Hall V. (2008). Porcine embryonic stem cells: A possible source for cell replacement therapy. *Stem Cell Review* **4:** 275-282.

Hanna J., Cheng A.W., Saha K., Kim J., Lengner C.J., Soldner F., Cassady J.P., Muffat J., Carey B.W., Jaenisch R. (2010). Human embryonic stem cells with biological and epigenetic characteristics similar to those of mouse ESCs. *Proceedings of National Academy of Sciences, USA* **107:** 9222-9227.

Hanna J., Markoulaki S., Mitalipova M., Cheng A.W., Cassady J.P., Staerk J., Carey B.W., Lengner C.J., Foreman R., Love J., Gao Q., Kim J., Jaenisch R. (2009). Metastable pluripotent states in NOD-mouse-derived ESCs. *Cell Stem Cell* **4:** 513-524.

He S., Pant D., Bischoff S., Gavin W., Melican D., Keefer C.L. (2005). Expression of pluripotency determining factors Oct4 and Nanog in preimplantation goat embryos. *Reproduction Fertility Development* **17:** 203.

He S., Pant D., Bischoff S., Melican D., Gavin W., Keefer C.L. (2004). Expression of embryonic stem cell (ESC) markers in preimplantation goat embryos. *Biology of Reproduction (Suppl.)* **1:** 212.

He S., Pant D., Schiffmacher A., Bischoff S., Melican D., Gavin W., Keefer C.L. (2006). Developmental expression of pluripotency determining factors in caprine embryo:novel pattern of Nanog protein localization in the nucleous. *Molecular Reproduction Development* **73:** 1512-1522.

Henderson J.K., Draper J.S., Baillie H.S., Fishel S., Thomson J.A., Moore H., Andrews P.W. (2002). Preimplantation human embryos and embryonic stem cells show comparable expression of stage-specific embryonic antigens. *Stem Cells* **20:** 329-337.

Huang B., Xie T.S., Shi D.S., Li T., Wang X.L., Mo Y., Wang Z.Q. and Li M.M. (2007). Isolation and characterization of EG-like cells from Chinese swamp buffalo (*Bubalus bubalis*). *Cell Biology International* **31:** 1079-1088.

Hubner K., Fuhrmann G., Christenson L.K., Kehler J., Reinbold R., De La Fuente R., Wood J., Strauss J.F. III, Boiani M., Scholer HR (2003). Derivation of oocytes from mouse embryonic stem cells. *Science* **300:** 1251-1256.

Humphrey R.K., Beattie G.M., Lopez A.D., Bucay N., King C.C., Firpo M.T., Rose-John S., Hayek A. (2004). Maintenance of pluripotency in human embryonic stem cells is STAT3 independent. *Stem Cells* **22:** 522-530.

Kaji K., Norrby K., Paca A., Mileikovsky M., Mohseni P., Woltjen K. (2009).Virus-free induction of pluripotency and subsequent excision of reprogramming factors. *Nature* **458:** 771-775.

Kanatsu-Shinohara M., Toyokuni S., Morimoto T., Matsui S., Honjo T., Shinohara T. (2003). Functional assessment of self-renewal activity of male germ line stem cells following cytotoxic damage and serial transplantation. *Biology of Reproduction* **68:** 1801-1807.

Kashyap V., Rezende N.C., Scotland K.B., Shaffer S.M., Persson J.L., Gudas L.J., Mongan N.P. (2009). Regulation of stem cell pluripotency and differentiation involves a mutual regulatory circuit of the Nanog, OCT4, and SOX2 pluripotency transcription factors with polycomb repressive complexes and stem cell microRNAs. *Stem Cells Development* **18:** 1093-1108.

Keefer C.L., Pant D., Blomberg L., Talbot N.C. (2007) Challenges and prospects for the establishment of embryonic stem cell lines of domesticated ungulates. *Animal Reproduction Science* **98:** 147-168.

Kirchhof N., Carnwath J.W., Lemme E., Anastassiadis K., Schöler H., Niemann H. (2000). Expression pattern of Oct-4 in preimplantation embryos of different species. *Biology of Reproduction* **63:** 1698-1705.

Kolber-Simonds D., Lai L., Watt S.R., Denaro M., Arn S., Augenstein M.L., Betthauser J, Carter D.B., Greenstein J.L., Hao Y., Im G.S., Liu Z., Mell G.D., Murphy C.N., Park K.W., Rieke A., Ryan D.J., Sachs D.H., Forsberg E.J., Prather R.S., Hawley R.J. (2004). Production of alpha-1,3-galactosyltransferase null pigs by means of nuclear transfer with fibroblasts bearing loss of heterozygosity mutations. *Proceedings of National Academy of Sciences, USA.* **101:** 7335-7340.

Kurosaka S., Eckardt S., McLaughlin K.J. (2004). Pluripotent lineage definition in bovine embryos by Oct4 transcript localization. *Biology of Reproduction* **71:** 1578-1582.

Lai L., Kolber-Simonds D., Park K.W., Cheong H.T., Greenstein J.L., Im G.S., Samuel M., Bonk A., Rieke A., Day B.N., Murphy C.N., Carter D.B., Hawley R.J., Prather R.S. (2002). Production of alpha-1,3-galactosyltransferase knockout pigs by nuclear transfer cloning. *Science* **295:** 1089-1092.

Li M., Pevny L., Lovell-Badge R., Snith A. (1998). Generation of purified neural precursors from embryonic stem cells by lineage selection. *Current Biology* **8:** 971-974.

Li P., Tong C., Mehrian-Shai R., Jia L., Wu N., Yan Y., Maxson R.E., Schulze E.N., Song H., Hsieh C.L., Pera M.F., Ying Q.L. (2008). Germline competent embryonic stem cells derived from rat blastocysts. *Cell* **135:** 1299-1310.

Martin G.R. (1981). Isolation of a pluripotent cell line from early mouse embryos cultured in medium conditioned by teratocarcinoma stem cells. *Proceedings of National Academy of Sciences*, USA **78:** 7634-7638.

Saito S., Ugai H., Sawai K., Yamamoto Y., Minamihashi A., Kurosaka K., Kobayashi Y., Murata T., Obata Y., Yokoyama K. (2002). Isolation of embryonic stem-like cells from equine blastocysts and their differentiation in vitro. *FEBS Letter* **531:** 389-396.

Nakagawa M., Koyanagi M., Tanabe K., Takahashi K., Ichisaka T., Aoi T., Okita K., Mochiduki Y., Takizawa N., Yamanaka S. (2008). Generation of induced pluripotent stem cells without Myc from mouse and human fibroblasts. *Nature Biotechnology* **26:** 101-106.

Nichols J., Smith A. (2009). Naive and primed pluripotent states. *Cell Stem Cell* **4:** 487-492.

Notarianni E., Galli C., Laurie S., Moor R.M., Evans M.J. (1991). Derivation of pluripotent, embryonic cell lines from the pig and sheep. *Journal of Reprod Fertil (Suppl).* **43:** 255-260.

Odorico J.S., Kaufman D.S., Thomson J.A. (2001). Multilineage differentiation from human embryonic stem cell lines. *Stem Cells* **19:** 193-204.

Ogawa T., Ohmura M., Yumura Y., Sawada H., Kubota Y. (2003) Expansion of murine spermatogonial stem cells through serial transplantation. *Biology of Reproduction* **68:** 316-322.

Okita K., Nakagawa M., Hyenjong H., Ichisaka T., Yamanaka S. (2008).Generation of mouse induced pluripotent stem cells without viral vectors. *Science* **322:** 949-953.

Park I.H., Zhao R., West J.A., Yabuuchi A., Huo H., Ince T.A., Lerou P.H., Lensch M.W., Daley G.Q. (2008). Reprogramming of human somatic cells to pluripotency with defined factors. *Nature* **451:** 141-146.

Piedrahita J.A., Mir B. (2004). Cloning and transgenesis in mammals: Implications for xenotransplantation. *American Journal of Transplant* **4** (Suppl 6): 43-50.

Reubinoff B.E., Pera M.F., Fong C.Y., Trounson A., Bongso A. (2000). Embryonic stem cell lines from human blastocysts: somatic differentiation in vitro. *Nature Biotechnology* **18:** 399-404.

Roberts R.M., Telugu B.P., Ezashi T. (2009). Induced pluripotent stem cells from swine (*Sus scrofa*): why they may prove to be important. *Cell Cycle* **8:** 3078-3081.

Rohwedel J., Guan K., Zuschratter W., Jin S., Ahnert-Hilger G., Fürst D.O., Fässler R., Wobus A.M. (1998). Loss of $\hat{a}_1$ integrin function results in a retardation of myogenic, but an acceleration of neuronal differentiation of embryonic stem (ES) cells in vitro. *Developmental Biology* **201:** 167-184.

Rohwedel J., Horak V., Hebrok M., Füchtbauer E.M., Wobus A.M. (1995). M-twist expression inhibits mouse embryonic stem cell-derived myogenic differentiation *in vitro. Experimental Cell Research* **220:** 92-100.

Sommer C.A., Stadtfeld M., Murphy G.J., Hochedlinger K., Kotton D.N., Mostoslavsky G. (2009) Induced pluripotent stem cell generation using a single lentiviral stem cell cassette. *Stem Cells* **27:** 543-549.

Schuldiner M., Yanuka O., Istkovitz-Eldor J., Melton D., Benvenistry N. (2000). Effects of eight growth factors on the differentiation of cells derived from human embryonic stem cells. *Proceedings of National Academy of Sciences, USA* **907:** 11307-11312.

Silva S.S., Rowntree R.K., Mekhoubad S., Lee J.T. (2008). X-chromosome inactivation and epigenetic fluidity in human embryonic stem cells. *Proceedings of National Academy of Sciences,* USA. **105:** 4820-4825.

Stadtfeld M., Nagaya M., Utikal J., Weir G., Hochedlinger K. (2008). Induced pluripotent stem cells generated without viral integration. *Science* **322:** 945-949.

Stahl O., Eberhard J., Jepson K., Spano M., Cwikiel M., Cavallin-Stahl E., Giwercman A. (2004). The impact of testicular carcinoma and its treatment on sperm DNA integrity. *Cancer* **100:** 1137-1144.

Suda Y., Suzuki M., Ikawa Y., Aizawa S. (1987). Mouse embryonic stem cells exhibit indefinite proliferative potential. *Journal of Cellular Physiology* **133:** 197-201.

Takahashi K., Yamanaka S. (2006). Induction of pluripotent stem cells from mouse embryonic and adult fibroblast cultures by defined factors. *Cell* **126:** 663-676.

Takahashi K., Tanabe K., Ohnuki M., Narita M., Ichisaka T., Tomoda K., Yamanaka S. (2007). Induction of pluripotent stem cells from adult human fibroblasts by defined factors. *Cell* **131:** 861-872.

Talbot N.C., Rexroad C.E.Jr., Pursel V.G., Powell A.M. (1993) Alkaline phosphatase staining of pig and sheep epiblast cells in culture. *Molecular Reproduction Development* **36:** 139-147.

Telugu B.P., Ezashi T., Roberts R.M. (2010). Porcine induced pluripotent stem cells analogous to naïve and primed embryonic stem cells of the mouse. *International Journal of Developmental Biology* **54:** 1703-1711.

Thomson J.A., Itskovitz-Eldor J., Shapiro S.S., Waknitz M.A., Swiergiel J.J., Marshall V.S., Jones J.M. (1998). Embryonic stem cell lines derived from human blastocysts. *Science* **282:** 1145-1147.

Thomson J.A., Kalishman J., Golos T.G., Durning M., Harris C.P., Becker R.A., Hearn J.P. (1995). Isolation of a primate embryonic stem cell line. *Proceedings of National Academy of Sciences, USA* **92:** 7844-7848.

Tillmann S.M., Meinecke B. (1996). Isolation of ES-like cell lines from ovine and caprine preimplantation embryos. *Journal of Animal Breeding and Genetics* **113:** 413-426.

Vackova I., Ungrova A., Lopes F. (2007). Putative embryonic stem cell lines from pig embryos. *Journal of Reproduction and Development* **53:** 1137-1149.

van Eijk M.J., van Rooijen M.A., Modina S., Scesi L., Folkers G., van Tol H.T., Bevers M.M., Fisher S.R., Lewin H.A., Rakacolli D., Galli C., de Vaureix C., Trounson A.O., Mummery C.L., Gandolfi F. (1999). Molecular cloning, genetic mapping, and developmental expression of bovine POU5F1. *Biology of Reproduction* **60:** 1093-1103.

Varas F., Stadtfeld M., de Andres-Aguayo L., Maherali N., di Tullio A., Pantano L., Notredame C., Hochedlinger K, Graf T. (2009). Fibroblast-derived induced pluripotent stem cells show no common retroviral vector insertions. *Stem Cells* **27:** 300-306.

Verma V., Gautam S.K., Singh B., Manik R.S., Palta P., Singla S.K., Goswami S.L., Chauhan M.S. (2007). Isolation and characterization of embryonic stem cell-like cells from in vitro-produced buffalo (Bubalus bubalis) embryos. *Molecular Reproduction and Development* **74:** 520-529.

Wang L., Duan E., Sung L.Y., Jeong B.S., Yang X., Tian X.C. (2005). Generation and characterization of pluripotent stem cells from cloned bovine embryos. *Biology of Reproduction* **73:** 149-155.

Warren L., Manos P.D., Ahfeldt T., Loh Y.H., Li H., Lau F., Ebina W., Mandal P.K., Smith Z.D., Meissner A., Daley G.Q., Brack A.S., Collins J.J., Cowan C., Schlaeger T.M., Rossi D.J. (2010). Highly efficient reprogramming to pluripotency and directed differentiation of human cells with synthetic modified mRNA. *Cell Stem Cell* **7:** 618-630.

Westfall S.D., Sachdev S., Das P., Hearne L.B., Hannink M., Roberts R.M., Ezashi T. (2008). Identification of oxygen-sensitive transcriptional programs in human embryonic stem cells. *Stem Cells Development* **17:** 869-881.

Wilmut I., Schnieke A.E., McWhir J., Kind A.J., Campbell K.H. (1997). Viable offspring derived from fetal and adult mammalian cells. *Nature* **385:** 810-813.

Wobus M.A. (2001). Potential of embryonic stem cells. *Molecular Aspects of Medicine* **22:** 149-164.

Wobus A.M., Boheler K.R. (2005). Embryonic stem cells: Prospects for developmental biology and cell therapy. *Physiological Review* **85:** 635-678.

Woltjen K., Michael I.P., Mohseni P., Desai R., Mileikovsky M., Hämäläinen R., Cowling R., Wang W., Liu P., Gertsenstein M., Kaji K., Sung H.K., Nagy A. (2009). piggyBac transposition reprograms fibroblasts to induced pluripotent stem cells. *Nature* **458:** 766-770.

Xu R.H., Chen X., Li D.S., Li R., Addicks G.C., Glennon C., Zwaka T.P., Thomson J.A. (2002). BMP4 initiates human embryonic stem cell differentiation to trophoblast. *Nature Biotechnology* **20:** 1261-1264.

Xu R.H., Peck R.M., Li D.S., Feng X., Ludwig T., Thomson J.A. (2005). Basic FGF and suppression of BMP signaling sustain undifferentiated proliferation of human ES cells. *Nature Methods* **2:** 185-190.

Xu Y., Zhu X., Hahm H.S., Wei W., Hao E., Hayek A., Ding S. (2010). Revealing a core signaling regulatory mechanism for pluripotent stem cell survival and self-renewal by small molecules. *Proceedings of National Academy of Sciences,* USA. **107:** 8129-8134.

Yadav P.S., Kues W.A., Herrmann D., Carnath J.W., Niemann H. (2005). Bovine ICM derived cell express the Oct4 ortholog. Molecular Reproduction and Development **72:** 182-190.

Yamanaka S. (2009). A fresh look at iPS cells. *Cell* **137:** 13-17.

Ye L., Chang J.C., Lin C., Qi Z., Yu J., Kan Y.W. (2010). Generation of induced pluripotent stem cells using site-specific integration with phage integrase. *Proceedings of National Academy of Sciences,* USA **107:** 19467-19472.

Ying Q.L., Nichols J., Chambers I., Smith A. (2003). BMP induction of Id proteins suppresses differentiation and sustains embryonic stem cell self-renewal in collaboration with STAT3. *Cell* **115:** 281-292.

Yu J., Hu K., Smuga-Otto K., Tian S., Stewart R., Slukvin I.I., Thomson J.A. (2009). Human induced pluripotent stem cells free of vector and transgene sequences. *Science* **324:** 797-801.

Yu J., Vodyanik M.A., Smuga-Otto K., Antosiewicz-Bourget J., Frane J.L., Tian S., Nie J., Jonsdottir G.A., Ruotti V., Stewart R., Slukvin I.I., Thomson J.A. (2007) Induced pluripotent stem cell lines derived from human somatic cells. *Science* **318:** 1917-1920.

❑❑❑

Chapter 22

Characterization of Mixed Microbial Signatures using Next Generation Sequencing

A.P. Kolte, A. Dhali, A.K. Samanta, S. Senani, U.B. Angadi
National Institute of Animal Nutrition and Physiology, Adugodi, Bangalore-560 030, Karnataka, India

Summary

Microbial signature or identity exploration in mixed microbial populations is based on amplification of 16S ribosomal DNA genes using universal primers and cloning and/or sequencing of the amplicons. The introduction of the Next Generation Sequencing (NGS) technologies has brought down the cost of sequencing per kb, facilitated sequencing of entire metagenomes to search the signatures of the microbes. Apart from the identity of the microbes, the data also provides opportunity for functional annotation of microbial genomic sequences and understanding the function of the metagenomes. The huge data generated from the NGS platform requires powerful bioinformatics and computational tools for analysis. The chapter introduces major NGS technologies and tools for processing the data for identifying microbial signatures from metagenome.

The unique capability of digesting ligno-cellulosic agricultural by-products by ruminants is vested by virtue of the variety of microbes (bacteria, fungi and protozoa) residing in the rumen (Miron *et al.*, 2001). The microbial consortia acquired during early stages of life, is dynamic yet characteristic for the species and type of feeding system. Most of our understandings on rumen microbes are based upon the knowledge generated by classical microbiological techniques of anaerobic culturing and counting of the organisms. In the past, microbial diversity was extensively studied using molecular techniques based on 16/18S RNA phylogeny. The 16S RNA gene contains 9 variable regions (V1-V9) which were used for differentiation of microbial species. But none of the variable regions are able to differentiate all the bacterial species, although, hypervariable regions *viz.*, V2 (137-242nt), V3 (433-497 nt), and V6 (986-1043 nt) contain maximum heterogeneity and thus have maximum discriminating power for analysis of bacterial groups (Chakravorty *et al.*, 2007). This technique is useful to glean the uncultivable microbial populations but suffer from the bias/inability of universal primers to amplify sequences from all microbes. Further, several artifacts including PCR generated chimeras and sequencing errors complicate the 16S RNA based analysis of mixed microbial samples (Quince *et al.*, 2009). Introduction of high throughput sequencing and availability of bioinformatics tools opened the new possibilities of studying these microbes directly from the rumen total DNA. Although the approach cannot overcome the limitation of sequencing errors and anomalies in the 16S RNA sequences submitted in the public databases, still the data can look into the phylogenetic as well as metabolic profile of the metagenome/microbial community.

1. What constitute the next generation sequencing methodologies?

Traditional sequencing is done by dye terminator method developed by Sanger. Although the method has been automated but the cost of the sequencing is so high that it is beyond the reach of many laboratories for large-scale applications. On the other hand next generation sequencing techniques gives the high throughput data in extremely low cost per base as compared to Sanger sequencing. There are four major platforms available for NGS, 1) the Roche Diagnostic Corporation marketed 454 Genome sequencer, 2) Illumina make HiSeq and two Applied Biosystems (Life Technologies) make 3) SOLiD and 4) Ion-Torent including some others are described in following text.

1.1 454 pyrosequencing

The 454 Life Sciences Corporation (now under Roche Diagnostics Corporation) had introduced the first commercially available next-generation sequencing instrument, 454 GS20. The GS20 machine was able to generate more than 2,00,000 sequences of 100 bps in 4 h, while the latest version of 454 sequencing system, the GS FLX^{+} is capable of generating over 10,00,000 sequences of 1000 bp in a 23 h run. The ability to generate 1000 bps reads is key advantage of the 454 sequencing system over other second-generation sequencing systems. Due to the longer read lengths, the 454 sequencing system often is the second-generation sequencing system of choice for sequencing large genomes (Velasco *et al.*, 2007; Wheeler *et al.*, 2008). This system uses fragmented DNA samples (few hundred bases) for sequencing as compared to good quality cloned DNA required for Sanger sequencing and obviated the need of sub-cloning of BAC clones. This advantage helped the system to be adopted quickly by the scientific community. The 454 sequencing system uses a sequencing-by-synthesis approach, in which the fragmented DNA is linked with adapters and the flanked DNA fragments are then captured on the surface of specially designed beads and amplified via emulsion PCR (Dressman *et al.*, 2003). The clonally enriched beads are loaded into picoliter wells where the actual sequencing reaction starts. Sequencing is performed via pyrosequencing, in which every addition of nucleotide to the growing strand results in the release of pyrophosphate. The released pyrophosphate generates a chemiluminescent signal via ATP sulfurylase and luciferase. The fluorescence intensity is captured and analyzed by high resolution CCD camera. The intensity is used to determine the number of nucleotides added during each incorporation event. The major limitation of the technology is sequencing of homopolymer tracts, where more than one nucleotide can be incorporated per cycle. In pyrosequencing the length of homopolymer bases must be inferred from the signal intensity which becomes less sensitive as the length of the homopolymer tract increases. As a result, insertion-deletion in homopolymer tracts represents the dominant error type for the 454 system. Longer homopolymers lead to higher error rates, as the number of insertion-deletion errors significantly increases after the 7th base in A/T homopolymer stretches (Wicker *et al.*, 2006).

1.2 Illumina

Solexa developed the second commercially available NGS platform, which was later acquired by Illumina. The latest version of the Illumina systems HiSeq 2000 and 2500 yields 3 billion sequences with single reads and 6 billion sequences with paired reads with 100 bp length. Clustered amplicons are generated by immobilizing adapter-flanked DNA fragments on a flow cell surface, coated by a dense lawn of covalently attached primers, whose sequences are complementary to the sequences of the adapters flanking the DNA fragments. A solid phase amplification protocol, also called "bridge amplification" (Fedurco *et al.*, 2006), generates up to 1,000 copies of each DNA fragment, grouped together into "clusters", with densities of up to 10 million clusters per square centimeter. After cluster formation, sequencing is performed using a sequencing-by-synthesis approach with reversible fluorescent terminator deoxyribonucleotides, in which each cycle consists of single-base extension followed by image acquisition after the release of a fluorescent signal which is indicative of the incorporated base. These nucleotides contain cleavable "blocking agents" at the 3′ hydroxyl position. Fluorescent labels and blocking agents are cleaved after single-base extension and imaging, allowing for the next cycle to occur (Turcatti *et al.*, 2008). Read lengths can be limited by several noise factors, including phasing, in which imperfections in single-base extension and cleavage chemistries accumulate at each cycle, leading to: (1) strands of various lengths within a DNA cluster, thus attenuating the signal delivered, (2) signal decay, as fluorescent signal intensities decrease as a function of cycle number and (3) fluorophore cross-talk, which becomes more preponderant in later cycles and can introduce substantial bias towards specific bases (Erlich *et al.*, 2008). In 2008, Illumina introduced new reagents that improved cleavage chemistry, thereby allowing longer read sequencing (up to 76 bps) and reducing the risk of errors. Currently, average error rate on the Illumina GA IIx platform is in the order of 0.5%.

1.3 SOLiD

The third commercially available NGS platform is developed by Applied Biosystems. It differs from the two previous platforms in that it uses sequencing-by-ligation approach (Shendure *et al.*, 2005) to sequence tens to hundreds of millions of adapter-flanked DNA fragments which are immobilized on the surface of paramagnetic beads and amplified via emulsion PCR (Dressman *et al.*, 2003). After breaking the emulsion, the clonally amplified beads are selectively recovered and deposited onto a glass slide array for sequencing. A universal primer whose last base is complementary to the nth position of the adapter sequence is hybridized to the array. At each cycle, a set of degenerate fluorescently labeled octamers, whose identity is correlated with the identity of the first 2 bases within the octamer, compete for ligation to the DNA fragment. After ligation and image acquisition, the octamer is chemically cleaved between position 5 and 6 to remove the fluorescent label, and subsequent cycles of octamer ligation, image acquisition and cleavage are performed, enabling sequencing of every 5th base, with the number of cycles determining the overall read length. A second round, in which the elongated primer is removed and a new universal primer whose last base is complementary to the $(n-1)^{th}$ position of the adapter sequence is added, followed by 3 more rounds of primer reset to complete the sequence of the DNA fragment. The SOLiD system features a two-base encoding mechanism, in which two adjacent bases, rather than a single base, are correlated with a fluorescent signal. Because each signal is used to label four possible di-nucleotides, the identity of a base is determined by analyzing the 16 dinucleotide combinations of two signals (color spaces) which result from two successive ligations. As a consequence, each base is interrogated twice, once as the first base and once as the second base, in two independent rounds of primer hybridization. This two-base encoding system allows sequencing errors to be promptly identified.

1.4 Ion Torrent

The equipment developed by ion torrent is rapid, compact and economical. The basic principle of the technology is similar to sequencing by synthesis. Uniqueness of this platform is conferred by incorporation of base to the growing chain results in release of pyrophosphate and a positively charged hydrogen ion, which is detected using semiconductor technology. It does not use the optics and light signal detection or the modified nucleotides for chain termination. The chemical reaction is performed in the microwells on the semiconductor chip with a sensor at the base of the microwells. Each microwell contains one molecule of DNA strand and a molecule of DNA polymerase is sequentially flooded with dNTP. Incorporation event, if any, is detected by change in the pH and incorporation of two or more nucleotides measured by greater change in the pH. The additive signal detection cannot be measured accurately as in pyrosequencing, which limits the use of this platform for homopolymer tract sequencing. The other disadvantage of the system is short read length and the throughput is much lesser than the current NGS platforms. The future versions may cover limitations by improving the chip design. Currently, due to short read length and limited throughput, the technology finds its applications for small microbe sequencing, microbial transcriptomics and amplicon sequencing.

1.5 Other technologies

Helicos Biosciences Corporation (http://www.helicosbio.com) developed true Single Molecule Sequencing (tSMS) technology. This technology is based on detecting synthesis reaction on single strand, eliminating the cluster formation or PCR amplification of the template. The DNA sample is fragmented and tagged with poly A linker, which is captured on the proprietary surface of flow cell and serves as template for sequencing reaction. The fluorescently labeled nucleotides are added and after synthesis and washing, signals are captured from the incorporated nucleotides using Heliscope. Fluorescent label is cleaved and next step proceeds. The advantage of the technology is that it does not require amplification step and thus avoids PCR induced bias and errors.

Pacific Biosciences (http://www.pacificbiosciences.com) has introduced a third generation sequencing technology in late 2010 that incorporates novel single molecule sequencing in real time. This SMRT (Single Molecule, Real Time) technology conduct, monitor and analyzes biochemical reactions at individual molecule level. The sequences are individual DNA strands are determined by capturing the signal before cleaving off the label for incorporation of next base. Unlike existing NGS platforms, the technology uses minimal reagents and there are no time consuming flushing scanning and washing steps. The platform does not require PCR amplification of the template. Main advantage of the technology is greater read lengths, average read length of 1000 bp and reported instances of 10000 bases.

Life Technologies has announced a third generation sequencing technology known as starlight originally developed by VisiGen Biotechnologies Inc. (USA). The technology features real time capturing of sequence data. Signal generated by growing DNA strand is due to FRET (Fluorescent Resonance Energy Transfer) from the fluorescent quantum dot nano-crystal coupled polymerase (FRET donor) and nucleotide gamma phosphate linked with one of the four FRET acceptors. The main advantage of the technology is capacity to sequence entire DNA template since the polymerase can be replaced, if it loses its activity. The expected speed of the system is 1 megabases per second.

2. Metagenomic sample coverage

Coverage in sequencing is defined as the mean number of times a nucleotide is sequenced. Thus 3X coverage means each nucleotide is sequenced to a mean number of 3 times. The short read sequencing necessitates higher coverage to ensure all the reads overlap and are unique to assemble the genomes. If one treats DNA shearing and sequencing as random events and the ability to detect and overlap between two truly overlapping reads does not vary between clones, then Poisson distribution model can be used to estimate the number of reads required to sequence entire genome. This model is given by Lander-Waterman equation (Lander and Waterman, 1988) which has the following equation:

$$C = \frac{L \times N}{G}$$

Where, L is the read length, N is the number of reads, G is the genome length and C is coverage as described above.

With a particular coverage the fraction of genome content sequenced can be represented by

$$P_0 = 1 - e^{-C} = 1\text{-}e^{-(LN/G)}$$

Or the number of reads required for sequencing P_0 fraction of the genome would be given by following formula

$$N = (-)\frac{\text{Log}(1 - \text{Po})}{L} XG$$

In an environmental sample containing *l* number of species, the metagenome size can be estimated by

$$Gm = \sum_{i=1}^{I} niGi$$

Where, G_i is the size of any given metagenome in *I* no of genome containing sample, and n_i is the number of copies of genome G_i. Since, the metagenomic sample contains numerous microbial species in different proportions. Therefore metagenome size G_m composed of genome sizes G_1 to G_k can be viewed as sum of fractions. Each component genome size Gi constitutes a fraction of G_m (Wooley *et al.*, 2010).

The species diversity in the sample can be estimated by using species-specific gene markers usually small ribosomal subunit DNA. Although, this sometimes cannot estimate adequate coverage of full diversity in species rich environment for less represented genomes. This has been established by rarefaction curve analysis (Countway *et al.*, 2005; Fierer and Jackson, 2006 and Youssef and Elshahed, 2008).

3. The quality of sequence

Each time DNA sequence data is obtained, it is measured to determine the bases of the DNA sample in an *in vitro* replication process which allows reading each base in the sequence. The measurements therefore have uncertainty, which is otherwise called as error probability. In Sanger sequencing, the error probabilities are represented in phred quality scores. The error probabilities are small fractions and decimal values with many leading zeros, these are converted into positive integers by the following formula

$$QV= -10 \log (p)$$

With this transformation, the probabilities becomes

1/100 = 20, 1/10000 = 40 and 1/1000000 = 60

In Sanger format, the phred quality scores from 0-93 are encoded by ASCII (American Standard Code for Information Interchange) 33-126. In Solexa format the scores are encoded form -5 to 62 using ASCII 59-126 and in later version Illumina format the scores from 0-62 are encoded by ASCII 54-126. In the SOLiD data the sequence is in color space and quality scores are same as Sanger's. The ASCII codes and corresponding character are given in Table 1. It is important to have easy access to quality values and error rates to troubleshoot issues with runs and samples.

Table 1 : ASCII codes used for encoding of quality values in sequence output files

Code	Character	Code	Character	Code	Character	Code	Character	Code	Character
33	!	52	4	71	G	90	Z	109	m
34	"	53	5	72	H	91	[	110	n
35	#	54	6	73	I	92	\	111	o
36	$	55	7	74	J	93	]	112	p
37	%	56	8	75	K	94	^	113	q
38	&	57	9	76	L	95	_	114	r
39	'	58	:	77	M	96	`	115	s
40	(	59	;	78	N	97	a	116	t
41	)	60	<	79	O	98	b	117	u
42	*	61	=	80	P	99	c	118	v
43	+	62	>	81	Q	100	d	119	w
44	,	63	?	82	R	101	e	120	x
45	-	64	@	83	S	102	f	121	y
46	.	65	A	84	T	103	g	122	z
47	/	66	B	85	U	104	h	123	{
48	0	67	C	86	V	105	i	124	|
49	1	68	D	87	W	106	j	125	}
50	2	69	E	88	X	107	k	126	~
51	3	70	F	89	Y	108	l	--	--

The quality values are primarily used for trimming the sequences and are ignored in the subsequent analysis. Quality filtering is required for trimming the sequences with low quality regions, which may otherwise terminate a long alignment due to mismatch. The poor quality regions are usually observed at the end of the sequences. These regions may complicate the overlap alignments used in sequence assembly. Since nucleotide blast against nucleotide database is an inherent step for annotation of the unidentified sequences. If a poor quality sequence is aligned, the alignment may terminate prematurely and provide incorrect estimate of significance score. The quality-adjusted sequence will always provide more accurate annotation.

4. Assessing sequence characteristics

The second generation sequencing files should be checked for sequence quality and other associated parameters. Although the software is integrated in the data processing pipeline of the sequencers, certain quality checks are desirable. A simple tool FAST QC is available at http://www.bioinformatics.bbsrc.ac.uk which can be used for this purpose as well. This tool computes basic statistics of the sequence reads including per base quality score, per base sequence content, per base GC content, per base N content, sequence length distribution, duplicate sequences, overrepresented sequences etc. These results give overall idea of the quality of the sequence reads generated by NGS. A similar tool SeqQC is available from http://www.genotypic.co.in.

The important quality checks performed on NGS data are

1. *Per base sequence quality*: The graph generated for per base sequence quality represents overview of range of quality scores across all the bases at each position of the sequence (Fig. 1).

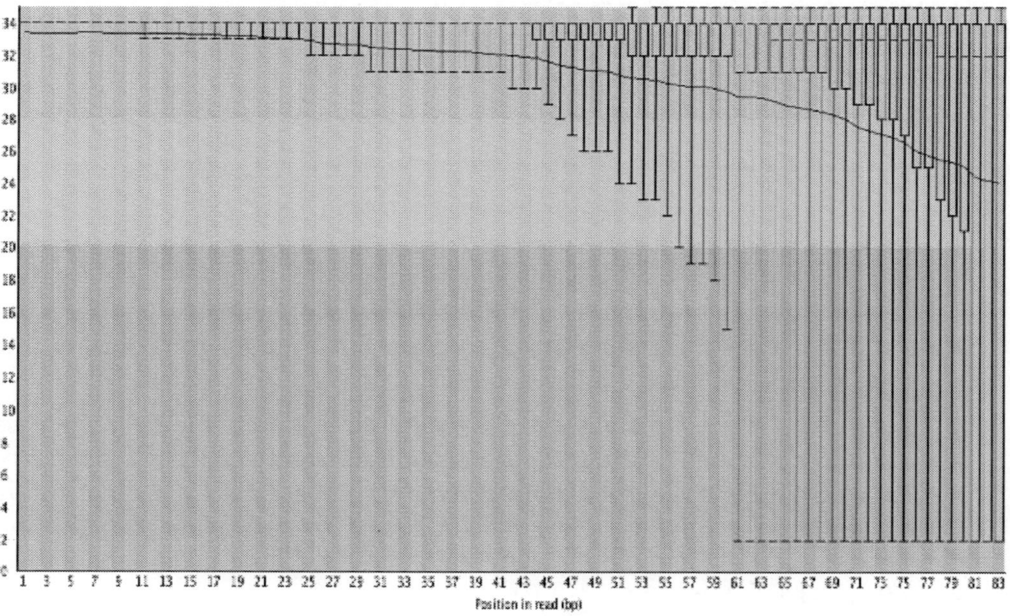

Fig. 1 : The x axis shows the base number and y axis represents quality scores. The quality scores at each read position are represented by box plot to show the distribution. The boxes represents the quality scores between inter quartile range 25-75%. The upper and lower bars represent 10% and 90 % point. Central red line shows median and the blue line represents the mean of the quality values. Higher the score, better the base call.

2. *Per sequence quality scores:* This graph is generated from the sequence data to show the average quality of a read and plotting the distribution of average quality values. A representative graph is shown in Fig. 2. The graph helps to understand whether low quality bases are positioned in a subset of data or spread uniformly throughout the sequence reads.

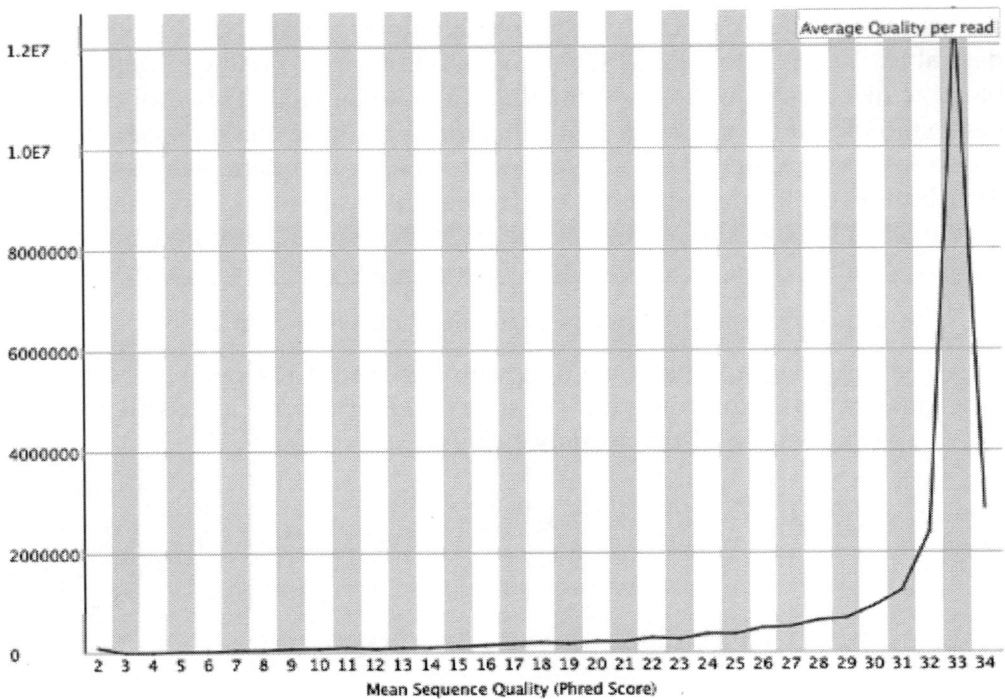

Fig. 2 : The x axis shows the quality scores and y axis represents the number of sequences.

There are always sequences with low quality scores in small subsets but this should be very small percentage of data. For a good quality data, the major peak should be after quality score 27.

1. *The per base N content analysis:* If the sequencer is not able to make base call with sufficient confidence, then it will normally call an N instead of the correct base. It is expressed in percentage of base calls at each position. It is common to observe a low percentage of Ns appearing near the end of the sequences. For good quality data, the Ns should be less than 5% at each read position.
2. *Per base sequence content analysis:* It plots the percentage of each base at each sequence read position. The graph should typically show four smooth lines around 25% unless the original sample is biased (typically miRNA and bisulphite sequencing data).
3. *Sequence duplication levels analysis* is performed to assess sequences with different degree of duplications. In diverse libraries, typically the sequences will appear only once and graph will show peak at one. A peak may be observed at 10 copies or more category representing dominant duplications or sequences from numerically dominant organisms in metagenomic sample.

5. Analyzing the sequence data for microbial assessment

Galaxy web server offers tools for analyzing large amount of sequence data (Taylor *et al.*, 2007) generated by NGS for finding microbial distribution (http://www.main.g2.bx.psu.edu). This site also supports sequence files or alignments performed elsewhere in tab delimited files. For microbial phylogeny, the alignments can be performed at CAMERA (Community cyber-infrastructure for Advanced Microbial Ecology Research and Analysis) web site or local BLASTx (Basic local alignment search tools) programs. Galaxy performs a homology-based search in the NR database (or other selected database) such as HTGs (High Throughput Genome) and WGS (Whole Genome Shotgun) and report results with taxonomic ranks for each matched sequence reads. The data can be further used for displaying taxonomic distribution of the microbes in the sequencing data. Since the homology search against total NR (Non redundant) database is computationally intensive, it is difficult to process the files on personal computer, although galaxy can be downloaded and installed locally. The local installation can be used for basic manipulations of the NGS data *viz.*, converting the fastq files from one format to another, splitting the large files before upload, looking at base quality distribution, combining fasta and qual files in case of 454 data into fastq format, and after trimming the poor quality reads converting the files into fasta format etc.

The galaxy web server has shared data and workflow links, where previously shared workflows are published. These workflows can work as reference to start with. Metagenomic workflow contains following steps modified from the Windshield splatter analysis (Koskovsky *et al.*, 2009) workflow:

1. Uploading data file on to the galaxy server.
2. Quality filtering of data files using the NGS QC and manipulation tools under the appropriate data platform. The data is filtered for minimal quality score, minimal sequence length (depending upon the sequenced length).
3. Converting the fastq files into fasta format before alignment.
4. Converting the fasta file into tabular format and adding a column for tagging base count.
5. Performing megablast against desired database (nr, HTGS or WGS). Specifying desired e value cutoff (preferably 0.00001), P value for identity cutoff and W value for best perfect match also called as word size. This process is computationally intensive and may take considerable time to complete.

6. Joining the files produced at sl no 4 and sl no 5 using join two databases tool.
7. Filtering the joined file using an expression c5/c15 >= 0.5, this step removes the suboptimal alignments where less than 50% of the sequences matched with the database entry.
8. Fetching taxonomic representation from the filter data. Discovery of taxonomic representation from metagenomic data employs LCA (Lowest Common Ancestor) for short reads ~100 bp.
9. Finding lowest diagnostic rank on the taxonomic representation data to get reads specific to ranks below kingdom level.
10. Summarizing the taxonomy on the above data and build a phylogenetic tree. The tree shows number reads assigned to each taxonomic rank/ node.

The phylogenetic tree generated on galaxy can be downloaded in pdf format for further use. The data of different phylogenetic ranks and read counts assigned to the respective rank can be downloaded from the galaxy server and used as input file on MEGAN metagenome analyser to compare multiple samples or to view the phylogeny at different level of taxonomy.

Metagenome analyzer (MEGAN) is a simple graphical user interface (GUI) program (Huson *et al.*, 2011) written in java. This program is suitable to run on a standard laptop with 2 GB RAM and uses output of any blast family programs. The MEGAN is used to estimate and interactively explore the taxonomical content of the data set, using the NCBI (National Center for Biotechnology Information) taxonomy. This program uses a simple algorithm that assigns each reads to the lowest common ancestor (LCA) of the set of taxa that hit in the comparison. As a result, species-specific sequences are assigned to taxa near the leaves of the NCBI tree, whereas widely conserved sequences are assigned to higher order taxa closer to the root. The results can be viewed in an interactive phylogenetic tree. Megan allows comparison of two or more datasets in single phylogenetic tree with proportions of each taxonomical interval in *pi* charts (Mitra *et al.*, 2010).

Several pipelines are introduced for functional profiling of the metagenomes. The MG-RAST (Metagenome Rapid Annotation using Subsystems Technology) server provides most comprehensive analysis of the metagenome data (Meyer *et al.*, 2008). Raw files uploaded will be processed on the MG RAST server. The results can be interactively viewed for phylogenetic as well as functional profile in terms of SEED (first annotation environment) categories and KEGG (Kyoto Encyclopedia for Genes and Genomes) (Aoki-Kinoshita and Kanehisa, 2007) pathway mapping to identify differences among the user samples and to compare results with pre-computed profiles from public metagenomes. The analysis tools on the web server allows to visualize the results in graphical format, generate PCA (Principal Component Analysis) for samples, generation of heat maps for comparative studies and p value analysis tool to compare the metagenomes and finding out statistical significance of the abundance in the samples.

The RAMMCAP (Rapid Analysis of Multiple Metagenomes with a Clustering and Annotation Pipeline) (Li, 2009) web tool is available at the CAMERA (Community cyber infrastructure for Advanced Microbial Ecology Research and Analysis) portal (Sheshadri *et al.*, 2007), which offers various functional profiling methods for analysis of single metagenomes. However, the comparison of different metagenomes needs to be performed on local installation of RAMMCAP. Web-CARMA, a web application for the functional and taxonomic classification of unassembled metagenomic reads (Gerlach *et al.*, 2009) also provides facilities for taxonomic profiling of metagenomes. A functional annotation of the sequences against Pfam (Protein Families Database) and GO (Gene Ontology) assignments can be obtained for offline comparison of different metagenomes. In addition to the above tools, there are several web based resources for comparative metagenome analysis but they do not support profiling of large amount of user supplied data (Goll *et al.*, 2010; Kottmann *et al.*, 2010). These tools require pre-computed sequence assignments from other web sites.

The CoMet web server (Li *et al.*, 2012) implements a complete pipeline for functional annotation and comparison of metagenomes. The combination of ORF (open reading frame) finding, fast Pfam domain detection and comparative statistical analysis with an easy-to-use web interface allows obtaining a quick overview of putative functional differences in a set of metagenomic samples. Although GO categories have only been used in few metagenomic studies so far, our results indicate the potential of GO terms for a comparative metagenome analysis.

Conclusions

The advent of second and third generation sequencing technologies has tremendously increased our abilities to sequence single and multiple genomes at affordable cost and in a short span of time. These technologies will be helpful in studying the function of various ecological niches through metagenomic analysis. The bioinformatics analysis tool are available to annotate and compare the multiple metagenomes will help in studying the community structure and function, finding new genes and enzymes, studying interactions with other ecological niches and understanding biology through systems approach. Although the computational requirements of such analyses are very high, but the publically available cloud computing resources will be a boon to the small laboratories and researchers.

References

Aoki-Kinoshita K.F., Kanehisa M. (2007). Gene annotation and pathway mapping in KEGG. *Methods in Molecular Biology* **396:** 71-91.

Chakravorty S., Helb D., Burday M., Connell N., Alland D. (2007). A detailed analysis of 16S ribosomal RNA gene segments for the diagnosis of pathogenic bacteria. *Journal of Microbiological Methods* **69:** 330-339.

Countway P.D., Gast R.J., Pratik Sava I., Caron D.A. (2005). Protistan diversity estimates based on 18s rDNA from seawater incubations in the western north atlantic. *Journal of Eukaryotic Microbiology* **52:** 95-106.

Dressman D., Yan H., Traverso G., Kinzler K.W., Vogelstein B. (2003). Transforming single DNA molecules into fluorescent magnetic particles for detection and enumeration of genetic variations. *Proceedings of National Academy of Sciences, USA* **100:** 8817-8822.

Erlich Y., Mitra P.P., delaBastide M., McCombie W.R., Hannon G.J. (2008). Alta-Cyclic: a self-optimizing base caller for next-generation sequencing. *Nature Methods* **5:** 679-682.

Fedurco M., Romieu A., Williams S., Lawrence I., Turcatti G. (2006). BTA, a novel reagent for DNA attachment on glass and efficient generation of solid-phase amplified DNA colonies. *Nucleic Acids Research* **34:** e22.

Fierer N., Jackson R.B. (2006). The diversity and biogeography of soil bacterial communities. *Proceedings of National Academy of Sciences, USA* **103:** 626-631.

Gerlach W., Junemann S., Tille F., Goesmann A., Stoye J. (2009). WebCARMA: a web application for the functional and taxonomic classification of unassembled metagenomic reads. *BMC Bioinformatics* **10:** 430.

Goll J., Rusch D.B., Tanenbaum D.M., Thiagarajan M., Li K., Methe B.A., Yooseph S. (2010). METAREP: JCVI metagenomics reports–an open source tool for high-performance comparative metagenomics. *Bioinformatics* **26:** 2631-2632.

Kottmann R., Kostadinov I., Duhaime M.B., Buttigieg P.L., Yilmaz P., Hankeln W., Waldmann J., Glockner F.O. (2010). Megx.net: integrated database resource for marine ecological genomics. *Nucleic Acids Research* **38:** D391-D395.

Lander E.S., Waterman M.S. (1988). Genomic mapping by fingerprinting random clones: a mathematical analysis. *Genomics* **2:** 231-239.

Li R.W., Connor E.E., Li C., Baldwin Vi R.L., Sparks M.E. (2012). Characterization of the rumen microbiota of pre-ruminant calves using metagenomic tools. *Environmental Microbiology* **14:** 129-139.

Li W. (2009). Analysis and comparison of very large metagenomes with fast clustering and functional annotation. *BMC Bioinformatics* **10:** 359.

Meyer F., Paarmann D., D'Souza M., Olson R., Glass E.M., Kubal M., Paczian T., Rodriguez A., Stevens R., Wilke A. *et al.* (2008) The metagenomics RAST server - a public resource for the automatic phylogenetic and functional analysis of metagenomes. *BMC Bioinformatics* **9:** 386.

Miron J., BenGhedalia D., Morrison M. (2001). Adhesion mechanisms of rumen cellulolytic bacteria. *Journal of Dairy Science* **84:** 1294-1309.

Quince C., Lanzén A., Curtis T.P., Davenport R.J., Hall N., Head I.M., Read L.F., Sloan W.T. (2009). Accurate determination of microbial diversity from 454 pyrosequencing data. *Nature Methods* **6:** 639-641.

Seshadri R., Kravitz S.A., Smarr L., Gilna P., Frazier M. (2007). CAMERA: a community resource for metagenomics. *PLoS Biology* **5:** e75.

Shendure J., Porreca G.J., Reppas N.B., Lin X., McCutcheon J.P., Rosenbaum A.M., Wang M.D., Zhang K., Mitra R.D., Church G.M. (2005). Accurate multiplex polony sequencing of an evolved bacterial genome. *Science* **309:** 1728-1732.

Turcatti G., Romieu A., Fedurco M., Tairi A.P. (2008). A new class of cleavable fluorescent nucleotides: synthesis and optimization as reversible terminators for DNA sequencing by synthesis. *Nucleic Acids Research* **36:** e25.

Velasco R., Zharkikh A., Troggio M., Cartwright D.A., Cestaro A., Pruss D., Pindo M., Fitzgerald L.M., Vezzulli S., Reid J., Malacarne G., Iliev D., Coppola G., Wardell B., Micheletti D., Macalma T., Facci M., Mitchell J.T., Perazzolli M., Eldredge G., Gatto P., Oyzerski R., Moretto M., Gutin N., Stefanini M., Chen Y., Segala C., Davenport C., Demattè L., Mraz A., Battilana J., Stormo K., Costa F., Tao Q., Si-Ammour A., Harkins T., Lackey A., Perbost C., Taillon B., Stella A., Solovyev V., Fawcett J.A., Sterck L., Vandepoele K., Grando S.M., Toppo S., Moser C., Lanchbury J., Bogden R., Skolnick M., Sgaramella V., Bhatnagar S.K., Fontana P., Gutin A., Peer Y., Salamini F., Viola R. (2007). A high quality draft consensus sequence of the genome of a heterozygous grapevine variety. *PloS One* **12:** e1326.

Wheeler D.A., Srinivasan M., Egholm M., Shen Y., Chen L., McGuire A., He W., Chen Y.J., Makhijani V., Roth G.T., Gomes X., Tartaro K., Niazi F., Turcotte C.L., Irzyk G.P., Lupski J.R., Chinault C., Song X.Z., Liu Y., Yuan Y., Nazareth L., Qin X., Muzny D.M., Margulies M., Weinstock G.M., Gibbs R.A., Rothberg J.M. (2008). The complete genome of an individual by massively parallel DNA sequencing. *Nature* **452:** 872-876.

Wicker T., Schlagenhauf E., Graner A., Close T., Keller B., Stein N. (2006). 454 sequencing put to the test using the complex genome of barley. *BMC Genomics* **7:** 275-285.

Wooley J.C., Godzik A., Friedberg I. (2010). A Primer on Metagenomics. *PLoS Computational Biology* **6:** e1000667.

Youssef N.H., Elshahed M.S. (2008). Species richness in soil bacterial communities: a proposed approach to overcome sample size bias. *Journal of Microbial Methods* **75:** 86-91.

Huson D.H., Mitra S., Weber N., Ruscheweyh H., Schuster S.C. (2011). Integrative analysis of environmental sequences using MEGAN4. *Genome Research* **21:** 1552-1560.

Mitra S., Gilbert J.A., Field D., Huson D.H. (2010). Comparison of multiple metagenomes using phylogenetic networks based on ecological indices, *ISME Journal* **4:** 1236-1242.

Koskovsky P.S., Wadhawan S., Chiaromonte F., Ananda G., Chung W., Taylor J., Nekrutenko A. (2009). Windshield splatter analysis with the Galaxy metagenomic pipeline. *Genome Research* **19:** 2144-2153.

❏❏❏

Chapter 23

Applications of Bioinformatics Tools to Understand the Structures and Functions of Proteins

U.B. Angadi, A.P. Kolte, A. Dhali, J. Ghosh
National Institute of Animal Nutrition and Physiology, Adugodi, Bangalore-560 030, Karnataka, India

Summary

An enormous protein and protein encoding genes sequence data is being accumulated in public databases. It is a challenge to the molecular biologist and computer professionals to decipher the structural, functional and evolutionary clues encoded in the language of those sequences. Tools for sequence, analysis, structure prediction and identification of evolutionary relatedness are essential to understand structures and functions of the proteins. In this chapter advances in databases, various approaches of sequence and structure analysis, prediction of structural information from protein sequences and protein-protein interactions using sequence and structural information to know functional pathways are discussed.

A central challenge in bioinformatics is the rationalization of the huge mass of sequence information with a view not only to derive more efficient means of data storage, but also for designing sharper analytical tools. Such tools are required to convert the sequence information into biochemical and biophysical knowledge and to decipher the structural, functional and evolutionary clues encoded in the language of those sequences. This language may be transformed into sentences represented by proteins, words by motifs and letters by amino/nucleic acids. Application of bioinformatics tools in protein analysis involves four major phases: 1) Creating a secondary database of sequences and structures of related proteins from primary databases using classification/clustering techniques, which includes publicly available primary and secondary databases and methodology creating secondary databases related to specific research domains; 2) Sequence alignment and similarity metrics which contains popular sequence aligning and similarity scoring techniques; 3) Predicting three-dimensional (3D) structure of unknown protein which comprises recent developments in protein structural analysis and predictions; 4) Indentify binding sites, protein-protein interactions and protein-RNA interaction to understand functional pathways, and interpret and decipher cell function using sequence and structural information.

1. Protein classification and databases

Due to concerted effort of many molecular biology laboratories throughout the world and the internet, sequence data in the public sequence databases can easily be accessed by anyone, anywhere and anytime. The first database was created immediately after the insulin protein sequence made available in 1956. Probably, the first published work on the biological sequence databases was 'Atlas of protein sequences and structures' in 1965 by Dayhoff, (Dayhoff *et al.*, 1978) which became the foundation for protein databases. After the second edition of the Atlas, 3D structures of protein were studied and the well-known protein data bank (PDB) was developed. It was the first protein structure database that had just 10 entries in 1972. Currently over 78,992 protein structure entries are there as on January 2012. Initially, the protein sequence databases were maintained by individual laboratories. Subsequently a consolidated protein sequence database Swiss-Prot was developed in 1986 and now this database has 5,34,242 entries as on January 2012.

The most important problem in computational biology is the structural and functional classification of protein sequences based on sequence homology. The two important outcomes of such categorical grouping are: 1) molecular analysis within a particular group, instead of individual protein sequence, which may provide valuable information on the protein structure, functional residues, and binding sites; and 2) the classified protein sequences reflect their structural, evolutionary, and functional relatedness. These relationships are embedded in hierarchical structure of protein classification.

In general, there are two types of biological databases based on source and quality.

1.1 Primary databases

These databases accept original data from researchers with little checking and validation. Examples of primary databases are GenBank, EMBL (European Molecular Biology Laboratory), DDBJ (DNA Data Bank of Japan), UniProt/Swiss-Prot, PDB, *etc.*

1.2 Secondary databases

Due to massive data in the primary databases, one cannot derive meaningful information from the primary databases. The sequence information is needed to be converted into biochemical and biophysical knowledge. To overcome these problems, secondary databases are either manually curated or semi-automatically generated from primary databases using analytical tools and these databases contain information such as the conserved sequences, signature sequences, common structures and active-site residues of protein families derived from a set of related sequences. Examples of secondary databases are PROSITE (Protein Sites), Pfam (Protein FAMilies), PRINTS (protein fingerPRINTS), SCOP (Structural Classification of Protein), CATH (Class Architecture Topology Homology) and Dali Domain Dictionary.

There are several secondary databases for structural classification of proteins, such as SCOP (Murzin *et al.*, 1995), CATH (Orengo *et al.*, 1997) and Dali Domain Dictionary (Holm and Sander, 1997) and, they have been developed to build protein domains in a hierarchical manner based on structural information which reflects structural, functional, and evolutionary relatedness. They employ different heuristics, similarity measures and degree of automation. The SCOP and CATH are the most widely used and active databases. The SCOP is curated manually, based on expert knowledge and, is accepted by many researchers as the gold standard for the analysis of structural, functional and evolutionary relatedness of proteins. This database contains extensive information relating to protein domains and structures. The proteins are well-organized in hierarchical classification at four main levels namely, classes, folds, superfamilies, and families. However, there are challenges in hierarchical protein classification, such as 1) availability of limited resources at the top level (folds) of hierarchy classification, 2) low level (family) of hierarchy based on sequence information, in which members may not be readily recognizable from sequences and 3) the need for the classified databases to be updated frequently to include the newly discovered protein in a timely manner. The SCOP is updated once in 6 months and the CATH is updated annually. In the CATH database, Class describes secondary structures, Architecture is summarized shape of protein, Topology reveals similarity in structures and functions, and homology depicts evolutionary relationship. *Dali* is an automatic structure comparison program to cluster proteins in hierarchical structure based on structural similarities; which yields a fold tree and provides a rich source of information for the study of both divergent and convergent aspects of molecular evolution.

On the other hand, the number of protein sequences and protein structures are constantly increasing. As per the release UniPortKB/Swiss-Port of 12th

Jan. 2012, there are 5,34,242 protein entries at www.expasy.ch, and as on Jan. 2012, there are 72,992 structures available at PDB (www.rcsb.org/pdb). In PDB, out of the available entries, only 38,221 proteins are classified till SCOP ASTRAL 1.75 (http://scop.berkelay.edu). Thus, a large number of proteins remain listed under the 'not a true class' level (Jain *et al.*, 2009; Liu and Rost, 2003). Hence, there is a greater need to develop more efficient, accurate, and automated classification methods. Manual classification cannot be completely replaced by automated methods and manual method still remains as the gold standard. However, the automated methods can be used as a preprocessing tool to help experts and to cope up with the pace with which new sequences and structures are generated.

Work on protein structural classification has been going on for over a decade. Many methods are currently available for the clustering of protein sequences into superfamilies and families. There are difficulties in classifying protein family/superfamily that share very weak similarities. In such cases, these methods fail to provide correct information about the classification of the sequence. Machine-learning algorithm classifier (Jain *et al.*, 2009; Angadi and Venktesulu, 2010, 2011) shows better results. But these approaches are based on what it learns from the classification already available in SCOP and not just on pair wise sequence alignment and similarity.

2. Sequence alignment and similarity metrics

Sequence alignment is a key factor in bioinformatics to identify homology in DNA/protein sequences. Sequence alignment and similarity scores are basic tools to analysis sequences, prediction of functions of genes and proteins, determine binding sites, structure formation, interaction among proteins/RNA and modulation of structures of protein.

A widely used class of alignment algorithms begins with the Needleman and Wunschi (1970) dynamic programming algorithm that can find the global alignment between two amino acid/nucleic acid sequences. Subsequently numerous heuristic algorithms were suggested, but those could not satisfy the biologists. Sellers (1974) developed a true metric measure of the distance between sequences. Sellers's work was generalized later by Waterman *et al.* (1976) to include multiple insertion/deletion. Smith and Waterman (Smith and Waterman, 1981) introduced a new algorithm with a different method of scoring similarity, aimed at finding optimum local aligned sub-sequences at the expense of the global score. Global algorithms are generally not sensitive to highly divergent sequences with some localized similarities within them. Alignment algorithms suffer from several inherent drawbacks. Firstly, the task of optimally aligning a set of strings is computationally very expensive. Secondly, alignment of an entire sequence can reveal only global similarity.

If the sequences under comparison are distantly related or if the relative order of their similar regions varies among sequences, then evolutionary relationships might only be detected as similarities over short stretches of residues. Efforts to overcome these drawbacks of sequence alignment led to devising the following new approaches.

The BLOCK database (http://blocks.fhcrc.org/; Henikoff *et al.*, 1995) approach is to look for small numbers (three for example) of amino acids or highly conserved positions separated by short fixed spacing and local alignment. Blocks are ungapped segments corresponding to the most highly conserved regions of proteins (Henikoff and Henikoff, 1992) and obtained by multiple alignments. This approach is used as a similarity measure for classifying sequences into families. The segments of fixed size with gapped substrings for sequence similarity score have been proposed by Angadi *et al.* (2008). In this method, segments with gaps are generated from a set of sequences using dynamic programming and leader (nearest neighbor) algorithm and frequency of these segments are used for calculating similarity score. The third type of approach is based on motifs. Motif is a sub-sequence that occurs frequently within a group of related proteins. It is a signature found in a set of related sequences and it characterizes a particular biochemical function. The problem of detecting all existing motifs is *NP-hard*. A reduction from the Longest Common Subsequences (LCS) problem can be used to prove this. Possible remedies include the use of heuristics (Smith and Waterman, 1981; Smith *et al.*, 1990; Lawrence *et al.*, 1993; Wang *et al.*, 1994; Bailey and Elkan, 1994; Buhler and Tompa, 2002; Price *et al.*, 2003) which offer enhanced performance, but at the expense of sacrificing the completeness of the results and/or the structural restriction of the patterns. Using the same approach, a new technique called GENETAL is proposed recently (Angadi and Venkatesulu, 2010). It provides conserved motifs from a set of sequences using evolutionary concept (Genetic algorithm). They employed GENETAL to cluster a set of sequences as feature extraction technique.

One way to overcome the difficulty that alignment algorithms have in identifying local similarities is to focus on the discovery of *patterns* shared by a set of related sequences. The *Pattern* is an arrangement of two or more amino acids occurring in a protein sequence. This is well illustrated by the PROSITE database of proteins *patterns* (Bairoch *et al.*, 1997). Here groups of functionally and evolutionarily related proteins are listed along with their *patterns* which can be used to distinguish each family from all other sequences in the Swiss-Prot protein sequences database. These *patterns* are extracted semi-manually. Several techniques for discovering *patterns* from a set of related sequences are described in literatures (Pesole *et al.*, 1992; Jonassen *et al.*, 1995; Bazma *et al.*, 1996; Sagot and Viari, 1995; Hertz and Stormo, 1999; Rigoutsos *et al.,* 2000) and practical use of these *patterns* have been demonstrated. These approaches have many drawbacks. They are basically a supervised machine learning technique to identify an unknown sequence whether it belongs to a particular group or not. Also the size of the set of sequences has profound impact on *pattern*. These methods tolerate no similarity measure between sequences, fails to diagnose sequences that contain subtle changes in the *pattern* and cannot be easily used as a similarity metric to search in a database or structural and functional analysis with interactions.

Dynamic programming approaches are impractical for finding similarity between large sized sequences due to high space and time complexity involved in searching large databases. Two main disadvantages in *pattern* approaches are: 1) Gaps and substitutions are not allowed in the conserved region; and 2) It is difficult to test the significance of the pattern. The BLOCK approach also does not take substitutions into account. These problems led to the development of BLAST (Basic Local Alignment Search Tool) and FASTA (FAST alignment). They use heuristic methods to approximate the optimal local similarity shared by two sequences. The FASTA was first described by Lipman and Pearson (1985). The original FASTP program was designed for protein sequence similarity searching. Later, it was extended to perform DNA: DNA searches, translate protein: DNA searches and also provides a more sophisticated shuffling program for evaluating statistical significance. The BLAST was proposed by Altschul and his team (Altschul *et al.,* 1990). They also have developed Gapped BLAST and PSI-BLAST (Position Specific Iterative BLAST) (Altschul *et al.,* 1997) programs. In PSI-BLAST, a method is introduced for automatically combining statistically significant alignments produced by BLAST into a position-specific score matrix and searching the database using this matrix. The PSI-BLAST is faster than the original BLAST and is able to produce gapped alignments. The BLAST programs are widely used tools for searching protein/DNA sequences in databases, sequence comparison and finding similarity score between pairs of sequences.

The BLAST protein sequence alignments use a substitution matrix to assign scores to amino acid matches or mismatches and a gap penalty for matching an amino acid in one sequence to the other. Several sets of BLOSUM (BLOcks of amino acid SUbstition Matrix) (Henikoff and Henikoff, 1992) and PAM (Point Accepted Mutation) (Dayhoff *et al.,* 1978) substitution matrices which have been named with numbers exist (PAM30, PAM70, PAM250, BLOSUM40, BLOSUM62, BLOSUM80 etc). Those named with higher numbers are designed for comparing closely related sequences, while those named with lower numbers are designed for comparing distantly related sequences. These matrices contain the substitution values for all pairs of 20 amino acids.

3. Prediction of protein 3D structure

Protein structure prediction is another important research area of bioinformatics. Protein sequence uniquely determines a structure in its native environment. This structural information is vital in understanding the function of a protein. The structural information of protein is classified into primary, secondary, tertiary and quaternary. The primary structure of a protein refers to the amino acid sequence of the polypeptide chain, which is formed during the process of protein biosynthesis and it is held together by covalent or peptide bonds. The secondary structure refers to highly regular local sub-structures defined by the patterns of hydrogen bonds between the peptide chains. The alpha helix and the beta strand are considered as the major secondary structures, which represent a way of saturating all the hydrogen bond donors and acceptors in the peptide backbone. Tertiary structure is the particular arrangement of secondary structure elements in three dimensional spaces. Domain is the unit of tertiary structure, which is composed of small number of secondary structure elements. Quaternary structure is a larger assembly of several protein molecules or polypeptide chains, usually known as subunit. The quaternary structure is stabilized by non-covalent interactions and disulfide bonds. Limited resources of structural information due to wet laboratory shortcomings lead to *in-silico* structural prediction using only sequence information. Currently a viable general solution for accurate prediction of 3D structure of protein remains an open problem. As of now, existing approaches are not up to the satisfactory level. But these can be used modeling 3D structure at *in-silico* level before taking work *in-vitro* and *in-vivo*, which saves a lot of time and expenses.

Determination of 3D structure of a protein is an important tool to understand their functions. Physicochemical approaches such as X-ray crystallography or NMR spectroscopy are used to determine 3D structures. However, these techniques have some limitations such as long processing time and high cost involvement. Therefore, computational methods have been developed to calculate 3D models from sequences. Prediction of 3D protein structures from amino acid sequences represents one of the most important problems in computational structural biology. Several efforts have been made since a decade in 3D structural prediction of protein from sequences. These approaches can be classified broadly into 3 categories based on the:

1. Laws of physics and dynamics
2. Knowledge of existing 3D structure of proteins and
3. Combination of merits of the previous two approaches

In the first approach, the state of minimal free energy is calculated based on the interaction between the molecules, within the molecules and solvents.

This energy influences the folding and conformational changes (Scheraga, 1996). Based on this approach, many versions of methods have been proposed such as AMBER (Case *et al.*, 2005), CHARMM (Brooks *et al.*, 2009) and GROMOS (Christem *et. al.* 2005). Simulation of folding of an immunoglobulin light chain-binding domain of protein has demonstrated using the REFINER method (Boniecki *et al.*, 2003). Usually 3D Cartesian coordinates are used to represent the protein 3D structure. This is unrealistic on some stages while modeling protein 3D structure. Hence torsion angles are used instead of Cartesian coordinates as degrees of freedom for protestation about single bond (Stein *et al.*, 1997; Parsons, 2005). Coarse-grained approach has also been introduced to reduce the number of degrees of freedom in which a smaller number of elements and interactions are considered (Lee, 1999).

The second approach is based on the existing 3D structure knowledge and sequences. Protein sequences are evolutionally related and thus structurally relevant to each other. Proteins usually retain the same 3D structure regardless of the several mutations and structure divergent is slower than sequence divergent. Based on this concept, the methods have been developed to align protein sequence of an unknown structure to known structure or template. Various versions of stand-alone and web based tool are available for modeling of protein 3D structure such as *ProRegIn* (Protein Regularity Index), FAMSBASE (Fully Automatic Modeling System dataBASE), SWISS-MODEL, MODELLER, CPHmodels (Protein Homology Models) (Nielsen *et al., 2010*), FAMS and ModWeb. The use of computational procedures for the prediction of the 3D structures was initiated by Huang *et al.* (1994) by introducing PrPC. The PrPC (Prion Protein) involved four major steps: 1) alignment of homologous sequences, 2) prediction of secondary structures, 3) packing of secondary elements to generate all plausible tertiary structures, and 4) selection and refinement of final structural models.

Thukral *et al.* (2006) developed a web-enabled tool *ProRegIn* based on the regularity in the Φ, Ψ dihedral angles of the amino acids that constitute loop regions by dividing the problem into three stages *viz.* secondary structure prediction, generation of plausible main chain loop dihedrals and side chain dihedral optimization. The SWISS-MODEL is a repository (http://swissmodel http://expasy.org/repository/) of 3D protein structure models generated by automated homology-modeling. This allows the users to assess the quality of the models to search for alternative templates and to build models.

"FAMSBASE", a fully automatic modeling system with relational database of comparative protein structure models for the whole genome of 41 species was presented in the GTOP database (Yamaguchi *et al.*, 2003). Jayaram *et al.* (2006) has described "Bhageerath" an energy based computer software suite for narrowing down the search space of tertiary structures of small globular proteins from primary and secondary structures. This is an automated encompasses with eight different computational modules.

The FAMSD (Fully Automatc Modelling System 3D structure prediction) (Kanou *et al.*, 2009) is based on a comparative modeling method which consists of the four steps similar to the method proposed by Huang *et al.* (1994): 1) generating and selecting sequence alignments between target and template proteins, 2) constructing 3D structure models based on each selected alignment, 3) selecting the best 3D structure model and 4) refining the selected model. PROTINFO (PROT INFOrmation) server was developed by Hung *et al.* (2005) using comparative modeling, fold generation and de novo methods for selection of final five conformers. Users can submit sequence and request for 3D structure.

Template-based modeling, the IntFOLD-TS/nFold (McGuffin and Roche, 2011) method was developed on the model quality assessment (QA), which generates numerous alternate models then ranked them in terms of global quality. CPHmodels-3.0 is a web server for predicting protein 3D structure by using single template homology modeling, employing a hybrid of the scoring functions with profile-profile scoring technique and a novel remote homology-modeling algorithm.

The third approach is a combination of the merits of the two approaches such as based on energy and existing knowledge. The SCRATCH (Cheng *et al.,* 2005) utilizes recursive neural networks, evolutionary information, fragment libraries and energy. The ASTRO-FOLD (Klepeis and Floudas, 2003) predicts tertiary structure based on overall deterministic framework coupled with mixed integer optimization.

The Center for Bioinformatics, University of Kansas USA has released many variants of 'iterative threading assembly refinement (I-TASSER)' (Yang, 2008). In which, C-scoring function is calculated based on the relative clustering structural density and the significance score of multiple threading templates. A strong correlation between C-score and structural similarity has been demonstrated.

4. Quaternary structure and protein-protein interaction

Quaternary structure is an assembly of multiple sub units/domains of proteins, which also referred to as multi-protein complexes since proteins are capable to form very firm complexes with other proteins, which indicates that proteins are evolved to bind on another protein. A new bioinformatics research area to address this complex problem of protein-protein interactions came into being in molecular biology. The protein-protein interaction initiates various molecular mechanisms to perform biological functions. Many methods and databases are available in this area at different levels of operation such as protein-protein, domain-domain, domain-motif and protein-RNA interactions. Protein complexes can be determined by X-ray crystallography or nuclear magnetic resonance. However, these techniques are expensive and time consuming. Moreover, recurrently experimental methods have reported false binding site due to experimental limitations. Therefore, *in-silico* prediction of protein-protein interaction can be used to save time and cost. These methods are useful in guiding biological experiments in order to confirm complexes and to predict functional pathway and biological networks. In other word, it helps to understand biological process at the cellular level. Mapping protein-protein interaction network may give new insights to understand biological process and problems.

Many such *in silico* methods proposed for protein-protein interaction studies are not up to the satisfaction of molecular biologists however some approaches have shown promise because of considerable prediction accuracy to understand cellular pathways. A fair number of protein-interaction databases are freely available to retrieve interaction information with graphical presentation. These databases can favor to determine and guide to elicit new molecular interactions and functional networks. A brief description of these methods and databases are given below:

1. Amos-Binks *et al.* (2011) have presented protein-protein interaction prediction engine (PIPE) based on machine learning techniques. In this method, known interaction has been used as training data to train engine and then applied method on test data sets. A novel method has been proposed by Hayashida *et al.* (2011) in which conditional random fields and mutual information between residues were used to model protein-protein interactions and domain-domain interactions. Li *et al.* (2011) developed a deeply buried atomic contacts (DBAC) method to predict binding hot spots using SVM (Support Vector Machine) machine learning technique and 3D structural information. In this method, different burial level numbers are used as input to the SVM to classify hot spot or non hot spot residues.

2. A phylogenetic framework, BindML, has been developed by La and Kihara, (2012) to capture critical sequence variations, which is essential for selection of residues for protein–protein binding. In this method, PDB structure of a target protein, a MSA (Multiple Sequence Alignment) of its family and target sequence are employed.

3. The DEPTH (Tan *et al.,* 2011) is a web server that computes depth and solvent-accessible surface area (SASA) values and predicts small-molecule binding cavities in proteins. It correlates with properties such as protein

stability, hydrogen exchange rate, protein–protein interaction hot spots, post-translational modification sites and sequence variability.

A domain-based approach has been proposed by Singhal and Resat (2007) based on multi-parameter optimization method using available PPI (protein-protein interaction) information derived from a quantitative scoring scheme for the domain-domain pairs. DOMINO (Ceol *et al.*, 2007) a relational database on domain–peptide interactions has been developed based on interaction of small protein modules. Intact (Hermjakob *et al.*, 2004) is a domain interaction MAP database of predicted and known interactions between protein domains. It integrates 5807 structurally known interactions and allows calculating domain interaction networks either for a domain of interest or for entire organisms.

4. The recent version of the IntAct 2012 (Kerrien *et al.* 2012), a web based molecular interaction database is curated from the literatures or from direct data depositions. It contains 2,75,000 binary interaction and has fast search facility and graphical presentation. Biological general repository for interaction datasets (BioGRID) database (Stark, 2011) contains 3,47,966 interactions. This is created from data sets and literatures. The web based accessible and downloadable microbial protein interaction database (MPIDB) holds 22,530 interactions among proteins of 191 bacterial species/strains (Goll *et al.*, 2008).

5. Kortemme *et al.* (2002) has developed a fast computational approach for the prediction of energetically important amino acid residues using Peter Kollman's "computational alanine scanning". It consists of a three-dimensional structure of a protein-protein complex, list of hot spots and amino acid side chains.

6. FoldX (Guerois *et al.*, 2002) has been developed to provide quantitative estimation of the importance of the interactions contributing to the stability of proteins and protein complexes based on various energy terms and machine learning technique. Similarly, EGAD, 'a genetic algorithm for protein design' (Pokala and Handel, 2005) is an energy function for protein design that can be used to study stability of proteins and protein complexes.

Conclusions

Bioinformatics tools can be used at *in-silico* experiment stage before *in-vivo* and *in-vitro* test experiments. These tools can save time and cost and guide to understand biological functions at cell level preceding the experiments at wet-lab. An enough number of bioinformatics tools have been developed based on different methods and databases are freely available. All the approaches have not been discussed in this chapter, because all tools are not effective for varying analytical applications. A particular tool may work better and give desired results than others in a specific situation but may not be suitable for another situation. This chapter would help the researchers for understanding the methodologies and applications of various bioinformatics tools for analyzing protein structure and functions. Nevertheless, development of bioinformatics techniques and tools is still an open research problem in computational biology and many more exciting developments in the field are yet to be experienced.

References

Altschul S.F., Gish W., Miller W., Myers E.W., Lipman D.J. (1990). Basic local alignment search tool. *Journal Molecular Biology* **215:** 403-410.

Altschul S.F., Madden T.L., Schäffer A.A., Zhang J., Zhang Z., Miller W., Lipman D.J. (1997). Gapped BLAST and PSI-BLAST: a new generation of protein database search programs. *Nucleic Acids Research* **25:** 3389-3402.

Amos-Binks A., Patuleav C., Pitre S., Schoenrock A., Gui Y., Green J.R., Golshani A., Dehne F. (2011). Binding site prediction for protein-protein interactions and novel motif discovery using re-occurring polypeptide sequences. *BMC Bioinformatics* **12:** 225 doi: 10.1186/1471-2105-12-225.

Angadi U.B., Venkatesulu M. (2011) Structural SCOP superfamily level classification Using Unsupervised Machine Learning. *IEEE Transaction on Computational Biology and Bioinformatics*. DOI:10.1109/TCBB.2011.114.

Angadi U.B., Venkatesulu M. (2010). FuzzyART for protein classification. *Journal of Bioinformatics and Computational Biology* **8:** 825-841.

Angadi U.B., Venkatesulu M., Patil S.S., Abraham Prabu P. (2008). Segment based clustering technique for classification of large set of DNA/protein sequence data. In: *Proc. National Conference on Advances in Applied Technology*, Kalasalingam University, Tamil Nadu, India, Feb 2008, pp 4-9.

Angadi U.B.,Venkatesulu M. (2010). GENETAL: A new technique for feature extraction from large set of biological sequences and its use in classification, *Journal of Computer Intelligence and Bioinformatics*. **3:** 49-61.

Bailey T.L., Elkan C. (1994). Fitting a mixture model by expectation maximization to discover motifs in biopolymers. In: *Second International Conference on Intelligent Systems for Molecular Biology*, Stanford University, Stanford, California, USA, Aug. 14-17, 1994, pp28-36.

Bairoch A., Bucher P., Hofmann K. (1997). The PROSITE database, its status in 1997. *Nucleic Acids Research* **25:** 217-221.

Boniecki M., Rotkiewicz P., Skolnick J., Kolinski A. (2003). Protein fragment reconstruction using various modeling techniques. *Journal of Computer-Aided Molecular Design* **17:** 725-738.

Brazma A., Jonassen I., Ukkonen E., Vilo J. (1996). Discovering patterns and subfamilies in biosequences. *International Conference on Intelligence System for Molecular Biology.* St. Louis, MO, USA, June 12-15 1996, pp 34-43.

Brooks B.R., Brooks C.L., Mackerell A.D. Jr., Nilsson L., Petrella R.J., Roux B., Won Y., Archontis G., Bartels C., Boresch S., Caflisch A., Caves L., Cui Q., Dinner A.R., Feig M., Fischer S., Gao J., Hodoscek M., Im W., Kuczera K., Lazaridis T., Ma J., Ovchinnikov V., Paci E., Pastor R.W., Post C.B., Pu J.Z., Schaefer M., Tidor B., Venable R.M., Woodcock H.L., Wu X., Yang W., York D.M., Karplus M. (2009). CHARMM: the biomolecular simulation program. *Journal Computational Chemistry* **30:** 1545-1614.

Buhler J.,Tompa M. (2002). Finding motifs using random projections, *Journal Computational Biology* **9:** 225-242.

Case D.A., Cheatham T.E., Darden T. Gohlke H., Luo R., Merz K.m., Onufriv A., Simmerlinng C., Wang B., Woods R.J. (2005). The Amber biomolecular simulation programs. *Journal Computational Chemistry* **26:** 1668-1688.

Ceol A, Chatr-aryamontri A., Santonico E., Sacco R., Castagnoli L., Cesareni G. (2007). DOMINO: a database of domain–peptide interactions. *Nucleic Acids Research* **35:** D557-D560.

Cheng, J., Randall,A.Z., Sweredoski,M.J. and Baldi,P. (2005). SCRATCH: a protein structure and structural feature prediction server. *Nucleic Acids Research* **33:** W 72-76.

Cho K, Kim D., Lee D. (2009). A feature-based approach to modeling protein-protein interaction hot spots. *Nucleic Acids Research* **37:** 2672-2687.

Christen M., Hunenberger P.H., Bakowies D., Baron R., Bürgi R., Geerke D.P., Heinz T.N., Kastenholz M.A., Kräutler V., Oostenbrink C., Peter C., Trzesniak D., van Gunsteren W.F. (2005). The GROMOS software for biomolecular simulation:GROMOS05. *Journal Computational Chemistry* **26:** 1719-1751.

Dayhoff M.O., Schwartz R. M., Orcutt B.C. (1978). A model of evolutionary change in proteins, Atlas of Protein Sequence and Structure, National. *Biomedical Research Foundation* **5:** 345-351.

Goll J, Rajagopala S.V., Shiau S.C., Wu H, Lamb B.T., Uetz P. (2008). MPIDB: the microbial protein interaction database. *Bioinformatics* **24:** 1743-1744.

Guerois R., Nielsen J.E., Serrano L. (2002). Predicting changes in the stability of proteins and protein complexes: a study of more than 1000 mutations. *Journal Molecular Biology* **320:** 369-387.

Hayashida H., Mayumi K., Jiangning S., Tatsuya A. (2011). Conditional random field approach to prediction of protein-protein interactions using domain information. *BMC Systems Biology* **5:** S8.

Henikoff S., Henikoff J. G., Alford W. J., Pietrokovski S. (1995). Automated construction and graphical presentation of protein blocks from unaligned sequences. *Gene-COMBIS* **163:** 17-26.

Henikoff S., Henikoff J.G. (1992). Amino acid substitution matrices from protein blocks. *Proceedings of National Academy of Sciences*, USA **89:** 10915-10919.

Hermjakob,H., Montecchi-Palazzi,L., Lewington,C., Mudali,S.,Kerrien,S., Orchard,S., Vingron,M., Roechert,B., Roepstorff,P., Valencia,A. Margalit H., Armstrong J., Bairoch A., Cesareni G., Sherman D., Apweiler R (2004). IntAct: an open source molecular interaction database. *Nucleic Acids Research* **32:** D452-D455.

Hertz G.Z., Stormo G.D. (1999). Identifying DNA and protein patterns with statistically significant alignments of multiple sequences. *Bioinformatics* **15:** 563-577.

Holm L., Sander C. (1997). Dali/FSSP classification of three-dimensional protein folds. *Nucleic Acid Research* **25:** 231-234.

Huang Z., Gabriel J.M., Baldwin M.A., Fletterick R.J., Prusiner S.B., Cohen F.E. (1994).Proposed three-dimensional structure for the cellular prion protein. *Proceedings National Academy of Sciences*, USA **91:** 7139-7143.

Hung L.H., Ngan S.C., Liu T., Samudrala R. (2005). PROTINFO: new algorithms for enhanced protein structure predictions. *Nucleic Acids Research*, **33:** W77-W80.

Jain P., Garibaldi J.M., Hirst J. D. (2009). Supervised machine learning algorithms for protein structure classification. *Computational Biology and Chemistry* **33:** 216-223.

Jayaram B., Bhushan K., Shenoy S.R., Narang P., Bose S., Agrawal P., Sahu D., Pandey V. (2006) Bhageerath: an energy based web enabled computer software suite for limiting the search space of tertiary structures of small globular proteins. *Nucleic Acids Research* **34:** 6195-6204.

Jonassen I., Collins J.F., Higgins D.G. (1995). Finding flexible patterns in unaligned protein sequences. *Protein Science* **4:** 1587-1595.

Kanou, K., Iwadate M. M., Hirata T., Terashi G., Umeyama H., Mayuko T. (2009). FAMSD: a powerful protein modeling platform that combines alignment methods, homology modeling, 3D structure quality estimation and molecular dynamics. *Chemical and Pharmaceutical Bulletin* **57:** 1335-1342.

Kerrien S., Aranda B., Breuza L., Bridge A., Broackes-Carter F., Chen C., Duesbury M., Dumousseau M., Feuermann M., Hinz U., Jandrasits C., Jimenez R. C., Khadake J., Mahadevan U., Masson P., Pedruzzi I., Pfeiffenberger E., Porras P., Raghunath A., Roechert B., Orchard S., Hermjakob H (2012). The 'Intact' molecular interaction database in 2012. *Nucleic Acids Research* **40:** D841-846.

Klepeis,J.L., Floudas C.A. (2003). ASTRO-FOLD: A combinatorial and global optimization framework for ab initio prediction of three-dimensional structures of proteins from the amino acid sequence. *Biophysics Journal* **85:** 2119-2146.

Kortemme T., Baker D. (2002). A simple physical model for binding energy hot spots in protein-protein complexes. *Proceedings National Academy of Sciences*, USA **99:** 14116-14121.

La D., Kihara D. (2012). A novel method for protein–protein interaction site prediction using phylogenetic substitution models. *Proteins* **80:** 126-141.

Lawrence C.E., Altschul S.F., Boguski M.S., Liu J.S., Neuwald A.F., Wootton J.C. (1993). Detecting subtle sequence signals: a Gibbs sampling strategy for multiple alignment. *Science* **262:** 208-214.

Lee J., Liwo A., Scheraga H.A., (1999). Energy-based de novo protein folding by conformational space annealing and an off-lattice united-residue force field: application to the 10-55 fragments of staphylococcal protein A and to apo-calbindin D9K. *Proceedings National Academy Sciences,* USA **96:** 2025-2030.

Li Z., Wong L., Li J. (2011). DBAC: A simple prediction method for protein binding hot spots based on burial levels and deeply buried atomic contacts. *BMC Systems Biology* **5:** S5.

Lipman D.J., Pearson W.R. (1985). Rapid and sensitive protein similarity searches. *Science* **227:** 1435-1441.

Liu J., Rost B. (2003). Domains, motifs and clusters in the protein universe. *Current Opinion in Chemical Biology* **7:** 5-11.

Luo Q., Pagel P., Vilne B., Frishman D. (2011). DIMA 3.0: Domain interaction map. *Nucleic Acids Research* **39:** 724-729.

McGuffin L.J., Roche D.B. (2011). Automated tertiary structure prediction with accurate local model quality assessment using the IntFOLD-TS method. *Proteins* **79:** 137-146.

Murzin A.G., Brenner S.E., Hubbard T., Chothia C. (1995). SCOP: a structural classification of proteins database for the investigation of sequences and structures. *Journal Molecular Biology* **247:** 536-540.

Needleman S.B., Wunsch C.D. (1970). A general method applicable to the search for similarities in the amino acid sequence of two proteins. *Journal Molecular Biology* **48:** 443-53.

Nielsen M., Lundegaard C., Lund O., Petersen T.N. (2010). CPHmodels-3.0 remote homology modeling using structure-guided sequence profiles. *Nucleic Acids Research* **38:** W576-W581.

Orengo C.A., Michie A.D., Jones S., Jones D.T., Swindells M.B., Thornton J.M. (1997). CATH - A hierarchic classification of protein domain structures. *Structure* **5:** 1093-1108.

Parsons J., Holmes J.B., Rojas J. M., Tsai J., Strauss C. E. (2005), Practical conversion from torsion space to Cartesian space for *in silico* protein synthesis. *Journal Computational Chemistry* **26:** 1063-1068.

Pesole G., Attimonelli M., Preparata G., Saccone C. (1992). A statistical method for detecting regions with different evolutionary dynamics in multi-aligned sequences. *Molecular Phylogenetics and Evolution* **1:** 91-96.

Pokala N., Handel T.M. (2005). Energy functions for protein design: adjustment with protein-protein complex affinities, models for the unfolded state, and negative design of solubility and specificity. *Journal of Molecular Biology* **18:** 203-227.

Price A., Ramabhadran S., Pevzner P.A. (2003). Finding subtle motifs by branching from sample strings. *Bioinformatics* **2***(Suppl.)*: ii149-ii155.

Rigoutsos I., Floratos A., Parida L., Gao Y., Platt D. (2000). The emergence of pattern discovery techniques in computational biology. *Metabolic Engineering* **2:** 159-177.

Sagot M.F., Viari A., Soldano H. (1995). A distance-based block searching algorithm. *In: Proc. International Conference on Intelligent System Molecular Biology.* Atelier de BioInformatique, Cambridge, United Kingdom, July 16-19, 1995, 322-331.

Scheraga H.A. (1996). Recent developments in the theory of protein folding: searching for the global energy minimum. *Biophysical Chemistry* **59:** 329-339.

Sellers P. H. (1974). On the theory and computation of evolutionary distances. *SIAM Journal on Applied Mathematics* **26:** 787-793.

Singhal M., Resat H. (2007). A domain-based approach to predict protein-protein interactions. *BMC Bioinformatics* **13:** 199.

Smith R.F., Smith T.F. (1990), Automatic generation of primary sequence patterns from sets of related protein sequences. *Proceedings National Academy of Sciences,* USA **87:** 118-122.

Smith T.F.,Waterman M.S. (1981). Identification of common molecular subsequences. *Journal Molecular Biology* **147:** 195-197.

Stark,C., Breitkreutz,B.J Chatr-Aryamontri A., Boucher L., Oughtred R., Livstone M.S., Nixon J., Van Auken K., Wang X., Shi X., Reguly T., Rust J.M., Winter A., Dolinski K., Tyers M. (2011) The BioGRID Interaction Database: 2011 update. *Nucleic Acids Research* **39:** D698–D704.

Stein E.G., Rice L.M., Brunger A.T. (1997). Torsion-angle molecular dynamics as a new efficient tool for NMR structure calculation. *Journal Magnetic Resonance* **124:** 154-164.

Tan K.P., Varadarajan R., Madhusudhan M.S. (2011). DEPTH: a web server to compute depth and predict small-molecule binding cavities in proteins. *Nucleic Acids Research* **39:** W242-W248.

Thukral L., Shenoy S.R., Bhushan K., Jayaram B. (2006). *ProRegIn*: A regularity index for the selection of native-like tertiary structures of proteins. *Journal of Biosciences* **32:** 71-81.

Wang J.T., Marr T.G., Shasha D., Shapiro B.A., Chirn G.W. (1994). Discovering active motifs in sets of related protein sequences and using them for classification. *Nucleic Acids Research* **22:** 2769-2775.

Waterman M.S., Smith T.F., Beyer W.A. (1976). Some biological sequence metrics. *Advances in Mathematics* **20:** 367-387.

Yamaguchi A., Mitsuo Suzuki I., Yura K., Kawakita S., Umeyama H., Go M. (2003). Enlarged FAMSBASE: protein 3D structure models of genome sequences for 41 species. *Nucleic Acids Research* **31:** 463-468.

Yang Z. (2008). I-TASSER server for protein 3D structure prediction. *BMC Bioinformatics* **9:** 40 doi:10.1186/1471-2105-9-40.

❑❑❑

Chapter 24

Nanobiotechnology in Animal Nutrition

A. Thulasi, D. Rajendran, S. Jash, S. Selvaraju, V. Lyju Jose, S. Velusamy, S.Mathivanan
National Institute of Animal Nutrition and Physiology, Adugodi, Bangalore-560 030, Karnataka, India

Summary

Nano biotechnology is an emerging bioscience tools which are used in agriculture, human health and nutrition. The potential application areas in animal science are growing at slow pace in physiology, nutritional and biotechnology research. This chapter deals with the description of various organic and inorganic nanomaterials, its digestion, absorption and metabolisms. Among the wide ranging applications, the use of nanotechnology in food/feed industry, poultry production including pathogen detection and removal are discussed along with the use of inclusion bodies as biological nanomaterials and the effect of nano selenium on rumen fermentation. More research attention is needed in this field to cater the benefit of these technologies in animal especially in nutritional science.

"Nanotechnology" is the creation of functional materials, devices, and systems through the manipulation of matter at a length scale of ~1–100 nm. At such a nanoscale, novel properties and functions occur because of size, the advantage of which is capitalized for application in pharmaceuticals and food/feed technologies. This emerging field is becoming important in the medical sciences (*e.g.*, nanomedicine), because it offers the possibility of examining biological processes in ways that were not possible previously. Nanotechnology offers a range of tools capable of monitoring individual cells at the level of individual molecules. It enables to monitor cellular and molecular function and to alter systems that are deregulated in disease. Nano biotechnology provides the tools to the researcher for changing the future of the feed technology as well. It is possible to produce feed; improve feed packaging, and develop special biosensors applying the tools of nanotechnology. The nano biosensors can monitor the feed safety and health of the crops, forest areas, fish ponds, and livestock (Mongillo, 2007). Smart nano sensors and delivery systems for feed are useful to the agricultural industry to combat viruses and other crop pathogens. In agriculture, nano catalysts are envisaged to be available which will increase the efficiency of pesticides and herbicides, allowing lower doses to be used. Nanotechnology may also be used to protect the environment through the use of alternative (renewable) energy supplies, and filters or catalysts to reduce pollution and clean-up existing pollutants (Food Safety Authority of Ireland, 2008) which has indirect bearings for the supply of human food or animal feeds. With vast potential areas of applications nano technology is still in its infancy for animal feed and nutritional studies. This chapter enumerates the possible areas in animal nutrition where advantages of these technologies can be utilized to help the researcher and policy makers.

1. Classification of nano materials

Nanoparticles can be classified into two broad categories, *viz.*, inorganic and organic (Fig. 1), based on their on the chemical characteristics, ability to carry different ingredients and react to different environmental conditions.

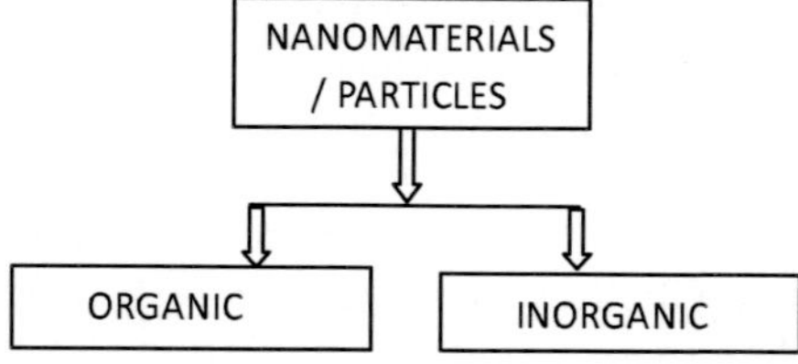

Fig. 1 : Classes of nanomaterials/particles based on the chemical properties

1.1. Organic nanomaterials

Organic nanomaterials include proteins, fat and sugar molecules. Nutraceuticals consisting of feed additives derived from plants are also organic nanomaterials used in feed. The nanoparticles incorporated into feeds include those engineered to provide encapsulation systems *e.g.*, micelles, liposomes, for delivery of feed ingredients and those tailored for use in feed packaging such as biosensors, identification markers, shelf-life extenders and antimicrobials. Organic nanoparticles are sometimes referred to as nanocapsules (when used as vehicles for delivery of essential nutrients or pharmaceuticals), are likely to be used to enhance the nutrient value of feed through improvement or alteration of feed functionality. These nanoparticles have been designed to deliver vitamins or other nutrients in feed without affecting the taste or appearance. Such nanoparticles encapsulate the nutrients and carry them via the gastrointestinal tract (GIT) into the bloodstream to increase their bioavailability.

1.2 Inorganic nanomaterials

Inorganic nanomaterials for applications in feed and feed additives include nano clay platelets for feed packaging; minerals such as silicon dioxide, calcium and magnesium; and silver nanoparticles for water purification or antimicrobial packaging or feed storage. Titanium dioxide, a feed colorant used as a UV protection barrier in feed packaging industry is an approved inorganic nanoparticles because it becomes transparent and also loses its ability to act as a feed colorant in its nano form The nanoparticles of silver are used as an antimicrobial agent. Nanosilver is used in fridge panels, storage boxes, packaging lines and other surfaces which come into contact with feed during manufacture. Feed storage bins are being produced with silver nanoparticles embedded in the plastic which kills bacteria from any feed that are stored in the bins and minimize the health risks.

2. Nanotechnology in nutritional sciences

In nutrition research, nanotechnology applications may assist with obtaining accurate spatial information about the location of a nutrient or bioactive food component in a tissue, cell, or cellular compartments. Ultrasensitive detection of nutrients and metabolite increases the understanding nutrient and biomolecular interactions in specific tissues. Such wonderful technologies have the potential to improve nutritional assessment and measures of bioavailability. They may help to identify and characterize molecular targets of nutrient activity and biomarkers of effect, exposure, and susceptibility. Gastrointestinal (GI) tract has always been chosen the preferred route of delivery for pharmacological or feed/food principles including nano particles. Therefore, one needs to understand the fate of nanoparticles when it is delivered through GI tract.

2.1 Digestion and absorption of nano particles

Nanoparticles can rout to the gastrointestinal tract (GIT) in many ways such as ingestion directly from food and water and from administration of therapeutic nano-drugs (*ingestion or swallow pathway*). Inhaled nanoparticles can also be swallowed and enter the GIT following clearance from the respiratory tract (*inhalation pathway*; Hoet *at al.*, 2004). Finally, oral or smart delivery into GIT (*oral pathway*); particle uptake in the GIT depends on diffusion and accessibility through mucus and contact with the cells of the GIT. Smaller the particle diameter faster is the diffusion through GIT mucus to reach the cells of intestinal lining, followed by uptake through GIT barrier to reach the blood (Hoet *et al.,* 2004). Very little information is available on the uptake of nanoparticles from the intestinal tract. Uptake occurs variously by passive diffusion across the mucosal cells, via active transport mechanisms (O'Hagan, 1996). Nanoparticles that are swallowed will sooner or later end up in the intestinal tract. It is not known clearly whether nano particle remain in the intestinal tract unabsorbed and excreted through feces as 'unwanted substance' or move into the body system readily. Existing evidences indicate that the particles smaller than 100 nm are absorbed in various tissues and organs. As a general rule, smaller the particles are, the more they are absorbed and deeper they can go into the body system. Insoluble nanoparticles (primarily inorganic, including man-made polymeric materials *e.g.,* polystyrene and carbon-based nanoparticles *e.g.,* fullerenes) might have a more restricted distribution. Following uptake from the GIT, nanoparticles can translocate via the lymph system to the liver and spleen, as demonstrated for polystyrene nanoparticles of 100nm or less (Jani *et al.,* 1990). Smaller particles that are capable of being taken up by the villus epithelium may directly enter the bloodstream, and are then predominantly scavenged by the liver and the spleen.

The intestinal uptake of inorganic, insoluble nanoparticles such as titanium dioxide and gold particles will be readily taken up across the intestinal barrier and hence are bioavailable than their micro or macro equivalents. Uptake is largely determined by particle solubility, charge and size. A number of experimental studies have demonstrated uptake of nanoparticles across the GIT following oral administration. Uptake of inert particles has been shown to occur trans-cellularly through the intestinal lining and to a lesser extent between epithelial cells (Jani *et al.,* 1990).

Organic nanoparticles such as casein micelles are likely to behave similarly to their micro or macro equivalents and can be predicted to be readily absorbed and highly bio-available. It is not understood whether higher molecular weight organic nanoparticles such as proteins, fats or carbohydrates are broken down to lower molecular weight entities in the GIT in the same way as the native molecules are, or taken up intact. However recent evidence showed that insulin encapsulated in vitamin B12-dextran nanoparticles are taken up from the GIT without degradation (Florence and Hussain, 2001).

2.2 Distribution, metabolism and excretion of nanoparticles

Few studies report the uptake and disposition of nanomaterials by the GIT, and most have shown that, dependent on size, nanoparticles either pass through the GIT without uptake into the body and are eliminated rapidly (Oberdörster *et al.,* 2005), or they cross the lining of the GIT and enter the blood stream, from where they relocate to other organs. Following uptake by the GIT, gold nanoparticles of less than 50 nm are shown to be trans-located to the blood stream and distributed all over the body (Hoet *et al.,* 2004). A recent study demonstrated that tissue distribution of gold nanoparticles after intravenous (IV) administration was size dependent with the smallest (10nm) particles showing widespread organ distribution (De Jong *et al.,* 2008). The absorption, distribution, breakdown and excretion of nanoparticles in the body will be dependent on physicochemical characteristics such as solubility, charge and size. Distribution/translocation of nanoparticles to body organs is expected to mirror that of their micro or macro equivalents, with small water-soluble or fat soluble organic nanomaterials such as lipid nanoparticles being widely distributed throughout the body. It can be anticipated that distribution and breakdown of such nanoparticles into constituent molecules occurs rapidly and efficiently, with subsequent clearance from the body.

3. Applications of nano technology in the feed industry

The application of nanotechnology for the feed industry include: 1) minor modifications of natural ingredients to enhance taste, palatability and sensory improvement such as flavor, color and texture; 2) enhancing nutrition quality of foods by stabilizing active ingredients such as nutraceuticals in feed matrices, packaging and product innovation to extend shelf-life, 3) increasing bioavailability of essential nutrients (Food Safety Authority of Ireland, 2008) by increasing absorption and targeted delivery of bioactive compound. The other applications envisaged are 4) developing biosensors for pathogen detection and diagnosis to improve feed safety; antimicrobials to kill pathogenic bacteria in feed. Nano-delivery of bioactive/nutrient ingredients in feedstuffs or *in vivo* in the animal is enabled through improved knowledge of feed materials at the nanoscale. The different nanomaterials that have the potential to be used for this purpose are nanocomposites, nanoclays and nanotubes. The nano products that would find applications are nanosensors, nanoimaging and nanochips and nanofilters. Similarly, the potential nano delivery systems are nanocapsules, nanocochleates, nanoballs, nanodevices, nanomachines and nanorobots.

4. Nano technology in poultry production

The future challenges of the poultry science research includes: increasing the feed efficiency; preparing the dynamic feed; controlling the macro and micronutrient absorption; tackling diseases outbreaks; targeted drug delivery; modifying the contents of the egg like full protein egg and cholesterol free egg; reducing the energy and protein wastage in unproductive physiological purposes there by increasing the feed efficiency; and reducing the price of the poultry meat. These all can be achieved through the application of nanobiotechnology and nano immunology to poultry research (Kannaki and Verma, 2006; Tzeng, 2008). Moreover, it will take more research and testing before the nanoparticle is ready to be used, in the distant future.

5. Biofunctionalized nanoparticles (BN) to remove enteric pathogens of poultry

Research is underway to develop a nanomaterial that can be given to chicken to remove *Campylobacter*. This bacterium does not harm the birds but when ingested by humans, they can cause cramps and blood diarrhoea. The idea is to add nanoparticles in chicken feed. When the feed is ingested the nanoparticles attach to *Campylobacter*, ensuring that it is excreted by chickens. Hence, the bird would be safe for human consumption. Nanoparticles would be specifically designed to attach on to molecules that exist on the surface of *Campylobacter* and removed from chicken before they reach humans (Kannaki and Verma, 2006).

It has been shown that presence of D-mannose inhibits the adherence of bacteria to both animal and human intestinal cells (Madigan *et al.*, 2000). *Campylobacter jejuni* attaches to the epithelial cells. This attachment of the bacterial cells is mediated by mannose-specific, lectin-like adhesions present on the bacterial surface which bind to mannose receptor sites (Madigan *et al.*, 2000. Biofunctionalized nanoparticles (BN) have been developed as an alternative to a natural material such as mannose (Taylor *et al.*, 2004; Luo *et al.*, 2005; Qu *et al.*, 2005). The BN have attracted interest as a treatment for enteric infection, serving as pathogen purging agents prior to transport and processing. The objective of BN development is to create an affinity for the bacterial adhesions. The BN are adhesion-specific to the enteropathogen *C. jejuni*. Preliminary research has shown that the BN have an affinity for the mannose receptor sites on the *Campylobacter* cell surface and that cell aggregation or attachment between the bacteria and BN may occur (Madigan *et al.*, 2000). The ability of these BN to adhere to *Campylobacter* cell surfaces will enable BN to compete with host cell receptors to reduce or eliminate the extent of bacterial colonization on the poultry intestinal wall. The BN synthesis is based on the self-assembly of organic polymers structured with intra-polymer binary pseudo-phase separation characteristics. These nano-particle structures consists of a hydrophobic polystyrene core, a hydrophilic tether such as polyethylene glycol, and sugars or peptides that are functionally identical to the host cell receptor groups that are bound by the pathogen's surface adhesions. By presenting the same functional groups from the surface of the nanoparticles, the BN should effectively compete with the mucosal lining of the gastrointestinal tract for microbial attachment. In addition, since the BN contain a relatively large surface density of functional sites, they should be able to agglutinate large numbers of pathogens, preventing them binding to their host enabling them to be expelled from the gastrointestinal system.

6. Vitamin and enzyme nano bioengineering

Nanotechnology has found application in the agri-food/feed sector also. Many vitamins and their precursors, such as carotenoids, are insoluble in water. But, when formulated as nanoparticles, these substances can easily be mixed with cold water which increases their bioavailability. Vitamin B_{12} absorption from the gut under physiological conditions occurs via receptor-mediated endocytosis. The ability to increase oral bioavailability of various peptides (*e.g.*, granulocyte colony stimulating factor, erythropoietin) and particles by covalent coupling to vitamin B_{12} has been studied (Russell Jones *et al.*, 1999; Russell Jones, 2001). For this intrinsic process, mucoprotein is required, which is prepared by the mucus membrane in the stomach and binds specifically to cobalamin. The mucoprotein then reaches the ileum where resorption is mediated by specific receptors.

In the future bio and gas nanosensors could gain importance. These sensors could be integrated into packaging materials to monitor the freshness of the food Enzymatic nano bioengineering can be a right answer where more efficient enzymes can be made through nano technology in order to make energy. Basically certain atoms of certain amino acids or the amino acids itself are engineered at nano scale to make the enzymes more efficient and rapid in degradation.

7. Use of vitamin E in nanomaterials

Vitamin E is a term describing all tocopherol and tocotrienol derivatives that exhibit the biological activity of alpha tocopherol. The structure of vitamin E is sensitive to light; heat and oxygen. Hence the stability of vitamin E in food is affected even when stored for relatively short periods of time. Natural sources of vitamin E include vegetable and soybean oils. Synthetic versions of vitamin E are less expensive, but have lower biological activity.

8. Functional or interactive feeds and other developments

Nanotechnology is making an impact on the development of functional or interactive foods/feeds, which respond to the body's requirements and can deliver nutrients more efficiently. Development of on demand feeds, which will remain dormant in the body and deliver nutrients to cells when needed, is on the anvil. A key element for this purpose would be the development of nanocapsules that can be incorporated into feed to deliver nutrients.

Other developments in feed processing include addition of nanoparticles to the existing feeds to enable increased absorption of nutrients. Additives which are easily absorbed by the body and can increase product shelf-life are being studied presently (http://www.biodeliverysciences.com/bioralnutrients,html). Colloid nanoceuticals of less than 5 nm diameter particles have been synthesized by BioDelivery systems International (http://smartwoman.royalbodycare.com/Nanotechnology Revolution.aspx) which would scavenge free radicals, increase hydration and balance body pH. This firm also developed a nano size powder combined with nutritional supplements that enhance the absorption of nutrients (http://www/nanotechnologyproject.org).

9. Nanoparticle based optical sensor technology to elucidate the mechanism of nutrient metabolism

One of the major applications of nano technology is to use it as a tool to elucidate the mechanism of nutrient metabolism and physiology. Probes encapsulated by biologically localized embedding (PEBBLE) are submicron optical sensors, designed for minimally invasive analyte monitoring in viable, single cells. The PEBBLE nanosensors are composed of matrices of cross-linked polyacrylamide, cross-linked poly (decyl methacrylate), or sol-gel silica, which have been fabricated as sensors for H^+, Ca^{2+}, K^+, Na^+, Mg^{2+}, Zn^{2+}, Cu^{2+} and some nonionic species (Buck *et al.,* 2004). A number of techniques have been used to deliver PEBBLE nanosensors into mouse oocytes, rat alveolar macrophages, rat C6-glioma, and human neuroblastoma cells (Buck *et al.,* 2004). Using gene gun injection as a delivery method, a sol gel-based PEBBLE nanosensor for reliable, real-time measurement of sub cellular molecular oxygen was inserted into rat C6 glioma cells. The cells responded to differing oxygen concentrations and provided real-time intracellular oxygen analysis. The PEBBLE contained oxygen -sensitive fluorescent indicator, Ru (II)-Tris (4,7-diphenyl- 1,10-phenanthroline) chloride ([Ru(dpp)3] 2+), and an oxygen-insensitive fluorescent dye, Oregon Green 488-dextran, as a reference for the purpose of ratiometric intensity measurements (Xu *et al.,* 2001).

10. Liposome technology

Liposomes are micelles which are used to encapsulate water and lipid soluble compounds (Taylor *et al.,* 2005). The dissolution of fat-soluble nutrients in water-based drinks is one of the key applications of liposomes. Liposome technology can be used to encapsulate enzymes, lactic acid bacteria extracts, recombinant microbes, prebiotics and antimicrobials. These can be produced in differing sizes (10–500nm) and engineered to have different stability and surface charge under different environmental conditions. Liposome technology can be used potentially to target specific sites within a feed product for enzymatic degradation.

10.1. Encapsulation based nanoparticle delivery system

A wide variety of encapsulation platforms, including nano-structured emulsions, water-in-oil-in-water or oil-in-water-in-oil double emulsions, solid lipid or biopolymer-based nanoparticles, and direct conjugation of phytochemicals to biopolymer side chains have been developed to encapsulate food constituents for enhanced delivery and bioavailability. With the aid of nanoencapsulation, *in vivo* absorption and circulation of bio-active food components appear to increase, which should assist n achieving the desired concentration and biological activity of these compounds. In an attempt to prove the anti-inflammatory activity of water insoluble dibenzoylmethane and a b-diketone analogue of curcumin in turmeric plant a polyphenol nanocapsules method was designed by (Wang X *et al.*, 2005) wherein a high-speed and high-pressure homogenized oil-in-water emulsions (using medium-chain triacylglycerols as oil and Tween 20 as emulsifier) was used in mouse ear inflammation model. This study demonstrated enhanced anti inflammatory activity. The similar technology is boon to the feed technologists and nutritionists for enhancing the supply of food/feed. However, it should be kept in mind that an increase in nutrient intake from an enhanced food supply may be beneficial, but need to monitor overconsumption and potential signs of toxicity more closely. Additionally, micronutrient imbalances may become more prevalent and drug-nutrient interactions will also require careful observation.

11. Bacterial recombinant protein inclusion body-based nanomaterials.

The formation of inclusion bodies (IBs) in bacteria, especially in *Escherichia coli*, has become one of the most common undesirable events when using these microbial cell factories to produce soluble recombinant proteins for both research and industrial applications (Marston, 1986; Georgiou and Valax, 1996; Martinez-Alonso *et al.*, 2010). Since IBs have been long considered a waste product, essentially formed by misfolded proteins, prone to aggregate, important efforts have been made to eliminate, or at least partially reduce, its formation. Gene dosage, promoter strength, mRNA stability, codon usage, culture temperature, protein and genetic engineering and over expression of folding modulators are examples of a vast list of parameters that needs to be modulated for avoiding IB formation (Martinez-Alonso *et al.*, 2009). The IBs are pure, mechanically stable protein deposits of a few hundred nm, size formed in bacteria during recombinant production of proteins, is an interesting biomaterial for tissue engineering purposes (Garcia-Fruitos *et al.*, 2009). The IB of a vast variety of bacterial materials are recently been used for nanotechnological or nanomedical purposes. Since the IB size, its chemical and mechanical properties can be tuned according to the conditions chosen to produce them (Garcia -Fruitos *et al.*, 2009). The production of this biomaterial is a fast, efficient, inexpensive, easily tunable and scalable process. IBs can become the material of choice for tissue engineering applications, avoiding important drawbacks such as immune rejection, pain, infection, short half-life and limited availability observed when using the existent materials (García-Fruitós, 2010).

Enzyme-based IBs are tested and it is observed that, enzymes embedded in such aggregates are also active. This observation not only corroborates the model regarding IB composition, but also opens a promising market in biocatalysis industry. Enzymes such as galactosidases (Garcia-Fruitos *et al.*, 2005; Garcia-Fruitos *et al.*, 2007), reductases (Garcia-Fruitos *et al.*, 2005), oxidases (Nahalka and Nidetzky, 2007), kinases, phosphorylases and aldolases have been produced as IBs and used successfully to catalyze specific reactions. The major advantage of IBs is that it can be easily removed from the reaction mixture by a simple centrifugation, allowing the possibility to reuse them in other reaction cycles (Nahalka *et al.*, 2006; Nahalka *et al.*, 2008; Nahalka, 2008). The high cost of the catalyst production, mass transfer problems occurring during the catalysis reaction and the loss of activity due to enzyme immobilization processes are important drawbacks in biocatalysis processes, the incorporation of IBs can draw an innovative and encouraging stage in the industrial catalysis market (Roessl *et al.*, 2010).

Nahálka and collaborators (2009) explored the possibility of using IBs with lectin activity in a hemaaglutination assay in order to design a cheap diagnostic tool for the characterization of glycoproteins. Their study revealed that IBs are a good alternative, to the expensive and cumbersome lectin microarrays, being able to be used for the design of an array of glycoproteins. The IBs, as proteinaceous nanoparticles, could also open the doors of an encouraging future in regenerative medicine, being these particulate aggregates a promising alternative (Garcia-Fruitos *et al.*, 2009; Garcia-Fruitos *et al.*, 2010; Díez-Gil *et al.*, 2010) to the classical materials used for tissue engineering purposes (Sengupta and Heilshorn, 2010; Tran and Webster, 2009; Villaverde, 2010). Further studies are needed to approach a universal alternative to obtain pure and functional IB with preserved morphology, regardless of the recombinant protein. The exploration of an improved strategy should take into account not only the selection of an appropriate lysis method, but also the design of the necessary washing steps to isolate native, undisturbed active protein nanoparticles. Thus, it seems that a new age of IBs has just started, which should necessarily go accompanied by an optimization of the IB isolation protocol. The IB's with suitable esterases could be put to use for improvement of fibre digestion in the rumen.

12. Application of nano selenium on rumen fermentation

Ruminal pH is an important indicator in reflecting the rumen microbial ecosystem. Lower pH has been appeared to have a negative effect on fibre digestion, by preventing the attachment of bacteria to plant cell walls. (With nano-selenium mean ruminal pH was in the optimum range for cellulolytic bacterial activity Faixová *et al.* (2007) found that Se supplementation could significantly increase rumen microbial population and activity. Similarly it has been observed that the Se supplementation could help development of some rumen ciliate species in young sheep (Shi *et al.*, 2011).

Nano-Se supplementation in sheep switched rumen fermentation pattern from acetate to propionate, and the increased propionate concentration resulted in the reduction in the ratio of acetate to propionate (Shi *et al.*, 2011). The urinary excretion of purine derivatives was used to measure microbial biomass supply. There was a decrease in the ruminal supply of nitrogen concentration and a quadratic increase in purine derivative excretion. This could be due to an enhanced microbial growth as rumen bacteria could have consumed more ammonia nitrogen.

13. Challenges and promises of nanotechnology

In food/feed technology nanomaterials are used for coatings foods and food packaging that serve as barriers to bacteria or that contains additional nutrients. Nutritional products claiming to use nanotechnology are currently available in the market. It is important to recognize the potential toxicity of nutrients that can be affected by a change in particle size. The properties of nanostructured materials that make them so attractive could potentially lead to unforeseen health or environmental hazards (Srinivas *et al.*, 2010). Some of these properties include high aspect ratio, bio-persistence, reactive surfaces and points that are capable of producing reactive oxygen species, composition and solubility. Coating the nanoparticle with biocompatible materials, however, has been shown to significantly reduce toxicity in some applications. Furthermore, little is known about the absorption and excretion of nanoparticles by experimental animals or in humans. The various challenges the application of this technology faces include higher exposure per unit mass; small size; large surface area ratio; different routes of exposure due to smaller size (*i.e.*, dermal penetration); different distribution to tissues by virtue of their different size or surface coating, chemistry, or particle charge; and novel properties of a nanoscale material that may alter absorption, digestion, metabolism, or excretion in the body.

Nanotechnology has the potential to transform the entire food industry by changing the way food is produced, processed, packaged, transported, and consumed. Applications in food packaging are very promising, because they can improve the safety and quality of food products. A nanocomposite is a multiphase solid material where one of the phases has one, two or three dimensions of less than 100 nanometers. The use of bionanocomposites for food packaging not only has the potential to protect the food and increase its shelf life but can also be considered more environmentally friendly. because such composites would reduce the requirement to use plastics as packaging materials, thus decreasing environmental pollution in addition to consuming less fossil fuel for their production. Zein, a prolamin and the major protein found in corn, has been an important material in science and industry because of its distinctive properties and molecular structure (Vinícius Müller *et al.*, 2011)). Novel approaches are expected to yield new applications for zein in the foods and biodegradable plastics industry. After solvent treatment, zein can form a tubular structure meshwork that is inert and resistant to microbes. Zein nanoparticles have been synthesized and examined as edible carriers of flavor compounds, for nanoencapsulation of dietary supplements.

14. Research areas of nanotechnology in nutrition

The major research areas in nanotechnology include

- The discovery of novel nutrient properties,
- Quantification and characterization of the properties of nutrients and their metabolites,
- Assessing nutritional status with special attention to target compartments and cells, targeting delivery of nutrients to cells and compartments,
- Developing new devices and hybrid structures for pathway repair as well as prevent and cure nutrient deficiencies in a more quantitative and timely fashion,
- Exploring epigenetic studies with emphasis on methylation and folate and one-carbon metabolism,
- Determination of critical cell nutrient signaling pathways,
- Examination of how nutrients/metabolites modulate cell signaling pathways and
- The effect of cell nutrient signaling on overall cell function.

The benefit nutrition research might get from applying or understanding nanotechnology include :

- Identifying sites of action (molecular targets) or bioactive food components; characterize biomarkers that effect exposure, response, and susceptibility to foods and their components;
- Identifying new target delivery systems for optimizing health; and improve food composition.

Little is known about the potential health risks of nano particles. More research on the toxicology of nanoparticles case-by-case basis and for general applicability, is also needed. Nanotechnology has the potential to advance the science of nutrition by assisting in the discovery, development, and delivery of several intervention strategies to improve health and reduce the risk and complications of several diseases.

Knowledge at the cellular and molecular levels has increased greatly, catalyzing a shift towards using more specific and targeted nano-therapies. With the recognition of the important multi-faceted roles carbohydrates play in many biological systems, tremendous advances have been made in recruiting sugar functionalized nanocomposites for biological applications. Glyco-nanomaterials have attracted a great deal of attention owing to their carbohydrate functionality, small sizes, polyvalency, biocompatibility, as well as beneficial optical, electronic and magnetic properties. In this review, we will summarize the development of glyco-nanotechnology and their applications in sensing, imaging and therapeutic interventions.

Nanotechnology could be a useful approach in designing bioreactors to improve product tolerance and in optically interrogating bioreactor membranes to evaluate stress.

14.1 New generation carbon nanotubes

A newer generation of nanomaterials is represented by carbon nanotubes. Nanotube membranes have significant potential for use in feed systems. Highly selective nanotube membranes can be used for analytical purposes as part of sensors for molecular recognition of enzymes, antibodies, various proteins, and DNA. Nanotube membranes can be tailored to separate molecules on the basis of their molecular size and shape and their chemical affinity. Membranes containing gold nanotubes with diameters of <1 nm were developed for the separation of molecules and for the transport of ions between solutions placed on either side of the membrane. The interior of the nanotubes was hydrophobic that could be applied in the future for the separation of food biomolecules with functional value (*e.g.*, proteins, peptides, vitamins, or minerals), which would be used for feed fortification or the manufacturing of dietary supplements or drugs.

15. Future directions

Nanotechnology offer methods to probe the function of key molecules using multiple modalities at the scale of single molecules in live cells. Quantum dots (QD) are used to examine activities that cannot normally be resolved under a microscope with conventional dyes and fluorescent labels. When excited by laser light, the QD nano crystals emit photons and shine more brightly and longer in duration than any conventional label. Two main QD-based technologies developed to investigate cellular function are: 1) QD imaging probes for imaging protein trafficking and endocytic events in live cells; and 2) ultrasensitive QD assays for studying protein expression and speci?c protein-protein interactions in limited cell samples (Vu *et al.*, 2005). In an experiment, a protein within rat cells that regulates the growth of nerve tissue was tracked using the peptide ligand b nerve growth factor (NGF) conjugated to QD surfaces (Vu *et al.*, 2005). The bNGF-QD, in their experiment were found to retain bioactivity, activate tyrosine kinase A (TrkA) receptors, and initiated a downstream cellular signaling cascades to promote neuronal differentiation in PC12 cells. Similar receptor-initiated activity of QD-immobilized ligand has wide-ranging implications for the development of molecular tools and therapeutics targeted at understanding and regulating cell function. It is possible that QD may soon be used to visualize drugs or nutrients as they move in cells and cellular compartments in living system. These QD-based technologies offer a means to probe specific inter-molecular interactions with significantly improved sensitivity and to relate these interactions with high- resolution in real time in live cells at the scale of single molecules.

Conclusions

Majority of commercial nanoparticles applications in medicine are geared towards drug delivery. In biosciences, nanoparticles are replacing organic dyes in the applications that require high photo-stability as well as high multiplexing capabilities. Nanobiotechnology seems to take charge as far as the use of ligno cellulosic nanofibres in plastic composites is concerned (Alemdar and Sain, 2008). It is envisaged that nano materials from renewable biowastes will be the main focus of future research. Supplementation of sheep with nano-Se increased ruminal VFA concentration and switched rumen fermentation pattern from acetate to propionate. *In situ* ruminal NDF degradation of *Leymus chinensis* and soy bean meal was improved by nano-Se(Shi *et al.*, 2011). Urinary excretions of purine derivatives and nutrients digestibility were also quadratically increased with increasing nano-Se supplementation. It is clear that Nano technology will soon find a place in improving fibre digestion in ruminants. As in other technologies applications of nanotechnology to feed would be beneficial to animals, improve the utilization of feed and the main objective would be to use the potential of nanotechnology to make feed safer.

References

Alemdar A., Sain M. (2008). Isolation and characterization of nanofibers from agricultural residues-wheat straw and soy hulls. *Bioresource Technology* **99:** 1664-1671.

Buck, S.M., Xu, H., Brasuel, M., Philbert, M.A., Kopelman, R., (2004) . Nanoscale probes encapsulated by biologically localized embedding (PEBBLEs) for ion sensing and imaging in live cells. *Talanta* **63:** 41-59.

Canham L.T. (2007). Nanoscale semiconducting silicon as a nutritional food additive. *Nanotechnology* **18:** 185704 (6pp).

De Jong W.H., Hagens W.I., Krystek P., Burger M.C., Sips A.J.A.M., Geertsma R.E. (2008). Particle size-dependent organ distribution of gold nanoparticles after intravenous administration. *Biomaterials* **29:** 1912-1919.

Díez-Gil C., Krabbenborg S., Garcia-Fruitos E., Vazquez E., Rodriguez- Carmona E., Ratera I., Ventosa N., Seras-Franzoso J., Cano-Garrido O., Ferrer-Miralles N., Villaverde A., Veciana J. (2010). The nanoscale properties of bacterial inclusion bodies and their effect on mammalian cell proliferation. *Biomaterials* **31:** 5805-5812.

Faixova Z., Faix S., Leng L., Vaczi1 P., Makova Z., Szaboova R. (2007). Haematological, blood and rumen chemistry changes in lambs following supplementation with Se-yeast. *Acta Veterinaria* **76:** 3-8.

Food Safety Authority of Ireland. (2008). The relevance of food safety of applications of nanotechnology in the food and feed industries, Court lower abbey street, Abbey, Dublin 1. www.fsai.ie

Florence, A.T., Hussain, N. (2001). Transcytosis of nanoparticle and dendrimer delivery systems: evolving vistas. *Advanced Drug Delivery Review* **50:** S69-S89

García-Fruitós E. (2010). Inclusion bodies: a new concept. *Microbial Cell Factories* **9:** 80-82.

Garcia-Fruitos E., Rodriguez-Carmona E., Diez-Gil C., Ferraz R.M., Vazquez E.s, Corchero J.L., Cano-Sarabia M., Ratera I., Ventosa N., Veciana J., Villaverde A. (2009). Surface cell growth engineering assisted by a novel bacterial nanomaterial. *Advanced Materials* **21:** 4249-4253.

Garcia-Fruitos E., Seras-Franzoso J., Vazquez E., Villaverde A. (2010). Tunable geometry of bacterial inclusion bodies as substrate materials for tissue engineering. *Nanotechnology* **21:** 205101.

Garcia-Fruitos E., Aris A., Villaverde A. (2007). Localization of functional polypeptides in bacterial inclusion bodies. *Applied and Environmental Microbiology* **73:** 289-294.

Garcia-Fruitos E., Gonzalez-Montalban N., Morell M., Vera A., Ferraz R.M., Aris A., Ventura S., Villaverde A. (2005).Aggregation as bacterial inclusion bodies does not imply inactivation of enzymes and fluorescent proteins. *Microbial Cell Factories* **4:** 27.

Georgiou G., Valax P. (1996). Expression of correctly folded proteins in *Escherichia coli*. *Current Opinion in Biotechnology* **7:** 190-197.

Hoet P., Bruske-Hohlfeld I., Salata O. (2004). Nanoparticles – known and unknown health risks. *Journal of Nanobiotechnology* **2:** 12-27.

Jani P., Halbert G.W., Langridge J., Florence A.T. (1990) Nanoparticle uptake by the rat gastrointestinal mucosa: quantitation and particle size dependency. *Journal of Pharmaceutical Sciences* **42:** 821-826.

Tzeng J. (2008). Nanotechnology to create intelligent poultry feed. http://www.worldpoultry.net

Kannaki T.R., Verma P.C. (2006,). The challenges of 2020 and the role of nanotechnology in poultry research. In: *Proc. National Seminar on Poultry Research Priorities to 2020* held on Nov 2-3, Izatnagar, Uttar Pradesh, India, pp 273-277.

Luo P.G., Tzeng T.R.J., Qu L., Lin Y., Caldwell E., Latour R.A., Stutzenberger F., Sun Y.P. (2005). Quantitative analysis of bacterial aggregation mediated by bioactive nanoparticles. *Journal of Biomedical Nanotechnology* **2:** 1-5.

Marston F.A. (1986). The purification of eukaryotic polypeptides synthesized in *Escherichia coli. Biochemical Journal* **240:** 1-12.

Martinez-Alonso M., Garcia-Fruitos E., Ferrer-Miralles N., Rinas U., Villaverde A. (2010). Side effects of chaperone gene co-expression in recombinant protein production. *Microbial Cell Factories* **9:** 64-69.

Martinez-Alonso M., Gonzalez-Montalban N., Garcia-Fruitos E., Villaverde A. (2009). Learning about protein solubility from bacterial inclusion bodies. *Microbial Cell Factories* **8:** 4-9.

Mongillo F.J. (2007) Nanotechnology 101. Greenwood Press, 88 Post Road West, Westport, CT 06881, USA.

Nahalka J. (2008). Physiological aggregation of maltodextrin phosphorylase from *Pyrococcus furious* and its application in a process of batch starch degradation to alpha-D-glucose-1-phosphate. *Journal of Industrial Microbiology and Biotechnology* **35:** 219-223.

Nahalka J., Gemeiner P., Bucko M., Wang P.G. (2006). Bioenergy beads: a tool for regeneration of ATP/NTP in biocatalytic synthesis. *Artificial Cells Blood Substitutes Biotechnology* **34:** 515-521.

Nahalka J., Mislovicova D., Kavcova H. (2009). Targeting lectin activity into inclusion bodies for the characterisation of glycoproteins. *Molecular BioSystems* **5:** 819-821.

Nahalka J., Nidetzky B. (2007). Fusion to a pull-down domain: a novel approach of producing Trigonopsis variabilis D-amino acid oxidase as insoluble enzyme aggregates. *Biotechnology and Bioengineering* **97:** 454-461.

Nahalka J., Vikartovska A., Hrabarova E. (2008). A crosslinked inclusion body process for sialic acid synthesis. *Journal of Biotechnology* **134:** 146-153.

Oberdörster G., Oberdörster E., Oberdörster J. (2005). Nanotoxicology: an emerging discipline evolving from studies of ultrafine particles. *Environmental Health Perspectives* **113:** 823-839.

O' Hagan D.T. (1996) The intestinal uptake of particles and the implications for drug and antigen delivery. *Journal of Anatomy* **189:** 477-482.

Qu L., Luo P.G., Taylor S., Lin Y., Huang W., Anyadike N.,. Tzeng T.R.J., Stutzenberger F., Latour R.A., Sun Y.P. (2005). Visualizing adhesion-induced agglutination of Escherichia coli with mannosylated nanoparticles. *Journal of Nanoscience and Nanotechnology* **5:** 319-322.

Roessl U., Nahalka J., Nidetzky B. (2010). Carrier-free immobilized enzymes for biocatalysis. *Biotechnology Letters* **32:** 341-350.

Schenk P.M., Thomas-Hall S.R., Stephens E., Marx U.C., Mussgnug Posten J.H.C., Kruse O., Ben Hankamer B. (2008). Second generation biofuels: high-efficiency microalgae for biodiesel production. *Journal BioEnergy Research* **1:** 20-43.

Sengupta D., Heilshorn S.C. (2010). Protein-engineered biomaterials: highly tunable tissue engineering scaffolds. *Tissue Engineering* **16:** 285-293.

Shi L., Yue W.X.W., Zhang C., Ren Y., Liu Q., Wang Q., Shi L. (2011) Effect of elemental nano-selenium on feed digestibility, rumen fermentation, and purine derivatives in sheep. *Animal Feed Science and Technology* **163:** 136-142.

Srinivas P.R., Philbert M., Vu T.Q., Huang Q., Kokini J.L., Saltos E., Chen H., Peterson C.M., Friedl K.E., McDade-Ngutter C., Hubbard V., Starke-Reed P., Miller N., Betz J.M., Dwyer J., Milner J., Ross S.A. (2010). Nanotechnology research: applications in nutritional sciences. *Journal of Nutrition* **140:** 119-124.

Taylor S., Qu L., Kitaygorodskiy A., Teske J., Latour R.A., Sun Y.P. (2004). Synthesis and characterization of peptide-functionalized polymeric nanoparticles. *Biomacromolecules* **5:** 245-248.

Taylor T.M., Davidson P.M., Bruce B.D., Weiss J. (2005). Liposomal nanocapsules in food science and agriculture. *Critical Reviews in Food Science and Nutrition* **45:** 1-19.

Tran N., Webster T.J. (2009). Nanotechnology for bone materials. *Wiley Interdisciplinary Reviews: Nanomedicine and Nanobiotechnology* **1:** 336-351.

Villaverde A. (2010). Nanotechnology, bionanotechnology and microbial cell factories. *Microbial Cell Factories* **9:** 53-56.

Müller V., Piai J.F., Fajardo A.R., Fávaro S.L., Rubira A.F., Muniz E.C.(2011). Preparation and characterization of zein and zein-chitosan microspheres with great prospective of application in controlled drug release. *Journal of Nanomaterials* Article ID 928728, p 1-6. doi:10.1155/2011/928728.

Vu T.Q,, Maddipati R., Blute T.A., Nehilla B.J., Nusblat L., Desai T.A. (2005). Peptide-conjugated quantum dots activate neuronal receptors and initiate downstream signaling of neurite growth. *Nano Letter* **5:** 603-607.

Wang X., Jiang Y., Wang Y.W., Huang M.T., Ho C.T., Huang Q. (2008) Enhancing anti-inflammation activity of curcumin through O/W nano-emulsions. *Food Chemistry* **108:** 419-424.

Xu H,, Aylott J.W., Kopelman R., Miller T.J., Philbert M.A. (2001) A real-time ratiometric method for the determination of molecular oxygen inside living cells using sol-gel-based spherical optical nanosensors with applications to rat C6 glioma. *Analytical Chemistry* **73:** 4124-4133.

❑❑❑

Chapter 25

Synthesis and Application of Nano Minerals in Livestock Industry

D. Rajendran, A. Thulasi, S. Jash, S. Selvaraju, S.B.N. Rao
National Institute of Animal Nutrition and Physiology, Adugodi, Bangalore-560 030, Karnataka, India

Summary

Bioavailability of the minerals can be enhanced by increasing the surface area. Nano minerals are used for enhancing the bioavailability in livestock. It can be synthesized by physical, chemical and biological means. The synthesized nano minerals are characterized by scanning electron microscope (SEM), transmission electron microscope (TEM), particle size analyser, X-ray diffraction (XRD) patterns, etc. Nanotechnology holds promise for medication and nutrition because materials at the nanometer dimension exhibit novel properties different from those of both isolated atom and bulk material. This chapter deals with synthesis of nano-minerals, characterization and application in livestock industry.

Minerals play a vital role in the livestock industry. Minerals perform digestive and biosynthesis process and growth of animals. Mineral are of two types, *i.e.*, major or macro-minerals [Calcium (Ca), Phosphorus (P), Magnesium (Mg), Sodium (Na), Potassium (K), Sulphur (S) and Chloride (Cl)] and trace or micro-minerals [Iron (Fe), Copper (Cu), Zinc (Zn), Cobalt (Co), Manganese (Mn), Iodine (I), Selenium (Se) *etc.*,]. Ca and P help in the increasing bone texture and tensile strength in growing animals. Ca play role in making animal physiologically and metabolically active, involved in transmission of nerve impulse, muscle contraction, blood coagulation, digestive secretion and hormonal balance in the body. Ca supplementation in milking animal improves milk production and reduces the cost of production. About 98% of Ca in the body is present in skeleton and remaining 2% in extracellular fluids. Impairment of Ca homeostasis in early stage of lactation leads to milk fever condition in milking animals. P is involved in component of cell wall and cell contents as phospholipids, phospho-proteins and nucleic acids. Mg is involved in many biochemical processes, including activation of phosphates and participation in carbohydrate metabolism. Its action is closely associated with Ca and P. The Na and K regulates cellular fluid volume, acid base equilibrium and active transport of nutrients across the cell membrane. Chloride is essential for the transport of carbon dioxide and oxygen. Sulphur is an integral component of essential amino acids (Suttle, 2010).

Other important minerals include Fe, Cu, Zn, Co, Mn, I, Se, are also involved in essential function of the body. The Fe is present in hemoglobin and is necessary for oxygen transportation to the cells. Copper plays role in the synthesis of hemoglobin, bone metabolism and heart functions. Copper deficiency results in anemia, retarded growth rate, reduced milk yield, diarrhea, de-pigmentation of hair and skin, increases risk to parasitism and susceptibility to infectious diseases. Zinc helps in maintaining the integrity of the skin, hoof, udder lining and protecting the mammary gland from infection. Zinc supplementation reduces stress on the animals and increases milk production. Cobalt deficiency results in loss of appetite, rough hair coat, stumbling gait, depressed growth in calves, degeneration of liver, anemia and reduced resistance to infection. The Mn deficiency causes skeletal abnormalities and reproductive inefficiency. Iodine functions like thyroxin, regulates metabolic rate of body. Iodine deficiency results in depressed immune response, so increases incidence of mastitis and respiratory diseases. Selenium supplementation in feed enhance fertility rate, improves immunity against infectious diseases and helps in increasing antibodies titer in immunized animals. Trace minerals in diet reduce early embryonic deaths, reduce incidence of cystic ovaries and increase the intensity of estrous symptoms. Zinc and Se in diet also reduce the incidence of mastitis in dairy animals. Overfeeding of minerals results in hormonal imbalance and affects the production performance of dairy animals. Mineral supplementation should be done keeping in view the physiological conditions of the animals (Suttle, 2010).

1. Minerals availability

The bioavailability of a mineral in a particular source is determined relative to its functional availability from a standard source. Use of a standard source allows expression of bioavailability in terms of relative biological availability (Ammerman *et al.*, 1995). Bioavailability can be affected by a number of factors including animal species, physiological state, previous nutrition, interactions with dietary nutrients and ingredients, choice of response criteria, choice of standard source, and chemical form and solubility of the mineral element

(Ammerman *et al.*, 1995). Among the factors, interaction between two minerals or more minerals can reduce bioavailability tremendously. O'Dell (1997) defines mineral interactions as "interrelationships among mineral elements as revealed by physiological or biochemical responses" and the interaction could be either positive (commonly synergistic) or negative (antagonistic). A high concentration of an antagonist element decreases the biologic effectiveness of its target element. The interactions between minerals can affect each component's bioavailability and two or more components may be affected simultaneously (Suttle, 2010). The following are the commonly encountered minerals interaction in domestic animals.

1. Copper-Molybdenum-Sulfur
2. Copper-Sulfur
3. Copper-Iron
4. Selenium-Sulfur

Several technologies are adopted to increase the bioavailability of the minerals, nano mineral is one among them. Nano minerals improve bioavailability due to the increase in the surface area. Further, nano-encapsulation technique avoids mineral-mineral or mineral-nutrient interaction and enhances their availability.

2. Synthesis of nano mineral particles

Since 1956, from the conception of idea by American physicist Richard Feynman, inspiration for the field of nanotechnology has started. Research on nano particles developed into an important field of modern research with potential effects in electronics to medicine and recently in agriculture and livestock industry. Nanotechnology can be defined as 'manipulation of (designing, synthesis) particle with dimensions less than a micron to that of individual atom'. Nanoparticles present a higher surface volume with decreasing size of the particle. Nanoparticles exhibit unique properties in terms of chemical, physical, photo-electrochemical and electronic properties when compared to their respective bulk materials. All these applications require customized synthesis methods for specific applications. Nanotechnology holds promise for medication and nutrition because materials at the nanometer dimension exhibit novel properties different from those of both isolated atom and bulk material (Albrecht *et al.*, 2006; Wang *et al.*, 2007). Nano-structured metal particles can be synthesized either by the "top down method", *i.e.*, by the mechanical grinding of bulk metals (physical method), or via "bottom-up method" which rely on the wet chemical reduction of metal salts (nucleation and growth of metallic atoms). Recently, integration of biological components in the formation of nano sized particles leading to the complete green synthesis of nanoparticles has emerged as novel method and gaining more importance among researchers (Durán *et al.*, 2005; Huang *et al.*, 2007; Ingle, 2008). For the synthesis of nanoparticulate metal colloids, a large variety of stabilizers, e.g. donor ligands, polymers and surfactants are used to control the growth of the initially formed nanoclusters and to prevent them from agglomeration.

2.1 Physical methods

There are many different physical methods for the preparation of metal nanoparticles. Physical methods of fabrication of nanoparticles traditionally involve those which employ low-temperature plasma, molecular beams, gas evaporation, cathode sputtering, shock waves, electro explosion, laser-induced electro-dispersion, supersonic jets and different versions of mechanical dispersion. Several methods have been developed during the last decade. The popular processes include electric arc-discharge, laser ablation, chemical vapor deposition, gas phase synthesis and ball milling-annealing methods.

2.1.1 Mechanical method (Ball milling)

A ball mill is a type of grinder used to grind materials into extremely fine powder in the form of nano mineral for efficient use in livestock industry (Koch, 1997; Siegel, 1991; Schaffer and McCormick, 1992; Bakker *et al.*, 1995). Controlled reactive ball milling has produced nano-sized particles of metal oxides, nitrides, hydrides and carbides at room temperature. Recently, high-energy ball milling (HEBM), has been developed which is very different from the traditional ball-milling technique. The major differences between conventional ball milling and the HEBM include: (1) the impact energy of HEBM is typically 1000 times higher than the conventional ball-milling energy. The dominant events in the conventional ball milling are particle fracturing and size reductions, which correspond to actually, only the first stage of the HEBM, (2) a longer milling time is generally required for HEBM to activate and complete the structural changes and chemical reactions. The HEBM requires the controls of milling atmosphere and temperature which are crucial to create the desired structural changes or chemical reactions. HEBM can cover most work normally performed by conventional ball milling. Therefore, conventional ball-milling equipment cannot be used directly to conduct any HEBM work and specially designed ball mills with a higher milling energy are used for HEBM purposes.

2.1.2 Physical vapour deposition (PVD)

Nano particle by PVD method can be synthesized (Cardenas *et al.*, 2007). The PVD is a process of transferring growth species from a source or target and deposit them on a substrate to form a film. Various methods have been developed for the removal of growth species from the source or target. The thickness of the deposits can vary from angstroms to mm. In general, those methods can be divided into two groups: evaporation and sputtering. In evaporation, the growth species are removed from the source by thermal means. In sputtering, atoms or molecules are dislodged from solid target through impact of gaseous ions (plasma). Each group can be further divided into a number of methods, depending on specific techniques applied to activate the source or target atoms or molecules and the deposition conditions applied (Cardenas *et al.*, 2007).

2.1.3 Gas phase synthesis of nano materials

Most gas-phase methods of nano particle synthesis involve atmospheric or low pressure evaporation of either powders or the pre formed semiconductor or the co-evaporation of the two elemental components, for example zinc and sulfur. Gold decorated silica nanoparticles by gas phase synthesis method have been produced (Adam *et al.*, 2011). However, the use of these techniques usually results in deposits of particles with larger size distributions, in some cases ranging from 10 to 200 nm.

2.2 Chemical methods

A broad particle size distribution is obtained from the physical methods. Traditional colloids are typically larger (>10 nm) and giving irreproducible catalytic activity. To avoid contamination during mechanical milling or other physical methods and to produce uniform nano sized particle, chemical method is adopted (Lane *et al.*, 2002).

Reduction of mineral salts by chemical methods is the most convenient ways to reduce the size of the particles. A key goal in the transition metal colloid area is the development of reproducible nanoparticles in opposition to traditional colloids. Generally nanoclusters should be or have at least: (i) specific size, 1-10 nm, (ii) well defined surface composition, and (iii) reproducible synthesis and properties,. Colloidal suspensions can be obtained by various methods leading to various particle size distributions. Nevertheless, whatever the method used, a stabilizing agent is always essential to prevent the colloids from aggregation. Five general synthetic methods are mainly used in the literature to synthesize transition metal colloids: (i) chemical reduction of transition metal salts, (ii) thermal, photochemical, or sonochemical decomposition, (iii) ligand reduction and displacement from organometallics and (iv) electrochemical reduction.

The synthesis of various types of nanoparticles through solution processes has several advantages. Formation of nanoparticles dispersed in a solvent is the most common approach and prefers several advantages, which include easiness of:

1. Stabilization of nanoparticles from agglomeration,
2. Extraction of nanoparticles from solvent,
3. Surface modification and application,
4. Processing control
5. Mass production.

Reduction of metal complexes in dilute solutions is the general method in the synthesis of metal colloidal dispersions, and a variety of methods have been developed to initiate and control the reduction reactions. The formation of monosized metallic nanoparticles is achieved in most cases by a combination of a low concentration of solute and polymeric monolayer adhered onto the growth surfaces. Both a low concentration and a polymeric monolayer would hinder the diffusion of growth species from the surrounding solution to the growth surfaces, so that the diffusion process is likely to be the rate limiting step of subsequent growth of initial nuclei, resulting in the formation of uniformly sized nanoparticles.

2.2.1 Influence of reducing agents in the synthesis of nanoparticles

The size and size distribution of metallic colloids vary significantly with the types of reduction reagents used during the synthesis. In general, a strong reduction reaction promotes a fast reaction rate and favors the formation of smaller nanoparticles. However, a slow reaction may result in either wider or narrower size distribution. If the slow reaction leads to continuous formation of new nuclei or secondary nuclei, a wide size distribution would be obtained. On the other hand, if no further nucleation or secondary nucleation occurs, a slow reduction reaction would lead to diffusion-limited growth of the nuclei would be controlled by the availability of the zero valent atoms. Metal nanoparticles have a tendency to agglomerate therefore, it is necessary to protect them using surfactants or polymers, such as cyclodextrin, poly vinyl pyrrolidone (PVP), poly vinyl alcohol (PVA), citrate or quaternary ammonium salts *etc.,* (Szczepanowicz *et al.,*2010).

2.2.2 Micro-emulsion method

Micro-emulsions are complex liquids with potentials for current and future application prospects. They consist of oil, water, surfactant and co-surfactant that form a clear solution. The amphiphilic nature of a surfactant, such as cetyl-tri-methyl ammonium bromide (CTAB) is commonly used to makes them miscible with water and oil. Micro emulsions can be either 'water in oil' (w/o) or 'oil in water' (o/w) stabilized by surfactant molecules with morphologies similar to those of micelles and reverse micelles where the interfacial tension is extremely low between the two phases. With these characteristics, microemulsions appear to be an ideal platform to bring together the metal precursor (*e.g.* water-soluble) and the reactant (*e.g.*, oil-soluble) to enable the reduction of the metal to occur. Generally, the size of micro emulsions is small and uniform. Hence, they can be regarded as a micro reactor for the synthesis of nanoparticles. As the water concentration alters, the system can change from a w/o to an o/w micro-emulsion. These systems offer a wide range of possibility and flexibility to carry out the synthesis. (Eastoe and Warne, 1996).

2.2.3 Green chemical synthesis

Recently nanoparticles are synthesized using eco-friendly chemicals, plant and fungal origin as reducing agents (Oremland *et al.*, 2004). Some of the chemicals used for the synthesis of nanoparticles are toxic and they cannot be directly used. To overcome these obstacles green chemistry method can be proposed for synthesis of metal nanoparticles. Eco-friendly chemicals such as glucose, starch, amino-acids and plant extract are used to synthesis metal nanoparticles. Alternatively sonochemical method and microwave synthesis are emerging methods for synthesis of nanoparticles in large scale and cost effective manner.

2.2.4 Stability of metal nanoparticles

One of the main characteristics of colloidal particles is their small size. Because of the small size of the particles, they often tend to fall out of the solution. These metallic nanoparticles are unstable with respect to agglomeration to the bulk. In most cases, this aggregation leads to the loss of the properties associated with the colloidal state of these metallic particles. For example, during catalysis, the coagulation of colloidal particles used as catalyst leads to a significant loss of activity. Thus the stabilization of metallic colloids and the means to preserve their finely dispersed state are the crucial aspects to be considered during their synthesis. In general the roles of the stabilizers are (i) prevention of uncontrollable growth of particles (ii) prevention of particle aggregation (iii) control of growth rate (iv) control of particle size and (v) allowing particle solubility in various solvents (Yang *et al.*, 2004).

2.2.5 Stabilization by ligands or the solvent molecules

One of the most frequently employed stabilizers for metal nanoparticles is the ligand notably called ligand stabilized metal nanoparticles. Ligands such as phosphines, thiols, amines, or carbon monoxide have been invariably used for the protection of various metal nanoparticles. Such type of stabilization occurs through coordination between the ligand moiety and metal nanoparticles. It has recently been reported that solvent molecules can stabilize the nanoparticles more efficiently (Zhou, 2005). Thus Ti and Ru nanoparticles were synthesized in tetrahydrofuran or thioethers without adding steric or electrostatic stabilizers.

2.2.6 Synthesis of zero valent iron (ZVI)

The zerovalent iron nanoparticles can be synthesized by chemical reduction of ferrous sulphate using $NaBH_4$ in presence of suitable stabilizing agent like polyvinylpyrrolidone. The reaction medium should be free from dissolved oxygen because iron nanoparticles easily oxidized to nonmagnetic Fe_3O_4. Recently it has been reported that green chemistry approach of synthesis of iron nanoparticles by green tea extract. The green nanoparticles can be directly used for the degradation of textile dyes and removal chloro-organic pollutants. Iron absorption is very limited in animals and varies among species. Hence it may be tried in animal science for better absorption through gastro intestinal tract for improving productivity.

2.3 Biological synthesis of nano minerals

The synthesis of nanoparticles involves usually the chemical and physical methods but those techniques have the dispute of hazardous. In order to minimize the toxicity, nano particle has been synthesized by biological means (Narayanan and Sakthivel, 2010). Recently, integration of biological components in formation of nano sized particles leading to the complete green synthesis of nanoparticles has emerged as novel method and gaining more importance among researchers. Biologically inorganic nano materials are produced either intra- or extracellular by employing microorganisms or plant derived materials. Various metal nanoparticles like silver, gold, cadmium, selenium, palladium, barium titanate and titanium has been successfully synthesized by biological methods. Among the various metal nanoparticles synthesized using biological method; noble metal nanoparticles such as silver and gold have been studied extensively (Huang *et al.*, 2007).

Microorganisms such as bacteria, actinomycetes, yeast and fungi are used for synthesis of various metal nanoparticles with different shape and size (Oremland *et al.*, 2004). Some well-known examples are: *Pseudomonas stutzeri, Magnetospirillum magneticum, Pseudomonas aeruginosa, Thermomonospora sp., Fusarium oxysporum, Candida glabrata, Schizosaccharomyces prombe, Penicillium fellutanum* and *Cladosporium cladosporioides.* Toward elucidating mechanism of nanoparticle formation, most of the literatures suggest the role of enzyme NADH dependent reductase and also by the high molecular weighed proteins released from the microorganisms. Biosynthesis of nanoparticles using microorganisms has some disadvantages beyond its successful synthesis of various metal nanoparticles. The difficulty in maintaining the culture and culture condition, exclusive media used for culturing, time period in formation of the nanoparticles and difficulty in nano particle product recovery are some of the reported disadvantages of the synthesis process using microorganisms (Narayanan and Sakthivel, 2010).

Overcoming all the above disadvantages, the synthesis of nanoparticles using plant materials offer numerous advantages. Simple synthesis procedures, mostly single step and one pot synthesis and easy product recovery from the final solutions. In addition the synthesis of plant materials are also eco-friendly, compatible for pharmaceutical and biomedical applications, cost effective, economic viability, non toxic and easily scaled up for large scale synthesis and also the less time consuming. Green nanoparticles have been synthesized using various plant species such as *Avena sativa, Azadirachta indica, Aloe vera, Alfalfa,* papaya fruit extract, lemongrass, *Sesbania drummondii,* latex of *Jatropha cutcas* (Shankar *et al.,* 2004).

The biomolecules present in these plants are acting as reducing agent and also as capping agent which favor the synthesis of size controlled nanoparticles through the biological synthesis method. The biomolecules like reducing sugars, phenolic compounds and protein molecules are reported to aid in reduction and proteins in capping the formed nanoparticles. Further detailed studies on the mechanism of nanoparticle synthesis in plants at the cellular level and the possible extracellular synthesis of nanoparticles using plant extract in large scale would revolutionize the field of plant biotechnology in nanoscience. This technology untaps the utilization of nanomaterial for agricultural purposes. These nanoparticles synthesized by various techniques have received special attention because they have found potential application in many fields such as catalysis, sensors, drug delivery systems etc. The green synthesized nanoparticles have wide application not only in the medical field like artificial implantations, diagnostic tools and biological research, it also applied in cosmetics, agriculture, environmental protection and in food industries. Using different plant sources such as *Azadirachta indica, Aloe vera* etc. for synthesizing nanoparticles will have a tremendous application in agricultural practices such as to increase the potentiality of fertilizers and insecticides and also in food preservation. Biological systems have large potency for the fabrication of nanoparticles which can be utilized for wide application areas. Desired size nanoparticles can be obtained by using products or live single celled microorganism to complex eukaryotes. Though many biological systems are identified to synthesize nanoparticles, the identification of key bio-components involved in reduction and stabilization will further help in the production of nanoparticles with desired shape and size. However, the elucidation of the exact mechanism of nano particle formation in biological methods needs much more experimental observations, so well-defined nanoparticles can be fabricated for application in livestock and feed industry (Narayanan and Sakthivel, 2010).

3. Characterization of nano minerals

The powders obtained after synthesis must be characterized for their size, shape, surface area, phase constitution, and micro-structural features. The crystalline size or grain size in nanoparticles can be determined with several techniques that rely upon the peak width in X-ray diffraction (XRD) patterns. The size and shape of powder particles may be determined accurately with direct methods of either scanning electron microscopy (SEM) for relatively coarse powders or transmission electron microscopy (TEM) for fine powders. In contrast to XRD, which gives a bulk-average value for grain size, observations of particle size via SEM/TEM give only values of an isolated sample area and, as such, may not be representative of the entire sample, vis-à-vis particle size distribution. The values of particle size should not be confused with crystalline size, as determined from XRD data (Rao and Biswas (2009).

4. Application of nano minerals in livestock industry

4.1 Nano mineral for animal production

Research works have been started to explore the efficacy of the nano minerals in livestock and agricultural industry (Subramanian and Tarafdar, 2011). Zhou and Wang (2011) concluded that supplementing diets with 0.30 mg/kg of nano-Se was effective in increasing the growth performance and feed conversion ratios of chickens, the Se content of tissues, and the quality of the meat. Recently Shi *et al.* (2011) concluded that the supplementation of Se improved growth performance and Se concentration in blood and tissues in growing male goat. Dietary supplementation of elemental nano-Se could be utilized more effectively when compared to inorganic or organic Se. The incorporation of different Se forms (sodium selenite, selenized yeast and elemental nano-Se) into growing goat diet increased Se concentrations in whole blood, serum and tissues.

The red elemental selenium has promising uses in the environmental protection from the pollution of the excessive selenium (Zhang *et al.*, 2001, 2004; Jia, *et al.*, 2005). Zhang *et al.* (2001) synthesized nano red elemental selenium (nano-Se) of size 5-100 nm and observed that nano-Se had a similar bioavailability in rat and much less acute toxicity in mice compared with selenite.

Zhou *et al.* (2009) reported that supplementation of nano selenium in crucian carp (*Carassius auratus gibelio*) has improved body weight than control group. Similarly, highest value ($P<0.05$) of selenium content in muscle was observed in nano selenium supplemented group. Shi *et al.* (2011a) observed that nano-Se supplementation in basal diet improved rumen fermentation and feed utilization. Nano-Se could also stimulate rumen microbial activity, digestive microorganisms or enzyme activity. The optimum dose of nano-Se was about 3.0 g/kg dietary DM in sheep.

Zha *et al.* (2009) reported that nano chromium (CrNano) supplementation significantly decreased serum concentrations of insulin and cortisol, increased sera levels of insulin-like growth factor I and immunoglobulin G, and enhanced the lympho proliferative response, and phagocytic activity of peritoneal macrophages. Similarly Zha *et al.* (2009a) reported that supplementation of Cr in the form of Cr-nano and CrPic might be an effective tool for enhancing the growth performance and carcass traits of broiler chicks in heat-stressed condition. Cr-nano seemed to have greater beneficial effects in comparison with CrPic.

It has been observed in cattle that the supplementation of nano zinc oxide had improved milk production in subclinical mastitis (Author's unpublished report). It was observed that increases in milk production, suppression of subclinical mastitis (reduction in somatic cell count) by nano zinc supplementation to dairy animal. It could be useful feeding strategies.

4.2 Nano mineral for improving immunity

Supplementation of nano zinc has drastically reduced SCC in subclinical mastitis cow and improved mastitis conditioned with increase in milk production than macro zinc oxide (Author's unpublished report). Similarly, Zhou *et al.* (2009) has observed that glutathione peroxidase (GSH-Px) activities in carp's plasma and liver of nano selenium group and selenomethionine were significantly improved with that of the control. Peng *et al.* (2007) suggest that Nano-Se should be most effective as a chemo-preventive agent at smaller particle size as it improves the activities of glutathione S-transferase. Antioxidant status was also improved by Se supplementation. Shi *et al.* (2011) concluded that supplementation of nano Se can improve growth performance, serum oxidant status and Se concentration in blood and tissues in growing male goat. The dietary supplementation of elemental nano-Se could be utilized more effectively in growing male goat when compared to inorganic or organic Se (Shi *et al.*, 2011).

4.3 Nano mineral for animal reproduction

Effect of nanoparticles on reproduction is scanty. However enormous scope is available to explore the effect of nano particles on reproduction. Nano sensors are available to study the causes of abortion. Nano anti-oxidant is one of the area to be explored to prevent retention of placenta and other reproductive problems after calving and also for improving infertility problems. Some of the nano particles need to be explored to include in the semen extender to improve the quality of the semen *e.g.*, Nano- Se, Nano Zn. The penetration of gold nano-particle into the sperm heads and tails was observed. After mixing the semen with a gold nano-particle solution, 25% of spermatozoa became non-motile (Wiwanitkit *et al.,* 2009). In goats, selenium deficiency resulted in abnormal spermatozoal mitochondria. Supplementation in goats nano-se enhanced the testis Se content, testicular and semen GSH-Px activity, protected the membrane system integrity and the tight arrangement of the mid-piece of the mitochondria (Shi *et al.,* 2010).

Conclusions

Nano minerals can be synthesized by physical, chemical and biological methods. In general biological methods are safe to use and can be efficiently exploited without further experiment on residual effect. Studies so far have indicated that the application of nano minerals in animal production, immunity and reproduction is promising. In animals nano-tubes are implanted under the skin to provide real time measurement of changes in the level of hormones in the blood. The nanotubes are used as a means of tracking animals in estrus because these tubes have the capacity to bind and detect the change in hormone at the time of estrous by near infrared fluorescence. The signal from this sensor will be incorporated as a part of a central monitoring and control system to actuate breeding. Microfluidics is used today in animal science to significantly simplify traditional *in vitro* fertilization procedures. It is being used in livestock breeding to physically sort sperm and eggs. Microfluidic and nanofluidic are the systems which analyse by controlling the flow of liquids or gases through a series of tiny channels and valves, thereby sorting them, much as a computer circuit sorts data through wires and logic gates. Application of nano-minerals is immense but the safety in application of nano-minerals needs to be assessed before it being applied in the livestock industry.

References

Adam M.B., Lei P., Calder S., Girshick S.L., (2011). Gas-phase production of gold-decorated silica nanoparticles. *Nanotechnology* **22:** 315603 doi:10.1088/0957-4484/22/31/315603.

Albrecht M.A., Evans C.W., Raston C.L. (2006). Green chemistry and the health implications of nano particles. *Green Chemistry* **8:** 417-432.

Ammerman C. B., Baker D. H., Lewis A. J. (1995). Bioavailability of nutrients for animals: amino acids, minerals, and vitamins. Academic Press, New York.

Bakker H., Zhou G. F., Yang H. (1995).Mechanically driven disorder and phase transformations in alloys. *Progress in Material Science* **39:** 159.

Cardenas G, Meléndrez M, Cruzat C, Díaz J. (2007). Synthesis of tin nanoparticles by physical vapour deposition technique (vd). *Acta Microscopica* **1:** 1-2.

Durán N., Marcato P.D., Alves O.L., De Souza G.I.H., Esposito E. (2005). Mechanistic aspects of biosynthesis of silver nanoparticles by several *Fusarium oxysporum* strains. *Journal Nano Biotechnology* **3:** 8. doi:10.1186/1477-3155-3-8.

Eastoe J. Warne B. (1996) Nanoparticle and polymer synthesis in microemulsions. *Current Opinion in Colloid and Interface Science* **1:** 800-805.

Huang J., Chen C., He N., Hong J., Lu Y., Qingbiao L., Shao W., Sun D., Wang X.H., Wang Y., Yiang X. (2007). Biosynthesis of silver and gold nanoparticles by novel sundried *Cinnamomum camphora* leaf. *Nanotechnology* **18:** 105-106.

Ingle A., Gade A., Pierrat S., Sonnichsen C., Rai M.K. (2008). Mycosynthesis of silver nanoparticles using the fungus Fusarium acuminatum and its activity against some human pathogenic bacteria. *Current Nano Science* **4:** 141-144.

Jia X., Li N., Chen J. (2005). A subchronic toxicity study of elemental nano-Se in Sprague Dawley rats. *Life Science* **76:** 1989-2003.

Koch C.C. (1997). Synthesis of nanostructured materials by mechanical milling: problems and opportunities, *Nanostructured Materials* **9:** 13-22.

Lane R., Craig B., Babcock W. (2002). Materials engineering with nature's building blocks. *AMPTIAC Newsletter Spring* **6:** 31-37.

Narayanan K.B., Sakthivel N.(2010) Biological synthesis of metal nanoparticles by microbes. *Advances in Colloid and Interface Science* **156:** 1-13.

O'Dell B. L. (1997). Mineral-ion interaction as assessed by bioavailability and ion channel function. In: *Handbook of nutritionally essential mineral elements.* (B.L. O'Dell R.A. Sunde, eds.). Marcel Dekker, New York p 23, pp 641-659.

Oremland R. S., Herbal M. J., Blum J. S., Langely S., Beveridge T. J., Jayan P. M, Sutto T., Ellis A. V. (2004). Structural and spectral features of selenium nanospheres produced by Se-respiring bacteria. *Applied Environmental Microbiology* **70:** 52-60.

Peng D., Zhang J., Liu Q., Taylor E.W. (2007). Size effect of elemental selenium nanoparticles (Nano-Se) at supranutritional levels on selenium accumulation and glutathione S-transferase activity. *Journal of Inorganic Biochemistry* **101:** 1457-1463.

Rao C.N.R., Biswas K. (2009). Characterization of Nanomaterials by Physical Methods. *Annual Review of Analytical Chemistry* **2:** 435-462.

Schaffer G. B., McCormick P. G. (1992). Mechanical alloying. *Material Forum* **16:** 91.

Shankar S.S., Ahmad A., Rai A., Sastry M. (2004). Rapid synthesis of Au Ag and bimetallic Au core-Ag shell nanoparticles by using neem (Azadirachta indica) leaf broth. *Journal of Colloids and Interface Science* **275:** 496-502.

Shi L. G., Xun W., Yue W., Zhang C., Ren Y., Liu Q., Wang Q., Shi L. (2011). Effect of elemental nano-selenium on feed digestibility, rumen fermentation, and purine derivatives in sheep. *Animal Feed Science and Technology* **163:** 136-142.

Shi L. G., Yang R. J., Yue W. B., Xun W.J., Zhang C.X., Ren Y.S., Shi L, Lei F.L. (2010). Effect of elemental nano-selenium on semen quality, glutathione peroxidase activity, and testis ultrastructure in male Boer goats. *Animal Reproduction Science* **118:** 248-254.

Shi L.G, Xuna W., Yue W, Zhang C , Ren Y , Shi L , Wang Q., Yang R ., Lei F. (2011). Effect of sodium selenite, Se-yeast and nano-elemental selenium on growth performance, Se concentration and antioxidant status in growing male goats. *Small Ruminant Research* **96:** 49-52.

Siegel R.W. (1991). Materials science and technology (R.W. Cahn, P. Haasen, E.S. Kramer, eds). VCH Weinheim, pp 583.

Subramanian K.S., Tarafdar J.C. (2011). Prospects of nanotechnology in Indian farming. *Indian Journal of Agricultural Sciences* **81:** 887-893.

Suttle N.F. (2010). The mineral nutrition of livestock. 4th ed, CABI Publishing. Oxford shire OX10 8DE, UK.

Szczepanowicz K., Stefan'ska J., Socha R.P. (2010). Preparation of silver nanoparticles via chemical reduction and their antimicrobial activity. *Physicochemcal Problem of Mineral Processing* **45:** 85-98

Wang H.L., Zhang J.S., Yu H.Q. (2007). Elemental selenium at nano size possesses lower toxicity without compromising the fundamental effect on selenoenzymes: Comparison with selenomethionine in mice. *Free Radical Biology & Medicine* **42:** 1524-1533.

Wiwanitkit V., Sereemaspun A., Rojanathanes R. (2009). Effect of gold nanoparticles on spermatozoa: the first world report. *Fertility and Sterility* **91:** 7-8.

Yang J., Deivaraj T.C., Too H.P., Lee J.Y. (2004). Acetate stabilization of metal nanoparticles and its role in the preparation of metal nanoparticles in ethylene glycol. *Langmuir* **20:** 4241-4245.

Zha L., Zeng J., Sun S., Deng H., Luo H., Li W. (2009). Chromium(III) nanoparticles affect hormone and immune responses in heat-stressed rats. *Biological Trace Element Research* **129:** 157-169.

Zha L.Y., Zeng J.W., Chu X.W., Mao L.M., Luo H.J. (2009a). Efficacy of trivalent chromium on growth performance, carcass characteristics and tissue chromium in heat stressed broiler chicks. *Journal of the Science of Food and Agriculture* **89:** 1782-1786.

Zhang J., Gao X., Zhang L., Bao Y.P. (2001). Biological effects of nano red elemental selenium. *Bio Factors* **15:** 27-38.

Zhang J.S., Wang H., Yan X., Zhang L.D. (2004). Comparison of short-term toxicity between nano-Se and selenite in mice. *Life Science* **75:** 447-459.

Zhou X., Wang Y. (2011). Influence of dietary nano elemental selenium on growth performance, tissue selenium distribution, meat quality, and glutathione peroxidase activity in Guangxi Yellow chicken. *Poultry Science* **90:** 680-686.

Zhou X.X., Wang Y.B., Gu Q., Li W.F. (2009). Effects of different dietary selenium sources (selenium nanoparticle and selenomethionine) on growth performance, muscle composition and glutathione peroxidase enzyme activity of crucian carp (*Carassius auratus gibelio*). *Aquaculture* **291:** 78-81.

Zhou Y (2005). Recent advances in ionic liquids for synthesis of inorganic nano-materials. *Current Nanoscience* **1:** 35-42.

❑❑❑

Chapter 26

Meta-Analysis : A New Statistical Tool to Synthesize Research Results

K.P. Suresh, R. Bhatta, S. Nandi, S. Mondal, G. Ravi Kiran, K.T. Sampath
National Institute of Animal Nutrition and Physiology, Adugodi, Bangalore-560 030, Karnataka, India

Summary

Research in animal nutrition and physiology, primarily requires processing and modeling of research data. In certain fields of research, the number of publications and results per publications is vast. Results from single classical experiment cannot be the basis for a large inference space because the conditions under which observations are made in a single experiment are generally very narrow. A single experimentation generally measures the effect of one or two variables while maintaining all other factors as constant as possible. Often these experiments are repeated by other workers/labs to verify the generalization and repeatability of the observations and sometime to challenge the range of applicability of observed results and conclusions. This leads to large number of similar studies being carried out and research papers published, even on a relatively narrow research domain. Often researchers are confused with the different results of similar research. In this context, there is a need to summarize the results across all the published studies. In this chapter the statistical methods dealing with the analysis of literature data, known as meta-analysis is presented.

The scientific investigation of animal nutrition and physiology seeks to provide the findings that can be confidently applied to improve the health, production and reproduction. The classical cycle of observation providing a hypothesis, testing the hypothesis and refinement of hypothesis by further testing can now be extended to include the investigation of hypothesis through production of estimates of effects and confidence in these effects using a series of existing studies. The objectives of this chapter are to introduce the concept of meta-analysis a systematic review and to discuss the rationale for this type of research and other general considerations.

1. Meta-analysis and systematic reviews

There are about 40,000 journals for sciences; the researchers are filling those journals at the rate of one article every 30 seconds. As results accumulate, it becomes increasingly difficult to understand what they tell us and becomes difficult to find the knowledge in this flood of information. Meta-analysis is a rapidly expanding area of research that has been relatively underutilized in animal nutrition and physiology research. Meta-analysis is defined as an analysis of a large collection of results from individual studies for the purpose of integrating the findings. It is a quantitative, formal, epidemiological study design used to systematically assess the previous research studies to derive the conclusions about the body of research. Outcomes from a meta-analysis may include more precise estimate of the effect of treatment or the risk factors for disease or condition than any individual studies contributing to the pooled analysis. Identification of source of variation in responses or heterogeneity of group of studies and generalization of responses can lead to more effective treatment or modification of management. Examination of heterogeneity is perhaps the most important task in meta-analysis. Major contributions include the development of protocol that provides the structure for literature search methods and analytical methods for evaluating the outcome of meta-analysis (Lean *et al.*, 2009). Meta-analysis places a less emphasis on significance testing and larger emphasis on determining the magnitude and precision of an effect of interest.

Meta-analyses are a subset of systematic review. A systematic review attempts to collate empirical evidence that fits pre-specified eligibility criteria to answer specific research question (Sauvart *et al.*, 2008). The key characteristics of a systematic review are 1) clearly stated set of objectives with predefined eligibility criteria for studies; 2) an explicit, reproducible methodology; 3) the systematic search that attempts to identify all studies that meet the eligibility criteria, an assessment of the validity of the findings of the included studies and systematic presentation. Systematic methods are used to minimize bias, thus providing more reliable findings from which the conclusions can be drawn and decisions made than traditional review methods. The benefits of meta-analysis include a consolidated and quantitative review of a large and often complex, sometimes apparently conflicting body of literature. Meta-analysis can be used to regulatory authorities to provide a quantitative evaluation of the efficacy of a product available for registration.

The hypothesis that can be raised in a meta-analysis may extend well beyond those examined in the original studies. Meta-analysis can be used to evaluate multivariable effects when compared to unavailable effect in individual studies.

The value of meta-analysis to address the marked increase in literature available to scientists and practitioners in most fields of scientific endeavor has been recognized. These methods have extended beyond the social sciences and human sciences where they were first developed, and span disciplines from astronomy to zoology. The number of publications in meta analysis had increased from 100 in 2000 to more than 1000 in 2008. Statistical techniques to combine results in randomized trials, economic evaluation and epidemiological studies have become more common, possibly because of the increasing size of the research literature and partly because of rigorous efficacy and safety standards.

Research in animal sciences, especially nutrition and physiology, increasingly requires processing and modeling of data generated through primary research. In certain areas of research, the number of publications and results per publications is increasing, thus periodically requiring quantitative summarization of literature data, for example, literature database on factors affecting the embryo yield, endocrine profiling of animals, nutritive requirements of livestock, effect of bypass protein on milk yield, effect of garlic on egg production and lipids etc. In such instances, statistical methods dealing with analysis of literature data, meta-analysis is more useful to provide the accurate information with low standard error (St Pierre, 2001; Cohen, 1988).

Research reviews can be arranged into four classes (Cooper, 1982; Jackson, 1980). The first type of review identifies and discuses new developments in a field. The second uses empirical evidences to highlight, illustrate or assess a particular theory or tentatively propose new theoretical frameworks. Third, a reviewer can organize knowledge from divergent lines of research. Meta-analysis belongs to fourth class of review, the integrative review. The integrative review is primarily interested in inferring generalizations about substantive issues from a set of studies having a direct bearing on those issues. A meta-analytic reviewer will typically collect a group of studies that investigate the same question through roughly similar procedures. Of course there would be little need for review if the convergence of hypothesis and research design produced identical results in all the studies.

Meta-analyses are conducted to assess the strength of evidence present on a disease, treatment or aspects of production or reproduction. One aim is to determine whether an effect exists is positive or negative and ideally to obtain a single summary estimate of the effect. The results of meta-analyses can improve precision of estimates of effect, answer questions not posed by individual studies, settle controversies arising from apparently conflicting studies and generate new hypothesis. In particular, an examination of heterogeneity is vital to the development of new hypothesis.

2. Individual or aggregated data

The majority of meta-analysis is based on a series of studies to produce a point estimate of an effect and measures the precision of that estimate. However, methods have been developed (Stewart and Clarke, 1995; Simmonds *et al.*, 2005) for the meta-analysis to be conducted on data obtained from the original trials. This approach is considered as gold standard in meta-analysis because it offers advantage over analyses using aggregated data, including the greater ability to validate the quality of data and to conduct appropriate statistical analysis. Further, it is easier to explore differences in effect across subgroups within the study population than with aggregated data. This approach relies on the co-operation between researchers who conduct relevant studies.

3. Study power

A major rationale of meta-analyses is to increase the statistical power of the hypothesis. Combining data from many published studies into a meta-analysis can explain some of the inconsistencies of these effects across a variety of experimental conditions. A meta-analysis provides additional statistical power (lower type II error) that can detect the significant differences in outcomes that are not statistically significant in individual studies and also provides the more precise point estimation and narrower confidence interval of the estimated effects (Jackson, 2006).

4. Empirical modeling of biological responses

For empirical modeling of biological responses of animals to nutritional practices or physiological conditions, the data extracted from many publications cover a much wider set of experimental conditions than those of each individual study and hence the conclusions and models derived from whole set have a much greater likelihood of yielding relevant predictions to decision makers. The meta-analytic activities have led to a new paradigm as a law of multiple responses to changes in feeding practices or physiological conditions. Significant progress can be made for the holistic researches like alteration in feeding practices impact feed efficiency, product quality, the environment, animal welfare etc using meta-analyses. Meta-analyses offer a mechanism of estimation that makes parameter estimation more precise and applicable to a broader range of conditions. Meta-analyses can also be used for external model evaluation.

5. Types of data and factors in meta-analyses

As in conventional statistical analysis, dependent variables in meta-analyses can be various types such as binary (present/absent, yes/no etc), counts of percentages, ordinal (poor, average, good and excellent) and continuous, which is the most frequent type in meta-analysis related to animal nutrition and physiology research. Independent factors (or variables) may be modeled using a fixed or random effect. In general, factors related to nutrition (grain type, dry matter intake etc.,) should be considered as fixed effect factors. The study effect can be considered either random or fixed. If a dataset comprised many individual studies from multiple research centers, the study effect should be considered random because each study is conceptually random outcome from a large population of studies to which inference is to be made. This is especially important if the meta-analysis has objective of empirical modeling of biological responses, or the collective summarizations of measurements, because it is likely that the researcher in those instances has a targeted range of inference much larger than the limited conditions represented by the specific studies.

6. Literature search

A sound meta-analysis is characterized by a thorough and disciplined literature search. A clear definition of hypothesis to be investigated provides the framework for such an investigation. It is important to obtain all relevant studies, because loss of even a single report can lead to bias in the study. Typically, published papers and abstracts are identified by a computerized literature search of electronic databases that can include Commonwealth Agricultural Bureau (CAB), Biological abstracts, Life sciences, Science Direct (www.sciencedirect.com), Scirus (www.scirus.com/srsapp), PubMed http://www.ncbi.nlm.nih.gov/pubmed), Agricola (Agricola.nal.usda.gov), ISI web of knowledge (http://isiwebofknowledge.com), Google Scholar (http:/scholar.google.com), http://cera.jccc.in a guide for online search and download articles and many more. Database searches should be augmented with hand searches of library for relevant articles, abstracts, books and conference proceedings. Cross-checking of references, citations, in review papers and communications with scientists who have been working in the relevant field are important methods used to provide a comprehensive search (Mandal *et al.,* 2009; Suresh *et al.,* 2009).

7. Inclusion or exclusion criteria and potential for bias

Studies are chosen for meta-analysis based on inclusion criteria. If there is more than one hypothesis to be tested, separate selection criteria should be defined for each hypothesis. Inclusion criteria are ideally defined at the stage of initial development of the study protocol. The rationale for the criteria for study selection used should be clearly stated. In practice, it may be necessary to revise the inclusion criteria for a meta-analysis after reviewing all of the studies found through the search strategy. Variation in studies reflects the type of study design, type and application of interventional products, etc, there are no standardized criteria for inclusion of studies in meta-analysis. Universal criteria are not appropriate because meta-analysis can be applied to a broad spectrum of topics. Published journals should be cross-checked with conference papers to avoid repetitions in presented data. The study design, including details of the method of randomization of subjects to treatment groups, criteria for eligibility in the study, blinding, method of assessing the outcome and handling of protocol deviations are important features defining study quality. When studies are excluded from a meta-analysis, reasons for exclusion should be provided for each excluded study. The inclusion of observational medical studies in meta-analysis led to considerable debate over the validity of meta-analytical approaches, as there was necessarily a concern that the observational studies were likely to be subjected to unidentified sources of confounding and risk modification (Greenland 1944a; Hedges and Olkin, 1985). Pooling such findings may not lead to more certain outcomes. Animal research has a distinct advantage over medical research in being more able to make use randomized controlled clinical trials and outcomes of animal experiment of similar hypothesis.

8. Data entry

Database on extracts from literature based results must be developed in a specified meta-analysis protocol. The structure and coding of the database must include numerous variables identifying the experimental objectives of all the experiments selected. Hence, numerous columns are potentially added to code each objective found in all the sources of experimental data. This coding is necessary so as to avoid the improper aggregation of results across the studies with very different objectives. During this coding phase, the analyst may chose to transform a continuous variable to a discrete variable with levels coded in a single column. Different criteria can guide the selection of classes, such as equidistant classes, classes with equal frequencies or probability of occurrence. The important point is that sum of these descriptive columns must entirely characterize the objective of all studies used.

9. Data filtering

There are at least three steps necessary to effective data filtering. First, the analyst must ensure that the study under consideration is coherent with the objectives of the meta-analysis. That is, the meta-analytic objectives dictate that some traits/ characteristics must be measured and reported. The second step consists of a thorough and critical review of each publication under consideration, focusing on the detection of errors in the reporting of the quantitative results. This underlines the importance of having a highly trained professional involved in this phase of the study. Verification of data entries is then another essential component to the process. In third step, it is important to ensure that a selected publication does not appear to be an outlier with respect to the characteristics and relations under considerations.

10. Testing the significance of homogeneity

In meta-analysis of several studies, it is usual to conduct a homogeneity test to determine if the effects measured by the studies are sufficiently similar to justify their integration. If each ith study produces an estimate of an underlying effect θ_i the homogeneity test is a test of hypothesis that the underlying effects are all equal. The effects can be measured by variety of statistics, among more important types of effect measures are simple means, correlation co-efficient, and for studies in which there are treatment and control arms, difference of sample means, standardized mean differences, odds ratio, and differences or ratios of binomial probabilities, which are referred to as risk differences and relative risks. Meta-analysis seeks to combine the results of several experiments in order to improve the accuracy of decisions. It is common to use a test for homogeneity to determine if the results of the several experiments are sufficiently similar to warrant their combination into an overall result. Cochran's Q statistic (Cochran, 1937; Glass, 1976) is frequently used for this homogeneity test. It is often assumed that Q follows a chi-square distribution under the null hypothesis of homogeneity.

The standard test for the equality of k variances was carried out. The k study-specific summary statistics shared a common mean θ. A statistical test for the homogeneity of study means is equivalent to testing,

$H_0:\theta = \theta_1 = \theta_2 = \ldots\ldots \theta_k$ against

H_1: At least one θ_i is different. Under H_0, for large sample sizes,

$$Q_w = \sum_1^k w_i (y_i - \hat{\theta}_{MLE}) \text{ Follows Chi-square with (k-1) degrees of freedom}$$

Where, $$\hat{\theta}_{MLE} = \frac{\sum w_i y_i}{\sum w_i} \text{ and } w_i = \frac{1}{s_i^2}$$

After testing for the significance of heterogeneity of studies based on chi-square test and Tau² (heterogeneity coefficient), fixed effect and random effect models were selected for integrating the results. When the Tau² value is zero, the Inverse variance method was used as fixed affect model, otherwise a random effect model by DerSimonian and Laird Method (DL method). The random effect model allows the study variation to extent some while integrating the results.

11. Fixed effect model

These models are used if the heterogeneity of studies is not statistically significant. One of the main fixed effect models pertinent to animal research is Inverse-Variance Method (IV-method)

Inverse-variance method

The Inverse-Variance Method was used to pool either binary, continuous or correlation data. This approach has wide applicability since it can be used to combine any estimate that has standard error available. The effect size or mean are combined to give a pooled estimate (denoted by θ) by calculating weighted average of the treatment effects from the individual studies as follows:

$$\theta_{IV} = \frac{\sum w_i \theta_i}{\sum w_i}$$

Where the weights w_i are calculated as,

$$w_i = \frac{1}{SE(\theta_i)^2}$$

That is, the weight for the ith study is equal to its precision of the estimate.

The standard error of θ_{IV} is given by,

$$SE(\theta_{IV}) = \frac{1}{\sqrt{\sum w_i}}$$

The heterogeneity statistic (denoted by Q_w) is given by,

$$Q_w = \sum w_i (\theta_i - \theta_{IV})^2$$

The Q_w follows chi-square distribution with (k-1) degrees of freedom, where k is the number of studies included in the meta-analysis.

12. Random effect model

These models are used if the heterogeneity of studies is statistically significant. One of the main random effect models pertinent to animal research is DerSimonian and Laird method (DL method).

DerSimonian and Laird method

The DerSimonian and Laird method of meta-analysis is based on the random effects model. Under the random effects model, the assumption of common effect is relaxed, and the effect size or mean θ_i are assumed to have a normal distribution with mean è and variance tau² (τ^2). The usual DL estimate for τ^2 is as follows:

$$\tau^2 = \frac{Q_w - (k - 1)}{\sum w_i - \frac{\sum w_i^2}{\sum w_i}}$$

Where Q_w is the heterogeneity statistic, and the weights w_i are calculated as in the I V Method, and k is the number of studies. The τ^2 is set to zero if Q_w<(k-1). In this approach, the weights for each study effect size w'_i are as given below.

$$w'_i = \frac{1}{SE(\theta_i)^2 + \tau^2}$$

The pooled estimate is given by,

$$\theta_{DL} = \frac{\sum w'_i\theta_i}{\sum w'_i}$$

With standard error,

$$SE(\theta_{DL}) = \frac{1}{\sqrt{\sum w'_i}}$$

The heterogeneity statistic and its test of significance is as given in the I V method (Normand, 1999; Williamson *et al.*, 2002; Cooper, 1982; Eugene *et al.*, 2004).

13. Mixed effect model

The mixed models are powerful tools for the analysis of clustered data, between and within study variability. Often, in this type of data, the observations in the same study are correlated to exhibit the heterogeneous variability (St.Pierre, 2001). In contrast, the regression analysis of such data, do not consider the correlation and heterogeneity variability in the data. Further, when the data is missing at random, regression method ignores the complete study for which any parameter is missing, while the mixed models are more robust in this condition, can accommodate the data that are missing at random (Runbin, 1976). The mixed models use the restricted maximum likelihood estimation (RMLE) to estimate the unknown variance-covariance method as compared to ordinary least squares method of estimation in regression method, which is robust for clustered and missing observation. The canonical form for mixed model is as follows,

$Yij = B_0 + B_1X_{ij} + B_2X_{ij}^{\ 2} + S_i + b_iX_{ij} + \varepsilon_{ij}$; i=1 to k, where k is the number of studies j=1 to n_i values, $B_0 + B_1X_{ij} + B_2X_{ij}^{\ 2}$ is fixed effect part of the model and $S_i + b_iX_{ij} + \varepsilon_{ij}$ is random effect part of the model and $€_{ij}$ is an unknown random error vector modeling the statistical noise. Mixed model can be implemented using SAS (2009) using PROC MIXED as follows.

```
proc mixed data = lact.datab noclprint noitprint;
class study;
model milk_=dcp dcp*dcp bw/solution outp=pred;
random intercept/type=un sub=study ;
run;
```

The above syntax expresses that the outcome Y(dependent variable) is modeled by fixed intercept which is implied in the model, a fixed slope, a random intercept clustered by study and random slope also clustered by study, type=un option in the random statement specifies an unspecified variance-covariance matrix. The variable "study" does not contain quantitative information and constitutes an additional variation source, it was therefore declared in the CLASS statement in the SAS code.

14. Application of meta-analysis in animal research: Cases studies

For better understanding on the concept three case studies on Meta-analysis are presented in this section. Effect of bypass protein on milk yield in Indian cattle (Suresh *et al.*, 2011), factors affecting the laboratory production of buffalo embryos (Suresh *et al.*, 2009) and deriving nutritive requirement for lactating cattle in India.

14.1 Effect of bypass protein on milk yield in Indian cattle: a meta-analysis

Twenty Indian studies pertaining to feeding of undegradable dietary protein (UDP) on milk production in lactating cows were selected. Based on inclusion and exclusion criteria to safeguard against the selection bias, only fourteen studies could be considered for conducting a meta-analysis. All the data included in the present study were from experiments conducted under iso-caloric diets and early to mid lactation with medium milk production (around 10 kg). The bypass protein intake was converted to UDP intake g/animal/day as input variable and milk yield was converted to 4% FCM (fat corrected milk) in order to achieve uniformity in study results. The UDP intake (g/animal/day) was categorized into 0-100, 101-200, 201-300, 301-400, 401-500 and 501-600. A database on UDP intake (g/animal/day), milk yield (kg) and fat % were developed based on the studies selected. The data were analyzed using the Meta-calculator, developed for the purpose.

The results indicated increase in milk yield as the UDP intake was increased. The amount of 4% FCM was 6.62 kg (SD: 0.43) at 0-100 g UDP intake and progressively increased to 10 kg when the UDP intake was >600 g/animal/day. The milk production response was observed to be quadratic *i.e.*, milk production increased with increasing UDP intake and thereafter milk production showed decreasing trend for unit increase in UDP levels (Fig. 1). From the meta-analysis of the data, it could be concluded that feeding of UDP is beneficial in increasing milk yield and the optimum level of UDP required for production of 10 kg 4 % FCM among Indian cattle is about 571 g/animal/day (Suresh *et al.*, 2011).

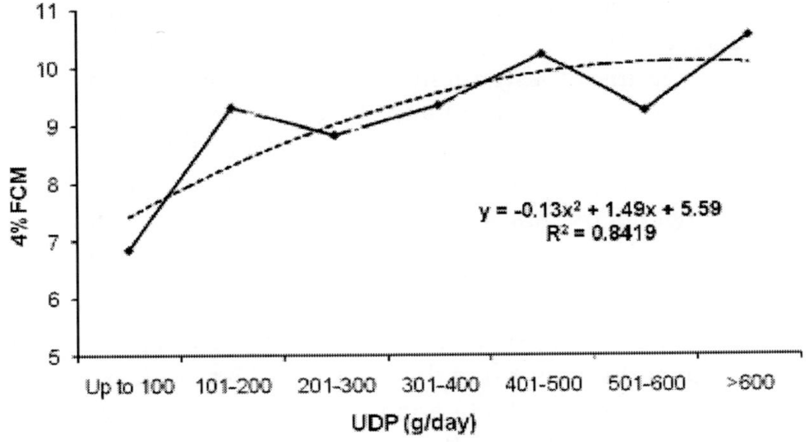

Fig. 1 : Meta –regression depecting the optimum level of UDP

14.2. Factors affecting laboratory production of buffalo embryos: a meta-analysis

Poor genetic makeup and reproductive failures limit the productivity of buffalo, an important species in India in terms of milk and meat production as well as draft. Assisted reproductive technologies like artificial insemination (AI), super-ovulation, *in vitro* fertilization (IVF), embryo transfer (ET) have been introduced to overcome these problems, to increase the number of offspring from selected females and to reduce the generation intervals in buffalo. Laboratory production of embryos (IVF technology) provides an excellent and cheap source of embryos for carrying out basic research on developmental physiology, farm animal breeding and for commercial application of the emerging bio-techniques like cloning and transgenesis. During the past two decades, considerable advancements have been made and more are still to come as a result of continuous scientific efforts. However, the rate of transferable embryo yield remains at a plateau. There are lots of variations exist in success rate among the laboratories hence, there is a need to analyze the conditions, protocols and factors that affect the successes rate of IVF in buffalo. A meta-analysis study was undertaken to analyse the factors affecting the successes rate in terms of maturation rate, fertilization rate and embryo yield in buffalo obtained in various laboratories. The idea was to analyze the present status of IVF in buffaloes identify the factors causing the inconsistencies between previous studies and to throw some lights on future direction of research in this field which can play a key role in planning new studies. About 100 literatures were searched and the study results were subjected to meta-analysis to determine the treatment variations without any bias. Various factors of maturation, cleavage and embryo yield were examined. Given a vast quantity of heterogeneous literature, the type of items that were collected include the characteristics on the report of the study (such as author, year and source), the study itself, research design (experimental or observational, treatment assignment mechanism or sampling mechanism, attrition rate or non-response rate) and the effect size (sample size, nature of outcome, estimates and standard error). For example, total 32 factors affecting *in vitro* embryo production in buffalo were considered (Suresh *et al.*, 2009). The extracts of results on 5 factors on the maturation, fertilization /cleavage and embryo production rate for all these factors are presented in Table 1.

By synthesizing, scrutinizing, tabulating, and perhaps integrating all relevant studies, meta-analysis allows a more objective appraisal, which can help to resolve uncertainties when the original research, classical reviews and editorial comments disagree. Meta-analysis is a scientific activity that borrows from both the expert review and the methodology of multi-centre studies.

14.3 Deriving nutritive requirement for lactating cattle in India: A meta-analysis

Articles published were sought using the on-line journal databases Web of Science (ISI, UK), CAB (CABI Publishing) and VET CDs. Articles were also found by cross-referencing citations in retrieved articles. No unpublished study was considered. About 41 peer reviewed studies with 753 lactating cattle of low & medium milk yielders, elaborating the body weight, milk yield, Dry matter intake (DMI), metabolizable energy intake (MEI), total digestible nutrient (TDN) and crude protein (CP) was extracted from studies.

Table 1 : Factors affecting maturation, fertilization and embryo yield in buffalo

S. No	Factors	Maturation rate	Cleavage/ Fertilization rate	Embryo yield
1	Serum	80.56± 0.06 (3127)	51.79±0.14 (2632)	16.08±0.09 (2310)
2	FSH+LH+E2	71.73± 0.16 (1662)	63.21±0.14 (2762)	18.27±0.10 (2639)
3	FSH	77.09± 0.23 (1779)	43.64±0.12 (1766)	19.51±0.17 (1384)
4	Cumulous investment (good)	69.49±0.28 (948)	59.95±0.35 (783)	25.79±0.29 (744)
5	Cumulous investment (moderate to good)	35.24±0.23 (988)	40.67±0.40 (855)	4.76±0.14 (779)

Numbers in bracket are sample size considered for meta-analysis, Mean ± SE

The criteria for selecting the studies were (i) Indian studies, (ii) lactating cattle and (iii) milk yield of 5 to 15 kg (4%FCM), and (iv) experiments conducted in normal conditions. The DM, CP, TDN and ME were converted to per animal per day as input variables and milk yield was converted to 4% FCM (fat corrected milk) in order to achieve uniformity in study results. Given a vast quantity of heterogeneous literature, the type of items that were collected include the characteristics on the report of the study (such as author, year and source), the study itself, research design (experimental or observational, treatment assignment mechanism or sampling mechanism, attrition rate or non-response rate). Descriptive statistical analysis was performed to standardize the data for outliers. Data was analyzed using the general linear model (Mixed models) and quadratic function analysis to understand the linear and quadratic relationship between the study variables. Mixed model by using the PROC MIXED (SAS 9.2) was performed to predict the nutrient requirements for different body weight and milk yield animals. The mixed model equations were developed for prediction of DM, TDN and CP requirement of Indian cattle were as follows:

$$DM = 3.4672 - 0.0061 * BW + 0.2872 * milk - 0.00913 * milk^2$$

$$CP = 28.5045 - 0.2755 * BW + 54.117 * milk - 1.8186 * milk^2$$

$$TDN = 1.6587 - 0.00454 * BW + 0.3106 * milk - 0.01062 * milk^2$$

Where, DMI is dry matter intake, CP is crude protein, TDN is total digestible nutrients, BW is the body weight. The results of prediction equations for deriving nutritive requirement is presented in Table 2.

Table 2 : Nutritive requirement of lactating Indian Cattle for different body weight and milk yield

S. No	Body weight (kg)	Milk yield (4% FCM)	DM (kg)	CP (kg)	TDN (kg)	ME (MJ)	Required % DCP in total diet	Required % TDN in total diet	Required ME/kg diet
1	300	5	8.5	0.51	4.8	71.3	6.0	55.9	8.4
2	300	6	9.1	0.61	5.3	80.0	6.7	58.8	8.8
3	300	7	9.6	0.70	5.9	87.8	7.3	61.1	9.2
4	300	8	10.0	0.78	6.3	94.6	7.7	62.9	9.4
5	300	9	10.4	0.84	6.7	100.4	8.1	64.3	9.6
6	300	10	10.8	0.90	7.0	105.3	8.3	65.3	9.8
7	350	5	8.9	0.54	4.8	71.3	6.2	53.7	8.0
8	350	6	9.5	0.66	5.4	81.4	7.0	57.1	8.6
9	350	7	10.1	0.77	6.0	90.5	7.6	59.7	9.0
10	350	8	10.6	0.86	6.6	98.4	8.1	61.8	9.3
11	350	9	11.1	0.93	7.0	105.3	8.4	63.3	9.5
12	350	10	11.5	1.00	7.4	111.0	8.7	64.4	9.7
13	400	5	8.9	0.57	4.5	67.8	6.4	50.8	7.6
14	400	6	9.6	0.70	5.3	79.4	7.3	54.9	8.2
15	400	7	10.3	0.82	6.0	89.8	7.9	58.0	8.7
16	400	8	10.9	0.92	6.6	98.9	8.5	60.4	9.1
17	400	9	11.4	1.01	7.1	106.7	8.8	62.2	9.3
18	400	10	11.9	1.09	7.5	113.2	9.1	63.4	9.5

15. Benefits of meta-analysis

The Benefits of meta-analysis include a consolidated and quantitative review of a large, and often complex, sometimes apparently conflicting body of literature. A substantial benefit of meta-analysis is the potential to investigate the new hypothesis using existing data, both through the development of a priori hypothesis and by examination of heterogeneity.

Conclusions

Meta-analysis cannot be thought of as a quick as easy way to pull a lot of studies together and come with a publication, but like any other study, requires an appreciable investment of time in planning and implementation. As with any scientific procedures, there are areas of controversy, like inclusion of studies with various amount of heterogeneity, selection of models of meta-analysis etc. In summary, a meta-analysis is an important and valuable tool for summarizing data from multiple studies. However, it is not an easy task and requires careful thought and planning to provide accurate and useful information.

References

Cochran W. (1937). Problems arising in the series of similar experiments. *Journal Royal Statistical Association* **4:** 102-118.

Cohen J. (1988). Statistical Power analysis for the behavioral sciences, 2nd edition. Lawrence Earlbaum Associates, Hillsdale, New Jersey, USA.

Cooper H., Hedges L.V. (1994). The Handbook of Research Synthesis. New York, Russell Sage.

Cooper H.M. (1982). Scientific guidelines for conducting integrative reviews. *Review of Educational Research* **52:** 291-302.

Eugene M., Archimede H., Sauvant D. (2004). Quantitative meta-analysis on the effects of defaunation of the rumen on growth, intake and digestion in ruminants. *Livestock Production Science* **85:** 81-91.

Glass G.V. (1976). Primary, secondary and meta-analysis of research. *Education Research* **5:** 3-8.

Greenland S. (1994). Invited commentary. A critical look at some some popular meta-analytic methods. *American Journal of Epidemiology* **110:** 290-296.

Hedges L., Olkin I. (1985). Statistical methods for meta-analysis. Orlando, Florida: Academic press.

Jackson D. (2006). The power of standard test for the presence of heterogeneity in meta-analysis. *Statistics in medicine* **25:** 2688-2699.

Jackson G.B. (1980). Methods of Integrative reviews. *Review of Educational Research* **50:** 438-460.

Lean I.J., Rabiee A.R., Dufield T.F., Dohoo I.R. (2009). Use of meta-analysis in animal health and reproduction: Methods and applications. *Journal Dairy Science* **92:** 3545-3565.

Mondal S., Suresh K.P., Nandi S. (2009). Endocrine Profiles of oestrous cycle in buffalo. A meta-analysis. *Asian-Australian Journal of Animal Sciences* **23:** 169-174.

Normand S. L. (1999). Tutorial in bio-statistics meta-analysis. Russell Sage Foundation. New York.

Sauvart D., Schmidely P., Daudin J.J., St Peirre N.R. (2008). Meta-analysis of experimental data in animal Nutrition. *Animal* **2-8:** 1203-1214.

Simonds M.C., Higgins J.P.T., Stewart L.A., Tierney J.F., Clarke M. J., Thompson S. G. (2005). Meta-analysis of individual patient data from randomized trials: A review of methods used in practice. *Clinical Trials* **2:** 209-217.

St Pierre N.R. (2001). Invited Review: Integrating Quantitative findings from multiple Studies Using Mixed Model Methodology. *Journal Dairy Science* **84:** 741-755.

Stewart L.A., Clarke M. J. (1995). Practical methodology of meta-analysis(overviews) using updated individual patient data. *Statistics in Medicine* **14:** 2057-2079.

Suresh K.P., Nandi S. Mondal S. (2009). Factors affecting laboratory production of buffalo embryos: A meta-analysis. *Theriogenology* **72:** 978-985.

Suresh K.P., Bhatta R., Mondal S., Sampath K.T. (2011). Effect of bypass protein on milk yield in Indian Cattle-a meta-analysis. *Animal Nutrition and Feed Technology* **11:** 19-26.

Williamson P.R., Smith C.T., Hutton J.L., Marson A.G. (2002). Aggregate data meta-analysis with time-to-event outcomes. *Statistics in Medicine* **21:** 3337-3351.

❏❏❏

Chapter 27

Remote Sensing Techniques for Estimation of Crop Residues and Biomass from Grasslands

K. Giridhar, S. Anandan
National Institute of Animal Nutrition and Physiology, Adugodi, Bangalore-560 030, Karnataka, India

Summary

Estimation of animal feed resources availability is an essential step in planning the strategies for improving the livestock productivity. The data from crop cutting experiments is useful to obtain grain to straw ratios of various crops, and the crop residues' production is indirectly estimated from the grain production data by using these ratios. As this traditional method is tedious, time consuming and prone to errors, remote sensing techniques are a better bet for the estimation of crop residues in the country. Vegetation Indices, derived from remote sensing data acquired at maximum vegetative growth stage, are indicative of crop growth, vigour and potential yield.

Once standardized, remote sensing techniques can be utilised to estimate production of residues from various crops as well as for the assessment of green fodder yield from the forage crops. Generation of timely and more precise production estimates of feed resources availability in the country will be of great help for better planning and management of livestock.

The production and productivity of livestock are closely linked to the feed resources availability, as feed is the major input factor in all livestock production systems. Efficient management of feed resources is of great importance for optimizing livestock production. Assessment of animal feed resources availability for any particular region and drawing an inventory of the resources available is a pre-requisite for planning any short term and long term strategies towards improvement of the animal husbandry activities (Raju *et al.*, 2002). In India, the livestock feed resources mostly include crop residues(dry fodder), green fodders and concentrates. Among them, the contribution from the dry fodder is the largest. Systematic and concerted efforts were made in the past two decades to estimate the availability of various feed resources, including the crop residues in the country.

1. Traditional method of estimating the crop residues' production

The availability of crop residues is assessed indirectly based on crop (grain) production by using appropriate conversion factors. The secondary data on crop production available from the Directorate of Economics & Statistics and Directorate of Agriculture is useful for this method. To validate the secondary data, limited primary data on major crop residues need to be collected from different states. Periodical checking of conversion factors can best account for the changes in varietal composition of major crops in the recent past. The availability of crop residues will be estimated from the grain production figures of cereal crops and pulses using the conversion factors based on grain to straw ratios. Since the systematic data of each district/state/agro-climatic zone and also, grain to straw ratio of each crop variety is difficult to obtain, many researchers use a widely accepted product to residue ratio for each crop. In view of the distinct differences in nutritive value of crop residues, the crop residues are generally categorized into four classes as:

- *Fine straw* : Crop residues from rice, wheat and finger millet
- *Coarse straw* : Crop residues from coarse cereals like jowar (Sorghum), bajra (pearl millet), maize and small millets
- *Haulms of legumes* : Crop residues from pulses and groundnut
- *Others* : Sugarcane tops

The evaluation of different methods for obtaining grain to straw ratios has shown that the 'crop cutting experiments (CCE)' data is the ideal one. These experiments are conducted every year for all the crops, for both irrigated and rainfed conditions. The statistical design adopted is multistage stratified random sampling, with taluk/block as strata, and villages within strata as primary sampling unit, and fields within each selected village as secondary sampling unit. The experimental plot is the unit of sampling (final sample selection). The allocation of experiments at district and taluk level is on the basis of proportion of area under crop varieties. The villages within the taluk or block are selected at random from timely reporting scheme villages. In each selected village, two experiments are conducted in two plots of specified size located at different survey numbers. The Directorate of Economics and Statistics is responsible for overall planning, analysis and publication of the results and the district statistical officer takes care of organizing the experiments at district level. The experiments so laid out are supervised by different agencies like the Agriculture department, Revenue department and Directorate of Economics and Statistics. The village accountants of revenue department and agricultural assistants from Agriculture department are the primary workers who select the plot as per the set procedure. They monitor the progress, facilitate supervision and record the fresh weights of both grain and straw after harvest. Data on at least 15 per cent of experiments planned for a specified crop or a minimum of four experiments are taken for the driage experiment on grain portion. The CCE data is used for estimating the production of all the crops in the country. As the estimation of grain yield is very important, all the necessary precautions are taken in the conduct of the CCE. However, the crop residues are not kept for drying to record their dry weights and driage coefficients. Hence, when the results from these experiments are pooled up at district, state and national level, the production figures for crop residues are not being reported, as the entire focus of this exercise is on generation of grain production figures only. To overcome this deficiency, a project was taken up to collect primary data on product to residue ratios of major crops through crop cutting surveys in all the principal states of the country by selecting two to three major districts in each of these states. The ratios for some of the important crops from major states (NIANP, 2010) are presented in Table 1.

Table 1 : Product to residue ratios of selected crops

State	Crop	Product to residue ratio
Punjab	Rice	1:1:36
Punjab	Wheat	1:1.23
Haryana	Rice	1:1.41
Haryana	Wheat	1:1.22
U.P	Rice	1:1.41
Uttarakhand	Rice	1:1.52
Bihar	Rice	1:1.52
Bihar	Wheat	1:1.24
Orissa	Rice	1:1.16
Kerala	Rice	1:1.15
A.P	Rice	1:1.14
A.P	Groundnut	1:1.35
Goa	Rice	1:1.43
West Bengal	Rice	1:1.16
M.P	Durum Wheat	1:1.37
Gujarat	Groundnut	1:2.21
Maharashtra	Jowar	1:1.61
Rajasthan	Jowar	1:1.22

The generation of state-wise residue conversion factors helped in improving the assessment of availability of various crop residues. However, as the crop varieties keep changing, it is essential to work out the grain to straw ratios periodically for better estimation of the availability of crop residues in different parts of the country.

2. Estimation of crop residues' production with remote sensing methods

The crop cutting survey method is tedious, time consuming and prone to errors. In the recent years, the remote sensing (RS) techniques are being used for estimation of acreage and production of various crops like rice, wheat, cotton etc., in our country. Dadhwal and Parihar (1985) made first attempt in India towards the use of satellite digital data for wheat acreage estimation in Karnal district of Haryana State. A project on 'crop acreage and production estimation (CAPE)' under the remote sensing applications with enlarged scope and objectives was formulated in 1986. The RS can provide information on important crop growth variables on a regional scale.

Vegetation indices are derived from remote sensing images and are one of the more popular and extensively studied products for assessing vegetation biomass. These indices are obtained by transformation of spectral bands of the electromagnetic spectrum, measured as reflectance from the earth's surface by earth observing satellites. These indices allow the spatial and temporal variation and relative contribution of vegetation properties such photosynthetic activity and canopy structure to be examined (Huete *et al.,* 2002). They can provide an unbiased representation of vegetation without regard to the soil type, land cover classification, or climatic condition. Since the early 1970s, a variety of vegetation indices have been proposed. These generally involve some combination of the red and near infrared (NIR) portions of the electromagnetic spectrum, specifically wavelengths in the 0.6 to 0.7ìm (red) and 0.75 to 1.1 ìm (NIR) ranges (Tucker *et al.,* 1983). In red range, much of the incident radiation is absorbed by leaf chlorophyll, whereas in the NIR range, the incident radiation is reflected by the leaf mesophyll cells. This provides a sharp contrast in the light reflectance back to the satellite that can be used for ratio or indexing (Brown *et al.,* 2006).

Vegetation indices derived from RS data acquired at maximum vegetative growth stage are indicative of crop growth, vigour and potential grain yield (Hooda *et al.,* 2006). Of the various vegetation indices, the 'normalized difference vegetation index (NDVI)' is the most used and accepted historically (Cracknell, 2001). The NDVI is a numerical indicator that uses the visible and near-infrared bands of the electromagnetic spectrum, and is adopted to analyze remote sensing measurements and assess whether the target being observed contains live green vegetation or not. It is computed from the red and NIR bands as follows:

NDVI = (ρnir - ρr) / (ρnir + ρr)

where, ρnir and ρr are the spectral reflectance values of the near-infrared and red wavelengths, respectively.

Generally, healthy vegetation will absorb most of the visible light that falls on it, and reflects a large portion of the near-infrared light. Unhealthy or sparse vegetation reflects more visible light and less near-infrared light. The NDVI values can range between -1 and +1. Increasing amounts of vegetation increase the index towards 1. This index has been used as surrogate to estimate leaf area index, vegetation biomass, and fraction of absorbed photosynthetically active radiation (Sellers, 1985). The experience gained over more than a decade of implementation of crop acreage and production estimation project has been used in formulating and implementing a project FASAL (Forecasting Agricultural output using Space, Agro-meteorology and Land-based observations), an integrated approach, to ensure nation–wide forecast of production of major crops. It uses inputs from the three types of observations, namely, field survey, weather and space to make multiple, in-season forecasts of desired coverage, accuracy, and timeliness (Dadhwal *et al.*, 2002). The FASAL is issuing multiple seasonal forecasts where the pre planting forecast is being taken care by Institute of Economic Growth, New Delhi and subsequent forecasts by Indian Meteorological Department and Space Applications Centre.

Due to the availability of quality satellite data and appropriate methodologies, estimations through these techniques are more objective, accurate and reliable. Hence, a study was taken up by National Institute of Animal Nutrition and Physiology, Bangalore in collaboration with National Remote Sensing Centre, Hyderabad for testing the feasibility of using remote sensing techniques to estimate the production of crop residues. As the first step, estimation of stover production is being tried out from *rabi* sorghum (jowar) in two districts i.e., Solapur (Maharashtra) and Kurnool (A.P). The LISS (Linear Imaging Self Scanner) sensor-III data of 'Indian remote sensing (IRS)' satellite with a spatial resolution of 24 m of November/December, corresponding to the optimal bio-window of jowar crop is chosen. During this period, the crop attains maximum vegetative growth, covering the canopy background fully. The data is analyzed for acreage estimation using maximum likelihood supervised classification. Ground truth is collected near synchronous to satellite pass from large contiguous and homogeneous sites of jowar grown under different physiographic conditions in both Solapur and Kurnool districts. The various steps involved in the acreage estimation are given in Fig. 1. The acreage and production data for these two districts is collected from the Department of Agriculture. After the area estimation, the major steps involved in the estimation of production from satellite imagery are superimposition of the crop mask, extraction of NDVI for jowar areas, studying the correlation between NDVI with crop parameters like leaf area index and the inversion of resulting relationship model. The flow chart for yield estimation is presented in figure 2. The estimates of acreage and stover production derived from satellite data will be compared with the data obtained from the Agriculture department to determine the accuracy of estimation.

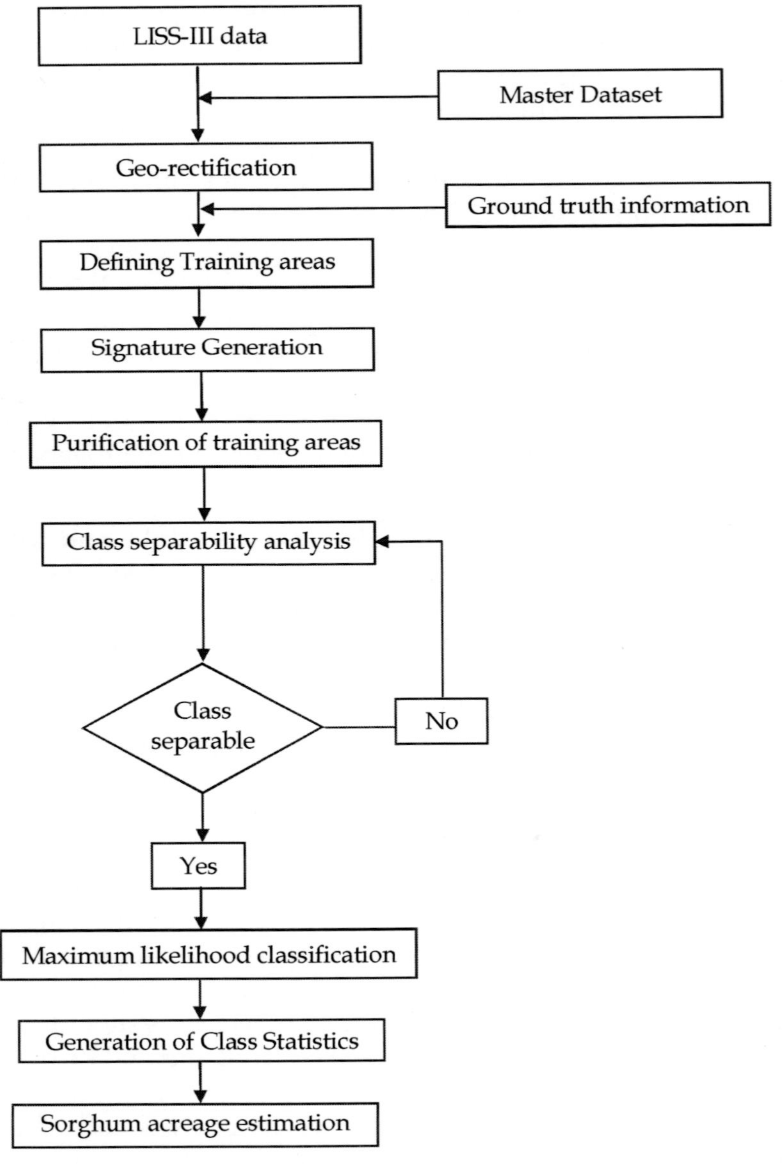

Fig. 1 : Flow chart of analysis of satellite data for sorghum acreage estimation

Once standardized, this technique can be extended to estimate production of residues from other major food crops and this information will be of great help in terms of better accuracy as well as the timeliness. As the information would be available much before the crop is harvested, it can greatly facilitate for taking informed decisions for addressing the feed surplus or shortage issues. The impact of natural calamities on feed availability of the livestock can be mitigated effectively with timely positive interventions.

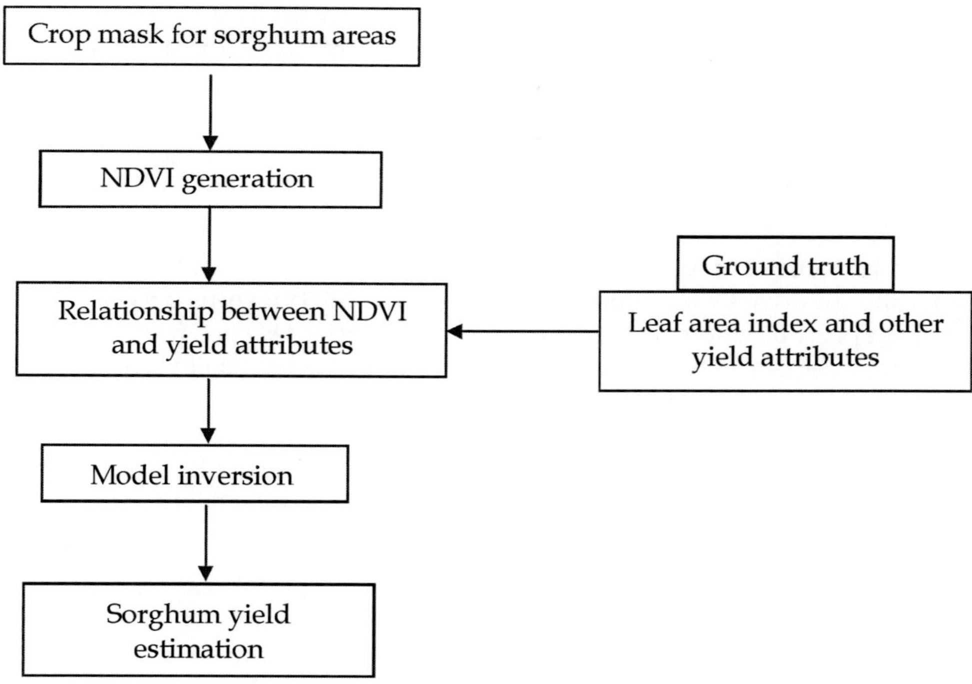

Fig. 2 : Flow chart for estimation of sorghum production

3. Estimation of biomass from grasslands

The field technique like quadrant method is an accurate method for assessing forage quality and quantity on grasslands. However, it requires a lot of time and resources for data collection, especially if data is needed on a periodical basis. The use of remote sensing imagery can be useful for assessing vegetation conditions in grasslands due to its wide aerial coverage, ability to examine remote or inaccessible areas, and the information availability at frequent time intervals than possible from field sampling. Since the 1970s, remote sensing imagery is in use for assessing the vegetation condition on rangelands. The approaches generally used for assessment of biomass using remote sensing imagery are:

1. Empirical models that predict the forage biomass based on a statistical relationship between the spectral bands or combination of bands in the image and vegetation biomass.
2. Process models that use remote sensing data as inputs for predicting the biomass.

In India, remote sensing data has been used for estimation of the extent of grasslands in various national parks. In New Zealand, forage yield in dairy pastures was predicted with over 90% accuracy by using a regression model that related NDVI and time of year to forage biomass (Mata *et al.*, 2007). Although much evidence exists that the application of biomass prediction on grasslands using remote sensing parameters is feasible, the extrapolation of these relationships to new areas is not always feasible or recommended. Generally, field data need to be collected for new areas or regions for developing the prediction equations.

Approaches for using remote sensing data to estimate forage quality generally involve the development of statistical relationships between remote sensing spectral band data and forage quality variables such as crude protein and forage digestibility. However, use of remote sensing data to estimate forage quality is not as extensive as that for the estimation of quantity. It is mostly related to the difficulties in obtaining forage quality information to use in empirical and modelling approaches. It is difficult to determine an appropriate sampling scheme to measure forage quality, especially when vegetation is highly heterogeneous.

Integration of field collected data, simulation model output, and remote sensing data into a 'geographical information system (GIS)' will help in generation of more comprehensive inventory of feed resources for better utility. A pertinent example of such an approach is the model developed by Stuth *et al.* (2005) for forage quantity assessment on a regional level for East Africa. This 'livestock early warning system (LEWS)' was developed to provide near real-time estimates of forage biomass and deviation from average conditions to provide pastoralists, policy makers, and other stakeholders with information on emerging forage conditions for making better risk management decision. The system combines field data collection from a series of monitoring sites, simulation model outputs, statistical forecasting, and GIS to produce regional maps of current and forecast forage conditions.

In the current Indian database, compared to crop residues and concentrates, the assessment of green fodder is the weakest link due to poor documentation on several aspects of green fodder i.e., area under fodder cultivation, productivity of various fodder crops, fodder biomass potential of different land categories etc. Till now, the estimation of green biomass from cultivated fodder and also, from different land categories is based on published literature that is quite old. Hence, the accuracy of such estimates is a matter of debate. With the advances in remote sensing techniques and the successful adoption of the same in different parts of the world, it should be possible to use and standardize them to quantify the green biomass availability from different land categories in Indian conditions. This would greatly help in assessing the green fodder availability precisely and improve the feeding of livestock and management of land resources in extensive and semi-extensive systems.

Further, even with regard to the assessment of dry fodder and concentrates, though the present approach of estimation based on the extraction ratios is reasonably good due to regular reporting of crop production data, such a data is not available immediately after the crop harvesting period. The common problem is that the final production data of crops is reported after a time lag of one to two years. For each crop, the average values of productivity and the extraction ratios are generally used to calculate the availability. The inter-state or inter-regional variations are not taken into consideration. However, by using remote sensing techniques, it will not only be possible to get timely data but also capture these regional differences. They can improve the precision of estimating dry fodder and concentrates. Although remote sensing can be powerful tool that can be applied to assess a wide range of resources, the technique needs to be standardized to suit our situation and the results have to be cross checked with the ground truth data for validation before their wider application.

Conclusions

Development of timely inventories of dry and green fodder in developing countries like India will facilitate efficient management of livestock feeding and better handling of the serious issues like feed shortage and surplus. The traditional method of estimating crop residues and biomass production from grass lands is laborious and time consuming. Therefore, there is an urgent need to apply the standardized remote sensing technique for the quick inventory assessment of the crop residues and biomass from the grass land for the livestock feeding. Developed countries have adopted this method however; developing countries need to tap the advantages of this recent technique which would help in efficient management of already available feed resources.

References

Brown M.E., Pinzon J.E., Didan K., Morisette J.T., Tucker C.J. (2006). Evaluation of the consistency of long-term NDVI time series derived from AVHRR, SPOT-Vegetation, SeaWiFS, MODIS, and Landsat ETM+ sensors. *IEEE Transactions on Geoscience and Remote Sensing* **44:** 1787-1793.

Cracknell A.P. (2001). The exciting and totally unanticipated success of the AVHRR inapplications for which it was never intended. *Advances in Space Research* **28:** 233-240.

Dadhwal V.K., Singh R.P., Dutta.S., Parihar J.S. (2002). Remote sensing based crop inventory: a review of Indian experience. *Tropical Ecology* **43:** 107-122.

Dadhwal V.K., Parihar J.S. (1985). Estimation of 1983-84 wheat acreage of Karnal district (Haryana) using Landsat MSS digital data. *Technical Note, IRS-UP/SAC/CPF/TN/09/85*. Space Applications Centre, Ahmedabad, India.

Hooda R.S., Yadav M., Kalubarme, M. H. (2006). Wheat production estimation using remote sensing data - an Indian experience. In: *ISPRS Archives XXXVI-8/W48 Workshop proceedings: Remote sensing support to crop yield forecast and area estimates*. November 30 December 1, 2006, Stresa, Italy.

Huete A., Didan K., Miura T., Rodriguez E. P., Gao X., Ferreira, L. G. (2002). Overview of the radiometric and biophysical performance of the MODIS vegetation indices. *Remote Sensing of Environment* **83:** 195-213.

Mata M., Clark D. A., Edirisinghe A., Waugh D., Minneé E. Gherardi S. G. (2007).Predicting accurate paddock average pasture cover in Waikato dairy farms using satellite images. *Proceedings of the 69th Annual NZ Grassland Association Conference* **69:** 23-28.

NIANP. (2010). *Annual report 2009-10*. National Institute of Animal Nutrition and Physiology, Bangalore, Karnataka.

Raju S.S., Anandan S., Angadi U.B., Ananthram K., Prasad C.S., Ramachandra K.S. (2002). Assessment of animal feed resource availability in Southern Karnataka region. *Indian Journal of Animal Sciences* **72:** 1137-1140.

Sellers P. J. (1985). Canopy reflectance, photosynthesis and transpiration. *International Journal of Remote Sensing* **6:** 1335-1372.

Tucker C.J., Vanpraet C., Boerwinkel E., Gaston A. (1983). Satellite remote-sensing of total dry-matter production in the Senegalese Sahel. *Remote Sensing of Environment* **13:** 461-474.

□□□

Chapter 28

Refined Approaches for Assessment of Feed Availability and Requirements

S. Anandan, S. Jash, U.B. Angadi, K. Giridhar
National Institute of Animal Nutrition and Physiology, Adugodi, Bangalore-560 030, Karnataka, India

Summary

Growing demand for livestock products coupled with shrinking natural resources calls for efficient management of all the inputs. Feed being the largest input, an efficient information system on feed availability and requirements can immensely help the policy makers, planners and developmental agencies in formulating and implementing effective schemes for livestock development. Assessing feed availability *vis-a-vis* requirements for a large country like India with diverse production systems and productivity is a challenging task. Added to the diversity, lack of proper documentation of various components of livestock production systems makes the task much more challenging. Existing system of assessment either through primary surveys or approaches based on secondary survey have certain limitations and there is a need to address these limitations to make the results much more reliable. Areas of refinements include assessing the non-feed uses of the feed resources, improvement in the precision of estimates of green fodder from cultivated fodder and other sources and assessing the requirements of different species of livestock as per the age categories and productivity. Further assessment of feed resources should not be a onetime exercise but it needs to be a regular activity as is being done for the food sector. This will not only ensure the timely updates on the recent position but would enhance the competitiveness of the livestock sector ensuring profitability and sustainability.

The growing demand for livestock products and need for economic and efficient production calls for better management of feed resources which account for 60-70% of the recurring cost of production. Consumption of livestock products is closely related to income levels and as the income levels in developing countries is growing rapidly over the last two decades; the consumption level of animal products has also increased (Steinfeld *et al.*, 2006). In most of the Asian countries, the demand for livestock products will outstrip the production levels and the demands are projected to grow by 2 to 3 times by 2050 (Devendra and Leng, 2011). As per the recent estimate, the consumption of livestock products in 2030 expressed as percentage increase of the 2000 consumption level in India for beef, milk, mutton, pork, poultry and eggs will be 51, 119, 85, 160, 844 and 280% respectively by (Robinson and Pozzi, 2011). The need for precise estimates of feed availability and requirements becomes all the more important when there is a shortage of feeds and the increasing feed costs and declining profits margins is a matter of concern. For a large country like India with diverse - production systems, livestock productivity, feeding practices and agro-eco regions coupled with poor documentation of the feeding practices and production systems makes the task of assessing feed resources much more difficult. The present chapter briefly discusses the need and utility of assessment, constraints, current approaches and their limitations and refinements for improving the precision of the estimates.

1. Need for assessment

Globally India ranks first in the milk production, third in egg and fish production, fifth position in broiler meat. Sustaining the present levels of production and catering to the growing demand for future from limited land and water resources will be a mammoth task. This effort would call for efficient management of all the inputs and feed is no exception. The first and foremost requirement for efficient management of any commodity is the information on its inventory (what is available and how much) and requirements which can be taken as a starting point based on which informed decisions can be taken for its optimal use. This is much truer for a commodity like animal feeds which on one hand is in short supply and on other hand is in great demand. Unlike the food sector where the government has reasonably good information system on the production of the grains and the reserve stocks against the requirements of the population, the information system on feed availability and requirements is underdeveloped or nonexistent (Ramachandra *et al.*, 2007, FAO, 2010). As a result, achieving food security is relatively easier to implement by taking appropriate interventions based on the information and a similar system needs to be developed for achieving feed security for the livestock sector. Although this is an important component of livestock production however, this has not received the due attention of the planners, policy makers and researchers alike. This in turn has resulted in the present situation where we are still struggling with multiple data from different agencies on the estimates of feed availability and requirements. For a large country like India with huge livestock population and production of livestock products, the information on the actual availability and requirements can provide the strategic information for realizing the full potential of our livestock wealth and improve our competitiveness in the global markets.

2. Utility of feed assessment

Feed assessment provides a realistic scenario based on which planners, policy makers and developmental agencies can develop meaningful plans, policies and schemes for livestock development. It is quite often observed that some of the ambitious schemes undertaken by different state governments and developmental agencies for livestock improvement by introducing elite animals of dairy/small ruminants have failed in spite of the good intentions and feed shortage has been one of the major factors. A realistic estimate of the feed availability would have probably helped them in identifying the appropriate regions and number of animals to be introduced resulting in better development. Correct assessment at regional or national level enables the local and national government in streamlining the export and import of feed resources as per the needs. Similarly the information on feed assessment can help the developmental agencies in tackling natural calamities like flood and droughts in sourcing the feed from the nearest surplus regions. This is much more true for a country like India where rainfed ecosystems accounts for 68% of the total cultivated area and supports 65% of the livestock population (Misra *et al* .,2009). Further with the help of powerful statistical tools and models the likely availability and demand for feeds under different production scenarios can be predicted (Gorti *et al.*,2012) which can greatly help the planners and policy makers in taking strategic initiatives and prepare for the future. Information on feed requirements and future demand can be very useful in determining the crops, land and water requirements for fulfilling these demands in sustainable manner. The information can be very handy for traders in chalking out their business strategy in locating their feed factories or setting up of farms in areas with sufficient feeds. It is more often easier to transport the livestock products to markets than transporting the feeds to farms located near markets. Additionally with intensification of the livestock systems more and more cereal grains are being used in feeding and monitoring the quantum of grains diverted for feed use is essential for achieving food security. Regular updating and refinement in feed assessment can be used to develop long term strategies for development of livestock sector, aid in exports by improving the competitiveness of livestock production systems and convincing aid agencies in seeking funds for developmental activities. Further the information on the feed availability and animals in different regions can greatly help the experts in evolving production systems that are best suited to different regions leading to economic production, competitiveness and environmental sustainability.

3. Constraints in assessment of feed resources

For a large country like India with different production systems, different agro eco regions, wide range of feed resources, diversity in breeds and productivity presents the greatest challenge in realistic assessment of feed resources. With regard to availability of feeds the greatest challenge is in terms of assessing the green fodder production, as the data on area under green fodder production and their productivity in different agro eco regions is either lacking or too little to arrive at realistic estimates. Similarly the green fodder availability from different categories of land like pastures, fallows, orchards and waste lands presents a greater challenge due to variation in the grass cover, soil types, rain fall and consequently the biomass production potential. Compared to greens, feed resources of crop origin are relatively easy as crop production data is available and updated at regular intervals and the extraction ratios for various byproducts are well documented. However there is a need to update the extraction ratios periodically and also properly document the non-feed uses of byproducts which is seriously lacking. Besides, a variety of agro industrial byproducts are used as feeds and the information on their availability is not documented.

Assessing the requirements of feeds for organized poultry is much easier than other species. This is mainly due to uniform productivity and feeding systems in poultry across the different regions. Unlike poultry, in ruminants the productivity of various breeds and the feeding systems varies across the different regions thus making the assessment difficult. The ruminant production system comprising of cattle, buffalo, sheep and goats represents the largest system accounting for the bulk of feed requirements and a realistic estimate of their requirements is must for arriving at the feed requirements.

The next important sector is aqua sector that is growing rapidly and accounts for reasonably good amount of concentrates share. The feeding systems varies from intensive to semi-intensive to extensive systems of production with poor recording of data on the proportions of different systems and consequently the concentrate requirements. Characterization of feeding systems and their proportions in different regions and the production life cycle of different animals is essential for realistic estimates of feed requirements which unfortunately have not been carried out till date. In addition to the major sectors like ruminants, poultry and aqua other minor sectors like pigs, equines, camels, yaks, mithuns etc. should also be considered to assess the feed requirement/availability to account for all the animals that utilize feed.

4. Different approaches for assessment of feed resources

The approaches for assessment of feed resources can be broadly classified into two categories: primary and secondary. In primary approach, the assessment is carried out by conducting a survey of the representative sample (village, taluk, district) area since it is not possible to cover the entire households. Ideally speaking the primary survey should be carried out on representative sample of the population, the questionnaire should be detailed enough to cover all the aspects and if possible measurements should be carried out to arrive at exact quantities and the survey should be spread across all the seasons to account for the seasonal variations. The household survey data can then be extrapolated to arrive at the feed demand and consumption at state, region or national level (Dikshit and Birthal, 2010). The major drawback of the primary survey is it is labor intensive, time consuming and requires a large work force to cover large area.

To overcome the limitations of the primary survey, secondary assessment has been resorted to by many workers (Ramachandra *et al.*, 2007; Gorti *et al.*, 2012). This is relatively easy and can be carried out in a short time to cover a large area provided all the information pertaining to feed resources is readily available and is accurate. Majority of the times the desired information for completing the secondary assessment is either lacking or incomplete making the results of the secondary surveys less reliable or accurate.

An ideal approach would be to use the combination of approaches wherein primary and secondary approaches are used together to arrive at the estimates with reasonable accuracy and in a short period of time. A limited primary survey of the representative systems and use of secondary approach based on the published information is a better approach. This when supplemented with the results of the primary survey findings can greatly improve the precision of estimates within a short span of time and with limited man power. It is likely that some of the information may not be able to be addressed by the primary survey and in those circumstances the opinion of the subject matter specialists/experts can be sought to get the desired information. The whole purpose of the exercise is that no gap or missing link should be there to ensure that all the related aspects are taken care to make the assessment as complete and as accurate as possible.

5. Suggested refinements in the assessment of feed resources

The refinements in assessment of feed resources should be a two way approach covering the feed availability estimates and the feed requirements.

5.1 Assessing feed availability

The first and foremost step to assess the feed availability is to have the complete inventory of feed resources used in a particular location or region for all the seasons. This will provide a good starting point from which the sources of feed resources can be traced back to a particular crop or commodity and the likely quantities available can be estimated. A good method of obtaining this information is to conduct a primary survey in representative areas spread across the different seasons to know the nature and quantity of feed resources used. The survey should be accompanied by measuring the quantities of feed and produce, as more often the information provided by farmer may not reflect the exact quantity. Further, this also gives the information on the feeding practices and productivity levels which can be used for precise estimates of feed requirements. A number of feed resources have multiple uses and it is essential to know the proportions of the commodity that is actually used for feeding as this can lead to correct estimate. For example in case of maize apart from feed use it is used by the distilleries and starch industry, hence it is essential to know the proportion of the maize that is used for livestock feeding. Similarly, we need to have the accurate information for all the resources on the proportion of the production that goes for feeding, to avoid overestimation of availability.

The major constraint in assessing the availability of greens is that there is no proper documentation on the area and type of fodder cultivated and their productivity (Ramachandra *et al.*, 2005). There is a need to identify suitable agency to carry out this exercise on regular basis as the information is vital for the livestock production systems. Similarly another area of concern is the availability of greens form pastures, fallow, waste lands and orchards which contribute substantially to the green fodder but have poor records to quantify. Biomass production can vary widely depending on the soil type, rainfall, grazing pressure, and other factors (Taku and Zheng, 2010). Recent advances in remote sensing technology enables in quantification of the green biomass from different categories of land and this techniques need to be adapted to our situations for precise quantification. In fact, this can go beyond the greens and can be used to estimate the grain and crop biomass production thus giving an advantage in terms of timely estimation well in advance before the resources becomes available for feeding.

Further, in regional feed assessments it is generally assumed that the feed resources produced within a region are consumed there itself and this doesn't happen in reality. There is lot of movement of concentrate feeds in and out of the region and of late even crop residues are transported across long distances to fulfill the demand in a region. There is a need to capture this information for better assessment of regional feed balances. Apart from inter-regional movement of feed there is export and import of feeds that are mainly dictated by the international prices and this needs to be accounted for in the feed assessment.

5.2 Assessing feed requirements

Assessing feed requirements is relatively easier than assessing feed availability. Since unlike feeds, the detailed information on availability of animal numbers and their age wise, and function wise categories are well documented and this provides a good starting point for proceeding with the calculations. While assessing the feed requirements, generally feeds are allocated to different categories of livestock to achieve maximum production potential (milk, growth) or fulfill the nutrient requirements as recommended by any standard. This type of approach generally inflates the requirements and may project a scenario which is far from the prevailing practice. In reality this does not happen and farmers generally tend to allocate feeds preferentially to the productive category and neglect some class of animals due to shortage of resources and economic considerations. There is need to work out the requirements using the actual feeding practices which can be obtained by either conducting primary surveys or in consultation with the experts and farming communities to arrive at the requirements based on the actual. Thus assessing the feed requirements should also include the assessments based on the prevailing practices in addition to the ideal requirements as this gives better information for the end users.

After working out the feed availability and the requirements the feed balance needs to be worked out and the feed balance needs to be related to the existing situations to judge its correctness. Any discrepancy with regard to the feed balance and the actual scenario demands a relook at the whole process, interact with the peers and experts to address the drawbacks and refine the approach accordingly.

5.3 Step wise approach for assessing feed availability

- Before proceeding on to the primary survey, it is desirable to have a fair idea about the different production systems and their proportions in the target area of the survey. This can be ascertained by interacting with the local organizations that work closely with the livestock sector. This gives a good start to design the questionnaire to address all the issues and ensure that number and type of clients chosen for survey is true representative of the system and in proportion to their share in the total system.
- The survey should be detailed enough to capture all the possible information - type of resources used for feeding, their quantities fed to each class of animals and source of these resources (home grown or purchased). Most of the times farmers are not aware of the quantity and it is always desirable to measure the quantity of feed offered and record the same instead of relying on the farmer's response.

- Many a times it may be difficult to quantify the feed resources in situations like grazing and in these cases it should be ensured that these resources are also accounted. Although it may not be possible to exactly quantify the biomass obtained during grazing, but based on the season, bio mass availability and duration of grazing, to begin with a fair estimated figure can be used and subsequently the same could be refined by taking the expert inputs and assessing the actual and using the corrected values.
- The type of resources and their quantities tend to differ with the seasons and it should be ensured that survey is carried out during the different seasons to get the seasonal scenarios and the total annual requirement.
- As most of the feed resources are of crop origin the extraction rates for major products and by products should be assessed locally and the local factors should be used for arriving at the feed availability and wherever it is not possible the factors can be adapted based on the expert inputs and published reports.
- Similarly for animals the production and production cycle has to be recorded during the primary survey. While some of the production parameters like milk yield are more easily recordable parameters like growth rate and body weights may not be recorded easily. This could be taken care by using spring balances for small animals like sheep, goat, calves etc and using body measurements for large animals like cattle and buffaloes for arriving at the body weights. Recording the productivity and production cycle (lactation length, age at calving, inter-calving interval, age of slaughter in meat animals) can be useful in arriving at the realistic estimates for feed requirements.
- After having assessed the feed availability and the feed requirements in a particular region it has to be fitted into the following equation

Net feed locally produced + imported feed = feed requirements of all the animals.

Where, net feed produced = total feed produced locally – locally produced feed sold outside the region, imported feed = feed imported from outside the region, and feed requirements of all the animals include the actual amount of feed fed by the farmers for maintenance and production purposes for the total species in a particular region.

The closeness of the availability *vis-a-vis* the requirements in the above equation would give us a fair idea about the precision of the assessment. A large difference in the values would indicate that the entire exercise has to be revisited and reviewed critically in consultation with the experts and the refinements carried out to arrive at a realistic estimate. Further, it should be clear that while assessing the feed availability and requirements it is not possible to gather/collect all the details and as a result there would always be an error component which is inevitable (Anandan *et al.*, 2005). The extent to which this error component would be accepted would largely depend on the scale of assessment (village, taluk, district, state, region or nation), quality of the information and the diversity of the production systems. Generally speaking an assessment for state or nation has a larger error component due to large diversity in the production system and limited information on several key components.

While assessing the requirements the standard practice is to allocate feeds to all categories of livestock as per the standard recommendation to enable the animal to achieve its maximum genetic potential and a result the requirements arrived are always on the higher side than what is practised by the farmers. The requirements arrived as per the prevailing practices are generally based on economic feeding where only productive animals are fed as per the requirements and the rest of the non productive animals are generally underfed due to shortage of resources or economic considerations.

Further, feed assessment is a continuous exercise that has to be carried out regularly to account for the changes in the availability and requirements of feeds. Regular updating not only provides the recent information that can immensely help the planners and policy makers in taking the right decision but also help in refining the methodological approach for better assessment.

Conclusions

Assessing livestock feed availability and requirements are an important exercise that can provide useful information for efficient management of feed resources that is increasingly becoming scarce and costly. The present approaches of assessment need to be refined in terms of i)the feed resources that are actually available for feeding rather than the potential availability ii) better precision for green fodder availability (area & productivity) and iii) requirements for livestock needs to be worked out for different age categories, productive functions and production systems. A combination of approaches using secondary data, inputs from the primary survey of representative households and wherever required using the expert inputs from the concerned to have the complete information with regard to all the resources and requirements is suggested. Regular assessments and relating the results of the findings to the actual scenario is the best indicator of the reliability of the assessment approach. Refining the approaches and updating the information on a regular basis is the best way to improve the efficiency of resource management of not only the feed but the entire livestock sector as it is a well established fact that the current production and productivity will be chiefly driven by feed in addition to the breed and management.

References

Anandan S., Raju S.S., Angadi U.B., Ramachandra K.S. (2005). Status of livestock and feed resources of Malnad Region in Karnataka. *Animal Nutrition and Feed Technology* **5:** 99-105.

Devendra C., Leng R.A. (2011). Feed resources for animals in Asia: Issues, strategies for use, intensification and integration for increased productivity. *Asian-Australasian Journal of Animal Science* **24:** 303-321.

Dikshit A.K., Birthal P.S. (2010). India's Livestock Feed Demand: Estimates and Projections. *Agricultural Economics Research Review* **23:** 15-28.

FAO. (2010). The State of Food Insecurity in the World 2010: Addressing food insecurity in protracted crises. *Food and Agriculture Organisation of the United Nations*, Rome, p 56.

Misra A.K., Rama Rao C.A., Saubramanyam K.V., Ramakrishna Y.S. (2009). Improving dairy production in India's rainfed agroecosystem: constraints and strategies. *Outlook Agriculture* **38:** 284-292.

Ramachandra K.S., Raju S.S., Anandan S., Angadi U.B. (2005). Animal feed resources and its impact on livestock production in India. *Indian Dairyman* **57:** 39-47.

Ramachandra K.S., Taneja V.K., Sampath K.T., Anandan S., Angadi U.B. (2007). Livestock feed resources in different agro-ecosystems of India: availability, requirement and their management. *National Institute of Animal Nutrition and Physiology*, Bangalore.

Gorti R.K., Suresh K.P., Sampath K.T., Giridhar K., Anandan S. (2012). Modeling and forecasting livestock and fish feed resources: Requirement and availability in India. National Institute of Animal Nutrition and Physiology, Bangalore, p 100.

Robinson T.P., Pozzi F. (2011). Mapping supply and demand for animal-source foods to 2030. Livestock production and health division (AGA) working paper. Food and Agriculture Organization of the United Nations, Rome *(In press).*

Steinfeld H., Gerber P., Wassenaar T., Castel V., Rosales M., de Haan C. (2006). Livestock's long shadow: Environmental issues and options. *Food and Agriculture Organization of the United Nations*, Rome.

Taku D., Zheng H Y. 2010. Regulation of plant biomass production. *Current Opinion in Plant Biology* **13:** 299-304.

❑❑❑

Chapter 29

Strategies for Transfer of Technology for Enhancing Livestock Production

Letha Devi, P. Khandekar
Economics, Statistics and Extension Section, NIANP, Adugodi, Bangalore-560 030, Karnataka, India

Summary

Improvement in livestock production is important for increasing the income of marginal and small farmers and landless labourers, given the uncertainties of agriculture. The livestock extension plays an important role to empower the farmers with appropriate knowledge and skills through informal education and training programs. Veterinarians or para-vets at the grass root level are considered as veterinary extension personnel. In the years to come, they will have to play an active role in acquisition, processing and delivering relevant information to the livestock farmers. The future extension thrust should be on marketing extension, farmwomen empowerment, facilitating formation of low-resource-base farmer's groups, private extension services and environmental extension for sustainability in farming. The research in extension needs to generate data on farming system, cost effectiveness of extension methods, accountability and extension federation for effective functioning of extension systems.

The livestock sector plays an important role in the rural economy of India next to land and irrigation; livestock is the single largest asset of rural farmers. Livestock provides draught power, milk, meat, eggs, wool etc., and thus ensuring regular additional income to farm families. About 75 percent of the Indian rural households have livestock, out of which nearly 80 percent is owned by resource poor farmers. Moreover, livestock and livelihood have an intimate relationship particularly in arid and semi arid areas. Seemingly, livestock production in India is largely associated with small holders and millions of rural households depend either directly or indirectly on livestock for their livelihoods. Livestock provides a major source of supplementary income for a large majority of rural households and provides sustenance during drought and other natural calamities.

Improvement in livestock production is an important pathway for increasing the income of marginal and small farmers and landless laborers, given the uncertainties of agriculture. The livestock extension education plays an important role in this context to empower the farmers with appropriate technological knowledge and skills through various informal education and training programs. This chapter briefs about livestock extension with a special reference to Indian livestock farming situation.

1. Purpose and significance

Livestock extension involves systematic and organized communication with livestock owners with a view to help them in such a way that the livestock owners acquire sufficient knowledge and skills necessary to increase production or reduce cost of production; develop positive attitude towards livestock development; identify problems, look for solutions, solve the identified problems; and evaluate the results within the farming system in which they are operating.

The subject matter delivered should be directly applicable to the livestock owners, for livestock development. This could be accomplished by designing the training program based on the needs of livestock owners. It is also important for the extension agencies to help the development of leadership among the livestock farmers. There are no means by which a large number of livestock owners, spread throughout length and breadth of the country, can be forced to practice animal husbandry in a specific way.

Livestock extension cannot operate in standalone situation and it needs the support of various other grass root level institutions and several groups of people. In addition to livestock extension, the other elements required for enhancing animal production are; remunerative market, assured water and electricity supply, local availability and accessibility of inputs such as feed, medicines, vaccines, technical services and equipments, transportation and storage facilities, timely credit supply, and appropriate policy on animal husbandry. The domain of knowledge covered by livestock extension are; technical problems such as selection of livestock, improved breeding, feeding, housing and management, farm records and organizational problems like importance of culling of animals, labour management, mechanization, credit and its repayment, farm plans, etc.

2. Historical background of livestock extension programs

The history of animal husbandry extension dates back to 1952, when the key village scheme was introduced. Later, a number of schemes or projects have been introduced to transfer the technologies and thereby improve livestock production (Govt. of India, Ministry of Agriculture, 1976).

2.1 All India key village scheme

The key village scheme (KVS) was a novel attempt with basic aim to bring about rapid improvement in the production potentiality of milch animals through improved breeding, effective health care, and scientific management and organized marketing facilities.

2.2 Intensive cattle development project (ICDP)

Government of India introduced ICDP in the year 1963, which was contemplated to locate the projects in the breeding tracts of indigenous breeds of cattle and buffaloes and in the milk shed areas of large dairy projects.

2.3 Operation Flood

The foundation for a viable, modern and self-sustaining dairy industry based on cooperative concepts was laid in 1970 in the form of Operation Flood. The National Dairy Development Board (NDDB) implemented this biggest dairy development project in three phases (Phase-I : 1970-1981, Phase-II : 1981-1985 and Phase-III : 1985-1996).

2.4 Dairy cooperatives

The first milk cooperative in Kaira district started with an initial collection of 250 litre and is now more popularly known as AMUL (Anand Milk Union Limited). Anand pattern is a three tier system of cooperative organization, with village level 'primary milk producers' cooperative societies', milk producers' union at district level and milk producers' federation at state level. At national level there is a 'national cooperative dairy federation'.

2.5 Technology mission on dairy development

The mission was launched in August 1988 and assigned 29 need based research program through research institutes of ICAR, state agricultural universities and NDDB. It also emphasized the optimization of resource use for cattle improvement in terms of breeding farms, bull mother farms, semen freezing and artificial insemination and, veterinary health care facilities available with the state animal husbandry departments and under Operation Flood.

2.6 Gaushalas

Gaushalas are the institutions to maintain the cattle, which are either donated by people or thrown out by farmers. These institutions are maintained basically to protect cows and are in existence for the last two centuries. They are being maintained in different parts of the country on account of religious and economic considerations. With the establishment of Central Council of Gosamvardhana in 1952, the gaushalas were reorganized.

2.7 Special livestock breeding program (SLBP)

This was launched in 1975-76, with objectives to provide employment opportunities to the weaker sections of the rural poor and to supplement their income and to increase production of the livestock products such as milk, eggs, wool. The program includes crossbred heifer rearing scheme and setting up of sheep, poultry and piggery production units.

The dairy development program in the country has gone through a metamorphic change from the initial 'key village scheme' and 'intensive cattle development project' aimed at the up-gradation of local cattle in selected tracts to a nationwide anti-poverty program as an instrument of social security in the rural India.

3. Livestock dynamics and challenges

The dynamic livestock situation poses several challenges to livestock extension services. Some of the challenges with which the extension personnel have to cope up with are:

1. How to reach millions of livestock owners spread all over the country, especially those who are thriving in complex, diverse and risk prone environment?
2. How to improve the living standards of rural livestock owners through farming especially when the pressure on land is increasing and common property lands are slowly fading out forcing the rural poor to maintain the animals on purchased fodders?
3. How to sustain the production of livestock products with decreasing area under fodder, increasing competition for feed resources and decreasing interests of the people in livestock farming?
4. How to face the emerging livestock development situation as a sequel to technological and development interventions?
5. How to take cognizance of the changes that are taking place in the society which include : occupational migration from farming to industry, spatial migration from rural to urban, shift from grazing to stall feeding, shift in focus from social to economic issue?

3.1 Gender issue and livestock development

The role and contribution of women to livestock development is very well recognized. Studies clearly revealed that women spend on an average about 5 to 6 h a day on various livestock activities which include cleaning of sheds, washing of animals, feeding and milking. They have fairly good control and accessibility on the income they get from the animals which is being used for children's education, household expenses, and treatment of sick people in addition to feeding of animals. The women especially below poverty line have been encouraged to organize themselves into women self help groups (WSHG) to bring about social and economic empowerment. These groups are being promoted by various government agencies such as NABARD, nationalized banks, DRDA and NGOs. As a result millions of WSHGs are formed and registered with livestock farming as the most sought after income generating activity. To reach and educate them on various aspects of livestock management in the context of very few or negligible women extension force in the country is the greatest challenge. Realizing the importance of gender and livestock development, the ICAR has incorporated this aspect as a teaching module in the post graduate program for veterinary extension students.

3.2 Information needs and client groups

Understanding and appreciating the information needs of different clients and providing quality extension services are central to the success, which necessitates quality manpower at different levels. The objectives of rearing animal may differ from region to region and within the region from farmer to farmer. The basic premise in development is that extension must be client centered. A technology which is useful to one group of farmers may not be useful or relevant to others. This is mainly because of variations in their socio-economic situation, type of animals, purpose of rearing animals, level of technology adoption, resource availability, market structure, extent of extension exposure or contact. Obviously the information needs of different groups of people differ and extension advisory service must take cognizance of these needs rather than promoting blanket recommendations.

3.3 Technology adoption

Putting a technology into practice by livestock farmers depends upon several factors. Adoption of recommended technologies depends upon the perceived technological characteristics (Rogers, 2003). For example, technologies related to disease prevention and control has got a limited observability of benefit by the farmers resulting in farmers' reluctance in vaccinating their cattle. There cannot be any technology which is devoid of negative consequences. It is necessary for the extension agent to provide the information on both positive and negative consequences of the technology to the livestock farmers which enable them to take appropriate decisions

(Table 1). However, this is possible if adequate information on the advantages and disadvantages of a particular technology in a particular social system are gathered through on farm trials. It is equally important for the extension agent to resist from the tendencies of painting a rosy picture of a technology to avoid future mistrust between him and the livestock farmer.

Table 1 : Consequences of technologies or practices

Sl.No.	Technology or practice	Positive consequences	Negative consequences
1	Vaccination	Protect the animal from disease	Reduction in milk yield vaccine failure
2	AI with exotic bull semen	Female calf	Male calf
3	Crossbred cow	Gives more milk provided it is managed properly.	Susceptible to diseases; Poor performance under poor management
4	Urea treatment of straws	Slight increase in milk production and at a low cost	Feed gets exhausted fast thereby requiring more dry fodder.

Source: Rao *et al.*,1995.

3.3.1 Factors influencing technology adoption

There are several factors affecting the adoption of a technology at field level, which can be analyzed using a fit approach. An example of a fit approach, applied to the case of urea treated straw is presented in Table 2.

Table 2 : An example of a "Fit" exercise for urea treated straw, meaning a listing of factors that determine the usefulness of this technology characteristic

Characteristics	Best fit case
Type of straw	works best with slender straws (rice, wheat, barley)
Availability of straw	good supplies are required relative to other feed
Type of animal	medium production capacity
Water availability	should be readily available
Green fodder availability	limited availability relative to straw
Cost and availability of urea	should be low cost and plentiful in supply
Cost and availability of (plastic) covering	low cost and good availability
Market price of milk	should be good enough to allow purchase of inputs like urea and polythene
Support service	should be good in initial stages of adoption

Source: Rao *et al.*, 1995.

3.3.2 Perceptual differences between researchers and farmers

The perceptions of researcher, extension worker and farmer about the same technology may vary as all look at the technology from a different perspective. An example is given in Table 3.

Table 3 : Perceptual differences between researchers and farmers object

Parameters	Researcher	Farmer	Extension worker	Policy maker
Local cow is a source of	Milk	Bull calves, dung	Milk	Milk
Gram husk	Poor feed	Good fed supplement	Poor feed	Poor feed
Early weaning of calves	Recommended	Bad practice since it weakens the calf	Recommended	Recommended
Nutritive value of paddy and wheat straw	No difference in the quality	Some like wheat straw, other prefer paddy straw	No difference in the quality	No difference in the quality
Criteria for feed evaluation	TDN and CP	Cost of feed and its effect on growth and fat yield	Feed responses on milk production	Possibility to earn foreign exchange
Reason for non-adoption of technology	Farmers ignorance and or ineffective extension	Technology is not relevant	Technology is not relevant	Technology is not relevant Farmers ignorance and or ineffective extension
New grain varieties	Grain yield	Grain and straw yield	More grain and may be more straw	To feed the growing population
Objective of research	To increase biological efficiency of milk production	To increase farm income	To increase milk as well as draught capacity of the animal	To increase milk supply to feed the growing urban population

Note: The readers may fill the gaps with question marks depending on their perceptions. It should be remembered that perceptions are perceptions, *i.e.*, they may differ between observers.
Source: Rao *et al.*, 1995.

3.4 Technology application: Assessment and refinement, demonstration and training

The technology application in the farmers' field is a pre-requisite for further steps in the process such as dissemination and adoption. It refers to assessment and refinement, demonstration, and training of the farmers. The 'technology assessment and refinement (TAR)' refers to the process or a set of activities undertaken before taking up new scientific information for its dissemination in a new productive system. It is expected that the situation prevailing at farm condition differs from that of experimental condition under which the scientist develops technologies resulting in performance gap and dissatisfaction. Therefore, the technologies need to be reviewed, assessed and refined in terms of specific needs, opportunities and constraints faced by the farmers in different production systems. Some of the reasons for low acceptance of technologies are not economically viable, not operationally feasible, not stable, not matching with the farmers' needs and not compatible with the farmers' overall farming systems. Therefore, the assessment and refinement of technology need to be site specific, holistic, farmer participatory, inter-disciplinary, interactive and gender sensitive.

3.5 Use of local leaders

A good veterinary extension agent must always try to get the support of local leaders/livestock owners in his extension work. In any extension organization there will be a small number of professional extension agents compared to the huge number of livestock owners to be reached. It is not possible for the extension agent to contact each and every livestock owner in his area of operation. This can be solved by engaging and encouraging local leaders in planning and implementing the extension programs. The local leaders assume responsibility for certain activities in the absence of extension agent, help to organize local extension programs, assist directly in the spread of new ideas and practices by demonstrating them in their fields, serve as point of contact between the agent and the livestock farmers.

4. National goals and extension strategies

Swanson (2008) outlined three important agricultural development goals at national level and the objectives of the extension and advisory system to accomplish the national goals. These national goals are: i) national food security, ii) improving rural livelihood to reduce poverty and food insecurity, and iii) the sustainable use of natural resources within the country.

To accomplish these goals, whether it is agriculture or livestock extension, needs to be focused on the following four objectives:

- *Technology transfer* for better production of food grains, milk, meat, eggs, fish
- *Human capital development*, by improving skills for farmer to increase farm income

- *Building social capital development* by organizing farmers into producer groups
- *Educating farmers* to utilize sustainable natural resource management practices

Livestock including poultry and fisheries get impacts due to natural disasters, policy changes, turbulent markets *etc.* Setting proper goals and appropriate objectives to realize these set goals is necessary for reducing poverty, malnutrition and diseases. It is in this context the extension services need to be innovative in their concept, objectives and approaches.

Many of the projects did not yield the expected results. The major cause of which is attributed to poor participation of the farmers. Stray attempts have been made by several organizations to improve the farmer participation in the development projects. Some of the approaches which focus on farmer participation are discussed below:

4.1 Livelihood approach

It is very well documented that livestock provided livelihood security to at least one fourth of our population. Research has clearly indicated the "asset role" being played by the livestock particularly bovines to the landless people whose livelihood depends to a great extent on the animals. Small ruminants and poultry are considered as important resources for rural poor and the income generated from these is quite substantial. Hence, while formulating the livestock development policies, the interests of these resource poor livestock owners must be taken into consideration.

4.2 Group approach

Extension approach needs to be changed from individual to group. Development of sustainable farming practices often requires collective decision making, whereas extension in the past mainly supported individual (Head of the family) decision making (van den Ban and Hawkins, 2004). NABARD's SHG bank linkage program boasts of over 26 lakh SHG and 3.9 crore households influencing the lives of over 160 million poor population. (NABARD, 2005). During the year 2006-7 alone, as many as 4,58,591 groups were credit linked. Out of this total population assisted through this group approach, 90% were 'women self help groups (WSHGs; Thorat, 2006). Livestock rearing projects account for about 25% of the total cost of the projects sanctioned to SHGs under 'swarna jayanthi gram swarojgar yojana'. There is enough evidence to show that as groups, the WSHGs could achieve social and economic empowerment with the involvement of government and non government institutions. However, the sustainability of these WSHGs is doubtful especially when the loans sanctioned have not been used for income generating activities, instead were used for unproductive purposes like house construction or repair, marriages, purchase of ornaments, repayment of previous loans etc. (Usharani, 2007).

4.3 Market driven approach

In this era of market economy, adoption of technologies is market driven rather than technology driven. With the available technologies, procurement, transportation and sale of livestock products are more difficult and complex than producing them. Although dairy sector has been doing quite well, not more than 20 % of the milk is being handled by the organized sector. Except in case of poultry eggs and chicken the marketing of other livestock products is totally in unorganized sector. Organized markets for livestock transactions literally do not exist. Unless the markets are improved with price fixation based on proper standards and grading it is difficult to encourage the livestock owners to adopt technologies to enhance production. Mosher (1966) highlighted five essentials for agricultural development which are quite relevant even today. These include: (i) markets for farm products, (ii) constantly changing technology, (iii) local availability of supplies and equipments, (iv) production incentives for farmers, and (v) transportation.

4.4 Entrepreneurial development approach

Farmers have got entrepreneurial abilities which enable them to try new methods of farming, which are usually described as innovators exist in almost all social systems and skill of the extension personnel lies in identifying as well as encouraging such people to enter into new ventures of livestock development. The experiences of these path finders could be profitably utilized to upscale for wider use. It is necessary to identify such entrepreneurs, prepare success stories and give wide publicity through various mass media channels to enable the interested people to emulate them.

4.5 Participatory approaches

Of late it is very well recognized that the farmers are considered as partners in development rather than as end users of technology. Evidences support that it is beneficial to involve the livestock farmers in developing, adopting and evaluating the technologies. Many of the extension programs were not successful due to poor participation of farmers and needs of the livestock farmers were not taken into consideration. The ICAR included on farm testing as one of the key activities of 'krishi vigyan kendras (KVKs)' for its obvious advantages. Livestock extension should aim at empowering farmers rather than making them just an agency for transfer of technology. It is necessary for the extension service providers to shift their approach from a fixed transfer of technology to more flexible and sustainable participatory extension to face the challenges in livestock development. Considering that more than 60 % of our livestock farmers are resource poor and depend heavily on public sector for their information needs as well as inputs and technical services, the extension personnel should be empowered and sensitized to meet the demands particularly by forging research-extension-education-farmer-market linkages. Technology must be developed based on the demand from the end users. Technologies which address the needs of the livestock farmers get adopted faster than those technologies which do not match their needs.

4.6 Multi-disciplinary approach

With the realization that problems in the field are usually multi dimensional which requires the expertise of different fields of knowledge, emphasis has to be given to multidisciplinary approach in formulating and implementing the research projects. The livestock extension issues revolve around livelihood, livestock, women, social groups, markets, economics of production and policies. With liberalization and fast changes in the societies the problems are becoming more and more complex.

4.7 Farming systems approach

It replaces the conventional single discipline based, commodity oriented approach. This approach considers the farm, the farm household and off-farm activities in a holistic way to take care not only of farming but also all aspects of nutrition, food security, sustainability, risk minimization, income and employment generation which make up the multiple objectives of farm households. Farming system considers interdependencies of the components under the control of members of the households as well as how these components interact with the physical, biological and socio-economic factors not under the household's control.

4.8 Participatory technology development (PTD) approach

This approach involves farmers and other stakeholders to engage in experiments so that they can learn, adopt new technologies and spread them to other farmers. In its purest form, PTD is a process in which farmers identify their problems for which solutions have been sought and prioritized define alternative solutions to be tested, decide design of experiment, implement them, decide monitoring, execute and evaluate the outcome. The objectives of PTD approach are to empower clients to develop and use livestock technologies, appropriately suite to the farm holdings, empower stakeholders, especially the marginalized ones, to make their own decision so that their capacity to make effective demands on research and extension organizations is strengthened. Those in turn improve the functional efficiency of formal research. The PTD encourages farmer experimentation, helps to tap ITKs, motivate the farmers and helps in rigorous testing of technologies. The outcome generation of technologies which suite diverse agro-ecologic and socio-economical situations and it complements laboratory-based research.

Despite its obvious advantages, farmers consider PTD as a time consuming process with the involvement of risk in subjecting their animals for experimentation. Similarly, the researchers are also bogged down with the perceptions that the results could be spoiled by mismanagement of factors outside the researchers' control and failure of technologies in farmers' fields may be construed as inadequacies of scientists.

4.9 Privatization of livestock extension services

In India, livestock extension is carried out mostly by the departments of animal husbandry (AHD) and to some extent by the milk unions, state veterinary/agricultural universities (SAUs), research institutions of ICAR, and NGOs. With the increase in pressure on the land and other resources and emphasis on efficiency on the use of resources, public spending on animal husbandry extension services is being questioned. Recognizing the limitations of public extension services in meeting the wide ranging demands for agricultural technology, it was suggested to promote private and community driven extension to operate competitively with pubic extension. The 'national commission on agriculture' (NCA, 1976) recommended that cattle owners should be charged for AI in areas where it is popular. However, it is being done by collecting nominal charges by the departments of animal husbandry, on cost basis by some of the Milk Producers' Cooperative Societies and NGOs. Similarly, the milk unions and AHDs are supplying cattle feed and vaccines on subsidy to milk producers. Some of the milk unions have implemented welfare measures like free cattle insurance, scholarships for children of the milk producers and accident insurance cover for the milk producers etc. In the case of poultry, which is being run more on commercial lines compared to other livestock, the animal husbandry extension services are more organized and the poultry farmers are charged for almost all the services such as vaccination, de-beaking, post mortem, diagnosis and treatment of chicks. Based on the study conducted on privatizing agricultural extension in India, Rasheed and Sadamate (2000) suggested that the public sector should concentrate on organizing educational programs for farmers, which are less attractive to the private agencies. The public sector should also take up the role as facilitator in the formation of farmers' groups, building linkages with other extension agencies and initiating paid consultancy services by maintaining a cadre of qualified staff at district and sub district levels and some of these services can later be entrusted to the farmers' groups. Private sector extension cannot completely substitute for public agencies in those circumstances where direct benefits do not assure to the firms involved, target populations are diffuse or remote, where infrastructure is inadequate and when production consists mainly of basic food grown by subsistence farmers. Research clearly indicated that investments in agricultural research and extension yield high returns. Ahuja *et al.* (2000) based on a study conducted in three states of India reported that, there is a significant demand for the delivery of veterinary services at home and the cattle owners including the poor are willing to pay to receive these services. The public extension service has still an important role to play in increasing the production of backyard poultry, which even today is the major contributor of egg and chicken production in the country. The AHDs continue to provide free inputs and technical services such as vaccinations to the backyard poultry.

4.10 Contract farming

Poultry production with layers and broilers has extended into contract farming wherein the poultry farmers agree to provide eggs or chicken of certain quality and adhere to the management practices indicated by an agency in return for an assured market. The agency is responsible for supply of chicks, vaccinations, and health care, feed and purchase the output, chicken or eggs. The farmers' responsibility is to provide land, sheds and labour for maintenance. Consequently, the small-scale broiler and layer farms could not withstand the competition from the large commercial farmers and vanished from the scene. As a result poultry production is highly commercialized and the role of public extension has become limited in this setup. Contract farming in poultry has been found successful in India due to the presence of strong backward linkages. Such contract has provision of coping up against production failure, remove grower risk through buyback guarantee and also supply inputs such as chicks, feed and medicine thus helped the poultry farmers raise quality chickens. Apparently, balanced contracts that benefit both parties in terms of assured markets, competitive price and guarantee against risk have resulted in the success of poultry contract farming. However, for smaller farmers, while contract may provide an opportunity to rise above subsistence farming, the risk of diversifying is likely to be higher (Gulati *et al.*, 2009). Studies also indicated that the contract broiler farming is exploitative to the small farmers as the contract is one sided and specifies standards for the output only. No quality standards are prescribed for the inputs supplied by the integrator which include chick, feed and medicines (Selvi and Rao, 2009).

4.11 Cyber extension and information communication technologies (ICTs)

Cyber extension refers to the process of extension done over cyber space or virtual space of interconnected networks over the globe which provides connectivity round the clock. In recent years cyber extension has gained popularity and successful cyber extension initiatives were taken up by both public and private sectors in India. The ICT encompasses all those technologies that enable the handling of information and facilitate different forms of communication among human actors, between human beings and electronic systems, and among electronic systems. With the technological advancement in an information society, the role of ICTs such as e-mail, cell phones, world wide web (www) and kiosks promise to provide innovative solutions to the problems of poverty and inequality by accelerating development through introducing transparency to the systems and operations. India with the highest English speaking population in Asia, has the highest number of information kiosks established across rural areas.

The newer technologies in communication system include 'geographic information system (GIS)', 'expert system (ES)', 'database (DBS)', 'compact-disc-read only memory (CD-ROM)', networks, electronic mail (e-mail), electronic bulletin boards (EBB)', 'on-line service (OLS)', 'electronic journals (EJS)', ICTs, kiosks, teleconferencing and 'electronic information retrieval system (EIRS)'. Some of the relevant technologies are discussed hereunder.

4.11.1 Geographic information system (GIS)

This is computer assisted methods and procedures for the capture, storage and analysis of data having location or geographic properties and the display of the results in the graphical form. The GIS can be positively explored to plan and implement ecologically sustainable, economically viable, socially acceptable transfer of technology programs for an equitable use of global land resources. Concern for the ecological issues in extension added a new dimension in the implementation of extension programs. Any project is assessed in terms of its sustainability, eco-friendliness and economic viability. Decisions are being made based on the information about natural resources and conditions in a particular location, whereas policy makers and project formulators were severely handicapped in this respect. This GIS dimension in the modern extension therefore, helps to overcome such difficulties in planning need based system specific extension programs.

4.11.2 Expert system

They are computer programs that emulate logic and problem solving proficiency of a human expert. Like human experts they can also use heuristics, a problem solving technique that uses experience based rules of thumb to arrive at appropriate solutions. Expert systems are advantageous in the sense that they bring performance to the expertise of an expert and at once they can be easily duplicated unlike in case of the human experts. Perhaps the most significant merit of expert systems is that they combine the expertise of several experts in the field. This is particularly useful for the present day context of multidisciplinary approach. When the experts are becoming more and more specialized and in a particular area of the field, such expert system helps us to get the entire knowledge of expertise in the field. Some of examples are COUNSELLER (to manage insects and diseases on wheat), GRAPES (a pest management system for grapes) and POMME (to manage disease and insects in apples) and 'poultry expert system'.

4.11.3 Tele and audio conferencing

Satellite communication has revolutionized the communication process and made the interaction among people possible located at different places at a point of time. Satellite technology links the communicator with his audience located at different places and makes the two way communication possible. A farmer in Haryana can directly interact with the group of experts available at AIR or Doordarsan studio or research institutes to clarify his doubts. Such type of tele or audio interacts are being used successfully by ICAR in linking the farmers with experts over a wide range of issues. The tele and audio conferencing is a boon to the extension communication as it facilitates direct interactions between the scientists, extension workers and farmers irrespective of their locations and distance.

4.11.4 ICT initiatives in livestock sector

Some of the successful ICT initiatives taken up under different projects in India are the 'warna wired village project' providing internet access to cooperative societies spread in 70 villages of Maharashtra, which provide information to the villagers by establishing networked booths in the villages. The 'Information village project' of 'M.S. Swaminathan research foundation (MSSRF)' established a hub of information network, in Villianur village, Pondicherry to cater to the information needs of the rural people by bringing the benefits of modern ICTs to rural families in Pondicherry. The department of animal husbandry and dairying (DAH&D)' has already established a 'local area network (LAN)' with 230 nodes at Krishi Bhawan, New Delhi with internet access through NICNET gateway. An 'ICT learning (e-Learning)' center has also been established to provide on line internet access. The 'dairy information and services kiosk (DISK)' is one of the successful initiatives taken up by 'Gujarat cooperative milk marketing federation ltd. (GCMFL)' with the help of Indian Institute of Management, Ahmedabad, which includes a complete history of milk cattle owned by the member farmers. The details are maintained in the system, which is being used at milk collection centers and in cooperatives to test the quality of the milk and making payment to farmers. It has resulted in the removal of incentives to those who adulterate milk, reduced the time for payments from 10 days to less than 5 min and instilled confidence in farmers on cooperative set up. The NDDB has established "AKASHGANGA" which provides total integrated solution for automatic milk collection. The Central Institute for Research on Goats (CIRG) has developed e-mail conference system for goat outreach on its goat-nic.in server using free software called 'majordoma' which is available on *www.greatcircle.com*. on a free Linux operating system. Three e-mail conferencing systems, *viz.*, mail to: *goat-net@cirg.nic.in*., *livestocknet@cirg.nic.in*. and *fishnet@cirg.nic.in*. have been launched by the institute to help information inflow among technologists, farmers, development officers and planners.

Under 'animal health project' funded by Department for International Development (DFID), Rajiv Gandhi College of Veterinary and Animal Sciences (RAGACOVAS) Pondicherry in collaboration with University of Reading, UK, has designed an interactive touch screen information kiosk. It has information on important cattle diseases in addition to management of cattle and methods of acquiring information. Livestock farmers can access the needed information on cattle management with the touch of the screen which had text and pictures with sound back-up. A similar attempt was made in developing a touch screen information kiosk on dairy cattle management by TANUVAS, Chennai. The RAGACOVAS also developed an Information kiosk on management of goats for the benefit of the goat keepers under 'rural innovation fund project' in collaboration with MSSRF.

4.11.5 ICT efforts of ICAR and Government of India

- IP-Telephony and video conferencing at ICAR Institutes/HQs
- V-SAT connectivity to 192 KVKs and eight zonal project directorates through ERNET-KVK, ICAR network
- Upgrading ICAR-ERNET network involving all ICAR Institutes and SAUs under ongoing NAIP project component
- Toll free number 1800-180-1551created by Ministry of Agriculture, Govt of India, can be used by farmers anywhere in the country to access the information on agriculture and allied subjects.

5. Globalization issues and livestock extension

Supply and demand forecasts for milk and meat in India by both International Food Policy Research Institute (IFPRI) and Govt. of India indicate that there will be modest surplus even in 2020 in spite of increase in local demand due to population growth, growing urbanization, increasing affluence and changing life styles, enabling limited but significant international trade. Since the livestock production system in India is entirely labor intensive, relying on the use of family labor, the local competitiveness depends on low opportunity costs for labor, the value captured from non-food farm outputs like crops residues and manure and the opportunity for capital accumulation in the form of livestock. Meat production in India, except in case of broiler industry and the meat from culled layers in organized farms, are all in the traditional production systems with a little investment. The international competitiveness of Indian livestock products-particularly milk and milk products assessed on the basis of 'nominal protection co-efficient (NPC)' indicates that ghee is slightly competitive while milk powders are not. Meat prices in India and their NPC indicate fairly high international competitiveness. However, they lose out on 'sanitary and phyto sanitary (SPS)' standards and have only limited markets confined to West, South and South East Asia. Ensuring quality standards and freedom from annual epidemics are pre-conditions of the guaranteed market access. Small holder production system often faces difficulties in capturing the economics of scale in marketing, input supply and services delivery. Livestock extension education plays an important role in this context to make the livestock products quality specific and cost effective. Livestock extension education has to play role in this direction by:

- Training of farmers and entrepreneurs on export quality standards and phyto sanitary requirements
- Training on 'fair average quality Standards (FAQ)' for livestock products
- Market intelligence through information technology and cyber extension
- Sensitization training to middle level extension functionaries to improve their technical and professional knowledge and skills
- Conducting 'livestock extension education' programs on 'good agricultural practices (GAP)', 'good laboratory practices (GLP)', 'good manufacturing practices (GMP)'.
- Capacity building in the areas of understanding WTO, SPS, legal issues of SPS, food safety, risk analysis, disease risk analysis, diagnosis *etc.* is the prime areas of importance for the livestock extension education system.

Conclusions

There are several sources to get the information on animal husbandry for farmers. These include state departments of animal husbandry, veterinary universities/animal science institutes of ICAR, research stations, milk cooperatives, KVKs, pharmaceutical companies, veterinary medical shops, progressive farmers and NGOs. However, para-vets or the veterinarians who are the grass root level service providers on animal husbandry are considered as veterinary extension personnel. The present day veterinarians are considered as the most reliable source of information on livestock in the villages but unfortunately their role as livestock advisor is marginalized by his role as clinician. But in the years to come, with an increase in the gap between information available and information to be utilized on technologies or make the information technology accessible to the livestock farmers, they have to play much more pro active role in acquisition, processing and delivering relevant information to the livestock owners. Government machinery has to provide adequate support to them as well.

'National sample survey organisation (NSSO)' survey indicated that 60 percent of the farmers do not access any source of information for advanced agricultural technologies. As a result, there is a wide adoption gap among farming community to achieve the vertical increase in production through optimum resource utilization. If this be the case with agricultural technologies, where there is a network on extension and lot of funds are being used for transfer of technologies, livestock extension has to give more emphasis for betterment of poor livestock farmers.

Research clearly revealed the yawning gaps in the knowledge levels of livestock owners which could be attributed to lack of livestock extension services in the country. Unlike in agriculture extension, there is a need to combine the education of livestock owners with the supply of quality inputs at right time to facilitate easy adoption of recommended practices by them. The future extension thrust should be on marketing extension, farmwomen empowerment, facilitating formation of low resource base farmer's groups, private extension services and environmental extension for sustainability in farming. The research in extension needs to generate data on farming system, cost effectiveness of extension methods, accountability and extension federation for effective functioning of extension systems.

References

Ahuja V., George P.S., Sunil R., McConnell K. E., Kurup M.P.G., Gandhi V., Dina Umali-Deininger, Cees de Haan. (2000). *Agricultural Services and the poor – a case of livestock health and breeding services in India.* Indian Institute of Management, Ahmedabad; The World Bank, Washington D.C. and The Swiss Agency for Development and Cooperation, Bern, Switzerland, pp 34-41.

Government of India. (2007). *Annual Report 2006-07.* Ministry of Rural Development, New Delhi, pp 11-15.

Government of India. (1976). *Report on national commission on agriculture, Vol.VII.* Ministry of Agriculture, New Delhi, pp 31-34.

Gulati A., Ganguly K., Landes R. M. (2009). *Toward contract farming in a changing agri-food system.* www.ncap.res.in/contract.

Mosher A.T. (1966). Getting agriculture moving: essentials for development and modernization. Praeger, New York, pp 94-97.

NABARD. (2005). *SHG bank linkage* program. http:// www.nabard.org.

Rao S.V.N., Patil B.R., Rangnekar D.V., Dey R.A., VanDenBan A.W. (1995). Farmers' perceptions of innovations. In: *Hand book for straw feeding systems – Principles and applications with emphasis on Indian livestock production* (K.Singh, J.B.Schiere, eds). Indo Dutch Project on Bio conversion of Crop Residues, ICAR, New Delhi and DTAP, Agricultural University, The Netherlands, pp 117-119.

Sulaiman R. V., Sadamate V.V. (2000). Privatizing agricultural extension in India. Policy Paper, National Center for Agricultural Economics and Policy Research, New Delhi, pp 12-16.

Rogers E.M. (2003). Diffusion of innovations. 5th Edition, Free Press, New York, pp 7-9.

Selvi R.K., Rao S.V.N. (2009). Farmers' perceptions on contract broiler farming. *Indian Journal of Poultry science* **44:** 243-248.

Swanson B.E. (2008). *Global review of good agricultural extension and advisory service practices.* Food and Agricultural Organisation of the United Nations, Rome, pp 9-11.

Thorat, Y.S.P. (2006). Microfinance in India: Sectoral issues and challenges. In: *Proceedings of policy conference towards a sustainable micro-finance outreach in India- experiences and perspectives,* New Delhi, pp 19-25.

Usharani R. (2007). Women empowerment through dairying – A study on women self help groups in Pondicherry. MVSc thesis, Rajiv Gandhi College of Veterinary & Animal Sciences, Pondicherry.

Van den Ban A.W., Hawkins H.W. (1996) Agricultural Extension, 2nd Edition, Blackwell Science, London.

Section - 4

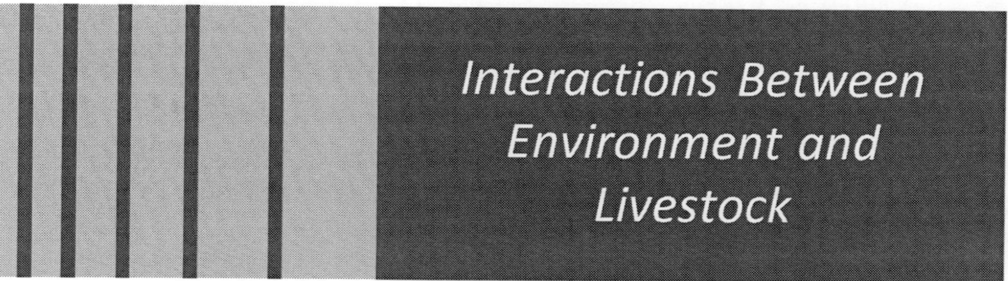

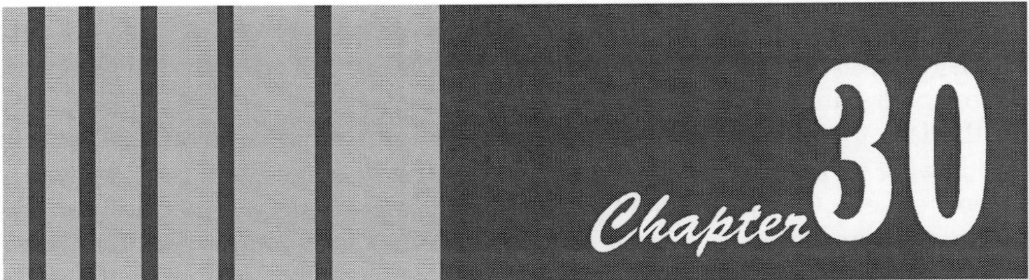

Climate Change, Enteric Methane Emission from Ruminants, their Estimation and Recent Strategies for Methane Mitigation

R. Bhatta[1], M. Kurihara[2], K.T. Sampath[1]

[1] National Institute of Animal Nutrition and Physiology, Adugodi, Bangalore-560 030, Karnataka, India

[2] National Institute for Livestock and Grassland Sciences, Tsukuba, Japan

Summary

Methane (CH_4) gas content of the atmosphere is increasing at 1% per annum. To stabilize CH_4 in the atmosphere, global CH_4 production needs to be reduced by 10–20%. Large ruminants produce some 15–20% of the global production of methane. Ruminants on low quality feeds possibly produce over 75% of the CH_4 from the world's population of ruminants. Supplementation to improve digestive efficiency in these animals could at times halve this CH_4 production per unit of feed consumed. Together with supplementation to improve efficiency of feed utilization and increase product output may thus reduce methane production per unit of milk or meat by a factor of 4–6. The dietary/nutritional strategy that improves productivity with no potential negative effects on livestock health and production and is cost effective has a better chance of being adopted. Other strategies (biotechnologies, additives) are promising but diversity and plasticity of functions of the rumen bacterial and methanogenic communities may be limiting factor for their successful application. Environmental impacts of strategies should also be taken into consideration. A global vision of production systems that considers all greenhouse gases emissions from the animal up to the farm scale as well as grassland use is essential. Further the sustainability of CH_4 suppressing strategies is an important issue.

The Intergovernmental Panel on Climate Change (IPCC) of the United Nations released a report in February 2007, that said global warming was 'very likely' - meaning an at least 90 per cent certainty–caused by human activity. That document forecasts that the average temperature will rise 1.8°C to 4°C by the year 2100 and sea levels will creep up by 17.8 cm to 58.4 cm by the end of the century. If polar sheets continue to melt, another rise of 9.9 cm to 19.8 cm is possible. The IPCC also found that snow cover since the late 1960s has decreased by about 10 per cent and lakes and rivers in the Northern Hemisphere are frozen over about two weeks less each year than they were in the late 1960s. Mountain glaciers in non-polar regions have also been in 'noticeable retreat' in the 20th century and the average global sea level has risen between 0.1 and 0.2 meters since 1900. In simple words, the world is getting warmer and the temperature is rising faster than ever. The IPCC predicts more floods, intense storms, heat waves and droughts. Its study forecasts a rise of 1.4 to 5.8°C in the global mean surface temperature over the next 100 years, with developing countries like India, most vulnerable.

It has been reported that methane (CH_4) promotes stratospheric ozone depletion (Blake and Rowland, 1988). The water vapor that is added to the stratosphere when CH_4 is oxidized may provide surfaces for heterogeneous reactions that destroy ozone. Worldwide initiatives such as the Kyoto Protocol demand that these emissions be reduced or at least prevented from further increase (Howden and Reyenga, 1999). Methane is a also major contributor to global warming with a 100-year global warming potential (GWP), 25 times than that of carbon dioxide (CO_2) (IPCC, 2001). Thus despite being present in the atmosphere at far lower concentrations (450 ppb) than CO_2, it was reported that CH_4 is responsible for approximately 20 per cent of the greenhouse gas effect (IPCC, 2001; 2007).

Increased understanding and improved quantification of CH_4 production in the rumen has implications not only for global environmental protection but also for efficient animal production. However, there appears to be uncertainty in the CH_4 estimation from livestock due to the limited availability of data to document the variability at the farm level and also due to the significant impact of diet on the enteric CH_4 production. The CH_4 mitigation strategies require robust prediction of emissions from rumen. There are many methods available which would be suitable for measuring CH_4 produced from the various stages of animal production. For the development of an accurate inventory, or to implement mitigation strategies, it is important that there be confidence in the accuracy of the CH_4 measurement technology. Methane emissions from livestock have been measured as part of the studies on ruminal fermentation, energy balance, evaluation of feed additives and most recently, to characterize and reduce the contribution of ruminants to the global CH_4 burden. Livestock CH_4 emissions have been measured using respiration calorimetry systems such as whole body chambers, head boxes, ventilated hoods and face masks (Johnson and Johnson, 1995). Data obtained from these techniques have been the foundation of the prediction equations used to generate mathematical models and countrywide and global inventories (Benchaar *et al.*, 1998; Mills *et al.*, 2001). To develop strategies to mitigate CH_4

emissions the precise quantification of CH_4 emissions from ruminants under a wide range of circumstances is very essential. However, several factors need to be considered in order to select the most appropriate technique such as the cost, level of accuracy required and the scale and design of the experiments to be undertaken. Selection of any technique depends on the accuracy as each one has its advantages and disadvantages. Screening of mitigation strategies may be evaluated using individual animal before large scale trials on groups of animals are carried out.

1. Consequences of global warming

Even given the moderate 0.8°C of global warming measured to date, the impacts can already be felt in every part of the world including India. For example, the summer extent of the ice mass in the Arctic Ocean has already shrunk by about half since the 1970s (Stroeve *et al.*, 2007). Since the ice is also thinning dramatically at the same time, the volume of ice declines even more rapidly (Kwok *et al.*, 2009). If warming should escalate unabated to 4°C or more, it might fundamentally change the earth system along with all its ecological resources and services. Global temperature differences on such a scale would roughly correspond to the difference between temperature at the peak of the last ice age 20,000 years of age and temperature today. In nut shell, global warming has the following consequences:

- The sea level rises due to the thermal expansion of sea water and the influx of melt water into the oceans and the warmer it becomes, the faster the sea level rises (Rahmstorf, 2007). Since, 1880, the global sea level has risen by around 20 cm. It could, however, rise by 50-150 cm by 2100 (Rahmstorf, 2007).
- Already, an increase in extreme weather events such as heat waves, droughts, extreme rain-fall events, floods and tropical storms has been observed in many regions (IPCC, 2007). A further rise of extreme weather events in the wake of additional warming is probable, depending on the type of event.
- Global warming in excess of 2°C threatens to accelerate the loss of genetic, species and ecosystem diversity, since many regions in the world will very rapidly enter climatic conditions not experienced for several million years. According to the IPCC (2007), this would place such an intolerable strain on nature's adaptive and regenerative capacity as to risk the irreversible loss of 20-30 % of animal and plant species and associated genetic resources. Ecosystems such as mangrove forests and coral reefs would suffer irreversible damage or destruction. Biodiversity loss would result in loss of ecosystem resources and services – e.g. the availability of clean drinking water and genetic resources which are also crucial functions for society's efforts to adapt to climate change.

2. Greenhouse gases and greenhouse effect

The IPCC included six gases which have high global warming potential (the CO_2 equivalence of a particular gas, when integrated over a time horizon of 100 years, is referred to as its Global Warming Potential) i.e. carbon dioxide (CO_2), methane (CH_4), nitrous oxide (N_2O), hydro fluorocarbons (HFCs), per fluorocarbons (PFCs) and sulphur hexafluoride (SF_6).

Three gases (carbon dioxide, methane and nitrous oxide) occur naturally in the atmosphere in small quantities (Fig. 1) and are being added continuously and therefore, their concentration is increasing due to human activities. The other three gases normally do not exist in the atmosphere, but are added due to industrial activities in small quantities, but these are sufficient to increase global warming substantially as these gases have very high GWP in comparison to CO_2. Greenhouse gases allow solar radiation to pass through the earth's atmosphere. But after the earth absorbs part of that radiation, it reflects the rest back. That's where the problem lies. Particles of greenhouse gas absorb the radiation, heating up and warming the atmosphere. The increasing levels of greenhouse gases are causing too much energy to be trapped–the so-called 'greenhouse effect' (IPCC, 2001).

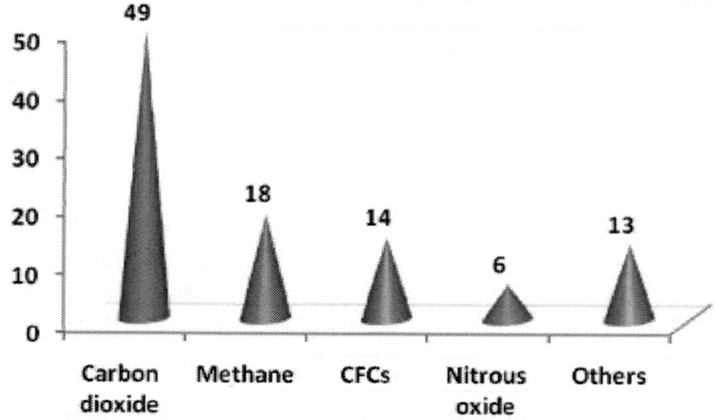

Fig. 1 : Relative contribution (%) of greenhouse gases to atmospheric warming (Source: World Resources Institute)

On a global scale, agriculture and in particular enteric fermentation in ruminants (predominantly cattle and small ruminants) produces between 21 and 25 per cent of the total anthropogenic emission of methane (Fig. 2). In India, out of the total 27 per cent GHG emission from agriculture sector, 40 per cent is estimated to be the contribution from its 485 million livestock which amounts to about 10.4 to 10.6 million tons, the major contribution coming from cattle and buffalo (92%) and rest from small ruminants (7%).

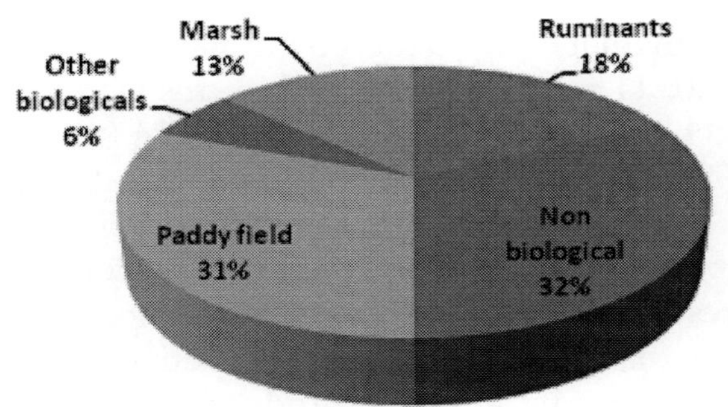

Fig. 2 : Relative contribution of biological resources to the global production of CH_4 (Tg per year) in the atmosphere (Bolle *et al.*, 1986).

3. Methanogenesis in the rumen

The primary digestive microorganisms (bacteria, protozoa and fungi) present in the rumen hydrolyze proteins, starch and plant cell wall polymers into amino acids and sugars. These simple products are then fermented to volatile fatty acids (VFA), hydrogen (H_2) and carbon dioxide (CO_2). Acetate, propionate and butyrate, which are the major VFA (Fig. 3), are then absorbed and utilized by the host animal. The major producers of H_2 are the organisms which produce acetic acid in the fermentation pathway. Acetate and butyrate production results in CH_4 production, while propionate formation serves as a competitive pathway for H_2 use in the rumen. Methane accounts for a significant energy loss to the ruminant animal, amounting to about 8% of gross energy at maintenance level of intake and falling to about 6% as the level of intake rises. The excreta of animals, if not properly managed also contribute significantly to greenhouse gases. However, the contribution of excreta to total greenhouse gas pool is less in India due to the practice of drying the dung for fuel use.

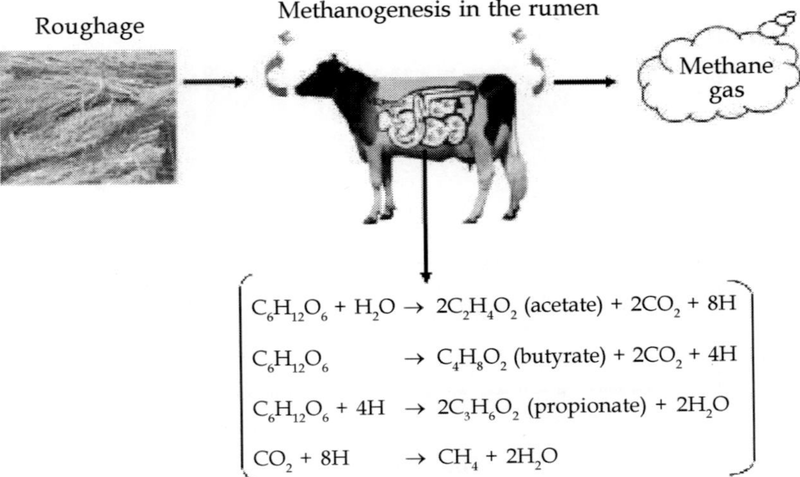

Fig. 3 : Schematic representation of methanogenesis in the rumen

Singh (2001) reported that methane production by Indian cattle, buffalo, sheep and goat were 76.7, 97.0, 11.6 and 10.1 g/head/d, respectively. The annual global methane production from livestock is about 80 Tg from enteric fermentation (Chynoweth, 1996) and India's contribution is about 11 Tg per year, which corresponds to 14% of the global influx of methane. The notable fact is that by 2012 India shall be bound by the restrictions of the Kyoto protocol that makes us mandatory to restrict our methane emission to a specified level and this might be much lower than the present level of methane emission. Therefore, for economic and eco-friendly livestock production, it is essential to minimize the production of methane and other gases to conserve nutrients and protect the environment (Bhatta *et al.*, 2008).

Methane is an important component of the increasing gases in the atmosphere and is the one most associated with animal agriculture (Bhatta *et al.*, 2005, 2006a). The rates of accumulation of methane and carbon dioxide in the world's atmosphere have changed dramatically in the last 10 years. Prior to this, the rise in world temperatures and composition of the atmosphere had changed little, but is now in what appears to be an exponential period (Fig. 4). Methane is accumulating at a fast rate, and is apparently responsible for a small proportion of the depletion of the protective ozone layer. Undoubtedly the contamination of the atmosphere with carbon dioxide, methane and other gases must be stabilized or the future of the earth is threatened.

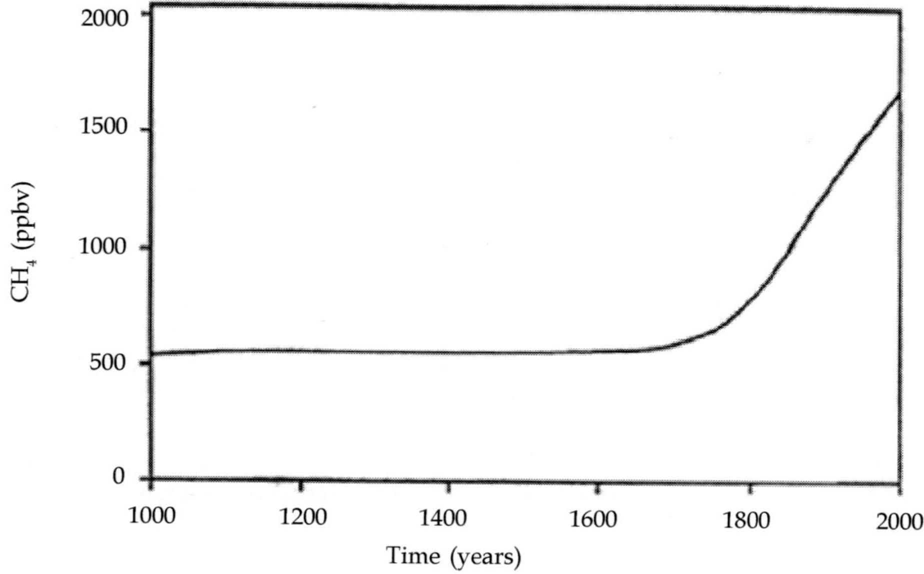

Fig. 4 : Trends in atmospheric methane accumulation (Khalil and Rasmussen, 1986)

4. Animal agriculture and the greenhouse effect

Animal production plays four important roles in the release of gases into the atmosphere (by Leng, 1991):

1. Fermentative digestion of ruminants produce methane in the rumen-direct
2. Proportion of the faecal materials decompose anaerobically -indirect,
3. CO_2 production from fossil fuels to provide the production and marketing infrastructure and inputs such as motorized transport, fertilizers, herbicides and insecticides-indirect
4. Clearing of forests and range lands, the timber on which was a natural sink for carbon dioxide-indirect

Table 1: Estimates of methane emissions from animals (adapted from Crutzen et al., 1986).

Animal type and region ($X10^{-6}$)		World Pop.	CH_4Prod. (kg/hd/yr)	Total CH_4 Prod.
Cattle:				
	Developed countries	573	55	31.8
	Developing countries*	653	35	22.8
Buffaloes		142	50	6.2
Sheep:				
	Developed countries	400	8	3.2
	Developing + Australia	738	5	2.4
Goats		476	5	2.4
Camels		17	58	1.0
Pigs:				
	Developed countries	329	1.5	0.5
	Developing countries	445	1.0	0.4
Horses		64	18	1.2
Mules & Asses		54	10	0.5
Humans		4670	0.05	0.3
Wild ruminants and large ruminants		100–500	1–50	2–6
Total				**76–80**

*includes Brazil and Argentina

** total estimate for emissions from domestic animals has an uncertainty factor of ± 15%

Ruminants in 'natural' production systems are inefficient and, in general, production increases depend on an expansion of numbers. There is a growing appreciation that efficiency per animal can be improved many fold with simple technology inputs which would have an impact on all four aspects of the contributions to global warming discussed above. The most important approach to be discussed in relation to the amelioration of greenhouse gas production by ruminants in Indian context is to increase the efficiency of animal production from available resources and develop the capacity to produce more from fewer animals.

The data obtained so far show an approximate even split of numbers of ruminant animals between the developing and developed countries; i.e. large ruminants contribute the greatest to world methane accumulation, and that other domestic and wild herbivores and man contribute an insignificant proportion. It is critical to note that it is the rates of methane production per unit of product produced over a life time which is important in identifying where it is possible to make major reductions in methane emissions.

Slow growth, low milk yield and poor reproductive performance results in poor feed conversion and a large methane output relative to product output. Methane output relative to product output of ruminants depends on two factors: the efficiency of fermentative digestion in the rumen and the efficiency of conversion of feed to product (e.g. milk, beef, draught power).

5. Effect of climate change on livestock

Climate change may have direct or indirect effects on livestock. The quantity and quality of the feed supplied to the animal is a major factor but as well as the direct relationship between the nutrition of the animal and its thermal environment, modifications to the seasonal availability of forage may have implications on animal production systems. For example, altered lambing times may be possible if patterns of spring forage growth change which would have implications for the marketing of finished lamb (Rowlinson, 2008).

5.1 Direct effects

The responses of animals to changes in environmental temperature and emphasizes the key difference between our ruminant and non-ruminant species in their comfort zones. Ruminants have wide comfort zones and high degree of thermal tolerance so it is likely that climate change resulting in an increase of a few degrees is not going to have a major effect on animal performance. The exceptions would be at the extremes. Areas currently characterized by low temperatures and high rainfall may become more favourable and be associated with a reduction in the mortality of young ones. At the other extreme, high summer temperature may be expected to present the dairy cow/buffalo with thermal stress and result in reduced intake and performance. Adaptations to management systems such as increased provision of shade and water should be adequate to counter this. By contrast the non-ruminant species have a very narrow comfort zones. This is one of the reasons pig and poultry enterprises have often been based on intensive housed systems in developed and developing countries. Higher environmental temperatures in winter may lead to a saving in heating costs for poultry buildings in layers and extra covering for goats. However, in the summer months the existing housing systems may not be able to cope with the increased thermal load. This may lead to an increased requirement for costly cooler systems especially in arid and semi-arid regions of Rajasthan (Rowlinson, 2008).

5.2 Indirect effects

Nutrition and feeding

Climate change can be expected to have several impacts on feed crops and grazing systems (Hopkins and Del Prado, 2007), like:

- Change in herbage growth brought about by change in atmospheric CO_2 concentration and temperature
- Changes in the composition of pastures, such as changes in the ratio of grasses to legumes
- Changes in herbage quality, with changing concentrations of water-soluble carbohydrates and N at given dry matter (DM) yields
- Greater incidences of drought, which may offset any DM yield increases
- Greater intensity of rainfall, which may increase N leaching in certain systems.

With regard to supply of feed, central to this consideration is an appreciation of what is fed to our livestock at present. Non-ruminant livestock will continue to receive diets consisting of maize and de-oiled cakes and with least cost ration formulation. A much greater threat is likely to be posed by the food: feed: fuel conflict providing reduced supplies. Ruminant diets differ in that there is a major forage component. In the case of extensive system like in sheep and goat, this may make up the entire diet whereas in more intensive dairy cattle or goat rearing systems the forage will be balanced by a more concentrated supplement. It is the source, quality and quantity of the forage component of ruminant's diet which is likely to be affected by climate change. The result may be either effects (advantageous or deleterious) on the existing forage species or a change to forage species not currently grown. With respect to our existing forage species, low environmental temperature is one of the major limitations to higher DM production. Thus any increase in temperature might be expected to have benefits on early season growth. If mean rainfall were to decline this would lead to soil moisture deficits which would require expenditure on irrigation unless reductions in DM yield were to be accepted. For existing species, the stage of maturity at which the crop is cut is major determinant of quality and in any altered climatic scenario the interplay between increasing quantity and declining quality would continue to be of major importance although the alterations in climate may be favorable to conservation and reduce losses during hay making. In many hill and upland areas which are currently characterized by low temperatures and water logged soils, climate change may be expected to lead to more favorable conditions and result in a shift towards more productive species with accompanying implications to animal production.

The other major possibility is that climate change will lead to a shift in the forage species grown in a country. For example elevated temperature may lead to an increase in the hectare of maize grown. This might be expected to result in improvements in both the quantity and quality of forage for ruminant livestock and could lead us towards the forage component of rations fed to dairy cattle elsewhere. In semi-arid regions of the country like Rajasthan, the palatable species of the plants might get replaced by non-palatable species in the pasture and might result in lower quantity of edible biomass for sheep on extensive system of rearing.

6. Methane measurement techniques

There are many methods available which would be suitable for measuring CH_4 produced from the various stages of animal production. However, several factors need to be considered in order to select the most appropriate technique like the cost, level of accuracy required and the scale and design of the experiments to be undertaken (Johnson *et al.*, 2001).

Methane sampling

There are many options available by which CH_4 emissions from ruminants could be measured. Selection of a technique depends on the accuracy as each one has its advantages and disadvantages. Screening of mitigation strategies may be best evaluated using individual animal before large scale tests on herds of animals are conducted (Johnson *et al.*, 2001).

6.1 Individual animal techniques

The classical standard for ruminant CH_4 measurement by nutritionists is the respiration chamber, or calorimeter. Respiration calorimetry techniques such as whole animal chambers, head boxes, or ventilated hoods and face masks have been used effectively to collect most of the available information concerning CH_4 emissions in livestock. The predominant use of calorimeters has been to measure gaseous exchange as part of energy balance measurements, CH_4 loss being a necessary part of this procedure. There are various designs of calorimeters (Blaxter, 1962), but the most common one being the open circuit calorimeter. The principle behind open-circuit indirect-respiration techniques is that outside air is circulated around the animal's head, mouth and nose and expired air is collected (Mclean and Tobin, 1987). The animal is placed in open-circuit respiration chamber for a period of several days, the inputs (feed, oxygen, CO_2) and outputs (excretion, oxygen, CO_2 and CH_4) were measured from the chamber.

The chamber should be well sealed and capable of a slight negative pressure (Fig. 5). This ensures that all leaks will be inward and not result in a net loss of CH_4. Air conditioning, dehumidification, feeders, waterers and a method by which faeces and urine could be removed are necessary in order to create a comfortable environment within the chamber. Animal movement and normal behaviour should be provided for as much as possible however, some degree of restraint is necessary within the chamber. Experimental factors that should be considered are a) restrictions to the animal's intake to ensure that the experiment can be reproduced, b) stresses on the animal from being in confinement, c) lack of environmental stresses on the animal (*e.g.*, lack of heat stress), d) lack of exercise e) experimental duration.

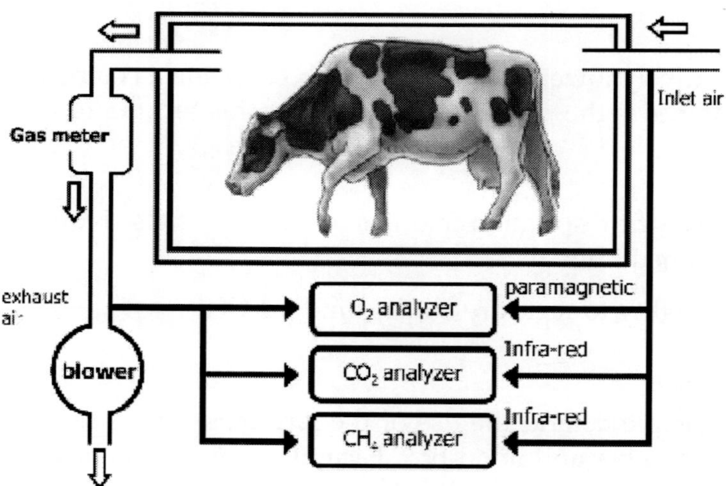

Fig. 5 : Open circuit respiration chamber for large ruminants. (Courtesy – Dr. Nishida, JIRCAS, Thailand)

Advantages

The technique has the ability to make accurate measurements of emissions including CH_4 from ruminal and hindgut fermentations.

Disadvantages

1. This technique is satisfactory for measuring CH_4 emission from dried diets; there are difficulties in deriving values that are applicable to the grazing ruminant. Grazing ruminant select their diet, maximum intakes in a chamber are considerably lower than in grazing animals.
2. The animal movement is restricted in the chamber.
3. Huge expenses is associated with the construction and maintenance of the chambers.

6.2 Head box

Head-box or a ventilated hood could also be used to quantify CH_4 emissions using the same principles as that of respiration chamber. This technique involves the use of an air-tight box (Fig. 6) that surrounds the animal's head. A sleeve or drape could be placed around the neck of the animal to minimize air leakage. The box must be big enough to allow the animal to move its head in an unrestricted manner and allows access to feed and water.

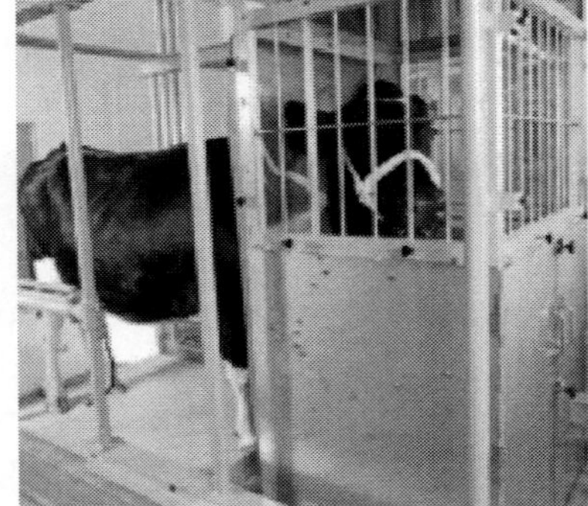

(National Institute of Livestock and Grassland Science- Japan)

Fig. 6 : A ventilated hood or head-box for large ruminants

Advantage

The relatively lower cost of the head box system as compared to a whole animal chamber is the primary advantage of this technique.

Disadvantages

1. Similar to the respiration chamber, use of a hood also requires a restrained and trained animal
2. The inability to measure all the hindgut CH_4

6.3 Face masks

The principle behind the use of the face mask is the same as that of the respiration chamber and hood-box. Face masks may also be used to quantify CH_4 production (Liang *et al.*, 1989).

Advantage

The primary advantage of this method is the simplicity and lower cost. They can also be used to collect the expired gas from the grazing animals periodically and estimate CH_4 production.

Disadvantages

The face mask, compared with chamber methods, underestimates heat production and likely CH_4 as well by an average 9.0 % (Liang *et al.*, 1989). It requires animal co-operation and eliminates its ability to eat and drink. Because of the normal daily variation in emissions, meaningful CH_4 emission measurements is difficult and hence short term measurements might lead to erroneous results (Johnson and Johnson, 1995).

6.4 Ventilated flow-through method with a face mask

In the face mask technique, the mask for the total collection of expired air has to be tightly sealed around the face of the animal, which may be stressful for the animal and also the Douglas-bag used for the collection of gas is not easy to handle. Kawashima *et al.* (2002) developed a ventilated flow-through method with a face mask (Fig. 7). The system consisted of four major components 1) main air flow system component 2) air-sampling component 3) gas analysis component 4) data record and calculation system.

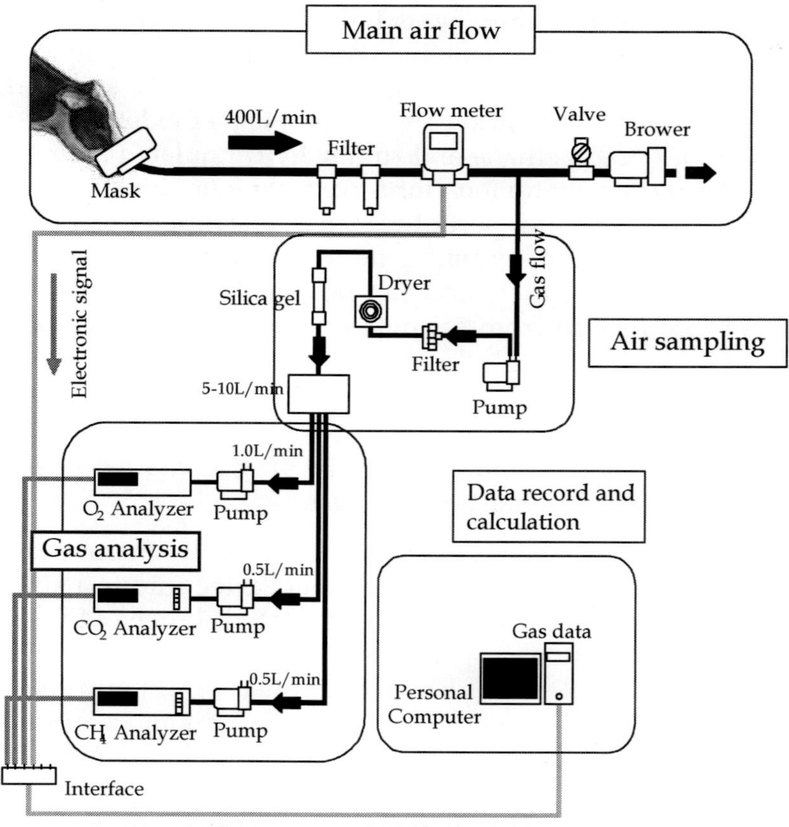

Fig. 7 : Ventilated flow-through assembly with a face mask (Courtesy – Dr. Nishida, JIRCAS, Thailand)

Three factors influence the accuracy of the CH_4 measurement in this technique viz. individual animal, daily difference and diurnal changes (Terada, 1999). The variance related to diurnal change was the largest among the three factors. It was suggested, based on these analyses that a respiration trial should be conducted for 2-3 days, 4-6 times a day with 4 experimental animals.

Calculation of methane production

The principle is based on the Brouwer's equation for measurement of heat production.

$$HP = 16.18\ V\ O_2 + 5.16\ V\ CO_2 - 5.90\ N - 2.42\ V\ CH_4$$

Where, HP: heat production (kJ); V O_2: oxygen consumption (liter); V CO_2: carbon dioxide production (liter); N: urinary nitrogen excretion (g); V CH_4: methane production (liter).

6.5 Tracer gas techniques

The rumen methane production can also be estimated by using the ERUCT technique (Emissions from Ruminants Using a Calibrated Tracer). The tracer can either be isotopic or non-isotopic. Isotopic tracer techniques generally require simple experimental designs and relatively straightforward calculations (Johnson and Johnson 1995). Isotopic methods involve the use of (^{3}H-) methane or (^{14}C-) methane and ruminally cannulated animals (Murray *et al.*, 1975). Using the continuous infusion technique, infusion lines deliver the labeled gas to the ventral part of rumen and sampling of gas takes place in the dorsal rumen. After determining the specific activity of the radio labeled CH_4 gas, total methane production can be calculated. It is also possible to measure CH_4 production from a single dose of injection of tracer (France *et al.*, 1993).

Disadvantage

The major limitation is the difficulty in the preparation of the infusion solution because of low solubility of CH_4 gas.

Non isotopic tracer techniques are also available for measurement of CH_4 production. Johnson *et al.* (2001) described a technique using sulphur hexafluoride (SF_6), an inert gas tracer. A calibrated source of SF_6 is placed in the rumen *per os* prior to an experiment. The source of SF_6 is a permeation tube, and the rate of release of SF_6 is controlled by a permeable Teflon™ membrane held in place by a porous stainless steel frit and a locking nut. The release rate of the gas permeation tube is calibrated at 39°C by regular weighing for a period prior to its insertion into the rumen. The tubes for sheep, typically 35 mm length by 11 mm in external diameter, are made from brass rods and weigh about 32 g.

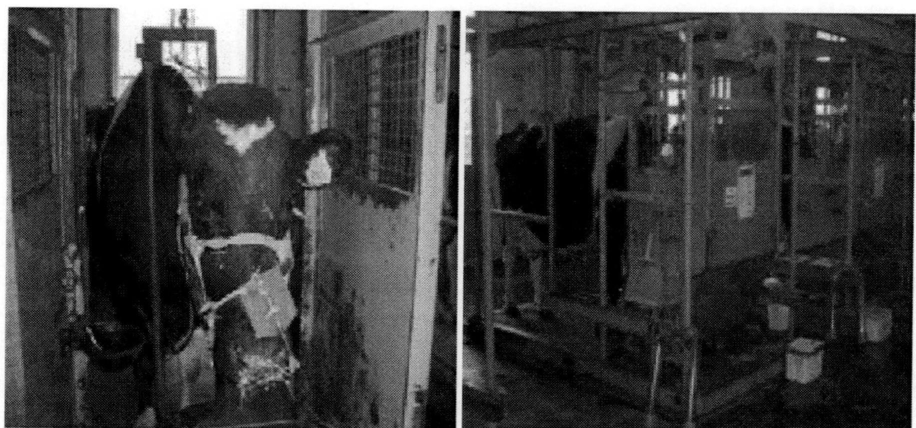

Fig. 8 : Sulphur hexafluoride tracer technique for methane estimation in vivo (Courtesy: National Institute of Livestock and Grassland Science – Japan)

The yoke is easily isolated for daily changing by means of a shut-off valve and quick connect fittings. Yoke volumes are typically 1.7 and 2.5 litre for sheep and cattle respectively, and the capillary system is designed to deliver half this volume during the collection period of 24 hours. An identical apparatus needs to be placed each day to collect an integrated background air sample. After collection of a sample the yoke is pressurized with nitrogen, and CH_4 and SF_6 concentrations are determined by gas chromatography.

Methane emission rate is calculated as follows

$$QCH_4 = QSF_6 \times [CH_4]/ [SF_6]$$

Where QCH_4 is the emission rate of methane in g/day; QSF_6 is the known release rate (g/day) of SF_6 from the permeation tube; $[CH_4]$ and $[SF_6]$ are the measured concentrations in the canister

Kurihara (personal communication) compared a set of 27 SF_6 measurement data where, each data was the average of 3-4 SF_6 measurements, with another set of 27 chamber data where, each data was the average of 2-3 chamber measurements from Holstein heifers or dry cattle and observed that the SF_6 estimates were 0.84 - 1.02 (mean = 0.99; P>0.1) of those in the chamber. Pinares-Patino (2000) in New Zealand found in an experiment with 10 sheep fed chaffed Lucerne hay that CH_4 production estimated from SF_6 was 0.95 chamber emission. Johnson *et al.* (1994) compared 55 measurements using the SF_6 technique with 25 chamber measurements of cattle, and showed that while the SF_6 estimates were 0.93 of those in the chamber, the difference was not significant. Boadi *et al.* (2002) compared estimates of CH_4 production using the SF_6 tracer technique (137.4 l/d) with an open circuit hood calorimeter (130.0 l/d) using yearling beef heifers and found no difference

(P = 0.24). However, Pinares-Patino (2000) in two experiments with sheep obtained SF_6 results that were extremely variable compared to chamber. McCrabb and Baker (cited by Ulyatt *et al.*, 1999) measured CH_4 production from 5 Friesian calves fed Rhodes grass (*Chlorisgayana*) hay, using both SF_6 and a confinement-type respiration chamber. The estimate of CH_4 production made with the respiration chamber (7.7 ± 0.67 l/h) was twice that (P<0.005) estimated using SF_6, either in pens (4.1 ± 0.35 l/h) or in the chamber (4.0 ± 0.46 l/h). SF_6 has also been used successfully as tracer to estimate the total CH_4 emission from all the cattle in a barn (Kaharabata and Schuepp, 2000).

Advantages

1. This technique allows the animal to move about and graze thus eliminates the necessity to restrain or enclose the animal.
2. The use of the tracer accounts changes in dilution associated with head or air movement and therefore it is also not necessary to sample directly from the animal's rumen or throat.

Disadvantages

1. This tracer technique does not measure all of the hindgut CH_4. Any CH_4 from the hindgut that is absorbed into the blood stream will be expired and collected but any CH_4 that escapes absorption and is released from the rectum is not collected.
2. It is necessary to train the animal to wear a halter and collection yoke/ canister.
3. The residues of SF_6 in meat and milk from farm animals is another issue
4. SF_6 is greenhouses gas itself, with a GWP 23, 900 times that of CO_2 and an atmospheric lifetime of 3,200 years (Machmuller and Hegarty, 2005).

Ethane (C_2H_6) has also been used as a marker to estimate CH_4 emission (Moate *et al.*, 1997; Mlbanzamihigo *et al.*, 2002) using essentially the same principle as SF_6. The major difference in the use of the two tracers is that ethane has to be bubbled from an external source into the rumen, and so is not suitable for use in grazing experiments. Hegarty *et al.* (2004) listed possibility of other markers for measuring enteric CH_4 emissions and approaches being considered (Table 2). Machmuller and Hegarty (2005) identified ethane and stable isotopes of methane as promising alternative tracer gases for the ERUCT technique.

Table 2 : Gases that could be used in the estimation of methane

Class	Tracer	Advantages	Disadvantages
Isotopes	$^{14}CH_4$, CH^3_4 radioisotopes	Very low detection limits	Radioactive so not useful in food chain
	$^{13}CH_4$ stable isotope	Little C transfer to other molecules OK for food chain	Very expensive
	CH^2_4 stable isotope	Cheap, safe, OK for food chain	Hydrogen transfer to other molecules
Noble gases	Argon	Low detection limit and moderate cost	High background concentration
	Xenon	Low background	High cost
	Krypton	Low background	Very high cost
Other Gases	Ethane	Availability	High detection limit
	Propane	Availability	High detection limit

7. Methane mitigation strategies

Challenges and opportunities for methane mitigation

Management of the H_2 production in the rumen is the most challenging factor to be considered when developing strategies to control ruminant CH_4 emissions (Joblin, 1999). It should therefore be possible to reduce CH_4 productions by inhibiting H_2 liberating reactions or by promoting alternative H_2-using reactions or routes for disposing of H_2 during fermentation (Fig. 9) (Boadi *et al.*, 2004).

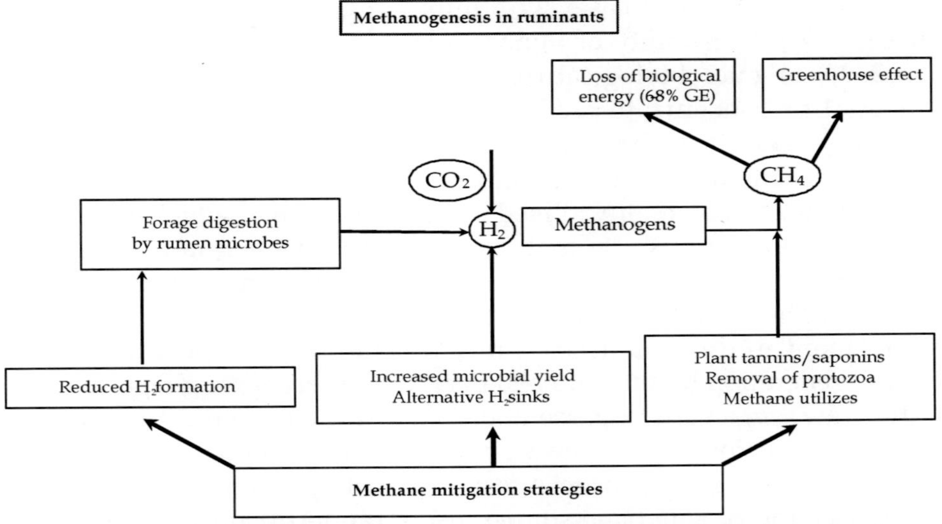

Fig. 9 : Schematic representation of methane mitigation strategies in ruminants

7A. Nutritional strategies for methane reduction

Johnson *et al.* (1996) reported that fermentation of cell wall carbohydrates produces more CH_4 than fermentation of soluble sugars, which produce more CH_4 than fermentation of starch. This is a consequence of decreased rates of ruminal fermentation and passage out of the rumen that favor a higher A:P ratio. On the contrary, high grain diets fed at high intake levels are associated with high rates of ruminal digestion and passage that favour higher propionic acid production. For e.g. when brewer's grain was added to timothy hay (60 parts) and corn (25) based diet, CH_4 output in goats was reduced by 10% (Bhatta *et al.,* 2005, 2007, 2008). Although increased grain component in ruminant rations reduce CH_4 production however, the challenge is the importance of ruminants in converting fibrous feeds unsuitable for human consumption to high quality protein in developing countries like India.

7.1 Feeding of oils and fats in the diet

Oil cakes are a better source of feed ingredients which can be included in the ration of animals to increase energy content and a rumen modifier. Some of the components of oils have anti-microbial activity and anti-fibrolytic activity and therefore, free oils cannot be fed beyond a certain level. Beauchemin and McGinn (2006) reported that adding canola oil at the rate of 4.6 % of DM intake inhibited methane emission by 32% and decreased methane emissions as a per cent of gross energy intake by 21%, but this decrease in methane emission was primarily attributed to reduced feed intake and lower total tract digestibility of feed, especially the fibre component.

7.2 Diet effect on methane production

Methanogenesis decreases with improving the quality of feed either by increasing the digestibility of lignocellulosic feeds by some chemical (Moss *et al.,* 2000) or microbiological treatment or by replacing these feeds with good quality concentrate feeds (Cecava *et al.,* 1990). The inhibition in methanogenesis is accompanied with increased propionate levels and decreased acetate to propionate ratios and better feed conversion efficiency. Improved nutritional quality of feed is one such method which can be used to inhibit methanogenesis. Animals grazing the lowest quality pasture will produce the highest amount of methane per unit product (Kirschgessner *et al.* 1995). The treatment of paddy straw with urea resulted in a significant improvement in digestibility of nutrients and a significant depression in methane generation by the animals. Even the different roughage sources like paddy straw, sugarcane bagasse and wheat straw caused different levels of methane production. Paddy straw supported more methane production than the other two roughage sources tested (Chatterjee *et al.,* 2005). Therefore, proper selection of roughage source in the ration of ruminant may help in reducing methanogenesis to some extent.

7.3 Stage of growth of the forage

McAllister *et al.* (1996) and Moss *et al.* (2000) noted that CH_4 production in ruminants tends to increase with maturity of forage fed, and CH_4 yield from the ruminal fermentation of legume forages is generally lower than the yield from grass forages.

7.4 Feeding frequency of the ration

It was observed that low frequency of feeding increased propionate, reduced acetic acid production and lowered CH_4 production in dairy cows. This was attributed to the lowering of methanogens as a result of high fluctuations in ruminal pH, since low frequency of feeding increase diurnal fluctuations in ruminal pH that can be inhibitory to methanogens. On the other hand, more frequent feeding was shown to increase the A: P ratio (Sutton *et al.*, 1986).

7.5 Use of complete feed blocks/ total mixed rations

Feeding complete feed blocks comprising 70 % roughage and 30 per cent concentrate ingredients could be an alternate approach as it ensures nutrient balancing leading to better productivity and lowering CH_4 production by 10 per cent. Similar effects have been observed when animals are provided total mixed rations blended with roughage and concentrate feeds. This approach could be best suited under our conditions as it helps in better utilization of unconventional feeds, reduces wastage and helps in lowering methane production.

7B. Manipulation of rumen fermentation

7.6 Feeding of Ionophores

Mathison *et al.* (1998) described Ionophores as highly lipophilic substances, which are able to shield and delocalize the charge of ions and facilitate their movement across the membranes. Their feeding have been associated with the selective reduction of gram-positive ruminococci, and the proliferation of gram-negative bacteria with the concurrent shift in the fermentation from acetate to propionate and decrease in CH_4 production (Newbold *et al.*, 1988).

7.7 Defaunation or removal of protozoa form the rumen

Defaunation, which is the partial/total elimination of protozoa from the rumen by dietary or chemical agents, has been shown to reduce ruminal CH_4 production by about 20-50% depending on the diet composition (Itabashi *et al.*, 1994). Protozoa in the rumen are associated with a high proportion of H_2 production, and are closely associated with methanogens by providing a habitat for up to 20% of rumen methanogens (Newbold *et al.*, 1995a). The reduced ruminal methanogenesis observed with defaunation can be attributed to factors such as a shift of digestion from the rumen to the hindgut (Van Nevel and Demeyer, 1996) or the loss of methanogens associated with protozoa during defaunation (Hegarty 1999). However, this process could lead to reduced digestibility of poor quality roughages not much suitable where agricultural crop residues are the major roughage source like in India.

7.8 Feeding of plants containing tannins and saponins

Tannins constitute one of the important secondary metabolites which have anti-microbial activity and are present widely in different groups of plants. More attention has been paid to condensed tannins (CT) in comparison to hydrolysable tannins (HT), perhaps due to lower risk of toxicity. Bhatta *et al.* (2006 b, c; 2009, 2010) confirmed that tannins suppress methanogenesis directly through their anti-methanoginic and indirectly through anti-protozoal activities. Samples containing both CT plus HT were more potent in reducing methanogenesis than those containing HT only. This was further confirmed through respiration chamber studies in goats (Bhatta *et al.*, 2010, 2012c).

Microbial activity in the rumen may be affected by the use of saponins. The microbial population increased by low saponins supply, but decreased when doses became excessive (Wallace *et al.*, 2002). The protozoal counts in rumen fluid decreased with higher saponin doses like with sarsaponin from *Y. schidigera*, quillaja saponin (Makkar and Becker, 1996) and with saponin rich plants or fruit pulp (Kamra, 2006).

At National Institute of Animal Nutrition and Physiology, Bangalore under the Outreach program on methane various tree leaves and medicinal and aromatic plants have been screened to assess their efficacy as methane suppressants. Promising results were obtained *in vitro* with some of the leaves tested. The data on protozoa count indicated that methane suppression recorded with plant tannins was not primarily due to their defaunation property (Bhatta *et al.*, 2012a, b).

7.9 Addition of propionate enhancers in the diet

As a result of growing awareness of the threat of microbial resistance to antibiotics, there is an increasing interest in alternatives to antibiotics as growth promoters (Moss *et al.*, 2000). Dicarboxylic acids such as fumeric and malic acids have been studied *in vitro* as feed additives in ruminant diets to reduce methane emissions. Reducing fumeric acid may provide an alternate electron sink for H_2 since H_2 ions are needed in this reaction.

7.10 Vaccination against methanogens

Researchers in CSIRO, Australia have vaccinated sheep with a number of experimental vaccine preparations against methanogens, so that the animals produce antibodies to methanogens. Methane production was reduced between 11 and 23 % in vaccinated sheep, with no long or short term adverse effects. Researchers anticipate that commercial vaccines will allow a 3 % gain in animal productivity and a 20 % reduction in CH_4 production. These vaccines were based on the cultivable methanogens. However, the work of Whitford *et al.* (2001) showed that most ruminal methanogens have not yet been cultivated.

7.11 Alternate hydrogen sink-reductive acetogenesis

In the gut of termites and rodents, acetogens convert excess H_2 to acetic acid, which is then utilized by the host (Joblin, 1999). However, in the rumen the number of acetogens is few and cannot compete effectively with methanogens for H_2 ions, because they have a lower affinity for H_2 than methanogens (Nollet *et al.*, 1998). Increasing the populations of acetogens through exogenous inoculations into the rumen could be useful for competing against methanogens (Joblin, 1999).

Conclusions

Mitigation of rumen CH_4 emission is essential and can be effectively achieved by strategies that improve the efficiency of animal production. The dietary/nutritional strategies that improves productivity with no potential negative effects on livestock health and production and are cost effective is a challenge for animal nutritionists. The approach for mitigation also depends on the production systems and agronomic practices in the region. Generation of a database on methane production under different production systems adopting a common protocol would be useful in drawing mitigation strategies. The possible strategies to mitigate methane emission from the livestock are: replacing non-productive or low productive livestock with high productive livestock, enhancing degradability of poor quality roughages (Bhatta *et al.*, 2005, 2008a), use of alternate hydrogen sinks, feed additives like Ionophores, plant secondary metabolites (Bhatta *et al.*, 2006b, 2009) and chemicals and the use of biotechnology techniques. The other strategies could be ration balancing and strategic supplementation of feeds. Mitigation of rumen CH_4 emission is essential and can be effectively achieved by strategies that improve the efficiency of animal production. The dietary/nutritional strategy that improves productivity with no potential negative effects on livestock health and production and is cost effective has a better chance of being adopted. The approach for mitigation also depends on the production systems and agronomic practices in the region.

References

Beauchemin K.A., McGinn S.M. (2006). Methane emissions from beef cattle: Effects of fumaric acid, essential oil, and canola oil. *Journal of Animal Science* **84:** 1489-1496.

Benchaar C., Rivest J., Pomar C., Chiquette J. (1998). Prediction of methane production from dairy cows using existing mechanistic models and regression equations. *Journal of Animal Science* **76:** 671-672.

Bhatta R., Uyeno Y., Tajima K., Takenaka A., Yabumoto Y., Nonaka I., Enishi O., Kurihara M., (2009). Difference in the nature of tannins on *in vitro* ruminal methane and volatile fatty acid production, and methanoginicarchaea and protozoal populations *Journal of Dairy Science.* **92:** 5512-5522.

Bhatta R., Enishi O., Takusari N., Higuchi K., Nonaka I., Kurihara M., (2008). Diet effects on methane production by goats and a comparison between measurement methodologies *Journal of Agricultural Science (Cambridge)* **146:** 705-715.

Bhatta R., Tajima K., Kurihara M., (2006b). Influence of temperature and pH on fermentation pattern and methane production in the rumen simulating fermenter (RUSITEC). *Asian Australasian Journal of Animal Sciences* **19:** 376-380.

Bhatta R., Tajima K., Takusari N., Higuchi K., Enishi O., Kurihara M. (2007). Comparison of *in vivo* and *in vitro* techniques for methane production from ruminant diets. *Asian Australasian Journal of Animal Sciences* **20:** 1049-1056.

Bhatta R., Enishi O., Kurihara M. (2006a). Measurement of methane production from ruminants-a review. *Asian Australasian Journal of Animal Sciences* **20:** 1305-1318.

Bhatta R., Baruah L., Saravanan S., Sampath K.T. (2010). Efficacy of plant phenolics from medicinal and aromatic plants on rumen fermentation, protozoal population and methanogenesis *in vitro*, Greenhouse Gases and Animal Agriculture Conference (GGAA2010) at Banff, Canada p 87.

Bhatta R., Baruah L., Saravanan S., Sampath K.T. (2012a). Effect of medicinal and aromatic plants on rumen fermentation, protozoa population and methanogenesis *in vitro*. *Journal of Animal Physiology and Animal Nutrition* (in press). DOI:10.111/j.1439-0396.2012.01285.

Bhatta R., Saravanan S., Baruah L., Sampath K.T. (2012b). Nutrient content, *in vitro* ruminal fermentation characteristics and methane reduction potential of tropical tannin-containing leaves. *Journal of the Science of Food and Agriculture* (in press).

Bhatta R., Enishi O., Yabumoto Y., Nonaka I., Takusari N., Higuchi K., Tajima K., Kurihara M., (2012c). Methane reduction and energy partitioning in goats fed two concentrations of tannin from *Mimosa sp. Journal of Agricultural Science* (Cambridge) (in press). DOI:10.1017/S0021859612000299.

Bhatta R., Tajima K., Takusari N., Higuchi K., Enishi O., Kurihara M. (2005). Comparison of sulfur hexafluoride tracer technique, rumen simulation technique and *in vitro* gas production techniques for methane production from ruminant feeds. In: Greenhouse gases and animal agriculture: An update. (C.R. Soliva, J. Takahashi, and M. Kreuzer, eds.), Elsevier International Congress Series 1293, Amsterdam, The Netherlands, pp 419-421.

Bhatta R., Tajima K., Uyeno Y., Enishi O., Kurihara M. (2006b). Effect of plant extracts as natural source of tannins on methane production in vitro. In: *Proc. international workshop on "Monsoon asia agricultural greenhouse gas emissions"*, March 7-9, Tsukuba, Japan, p 67.

Bhatta R., Tajima K., Uyeno Y., Enishi O., Kurihara M. (2006c). Effect of plant extracts as natural source of tannins on methane production *in vitro*, International Workshop on Monsoon Asia Agricultural Greenhouse Gas Emissions (MAGE), March 7-9, Tsukuba, Japan, p 67.

Blake D.R., Rowland F.S. (1988). Continuing worldwide increase in tropospheric methane, 1978 to 1987. *Science* **239:** 1129-1131.

Blaxter K.L. (1962). *The Energy Metabolism of Ruminants*. London, Hutchinson.

Boadi D., Benchaar C., Chiquette J., Masse D. (2004). Mitigation strategies to reduce enteric methane emissions from dairy cows: update review. *Canadian Journal of Animal Science* **84:** 319-335.

Boadi D.A., Wittenberg K.M., Kennedy, A.D. (2002). Validation of the sulphur hexafluoride (SF_6) tracer gas technique for measurement of methane and carbon dioxide production by cattle. *Canadian Journal of Animal Science* **82:** 125-131.

Bolle H.J., Seiler W., Bolin B. (1986). Other greenhouse gases and aerosols; assessing their role for atmospheric radioactive transfer. In: *The greenhouse effect, climatic change and ecosystems* (B. Bolin, B.R. Doos, B. Warrick and D. Jager, eds), John Wiley and Sons: New York.

Cesava M.J., Merchen N.R., Gay L.C., Berger L.L. (1990). Composition of ruminal bacteria harvested from steers as influenced by dietary energy level, feeding frequency and isolation techniques. *Journal of Dairy Science* **73:** 2480-2488.

Chatterjee P.N. (2005). Influence of diet and plant secondary compounds on methanogenesis and rumen fermentation pattern. *Ph D. Thesis*, IVRI Deemed Univ., Izatnagar, India.

Cynoweth D.P. (1996). Environmental impact of biomethanogenesis, monitoring and assessment, Kluwer Academic Publishers. The Netherlands **42:** 3-18.

France J., Beever D.E., Siddons R.C. (1993). Compartmental schemes for estimating methanogenesis in ruminants from isotope dilution data. *Journal of Theoretical Biology*. **164:** 207-218.

Hegarty R.S., Gerdes R. (1998). Hydrogen production and transfer in the rumen. *Recent Advances in Animal Nutrition* **12:** 37-44.

Hegarty R.S., Goopy J.P., Herd R.M., McCorkell B. (2007). Cattle selected for lower residual feed intake have reduced daily methane production. *Journal of Animal Science* **85:** 1479-1486.

Hegarty R.S., Machmueller A., Waghorn G.C. (2004). Can tracers other than SF_6 be used to measure enteric methane emissions from individual animals. Clarkson, T. S. (comp.) In: *Proc. workshop on "The science of atmospheric trace gases."* NIWA Technical Report **125:** 139.

Hopkins A., Del Prado A., (2007). Implications of climate change for grassland in Europe: impacts, adaptations and mitigation options- a review. *Grass and Forage Science* **62:** 118-126.

Howden S.M., Reyenga P. J. (1999). Methane emissions from Australian livestock: implications of the Kyoto Protocol. *Australian Journal of Agricultural Research* **50:** 1285-1291.

IPCC (Intergovernmental Panel on Climate Change) (2007). Impacts, adaptation and vulnerability.Summary for policy makers. Online at Error! Hyperlink reference not valid.

IPCC (Intergovernmental Panel on Climate Change) (2001): The scientific basis. Contribution of working group I to the third assessment report of the intergovernmental panel on climate change. Cambridge Press.

Itabashi H., Washio Y., Takenaka A., Oda S., Ishibashi J. (1994). Effects of controlled fauna on methanogenesis, fibre digestion and rate of growth of calves. *Proceedings of the Society of Nutrition and Physiology* **3:** 179-184.

Joblin K. (1999). Ruminal acetogens and their potential to lower ruminant methane emissions, *Australian Journal of Agricultural Research* **50:** 1307-1313.

Johnson D.E., Johnson K.A., Ward G.M., Branine M.E. (2000). Ruminants and other animals. In: *Atmospheric methane: Its role in the global environment*, (M.A.K. Khalil, ed), Springer-Verlag, Berlin Heidelberg, pp 112-133.

Johnson K.A., Huyler M., Westberg H., Lamb B., Zimmerman P. (1994). Measurement of methane emissions from ruminant livestock using a SF_6 tracer technique. *Environmental Science and Technology* **28:** 359-362.

Johnson K.A., Johnson D.E. (1995). Methane emissions from cattle. *Journal of Animal Science* **73:** 2483-2492.

Johnson, K. A., Westberg, H. H., Lamb B. K., Kincaid, R. L. (2001). The use of sulphur hexafluoride for measuring methane emissions from farm animals. In: *Proc. 1st international conference on greenhouse gases and animal agriculture,* Obihiro, Hokkaido, Japan, pp 72-81.

Kaharabata S. K., Schuepp P. H. (2000). Estimating methane emissions from dairy cattle housed in a barn and feedlot using atmospheric tracer. *Environmental Science and Technology* **34:** 3296-3302.

Kamra D.N., Patra A.K., Chatterjee P.N., Kumar R., Agarwal N., Chaudhary L.C. (2008). Effect of plant extract on methanogenesis and microbial profile of the rumen of buffalo: a brief overview. *Australian Journal of Experimental Agriculture* **48:** 175-178.

Kawashima T. (2001). Measurement of methane production from ruminants by ventilated flow-through method with a face mask. In: *Proc. Tsukuba workshop on "Development of new monitoring method for methane emission from ruminants", NILGS,* Japan, pp 16-19.

Khalil M.A.K., Rasmussen R.A. (1986). Trends of atmospheric methane: past, present and future In: *Proc. Symposium on "CO_2 and other Greenhouse gases"*. Brussels, Belgium.

Kirchgessner C.U., Patil C.K., Evans J.W., Cuomo C.A., Fried L.M., Carter T., Oettinger M.A. Brown J.M. (1995). DNA-dependent kinase (p350) as a candidate gene for the murine SCID defect. *Science* **267:** 1178-1183.

Kwok R., Cunningham G.F., Wensnahan M., Rigor I., Zwally H.J., Yi D. (2009). Thinning and volume loss of the Arctic Ocean sea ice cover: 2003–2008, *Journal of Geophysical Research* **114:** 526-538.

Liang J.B., Terada F., Hamaguchi I. (1989). Efficacy of using the face masks technique for the estimation of daily heat production of cattle. In: *Energy metabolism of farm animals.* (Y. Van Der Honing and W. H. Close, eds.) Pudoc, Waginingen, the Netherlands.

Machmuller A., Hegarty R.S. (2005). Alternative tracer gases for the ERUCT technique to estimate methane emission from grazing animals. In: *2nd International Conference on Greenhouse Gases and Animal Agriculture*, Zurich, pp 365-368.

Makkar H.P.S., Becker K. (1996) Nutritional value and antinutritional components of whole and ethanol extracted *Moringa oliefera* leaves. *Animal Feed Science Technology* **63:** 211-228.

Makkar H.P.S., Blummel M., Becker K. (1995). Formation of complexes between polyvinyl pyrrolidones or polyethylene glycols and tannins, and their implication in gas production and true digestibility in *in vitro* techniques. *British Journal of Nutrition* **73:** 897-913.

Marc F., Whitford Ronald M.T., Robert, J. F. (2001) Phylogenetic analysis of methanogens from the bovine rumen. *BMC Microbiology* 1:5, http://www.biomedcentral.com/1471-2180/1/5.

Mathison G.W., Okine E.K., McAllister T.A., Dong Y., Galbraith J., Dmytruk O.I.N. (1998). Reducing methane emission from ruminant animals. *Journal of Applied Animal Research.* **14:** 1-28.

Mbanzamihigo, L. V., Fievez, C., da Costa Gomez, F., Piattoni, L., Carlier, Demeyer, D. (2002). Methane emissions from the rumen of sheep fed a mixed grass-clover pasture at two fertilisation rates in early and late season. *Canadian Journal of Animal Science* **82:** 69-77.

McAllister T.A., Okine E.K., Mathison G.W., Cheng K.N., (1996). Dietary, environmental and microbiological aspects of methane production in ruminants. *Canadian Journal of Animal Science* **76:** 231-243.

McLean J.A., Tobin G. (1987). Animal and human calorimetry. Cambridge university press. New York.

Mills J.A.N., Dijkstra J., Bannick A., Camel S.B., Krebreab E., France J. (2001). A mechanistic model of whole-tract digestion and methanogenesis in the lactating dairy cow: model development, evaluation and application. *Journal of Animal Science* **79:** 1584-1597.

Moate C.P., Dunn J.L., Bates C.A., Liu Y.M. (1997). An analytical model for the H X (h + g) Jahn- Teller system. *Journal of Physical Condensed Matter* **9:** 6049-6060.

Moss A.R., Jouany J.P., Newbold J. (2000). Methane production by ruminants: its contribution to global warming. *Annals of Zootechnica* **49:** 231-253.

Murray R.M., Bryant A.M., Leng R.A. (1975). Measurement of methane production in sheep. In: *Tracer studies on non-protein nitrogen for ruminants II.* International Atomic Energy Agency. Vienna.

Newbold C.J., El Hassan S.M., Wang J., Ortega M.E., Wallace R. J. (1997). Influence of foliage from African multipurpose tree on activity of rumen protozoa and bacteria. *British Journal of Nutrition* **78:** 237-249.

Nollet L., Mbanzamihigo L., Demeyer D., Verstrete W. (1998) Effect of addition of *Peptostreptococcus productus* ATCC 35244 on the reductive acetogenesis in the ruminal ecosystem after inhibition of methanogenesis by cell-free supernatant *Lactobacillus plantarum* 80. *Animal Feed Science and Technology* **71:** 49-66.

Pinares-Patiño C. (2000). Rumen function and digestion parameters associated with differences between sheep in methane emissions when fed chaffed lucerne hay. *Journal of Agricultural Science Cambridge* **140:** 205-214.

Rahmstorf S. (2007). A semi-empirical approach to projecting future sea-level rise. *Science* **19:** 368-370.

Rowlinson P. (2008). Livestock and Global climate change, (P. Rowlinson, M. Steele and A. Nefzaoui, eds), Cambridge University press, pp 61-63.

Singh G.P. (1997). Effect of greenhouse gases on climate change and Indian ruminant livestock. *Current Science* **72:** 441-446.

Stefan R. (2007). A semi-empirical approach to projecting future sea-level rise. *Science* **315:** 368-370.

Stroeve J., Holland M.M., Meier W., Scambos T., Serreze M. (2007) Arctic sea ice decline: Faster than forecast. *Geophysical Research Letters* **34:** 1-5.

Sutton J.D., Hart I.C., Brostel W.H., Elliot R.J., Sehuller E. (1986). Influence of plane of nutrition and diet composition on rumen fermentation and energy utilization by dairy cows. *British Journal of Nutrition* **56:** 181-192.

Terada F. (1999). Methane emission from ruminant animals. In: Studies on the evaluation of estimation of anthropogenic sources and sinks of greenhouse gases. *Final report of global environment research fund, Environment agency* pp 157-162 (Jpn).

Van Nevel C.J., Demeyer D.I. (1996). Effect of pH on biohydrogenation of polyunsaturated fatty acids and their Ca-salts by rumen microorganisms *in vitro*. *Archives of Animal Nutrition* **49:** 151-157.

❏❏❏

Chapter 31

Abiotic Stress in Livestock Production System : Recent Development

K.S. Roy, J. Ghosh, S.C. Roy, A. Dhali, A. Mech
National Institute of Animal Nutrition and Physiology, Adugodi, Bangalore-560 030, Karnataka, India

Summary

The abiotic stress plays a vital role in lowering the efficiency of reproductive and productive performance of livestock under the present global climate change scenario. It affects livestock in terms of weight gain, meat quality, milk production, reproduction, compromised immune systems to make animals vulnerable to diseases and finally reduces the survival rate in young stocks. During summer lack of feeds and fodders is another major contributing factor for occurance of stress. Therefore, dietary corrections are required to increase intake and alter levels of nutrients to improve the feed conversion efficiency. There are wide differences existing on thermo-adaptability between species and breeds of animals. Genetic differences of thermo-tolerance extend to the cellular levels are due to the acquisition of certain genes. Deleterious effects of elevated temperature on cellular function are less in cells of *indicus* cattle than in European cattle. A concrete understanding on effects of abiotic stress, particularly the heat stress require congregation of a lot of information on cooling cycle, reproductive phenomena and productive efficiency; and also require a constant monitoring, documentation, evaluation and strategic research on these area to have a climate resilient livestock production system for our national need.

The cumulative effect of abiotic stress reduces the efficiency of reproductive and productive performance of livestock. Different environmental factors, like ambient temperature, relative humidity, radiant energy and metabolic heat associated with maintenance and productive processes are the major contributor to heat stress. When livestock face difficulty for coping up with stress, their productivity gets affected in terms of weight gain, meat quality, milk production, reproduction, and compromised immune systems, occurrence of diseases, maladaptive behaviors that execute negative impact on animal and finally lower survival rates in offspring. During summer lack of feeds and fodders are other important contributing factors for manifestation of stress. We need to have more critical information on total dietary needs of livestock during hot environment. Dietary emphasis should be given to increase intake or to alter levels of different nutrients to improve the conversion of feed units into production units. There are wide differences of thermo-adaptability existing in between species and breeds of animal. It is interesting to note that the cattle from Indian origin (*Bos indicus)* are better capable to regulate body temperature in response to heat stress than the cattle from European origin (*Bos taurus*). Genetic differences in thermo-tolerance extend to the cellular level, as well as deleterious effects of elevated temperature on cellular function are less for cells from *indicus* cattle than cells from Angus and Holstein. Genetic adaptations that have developed in *indicus* cattle during its evolution is the acquisition of genes for thermo-tolerance. In the recent time of paradigm shift in global climatic change a constant monitoring, documentation and strategic research is needed to cope up with the upcoming situation of sustenance and augmentation of livestock production in India and all over the world.

1. Defining stress

Stress is defined as a complex multi-dimensional phenomenon promoted by several noxious or unpredictable stimuli that cause a physiological response aimed at maintaining or recovering the body homeostasis (Moberg, 2000). Generally, heat stress is the outcome of animal's inability to dissipate sufficient amount of heat to maintain homoeothermy. The "abiotic stress" mainly refers to the meteorological elements, which causes distress to the animal as a whole. The most important ones are environmental temperature, air humidity and solar radiation. Air movement has a heating effect only when air temperature is above body surface temperature, which occurs rarely. The animal can defend itself against heat by behavioral means, reducing body insulation, increasing evaporation, lowering heat production and increasing the reflectance of the hair coat to solar radiation. Different environmental factors, like ambient temperature, relative humidity, radiant energy and metabolic heat associated with maintenance and productive processes, are the major contributor to heat stress. When livestock face difficulty for coping up with stress their productivity gets affected in terms of weight gain and meat quality, milk production, reproduction, compromised immune systems which makes animal vulnerable to diseases, maladaptive behaviors that negatively impact the animal and finally lower survival rates in young. Whatever animal perceives, the response begins with the activation of the sympathetic nervous system (SNS) and the hypothalamic-pituitary-adrenal system (HPA). Several other functions of the animal also get involved such as immune systems and metabolic pathways. As a final result of the adaptive modifications the homeostasis of animal body worsens as a whole.

2. Adaptation to stress

Adaptation is often used as a term for the characters or traits observed in animals that are the result of selection. But it could be defined as a process or the means by which the frequency of genes that code for traits affecting fitness gets adjusted by natural selection when interacted with environmental phenomena. It can be best described as short-term compensatory changes in response to environmental disturbance. The changes that occur in cattle during climatic stress are compensatory and are directed for maintaining or restoring thermal balance. These include sweating, rapid respiratory rate, greater vasodilation with increased blood flow to the skin surface, reduced rate of metabolism, decreased DM and nutrient intake and altered water metabolism.

2.1 Endocrinological changes during heat stress

The plasma growth hormone concentration and growth hormone secretion rate declined with hot temperatures (35°C). Growth hormone (GH) content in milk of low, medium, and high production groups declined when 'temperature-humidity index (THI)' exceeded around 72, possibly reflecting suppressed production of growth hormone so that metabolic heat production is reduced. The thyroid hormones reduce in response to heat stress, which is probably an attempt to decrease the metabolic heat production in the cow. Greater plasma content of epinephrine and norepinephrine with high ambient temperatures is an indicator of stress response and reduces rate of passage of digesta in the digestive tract so as to decrease metabolic rate. The level of prolactin was found to rise tremendously under heat stress in buffaloes (Roy and Prakash, 2009a,b). Cortisol response to heat stress challenge is often variable, but workers evaluating the effects of increasing fiber content of the diet on the response to hot, humid weather reported a linear increase in plasma cortisol with increasing fiber content of the diet.

2.2 Nutritional changes during heat stress

It has been observed that feed dry matter intake (DMI) starts to decline and maintenance expenditure increase when environmental temperatures exceed 25°C. Milk yield and total digestible nutrients (TDN) intake decline slightly when the THI exceed 72 and decline sharply when THI exceed 76. Milk yield declines when body temperature exceed 38.9°C, and, for each 0.55°C increase in rectal temperature, milk yield and intake of TDN (total digestible nutrient) decline 1.8 and 1.4 kg, respectively. Water is the most critical nutrient for cattle and other livestock; and the need is intensified for those subjected to hot climatic conditions. Water losses through the lungs increased gradually and losses from the skin increased sharply as ambient temperature increased from about 16°C to 35°C. Cows acclimatized to 21.1°C and then exposed to 32.2°C for 2 weeks showed increased water consumption by 110%, and water losses from the respiratory tract and from the skin surface increased by 55% and 177% at the higher temperature. Feeding excessive quantities of nutrients like crude protein, can contribute to reduced efficiency of energy utilization and potentially adding up to stress levels in animal. So, a thorough understanding of dietary modifications is necessary to minimize heat stress.

2.3 Endocrine indicators

During stressful situations two main endocrine systems are activated that promotes the release of several hormones: catecholamines (*viz.*, epinephrine, nor-epinephrine), corticotrophic-releasing hormone, adreno-corticotrophin, corticosteroids (cortisol being the major). Unfortunately, most of these hormones show a very short spike in the blood after occurrence of stress events, revealing their unreliability in measuring chronic stress conditions.

2.3.1 Cortisol

The basal level of cortisol and its variation after adeno-corticotrophin hormone (ACTH) challenge is a possible candidate for chronic stress evaluation in animal system. Although an increase in cortisol occurs after any acute stress, it shows marked and more prolonged variations before and during stress that seems reasonably related to maladaptation. In fact high levels of cortisol seem to be maintained when there is a failure to restore homeostasis or after repeated stress. However, some contradictory results emerge from the literature relating to farm animals. Hyper-reactivity in animals under chronic stress after ACTH challenges supports the relationship between high basal cortisol levels and chronic stress. Undoubtedly, the interpretation of the basal blood cortisol is not easy because it is affected by a variety of other factors, including circadian rhythms, sampling, restraint, stage of lactation, coitus and nursing, milking, degree of habituation, other hormones (*e.g.*, vasopressin increase ACTH secretion), infections and endotoxin.

2.3.2 β-endorphin

The β-endorphin is a cleavage product of proopiomelanocortin, a precursor of ACTH, formed in the anterior pituitary. It is supposed that β-endorphin produces a major effect in the CNS, where it interacts with the opiate receptors. As â-endorphin is involved in pain, cerebral ageing, behavior with respect to feelings, food intake and emotions; so it can be a good indicator of chronic stress evaluation. Although β-endorphin seems to reduce perception of pain, similar to drugs such as morphine and codeine, more data are needed to clarify the effective relationship between β-endorphin and chronic stress, for a better interpretation of its basal levels.

2.4 Heat shock proteins (HSPs)

These evolutionary ancient families of molecules are essential for survivals of all prokaryotic and eukaryotic cells. On expression, they play an important role in protection and maintenance of vital cellular functions. At the cellular level, the cells respond to stresses by the production of a specific set of proteins called heat shock or stress proteins (Lindquist, 1986). A variety of factors, including heat stress, heavy metals, amino acid analogues, inhibitors of energy metabolism, chelating agents and infection with certain viruses, are capable of inducing the synthesis of these proteins. The definite function for heat stress proteins is unknown, but they are thought to help the cell to survive during the stress (Li and Werb, 1982). Animals have been shown to acquire thermo-tolerance by exposure to a conditioning body heat dose (Li *et al.*, 1983); hyperthermia of whole animals induces the synthesis of stress proteins (Dean and Atkinson, 1985; Rodenhiser *et al.*, 1985). During steady state conditions, HSPs fulfill a variety of functions like intracellular assembly, folding and translocation of oligomeric proteins. Under conditions of cellular stress they act as a cytoprotective agent by binding to misfolded proteins and protect them from denaturation; and thus elevated HSPs repair protein damage and facilitate normal cell growth.

HSPs are immunodominant molecules and because of their conserved nature along with their inherent immunogenecity they might act as auto antigens that are capable of initiating and driving inflammatory process (Kaufmann, 1990). Immune recognition of cross-reactive heat shock protein epitopes provides a link between infection and autoimmunity. The lymphocytes isolated from various animals were heat stressed *in vitro* and responded by synthesizing heat stress proteins. The most studied of these proteins have molecular weights of approximately 90, 70 and 27 kDa and are referred to as HSP90, HSP70 and HSP27 *etc.* These wide ranges of HSPs are the confirmatory physiological biomarkers for stress determination. And the most important protein in this group is HSP70.

The expression of HSP 70 is strictly stress inducible and can only be detected following a significant stress upon the cell or organism (Ito *et al.*, 1999). The HSP70 has been studied in variety of medically relevant models or conditions such as hyperthermia, hypertension, toxic exposure to chemical agents, hypoxia, ischemia, inflammation, autoimmunity, apoptosis, cancer, organ transplantation, bacterial and viral infections. In the field of medico-clinico-pathological study (*e.g.*, treatment of tumor, cancer *etc.*) HSP gives specific "cancer fingerprint" and at present vaccination against cancer is possible. Current research is aimed at investigating HSP70 as a cytoprotective therapeutic agent as well as a sensitive biomarker for monitoring cellular tress or perturbation in homeostasis.

2.5 Physiological indicators

Acute stress affects the physiological parameters such as heart rate, heart rate variability, respiration rate and transpiration. Between these parameters, the measure of the heart rate variability (HRV) seems a promising approach for evaluating stress (acute and chronic) and for emotional states in human (Appelhans and Luecken, 2006) and farm animals (von Borrel *et al.*, 2007). The HRV measures continuous interplay between sympathetic and parasympathetic influences on heart rate, which determine the typical irregular time intervals between consecutive heart beats. Therefore, according to Appelhans and Luecken (2006), HRV represents the different capacity for regulated emotional response. In animals, HRV is proposed as an index of maladaptation for an expected future flight response, which could remain modified for several days during a psychological stress.

3. Effects of heat stress on reproduction

3.1 Effect of heat stress on estrus activity, hormone function, and follicular development

Heat stress reduces the length and intensity of estrus in cows and other species. During summer, motor activity and other manifestations of estrus are reduced and incidence of anestrous and silent ovulations are increased in cattle and buffaloes (Gwazdauskas *et al.*, 1981; Nebel *et al.*, 1997; Roy and Prakash, 2009a,b). Heat stress impairs follicle selection and increases the length of follicular waves, thus reducing the quality of oocytes and modulating follicular steroidogenesis. Summer heat stress has been shown to increase the number of subordinate follicles while reducing the degree of dominance of the dominant follicle and decreasing inhibin and estrogen levels. The heat stress induced increase in duration of follicular dominance has been associated with a reduced fertility in beef heifers. Study showed that there is an increase in twinning rates in dairy cows during summer versus winter (Ryan and Boland, 1991). Summer heat stress reduces follicular dominance allowing more than one dominant follicle to develop, explaining the increased twinning seen in summer months. The follicle destined to ovulate emerges 40 to 50 days prior to ovulation (Roth *et al.*, 2001). Therefore, heat stress occurring at any time during this period can compromise follicular growth and steroidogenic capacity. In addition, either due to direct actions of elevated temperature or alterations of follicular function, the oocyte has the potential to be compromised.

3.2 Effect of heat stress on oocytes, fertilization, and early developing embryos

Generally during summer, heat stress reduces pregnancy and conception rate, which can carry over into the fall months (Wolfenson *et al.*, 2000). It has been found that the oocytes obtained from dairy cows during the summer heat stress period had reduced developmental competence *in vitro* (Rocha *et al.*, 1998). When superovulated donor heifers were exposed to heat stress for 16h beginning at the onset of estrus, there was no effect on fertilization rate. However, there were a reduced number of normal embryos recovered seven days after estrus (Putney *et al.*, 1988a). This illustrates that a brief heat stress can still affect oocyte competence within the preovulatory follicle. In addition, exposure of cultured oocytes to elevated temperatures during maturation decreased cleavage rate and the proportion of oocytes that become blastocysts (Edwards and Hansen, 1997). Heat stress can also affect the early developing embryo. When heat stress was applied from day 1 to day 7 after estrus, there was a reduction in quality and stage of development of embryos flushed from the reproductive tract on day 7 after estrus. In addition, embryos collected from superovulated donor cows in summer months were less able to develop in culture than embryos collected from superovulated cows during fall, winter and spring months. An earlier study showed that heat stress caused a greater reduction in embryo development when applied at 2-cell stage than the morula stage or at day 3 following fertilization than at day 4 (Ju *et al.*, 1999).

4. Cellular and molecular changes during abiotic stress

4.1 Cellular resistance to heat stress

The hyperthermia resulting from heat stress can compromise cellular function and result in physiological changes unfavorable to animal production. This is particularly true for reproduction, like elevations in testicular temperature impede spermatogenesis and culture of oocytes and embryos at temperatures characteristic of those experienced by heat-stressed cows can compromise subsequent embryonic development (Roth and Hansen, 2004). There is evidence that cattle evolved in hot climates have acquired genes that protect cells from the deleterious actions of elevated temperature. Genetic resistances to cellular effects of elevated temperature are seen in both *B. indicus* as well as two breeds of *B. taurus*, the Senepol and Romosinuano. Thus, decrease in lymphocyte viability caused by heat shock was greater for lymphocytes from Angus cows than for lymphocytes from Brahman (*B. indicus*) and Senepol cows. Likewise, lymphocytes from Brahman and Senepol cows were more resistant to heat-induced apoptosis than lymphocytes from Angus and Holstein cows. Short-term exposure of embryos to elevated temperature causes a less severe reduction in development for Brahman and

Romosinuano embryos than for Angus or Holstein embryos. There were also differences between Brahman and Holstein in endometrial responses to culture at elevated temperature. There are genetic differences in cellular resistance to elevated temperature in cattle is the first example in endotherms of genetic adaptations in cellular resistance to elevated temperature. It is possible that the same gene or genes conferring cellular thermo-tolerance are present in Brahman, Senepol, and Romosinuano, especially because of the contribution of *B. indicus* genotypes to these cattle breeds (Magee *et al.*, 2002). An alternative explanation is that distinct thermo-tolerance genes are present in the different genotypes. Identification of the genes conferring cellular thermo-tolerance offers the possibility of transferring these genes to heat-sensitive breeds to improve reproduction and other physiological systems compromised by hyperthermia. At present, little is known regarding the molecular basis for the improved cellular resistance to elevated temperature in thermo-tolerant cattle. There were no significant differences between Brahman, Senepol and Angus in the amount of heat shock protein 70 (HSP70) in heat-shocked lymphocytes, although the non-significant tendency for lower amounts in Brahman and Senepol may indicate that protein denaturation in response to elevated temperature (one of the signals for HSP70 synthesis) is reduced in Brahman and Senepol. The capacity for transcription in response to elevated temperature seems to be important for expression of genetic differences because there were no differences between Brahman and Holstein embryos in resistance to elevated temperature at the two-cell stage, a time when the embryonic genome is largely inactive (Memili and First, 2000). Not only the genetic differences in cellular resistance to elevated temperature are expressed at the two-cell stage, a time when embryos are very sensitive to elevated temperature, but the cellular thermo-tolerance of crossbred embryos is dependent upon the genotype of the oocyte and not the spermatozoa. Embryos produced by insemination of Brahman oocytes with Angus spermatozoa were more thermo-tolerant than embryos produced by insemination of Holstein oocytes with Angus semen. In contrast, there were no differences in thermo-tolerance between Brahman × Holstein embryos and Angus × Holstein embryos. These results indicate that either genes conferring thermo-tolerance are paternally imprinted (only the maternal allele being expressed) or that thermo-tolerance in embryos depends upon some genetically-controlled factor produced in the oocyte. Data by Turner (1982) suggested that regulation of body temperature is the most critical factor for genetic differences in reproductive function during heat stress since the depression in fertility per unit increase in body temperature was the same for *B. indicus* × *B. taurus* crossbred cows as for Hereford × Shorthorn cows.

4.2 Exploitation of indigenous genotypes to increase thermo-tolerance in cattle

The Brahman cattle exposed to heat stress experience less severe alterations in feed intake, growth rate, milk yield and reproduction than do cattle from *B. taurus* breeds that are not adapted to warm climates. In addition to being thermo-tolerant, Brahman cattle are tick resistant and efficient at digesting poor quality forages. Not surprisingly, much use has been made of Brahman genotypes to develop cattle for beef and dairy production in the tropics and semi-tropics. However, other genetic characteristics of Brahman cattle that limit their usefulness as beef and dairy animals include poor meat tenderness, low milk yields and lactation persistency, a long prepubertal period, short duration of estrus and poor temperament. In dairy cattle systems, utilization of Brahman crossbreds in hot climates becomes more beneficial relative to purebred European breeds as the overall level of feed resources and other inputs decline. An alternative scheme to crossbreeding for utilizing the Brahman genotype for livestock production in hot climates is to incorporate those Brahman genes that confer thermo-tolerance into European breeds while avoiding undesirable genes. Olson *et al.* (2003) have identified a phenotype characterized by development of a very short, sleek hair coat that is inherited as if controlled by a single dominant gene. Cattle inheriting the *slick hair* gene are better able to regulate body temperature and for Carora, have higher milk yields. Identification of specific gene loci conferring thermo-tolerance in Brahman cattle could be followed by crossbreeding and selection for the favorable allele using phenotypic traits or molecular markers. Efforts have been made to identify specific loci in Brahman crossbreds that affect carcass and growth traits (Casas *et al.*, 2003) but no effort has been made for identifying genetic markers for thermo-tolerance. Care must be taken in doing so to avoid inadvertent selection of genes for reduced production since genes causing low feed intake and low milk yield would increase thermo-tolerance. This problem could be avoided by identifying candidate genes known to be involved in thermo-tolerance (Taylor *et al.*, 1998). The advent of molecular genetics, marker assisted selection, and transgenics makes the strategies technically feasible. However, realization of the promise these technologies offer awaits intensive research into the molecular basis for thermo-tolerance in cattle. Almost nothing is known about specific genes controlling heat resistance in Brahman cattle and indeed, our understanding of the physiological basis for thermo-tolerance in these cattle is still incomplete. There is a compelling need to use modern methods to further define the physiological and cellular basis for thermo-tolerance in Brahman cattle and to identify the genes responsible. Once this is accomplished, the complete armamentarium of modern genetics can be brought to bear to exploit the Brahman genome for livestock production.

The utilization of thermo-tolerant breeds has been exploited by beef industry in many of the countries with a hot climate. Additionally, *in vivo* and *in vitro* embryo transfer has been increasing in tropical countries like Brazil, particularly in the Nelore breed (*B. indicus*, over 90 million animals are in Brazil). European breeds usually predominate in the dairy industries of tropical and subtropical regions because of the higher milk yields as compared to Brahman cattle. Utilization of Brahman crossbred in hot climates may become more beneficial relative to purebred European breeds as the overall level of feed resources and other inputs decline and cause great economic gain.

4.3 Embryonic susceptibility to heat stress

In most mammals, the effects of heat stress are most pronounced from estrus until insemination, and during the first cleavage stages of embryonic development. The effects of heat stress on embryonic mortality decrease as pregnancy progresses, and become minimized by three days after estrus in cows. Several *in vitro* studies have confirmed that bovine embryos become resistant to heat stress as they become more developed. According to Edwards and Hansen (1997), there are at least two possibilities to explain why embryos become more thermo-tolerant as development proceeds. One possibility is that a larger embryo with more cells is better able to survive the loss of a fraction of its cells than embryos with a smaller number of cells. If one assumes hypothetically that the effect of heat shock is to alter the function of 50% of the blastomeres, a two-cell embryo would be left with only one blastomere to form a viable embryo, whereas a morula or blastocyst would have 30–50 viable blastomeres to continue development. The second possibility is that embryos acquire mechanisms of thermo-protection during development, such as production of heat shock proteins and glutathione.

4.4 Contribution of male and female gametes genotypes for development of thermo-tolerance

The *Bos indicus* embryos exposed to heat shock at early stages of development are better able to survive as compared to *B. taurus* embryos. More recently, the effect of heat stress on embryonic development in culture was evaluated in Nelore (*B. indicus*) and crossbred (indicus versus taurus) oocytes fertilized with Nelore or Angus (*B. taurus*) spermatozoa. The decrease in blastocyst development rates caused by exposure to 41°C during 12 h was more evident when the heat shock was applied at earlier stages of development, particularly for embryos that had a predominant *taurus* genotype. It has been observed that the Nelore embryos are better able to survive under heat stress at early stages of development and more capable of initiating pregnancies following heat stress than Angus embryos. The fact that embryo genotype determines resistance to heat shock leads to the query as to whether embryos sired by thermo-tolerant breeds exhibit the same resistance to heat shock or not. And this is a query of practical importance because, if true, one could conceivably increase pregnancy rates during heat stress by insemination with semen from thermo-tolerant breeds. Embryos produced by insemination of Brahman oocytes with Angus spermatozoa were more thermo-tolerant than embryos produced by insemination of Holstein oocytes with Angus semen (Hernández-Cerón, 2004). In contrast, there were no differences in thermo-tolerance between Holstein-Brahman embryos and Holstein-Angus embryos. The results regarding the contribution of oocyte were obtained by Eberhardt *et al.* (2005) using *B. indicus* (Nelore) or *B. taurus* (Holstein) oocytes fertilized with Nelore or Angus (*B. taurus*) semen, i.e., the deleterious effect of heat shock (decline in blastocyst rate) was less pronounced in Nelore as compared to Holstein or crossbred embryos.

4.5 Contribution of male and female gametes for embryonic development and survival under heat stress condition

The spermatozoa as well as oocyte contribute in the ability of embryos to resist effects of heat stress. However, an interpretation obtained by Pegorer, (2007) is that higher pregnancy rates observed in Holstein cows inseminated with Gir(Gyr) breed as compared to Holstein sires is caused by the beneficial effect of heterosis. Although Fisher *et al.* (2000) did not find any evidence for heterosis for embryo development *in vitro*, it may be present in vivo. If that is the case, the results above would be the first to support this concept. Another interesting aspect of the importance of sperm on fertility and embryonic development is the observation that individual bulls differ in their ability to fertilize oocytes following IVF (*in vitro* fertilization) procedures and that there is a strong male effect on the development of fertilized oocytes. Under conditions for bovine IVF, approximately two-thirds of oocytes fail to reach the blastocyst stage. The factors responsible for this relatively poor development are unknown; however, the intrinsic quality of the oocyte is thought to be of critical importance in determining the developmental outcome. It has been demonstrated that there is a clear relationship between the time of the first cleavage of a bovine oocyte *in vitro* and its developmental ability, with the earliest-cleaving oocytes being more likely to develop to the blastocyst stage than those that cleave late. According to Gutie´rrez-Adan *et al.* (2004), genes that may be stress induced such as sarcosine oxidase, mitochondrial Mn-superoxide dismutase, apoptosis regulator box-α, interferon-τ, and glucose-6-phosphate dehydrogenase were highly transcribed in embryos produced *in vitro* and in embryos with slow developmental speed. Conversely, transcripts from genes related with metabolism, growth, and differentiation (glucose transporter-5, connexin 43, insulin-like growth factor-II, and insulin-like growth factor-I receptor) were detected in higher amounts in *in vivo* produced embryos and in embryos with fast developmental speed. Upon entry into the oocyte, the sperm chromatin undergoes extensive remodeling resulting in the reorganization of the paternal genome into the male pronucleus. The female and male pronuclei undergo a round of DNA synthesis before entering the first mitosis, culminating in the first cleavage to a two-cell embryo. There is evidence that in cattle the sire can affect the timing of the onset and duration of this DNA replication during the first cell cycle, and thereby ultimately affect the timing of the first cleavage division (Barros *et al.*, 2006).

5. Strategies to improve reproduction during heat stress

5.1 Improving reproduction by cooling dry cows

Most of the time dry pregnant cows are provided little protection from heat stress (HS) because they are not lactating, and it is incorrectly assumed that they are less prone to heat stress. Stress during this period due to abrupt physiological, nutritional, and environmental changes have a critical influence on postpartum cow health, milk production, and reproduction. The dry period is particularly crucial since it involves mammary gland involution and subsequent development, rapid fetal growth, and induction of lactation. Heat stress during this time period can affect endocrine responses that may increase fetal abortions, shorten the gestation length, lower calf birth weight, and reduce follicle and oocyte maturation associated with the postpartum reproductive cycle. It takes approximately 40 to 50 days for antral follicles to develop into large dominant follicles and ovulate (Roth *et al.*, 2001). If heat stress occurs during this time period, both the follicle and oocyte inside the follicle become damaged. Once ovulation occurs, the damaged oocyte has reduced chances of fertilizing and developing into a viable embryo. Cooling dry cows may reduce heat stress effects on the antral follicle destined to ovulate 40 to 50 days later, which coincides with the start of most breeding periods, and possibly increases first service conception rates. The greatest opportunity to reduce the negative effects of heat stress during both the pre- and postpartum periods is through cooling.

5.2 Improving lactating dairy cow reproduction during heat stress

The genetic selection for milk production has increased metabolic heat load per cow. This has considerably increased the lactating dairy cow's susceptibility to heat stress. In addition, the first several days to weeks following calving, the cow is vulnerable to infectious diseases and metabolic disorders. These stress factors, coupled with physiological, nutritional, and environmental changes occurring at calving, can reduce reproductive performance.

5.3 Reducing negative effects of postpartum heat stress

Two major strategies are to minimize heat gain by reducing solar heat load and maximize heat loss by reducing air temperature around the animal or increasing evaporative heat loss directly from animals. Locating where heat stress is occurring on the dairy facility by identifying hot spots is the key to implement the proper cooling or management strategy to eliminate these hot spots. Providing enough shade and cow cooling is vital for proper cow comfort. There should be at least 38 to 45 square feet of shade per mature dairy cow to reduce solar radiation. Spray and fan systems should be used in the holding pen, over feeding areas, over the feeding areas in some free-stall barns, and under shades on dry-lot dairies in arid climates. Exit lane cooling is an inexpensive way to cool cows as they leave the parlor. Providing enough access to water during heat stress is critical. Water needs increase 1.2 to 2 times during heat stress conditions. Lactating cows require 130 to 170 L of water/day. The holding pen is often an area of elevated heat stress conditions. Cows are crowded into a confined area for several minutes to hours. Cows should not spend more than 60 to 90 minutes in the holding area. In addition, provide shade, fans, and sprinklers in the holding pen. It is interesting to know that the cow's warmest body temperature occurs between evenings to midnight.

5.4 Nutritional modifications

The effects of nutrition on reproduction are well documented. Reducing metabolic diseases will further enhance our ability to improve reproduction during the summer months. Some simple feeding and nutritional strategies can be implemented to reduce the negative effects of summer heat stress on reproduction. The maintenance requirement of lactating dairy cows increases substantially as environmental temperature increases. When possible, the number of feedings should be increased in order to increase DMI. In addition, feeding during cooler parts of the day, and increasing moisture content in the ration from an average of 35 to 40% to an average of 45 to 50% are two more strategies The heat stress cow is prone to rumen acidosis, and many of the lasting effects of warm weather such as laminitis, low milk fats, etc. Obviously, fiber quality is important all the time, but it is paramount during the summer as it has some buffering capacity and stimulates saliva production. Furthermore, dietary -HCO_3 may be a valuable tool to maintain a healthy rumen pH. Feeding dietary fat in the form of rumen bypass fat remains an effective strategy of providing extra energy during a time of negative energy balance. Compared to starch and fiber, fat has a much lower heat increment in the rumen and thus provides energy without a negative thermal side effect. A safe and effective method of maximizing rumen propionate production is with monensin. Having a negative dietary cation-anion difference (DCAD) during the dry period and a positive DCAD during lactation is a good strategy to maintain health and maximize production. It appears that keeping the DCAD at a healthy lactating level (approximately +20 to +30 meq/100 g DM) remains a good strategy during the warm summer months (Wildman *et al.*, 2007). Unlike humans, cattle utilize potassium (K+) as their primary osmotic regulator of water secretion from their sweat glands. As a consequence, K+ requirements are increased (1.4 to 1.6% of DM) during the summer, and this should be adjusted for in the diet. In addition, dietary levels of sodium (Na+) and magnesium (Mg+) should be increased, as they compete with potassium (K+) for intestinal absorption.

5.5 Changes in reproductive protocol

The judicious observation for estrus two to three times daily for 20 to 30 min, can increase the number and accuracy of cows detected in estrus. Using teaser bull and tail head paint is the most popular estrus detection aid and should be applied in adequate amounts with easily observable colors. Several technologies are available to improve identification of estrus. The Heat Watch® (Cow Chips, LLC, Denver, CO) system records the number and times mounted during estrus through the use of a radio-telemetric pressure transducer placed on the tail head to transmit information to a computer. Pedometers can also be used to measure the increased amount of activity associated with estrus. The use of fixed timed artificial insemination (TAI) to avoid the deleterious effects of reduced estrous detection has been well documented. Utilizing some type of TAI along with Ovsynch, either coupled with or without estrus detection, can improve fertility during the summer (Roy and Prakash, 2009b).

5.6 Probable solutions for improving summer fertility

The use of embryo transfer can significantly improve pregnancy rates during the summer months (Drost *et al.*, 1999). Embryo transfers can bypass the period (*i.e.*, before day 7) in which the embryo is more susceptible to heat stress. Nevertheless, embryo transfer is not a widely adopted technique. Improvements need to be in made in the *in vitro* embryo production techniques, embryo freezing, timed embryo transfer, and lowering the cost of commercially available embryos before this becomes a feasible solution. The maternal reproductive system under summer stress plays an important role successful execution of fertility. Putney *et al.* (1988b) studied that the heat stress conditions decreased protein synthesis and secretion of interferon-tau by 71% in embryos; however, endometrial secretion of $PGF_{2\alpha}$ and embryo secretion of PGE2 increased in response to HS by 72%. Collectively, these studies demonstrate that both the embryo and the uterine environment can be disrupted due to HS inhibiting the embryo's ability to secrete interferon-tau (signal to block CL regression) and maintain pregnancy and (or) manipulating production of important proteins from the uterine lining. However, selecting particular genes that control traits related to thermo-tolerance makes it possible to select for thermal resistance without inadvertently selecting against milk yield (Hansen and Arechiga, 1999). The traits that could possibly be selected for include coat color, genes controlling hair length, and genes controlling heat shock resistance in cells. In addition, genetic modification or altering biochemical properties of the embryo before embryo transfer may be possible to improve thermal resistance and increase summer fertility. There may be feed additives which can partially alleviate heat stress through increased heat dissipation, thereby lowering internal body temperature. The resulting management changes could reduce the negative effects of heat stress on reproduction.

Conclusions

The development and use of improved cooling system for cow shed is still the most profitable and effective way to improve production and reproduction during the summer months. Dry cows are also susceptible to heat stress and should be provided some type of cooling to improve subsequent fertility after calving. Postpartum heat stress can significantly decrease pregnancy rates with impacts lingering well into the fall months. Strategies to reduce negative effects of heat stress on fertility, such as enhanced cooling, ration adjustments, and reproductive protocol changes will improve dairy farm profitability to a great extent. The different reproductive technologies such as artificial insemination, TAI, and *in vivo* and *in vitro* embryo production can be used to exploit both sperm and oocyte genotypes to produce crossbred animals that are more thermo-tolerant than purebred exotic breeds. These available biotechnologies can be used to avoid or minimize the effects of heat stress at critical periods, i.e. during fertilization and early embryonic development. In this regard, sperm from thermo-tolerant sires can be used to increase pregnancy rates in breeds more susceptible to high temperatures. The strategies for combating imminent abiotic stress are to develop a livestock population having high frequency of better adaptive genes for stress and heat tolerance. There are number of genes that are involved in the thermoregulation and homeostatic mechanism of mammals. The approach of identifying high THI-tolerant animals and targeting the candidate genes through subtractive hybridization, DDRT-PCR analysis, gene expression microarrays, SNPs or recent times next generation sequencing data are no most evident to face the eventuality. Once the candidate genes are identified markers can be developed that can be included in the breeding programme to take care for adaptive tolerance in livestock species. Molecular mechanism of animal behavior (stress, reproduction, lactation, growth, feeding, shelter seeking etc.) with advanced tools of stress physiology, genetic engineering, biotechnology and on field study through telemetry gadgets facility will definitely produce valuable output of research to augment the reproduction, production and sustainability of livestock under this diversified abiotic stress condition and continuous global climate change scenario.

References

Appelhans B., Luecken L.J. (2006). Attentional processes, anxiety, and the regulation of physiological reactivity. *Anxiety, Stress, and Coping* **19:** 81-92.

Barros C.M., Pegorer M.F., Vasconcelos J.L., Eberhardt B.G. Monteiro F.M. (2006). Importance of sperm genotype (*indicus* versus *taurus*) for fertility and embryonic development at elevated temperatures. *Theriogenology* **65:** 210-218.

Casas E., Shackelford S.D., Keele J.W., Koohmaraie M., Smith T.P., Stone, R.T., (2003). Detection of quantitative trait loci for growth and carcass composition in cattle. *Journal of Animal Science* **81:** 2976-2983.

Dean R. L. and Atkinson, B.G. (1985). Synthesis of heat shock proteins in quail red blood cells flowing brief, physiologically relevant increases in whole body temperature. *Comparative Biochemistry and Physiology* **81B:** 185.

Drost M., Ambrose J.D., Thatcher M.J., Cantrell C.K., Wolsdorf K.E., Hasler J.F., Thatcher W.W.(1999). Conception rates after artificial insemination or embryo transfer in lactating dairy cows during summer in Florida. *Theriogenology* **52:** 1161-1167.

Eberhardt B.G., Satrapa R.A., Capinzaiki R.L., Barros C.M. (2005). Influence of the breed of bull and the breed of cow on the resistance of bovine embryos to heat shock *in vitro*, at early stages of development. *Acta Scientae Veterinariae* **33:** 362.

Edwards J.L., Hansen P.J. (1997). Differential responses of bovine oocytes and pre-implantation embryos to heat shock. *Molecular Reproduction and Development* **46:** 138-145.

Fisher A.F., Bernal D.P., Gutierrez-Robayo C., Rutledge J.J. (2000). Estimates of heterosis for *in vitro* embryo production using reciprocal crosses in cattle. *Theriogenology* **54:** 1433-1442.

Gutie´rrez-Adan A.D.R., Fair T., Moreira P.N., Pintado B., de la Fuente J., Boland M.P. (2004). Effect of speed of development on mRNA expression pattern in early bovine embryos cultured in vivo or *in vitro*. *Molecular Reproduction and Development* **68:** 441-448.

Gwazdauskas F.C., Thatcher W.W., Kiddy C.A., Paape M.J., Wilcox C.J. (1981). Hormonal patterns during heat stress following PGF2a-tham salt induced luteal regression in heifers. *Theriogenology*. **16:** 271-285.

Hansen P.J., Arechiga C.F. (1999). Strategies for managing reproduction in the heat-stressed dairy cow. *Journal of Animal Science 77(Suppl 2)*: 36-50.

Hernández-Cerón J., Chase C.C. Jr, Hansen P.J. (2004). Differences in heat tolerance between preimplantation embryos from Brahman, Romosinuano and Angus breeds. *Journal of Dairy Science* **87:** 53-58.

Ito H., Shimojo T., Fujisaki H., Tamamori M., Isiyama S., Adachi S., Abe S., Marumo F. and Hiroe M. (1999). *Life Sciences* **64:** 755-761.

Ju J.C., Parks J.E., Yang X. (1999). Thermo-tolerance of IVM-derived bovine oocytes and embryos after short-term heat shock. *Molecular Reproduction and Development* **53:** 336-340.

Kaufmann, S. (1990). Heat shock proteins and the immune response. *Immunology Today* **11:** 129-136.

Li G.C., Werb Z. (1982). Correlation between synthesis of heat shock proteins and development of thermo-tolerence in Chinese hamster fibroblasts. *PNAS,* USA **79:** 3218.

Li G.C., Meyer J.L., Mak J.Y. and Hahn G.M. (1983). Heat induced protection of mice against thermal death. *Cancer Research* **43:** 5788.

Lindquist, S. (1986). The heat shock response. *Annual Review of Biochemistry* **55:** 1151-1191.

Magee D.A., Meghen C., Harrison S., Troy C.S., Cymbron T., Gaillard C., Morrow A., Maillard J.C., Bradley D.G. (2002). A partial African ancestry for the creole cattle populations of the Caribbean. *Journal of Heredity* **93:** 429-432.

Memili E., First N.L. (2000). Zygotic and embryonic gene expression in cow: a review of timing and mechanisms of early gene expression as compared with other species. *Zygote* **8:** 87-96.

Moberg G.P. (2000). Biological response to stress: Implications for animal welfare. In: *The Biology of Animal Stress.* (G.P. Moberg, J.A. Mench, eds). CAB International, Wallingford, UK, pp 1-21.

Nebel R.L., Jobst S.M., Dransfield M.B.G., Pandolfi S.M., Bailey T.L. (1997). Use of radio frequency data communication system, HeatWatch®, to describe behavioral estrus in dairy cattle. *Journal of Dairy Science* **80**(*Suppl.*1): 179.

Olson T.A., Lucena C., Chase Jr., C.C., Hammond A.C. (2003). Evidence of a major gene influencing hair length and heat tolerance in *Bos taurus* cattle. *Journal of Animal Science* **81:** 80-90.

Pegorer M.F., Vasconcelos J.L.M., Trinca L.A., Hansen P.J., Ciro M., Barros C.M. (2007). Influence of sire and sire breed (Gyr versus Holstein) on establishment of pregnancy and embryonic loss in lactating Holstein cows during summer heat stress. *Theriogenology* **67:** 692-697.

Putney D.J., Drost M., Thatcher W.W. (1988a). Embryonic development in superovulated dairy cattle exposed to elevated ambient temperature between days 1 to 7 post insemination. *Theriogenology* **30:** 195-209.

Putney D.J., Malayer J.R., Gross T.S., Thatcher W.W., Hansen P.J., Drost M. (1988b). Heat stress-induced alterations in the synthesis and secretion of proteins and prostaglandins by cultured bovine conceptuses and uterine endometrium. *Biology of Reproduction* **39:** 717-728.

Rocha A., Randel R.D., Broussard J.R., Lim J.M., Blair R.M., Roussel J.D., Godke R.A., Hansel W. (1998). High environmental temperature and humidity decrease oocyte quality in Bos taurus but not in *Bos indicus* cows. *Theriogenology* **49:** 657-665.

Rodenhiser D., Jung J.H.J., Atkinson B.G. (1985). Mammalian Lymphocytes: Stress induced synthesis of heat shock proteins *in vitro* and *in vivo*. *Canadian Journal of Biochemistry and Cell Biology* **63:** 711.

Roth Z., Hansen P.J. (2004). Sphingosine-1-phosphate protects cultured bovine oocytes from physiologicallyrelevant thermal stress. *Reproduction Fertility and Development* **16:** 282 (*Abstr.*).

Roth, Z., Arav, A., Bor, A., Zeron, Y., Braw-Tal, R., Wolfenson, D. (2001). Improvement of quality of oocytes collected in the autumn by enhanced removal of impaired follicles from previously heat-stressed cows. *Reproduction* **122:** 737-744.

Roy K. S., Prakash B. S. (2009a). Changes in endocrine profiles during ovsynch and ovsynch plus norprolac treatment in Murrah buffalo heifers at hot summer season. *Tropical Animal Health and Production* **41:** 677-687.

Roy K. S., Prakash B. S. (2009b). Pattern of plasma progesterone, estradiol-17â and total estrogen profiles in relation to estrous behavior during ovsynch treatment in Murrah buffalo heifers; *Journal of Animal Physiology and Animal Nutrition* **93:** 486-495.

Ryan, D.P., and M.P. Boland. (1991). Frequency of twin births among Holstein X Friesian cows in a warm dry climate. *Theriogenology* **36:** 1-10.

Taylor J.F., Coutinho L.L., Herring K.L., Gallagher Jr., D.S., Brenneman R.A., Burney N., Sanders J.O., Turner J.W., Smith S.B., Miller R.K., Savell J.W., Davis S.K. (1998). Candidate gene analysis of GH1 for effects on growth and carcass composition of cattle. *Animal Genetics* **29:** 194-201.

Turner H.G. (1982). Genetic variation of rectal temperature in cows and its relationship to fertility. *Animal Production* **35:** 401-412.

von Borrel E., Langbein J., Despres G., Hansen S., Leterrier C., Marchant-Forde J., Marchant-Forde R., Minero M., Mohr E., Prunier A., Valance D., Veissier I. (2007). Heart rate variability as a measure of autonomic regulation of cardiac activity for assessing stress and welfare in farm animals- A review. *Physiology and Behaviour* **92:** 293-316.

Wildman C.D., West J.W., Bernard J.K. (2007). Effect of dietary cation-anion difference and dietary crude protein on performance of lactating dairy cows during hot weather. *Journal of Dairy Science* **90:** 1842-1850.

Wolfenson D., Roth Z., Meidan R. (2000). Impaired reproduction in heat-stressed cattle: basic and applied aspects. *Animal Reproduction Science* **60/61:** 535-547.

❑❑❑

Section - 5

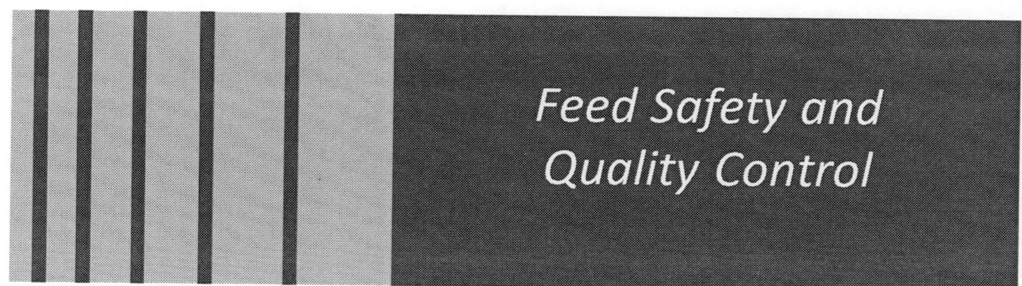

Chapter 32

Recent Advances in Mycotoxin Research in Poultry

R.U. Suganthi, M. Sridhar, A. Mech, T. Vandana, K.S. Prasad
National Institute of Animal Nutrition and Physiology, Adugodi, Bangalore-560 030, Karnataka, India

Summary

Chicken is a major source of protein in the world, with billions of birds used in meat and egg production each year. However one of the problems of poultry industry is the occurrence of mycotoxins in feed. Mycotoxins are toxic secondary metabolites produced by fungi (molds) that cause an undesirable effect (mycotoxicosis) when birds are exposed. Among hundreds of mycotoxins, the primary classes of mycotoxins are aflatoxins, ochratoxins, trichothecenes, zearalenone and fumonisins. They exert a wide range of effects in poultry and the susceptibility of poultry to different mycotoxins varies. So far the toxic effects of mycotoxins were studied in terms of alteration in blood parameters and performance parameters. Application of DNA microarray and other advanced molecular biology tools resulted in unveiling the molecular mechanisms of mycotoxin action in poultry. The toxic effects of mycotoxins, their mode of action, prevention and counteraction of toxicity are discussed in detail in this chapter.

Birds are part of the diapsid branch of vertebrates that split from the synapsid line (including mammals) over 310 million years ago. Modern birds (*Ornithurae*) evolved from therapod dinosaurs in the middle of the Mesozoic era. The chickens kept by the Harappan culture (2500-2100 BC) of the Indus valley are considered as the main source for subsequent global dispersal of domestic animals. The red jungle fowl is the nearest ancestor to the domestic chicken. For more than 8 millennia, the chicken has flourished as a domesticated livestock species deeply integrated into human culture. It is hypothesized that chickens were utilized primarily for religious ceremonies and sporting purposes and, in fact eating chicken was likely taboo in many cultures (Cogburn *et al.*, 2007). Until the middle of the last century most chicken breeds were raised in fairly small flocks for meat and eggs. Presently chicken is a major source of protein in the world and billions of birds are used in meat and egg production every year. Several breakthroughs in poultry science and technology have led to the development of genetically superior breeds capable of higher production, even under adverse climatic conditions that offer opportunities for overseas entrepreneurs to expand export and import of poultry products on a large scale. A relatively strong growth for the egg and poultry meat industry for the next two decades is predicted in India both in urban and rural areas. In spite of various advances in poultry, one of the problems industry faces is the occurrence of mycotoxins in poultry feed. The importance of mycotoxins as one of the major detractor of poultry productivity and also of product quality, now becomes more relevant than ever due to the growing awareness for food quality and safety (Manafi, 2011). Mycotoxin contamination of food and feed is a global phenomenon. The climatic conditions, pre and postharvest practices and the storage conditions in different regions of the world favors growth of different mycotoxic fungi and in turn the mycotoxins. However, in the present scenario, no part of the world could be suggested as mycotoxin free because of the international trade policies that have led to import and export of food and feed between countries. The Council for Agricultural Sciences and Technology in USA has recorded an annual crop losses of $932 million due to mycotoxin contamination and additional losses of $466 million in efforts to prevent or reduce contamination (Richard *et al.*, 2003).

1. Mycotoxins

Mycotoxins are toxic secondary metabolites produced by fungi (molds) that cause an undesirable effect (mycotoxicosis) when birds are exposed. They were first identified in 1962 after the outbreak of Turkey-X-disease which claimed the lives of 100,000 turkey poults near London, England. When the causative agent was traced, it was linked to a peanut (groundnut) meal contaminated with secondary metabolites from *Aspergillus flavus* (aflatoxins). Soon various mycotoxins were identified by scientists and the period between 1960 and 1975 has been termed the mycotoxin gold rush. Around 300 to 400 compounds are now recognized as mycotoxins. Among them, the primary classes of mycotoxins which pose threat to human and animal health are aflatoxins, ochratoxins, zearalenone, trichothecenes, fumonisins, and the ergot alkaloids. (Blount, 1961; Chukwaka *et al.*, 2010).

1.1 Occurrence of mycotoxins

Toxigenic fungal spores are present everywhere in soil, air and water. When conditions are favorable, they germinate, grow and produce the toxin.

Factors that influence the mycotoxin production include: temperature, moisture, oxygen, substrate aeration, inoculum concentration, microbial interaction, mechanical damage and insect infestation. The toxins are produced as a result of high moisture in the field, during harvest and storage (Leeson *et al.*, 2001).Various agricultural commodities including, cereals (maize, sorghum, pearl millet, rice, and wheat), oilseeds (peanut, soybean, sunflower, and cotton) and tree nuts (coconut, almonds, pitachio, and walnuts) are contaminated by mycotoxins (Farombi, 2006; Murphy *et al.*, 2006). Mycotoxin problem is of special significance in developing countries like India because of favorable climatic conditions and poor harvest and storage practices that favor the growth of fungi and thus the increased production of mycotoxins in feed (Gowda *et al.*, 2002; Williams *et al.*, 2004; Umaya *et al.*, 2010). Consumption of such contaminated feed leads to deleterious effects in animals and there are number of studies indicating the toxic effects of mycotoxins in poultry.

2. Common mycotoxins and their toxicity

The mycotoxins that affect poultry are aflatoxins, ochratoxins, trichothecenes and fumonisins. Mycotoxins and their metabolites affect the normal functions and susceptibility of poultry to these mycotoxins depends on age, dose and species. An area of science termed, "toxicogenomics" has been evolved which studies the response of a whole genome to toxicants or environmental stressors involving genomic-scale mRNA expression (transcriptomics), cell and tissue-wide protein expression (proteomics), metabolite profiling (metabolomics) and bioinformatics (Burczynski *et al.*, 2000; Lee *et al.*, 2005). Toxicogenomic-based investigations are applied to understand the mode of action of chemicals and other environmental stressors on biological systems. Such studies have provided useful information on the genes involved in metabolism of mycotoxins; metabolic pathways altered by them; and the concentration at which the mycotoxin influences gene expression in metabolic organs. Mycotoxins, their metabolism and toxicity with special reference to toxicogenomics in poultry are discussed in the following sections.

3. Aflatoxins

Among various mycotoxins, aflatoxins are reported to be predominant in Indian poultry feeds (Umaya and Parvatham, 2009). Chemically, aflatoxins (AFs) are a group of difuranocoumarin derivatives and the major types of aflatoxins are aflatoxin B1 (AFB1), B2 (AFB2), G1 (AFG1) and G2 (AFG2). Among the aflatoxins, AFB1 is the most toxic and most prevalent compound, followed by G1, B2 and G2 with decreasing toxicity (Murphy *et al.*, 2006). Poultry, especially turkeys, are extremely sensitive to the toxic effects of AFB1 (Rawal *et al.*, 2010). The manifestation of chronic or acute toxicosis in broilers depends on strain, duration of exposure and rate of metabolism of aflatoxin to less toxic metabolites (Kermanshahi *et al.*, 2009; Shabani *et al.*, 2010). Aflatoxin primarily affects liver, kidney and immune system and leads to reduction in performance and mortality. Some of the metabolites formed during the metabolism of AFB1 are transmitted to edible animal products, liver, muscle (Bintvihik and Davitiyananda, 2002) and eggs, which exert immunosuppressive, embryotoxic and teratogenic effects. The AFB1 is a class 1 carcinogen and is one of the etiological factors of human hepatocellular carcinoma (Celik *et al.*, 2000; Oliveira *et al.*, 2000).

3.1 Aflatoxin metabolism

Aflatoxins are metabolized by liver in two phases: phase I and phase II. The phase I involves biotransformation and phase II involves conjugation of the resulting phase I metabolites to more water soluble compounds and excretion from the body.

a) Phase I metabolism of aflatoxin

The cytochrome P450 (CYP) enzymes (mixed function oxidases) are mainly involved in phase I metabolism of aflatoxin. Cytochrome P450 enzymes are classified into families identified by a number (*e.g.*, 1, 2, 3, and 4), subfamilies identified by a letter (*e.g.*, 2A, 2B, 2D, and 2E), and specific members identified by another number (*viz.*, CYP2E1 and CYP2A6; Diaz *et al.*, 2010). They aid in hydroxylation, epoxidation, dehydrogenation, nitrogen dealkylation, and oxidative deamination of carcinogens (Parkinson, 2001). The AFB1 is metabolized by cytochrome P450 enzymes to AFB1-8, 9-exo-epoxide (AFBO).The AFB1 is not toxic as such, but requires metabolic conversion to the reactive and electrophilic exo-AFBO by P450s to exert its toxicity (Guengerich *et al.*, 1996). In quails and chickens, AFB1 is bioactivated into its toxic epoxide by CYP1A1 and CYP2A6. Turkey liver P450s are especially efficient towards AFB1 bioactivation compared to other poultry species. Turkey liver microsomes bioactivate aflatoxins 1.8 and 3.5 times more than quail and chicken liver microsomes respectively (Lozano and Diaz, 2006). Young birds bioactivate aflatoxins more actively than the older birds (Klein *et al.*, 2002). In turkey liver, AFB1 is metabolized to AFB1-8, 9-epoxide (AFBO) by CYP1A5 and CYP3A37. Although both CYP1A and 3A isoforms oxidize AFB1, there are conflicting reports on their relative importance. In humans, CYP1A2 and CYP3A4 are mainly responsible for the conversion of AFB1 to its epoxide (Vleet *et al.*, 2002; Kamdem *et al.*, 2006). Biotransformation of AFB1 may also result in the production of more polar metabolites, aflatoxin M1 (AFM1), aflatoxin Q1 (AFQ1) and aflatoxin P1 (AFP1) which are considered as detoxification products. Reduction of AFB1 via cytosolic reductase produces aflatoxicol (AFL) and it is not a detoxification product, as it can be converted back to AFB1 by a microsomal dehydrogenase, which prolongs the in vivo half-life of the original toxin (Rawal *et al.*, 2010).

The AFBO formed may be hydrolysed to form AFB1-8,9-dihydrodiol (AFB1- dhd) either by the enzyme epoxide hydrolase or spontaneously or may be conjugated with reduced glutathione (GSH). The former rearranges to a dialdehyde which is able to bind to proteins at lysine residues. However, an aflatoxin aldehyde reductase (AFAR) has been identified which protects against di-aldehyde, by catalyzing its reduction to a di-alcohol.

b) Phase II metabolism of aflatoxin

Phase II biotransformation reactions include glucuronidation, sulfation, acetylation, methylation, and conjugation with glutathione and amino acids. Conjugation converts the compound being metabolized into a highly hydrophilic form that can be readily excreted in urine through the kidneys or with bile out of the body.

Conjugation of AFBO with GSH through glutathione S-transferase (GST) is a detoxification step and this protects against the genotoxicity of AFB1 (Tiemersma *et al.,* 2001).Avian GSTs comprise a complex isoenzyme system and five groups of GST subunits (designated CL1 to CL5) are present in liver of white Leghorn chicks (Chang *et al.,* 1990). In domestic chicken, four classes of GSTs namely, α (Chang *et al.,* 1990), μ (Sun *et al.,* 1998), τ (Hsiao *et al.,* 1995) and σ (Thomson *et al.,* 1998) are present and the α-class GSTs are *cGSTA1, cGSTA2, cGSTA3* and *cGSTA-CL.3*. The α-class GST gene cluster in turkeys consist of six forms - tGSTA1.1, *t*GSTA1.2, tGSTA1.3, tGSTA2 , tGSTA3 and tGSTA4 (Kim *et al.,* 2010). The avian μ-class GST exists as cGSTM1-1, rGSTM3-3, rGSTM1-1 and hGSTM2-2 (Sun *et al.,* 1998; Kim *et al.,* 2010). Conjugation of the epoxide by GSH is the major, rate-limiting determinant in species susceptibility to AFB1, regardless of the extent of P450-mediated bio-activation. Though different types of GSTs are present, the deficiency or absence of a functional GST with affinity towards AFBO appears to be a major reason for the extreme susceptibility of poultry to AFB1 (Klein *et al.,* 2000).

The electrophilic metabolite, AFB1-8, 9-exo-epoxide formed from AFB1 can induce mutations by alkylating DNA, principally at the N^7 position of guanine forming the 8, 9-dihydro-8-(N^7-guanyl)-9-hydroxy-AFB1. The AFB1-DNA adduct thus formed disturbs function of the specific gene. In addition, AFBO can bind to proteins and other critical cellular nucleophiles and alter cell function. Further, AFB1-8, 9-dihydrodiol can react strongly with proteins and cause cytotoxicity (Klein *et al.,* 2003). Gene expression analysis by microarray indicates up regulation of cytochrome P450 genes and down regulation of epoxide hydrolase and glutathione-S-transferase genes in liver of broilers fed 2 ppm aflatoxin (Yarru *et al.,* 2009). The up regulation of genes responsible for activation of aflatoxin and down regulation of genes involved in detoxification of aflatoxin metabolites is associated with the toxic effects of aflatoxin in birds.

3.2 Oxidative stress and aflatoxin toxicity

Under normal metabolism of cells, reactive oxygen species (superoxide radical, hydroxyl radical and hydrogen peroxide) are formed. Aerobic organisms possess defense systems for converting reactive oxygen species into less harmful or harmless compounds formed within the cells, *i.e.*, antioxidants. Reactive oxygen species target polyunsaturated fatty acids and form lipid hydroperoxides, which are finally decomposed to form reactive lipid aldehydes (lipid peroxidation process). Oxidative damage in the cell or tissue occurs when the concentration of reactive oxygen species generated exceeds the antioxidant capability of the cell or when the antioxidant capacity of the cell decreases. Levels of non-enzymatic antioxidants *viz.*, glutathione, ascorbic acid and enzymatic antioxidants *viz.*, glutathione peroxidase (GPx), catalase and superoxide dismutase (SOD) are the main determinants of the antioxidant defense mechanism of the cell. The SOD is a family of metallo-enzymes which dismutate endogenous cytotoxic superoxide radicals to hydrogen peroxide. The hydrogen peroxide produced by SOD is further removed by catalase. The different GPx enzymes remove both hydrogen peroxide and lipid peroxides by catalyzing the conversion of lipid hydroperoxides to hydroxy acids in the presence of reduced glutathione (Umaya and Parvatham, 2009).

Aflatoxins cause formation of reactive oxygen species including superoxide radicals, hydroxyl radicals and hydrogen peroxides which reacts with guanine residues in DNA to form 8-hydroxydeoxyguanosine (Shen *et al.*, 1995; Bedard and Massey, 2006). It also induces expression of inducible nitric oxide synthase and in turn nitric oxide (NO), peroxynitrite, nitrogen dioxide or nitrate which cause protein and DNA damage (Ozen *et al.*, 2009). Elevated levels of lipid peroxidation products and decreased levels of antioxidants are reported in aflatoxin fed animals (Umaya and Parvatham, 2009). In support of these earlier findings, microarray analysis of liver samples of aflatoxin treated (2ppm) birds show down regulation of the genes encoding SOD and GPx (Yarru *et al.*, 2009) and confirm oxidative stress during aflatoxicosis.

3.3 Aflatoxicosis and cellular functions

Carbohydrates, fats and proteins present in feed are catabolized by various metabolic pathways to provide energy to the cells. The mitochondria, the power house of the cell possess electron transport chain and are involved in production of high-energy phosphate by the process termed oxidative phosphorylation. The immune system of the organism (humoral and cell mediated immunity) protects the birds from infections and during injury, blood clotting mechanism protects the birds from blood loss. All the functions of the body are thus well organized. Studies indicate reduction in activities of specific enzymes involved in digestion of carbohydrates, proteins, lipids nucleic acids and the absorption of essential nutrients in birds fed aflatoxin contaminated feed (Abousadi *et al.*, 2007). Earlier studies indicate biochemical, hematological, reproductive and pathological changes during aflatoxicosis in poultry (Ortatatli and Oguz, 2001; Iheshiulor *et al.*, 2011). Further, aflatoxicosis in poultry has also been associated with liver damage, immunosuppression, poor performance and mortality. Microarray data of liver of broilers fed 2ppm aflatoxin shows alteration in expression of genes related to various functions of the cell. The genes involved in electron transport (adrenodoxin mitochondrial precursor (adrenal ferredoxin, cytochrome P450 2C5, cytochrome P450 2P3, and NADH-cytochrome b5 reductase), transport of long chain fatty acids into mitochondria (carnitine palmitoyl transferase gene), immune function (ovomucoid precursor, Interleukin 10 receptor , Interleukin 6 receptor, Mitogen-activated protein kinase 2 genes), translation (ribosomal protein17a, ribosomal protein 130, ribosomal protein 135, ribosomal protein 15), growth (Insulin like growth factor gene) and coagulation (coagulation factor IX, coagulation factor X precursor-Stuart factor) are down regulated by aflatoxin (Yarru *et al.*, 2009). On the other hand, genes associated with cell proliferation (peroxisome proliferator-activated receptor alpha, nuclear receptor subfamily 1d, bHLH transcription factor, ornithine decarboxylase, histone deacetylase 2, transcription factor Sox-9, v-jun sarcoma virus 17 oncogene homolog and alpha-fetoprotein enhancer-binding protein), carbohydrate metabolism (glycogen synthase 1, lactate dehydrogenase H subunit, pyruvate dehydrogenase complex E1 component, malic enzyme 1 NADP(+)-dependent cytosolic) and protein metabolism (muller glia protein tyrosine phosphatase 2, LIM domain kinase 2, muller glia protein tyrosine phosphatase 2, presenilin 1, hepatocyte growth factor-like/macrophage stimulating protein, hect domain and RLD 4) are down regulated by aflatoxin. During aflatoxicosis, the alterations in gene expression patterns are reflected by the biochemical and performance parameters of broilers (Yarru *et al.*, 2009). Altogether, aflatoxin affects cellular functions and cause reduction in growth rate in poultry (Celik *et al.*, 2000; Murray *et al.*, 2000).

3.4 Effects of aflatoxin on FCR: meta-analysis

In poultry industry the term feed conversion ratio (FCR) is very important and any factor that affects FCR affects the profit of the farmers and industry. A number of studies have been carried out worldwide to study the effect of aflatoxin on FCR but the results are not homogenous. To arrive at an appropriate conclusion, Umaya *et al.,* (2011) did a statistical meta-analysis, which systematically assesses large collections of research results obtained from individual studies, integrates the findings and derives the conclusions. This study combined research results of ten publications on feed conversion ratio of broilers which were fed with aflatoxin from first day to six weeks of age and is summarized below. The effect size (d = the standardized difference of means of control and experimental groups) of 0.5 and above in their study was considered statistically relevant (Umaya *et al.,* 2011).

a) During 1-3 weeks of age

Aflatoxin feeding at 0.6ppm dose (Diaz and Sugahara, 1995) decreases FCR at the end of first week of age. In contrary some reports indicate no change in FCR by feeding aflatoxins (0.5- 3.0ppm) in diet up to 1 week of age (Celik *et al.,* 2005). Oguz and Kurtoglu (2000) did not observe any reduction in FCR after feeding 2.5ppm aflatoxin B1 for 2 weeks. The reports on effect of aflatoxin on FCR at three weeks of age of broilers are contrary. A significant increase in FCR by 17% to 24% is shown in chicks fed a diet containing 2.5 ppm aflatoxin (Huff *et al.,* 1986; Oguz 1997) and 5.0 ppm aflatoxin (Diaz and Sugahara, 1995) from 1 to 21days of age. The meta-analysis indicated negligible (d = 0.2), moderate (d=0.57) and large effect (d=2.76) of aflatoxin on FCR at the end of first, second and third weeks of age of broilers, respectively.

b) During 4-6 weeks of age

In vivo studies in broilers showed a reduction in FCR in day old birds fed 0.1 ppm for 5 weeks or 8 weeks (Verma *et al.,* 2004), 0.5 ppm and 1.0 ppm aflatoxin for 4 weeks (Celik *et al.,* 2005) and 2.0 ppm aflatoxin for seven weeks (Pandey and Chauhan, 2007; Shabani *et al.,* 2010). But there are contrary reports that do not indicate any negative effect of feeding 0.5 and 1.0 ppm AF for six weeks (Edrington *et al.,* 1997; Kermanshahi *et al.,* 2009). Meta-analysis indicated adverse effect of aflatoxin on FCR at the end of fourth (d = 8.36), fifth (d = 1.77) and sixth weeks of age of broilers (d = 3.79).

The adverse effect observed during third to six weeks of age of broilers, the crucial period of weight gain is a matter of apprehension to poultry farmers. Many a times, under the field conditions, birds are exposed to low levels of aflatoxins; chronic exposure of poultry to aflatoxins without clinical symptoms is a major concern in the poultry industry as the diagnosis and treatment are difficult. Hence it is essential to take appropriate measures to protect broilers from one day of age to prevent losses due to aflatoxin.

3.5 Action levels for aflatoxin

Action levels and tolerances are established based on the unavoidability of the poisonous or deleterious substances and do not represent permissible levels of contamination where it is avoidable. The action level for aflatoxin given by FDA for various commodities is given in Table 1.

Table 1 : FDA action level for aflatoxin in various commodities

Commodity	Action level (ppb)
Animal feeds	
Corn and peanut products intended for finishing (*i.e.*, feedlot) beef cattle	300
Cottonseed meal intended for beef, cattle, swine, or poultry (regardless of age or breeding status)	300
Corn and peanut products intended for finishing swine of 100 pounds or greater	200
Corn and peanut products intended for breeding beef cattle, breeding swine, or mature poultry	100
Corn, peanut products, and other animal feeds and feed ingredients but excluding cottonseed meal, intended for immature animals	20
Corn, peanut products, cottonseed meal, and other animal feed ingredients intended for dairy animals, for animal species or uses not specified above, or when the intended use is not known	20
Brazil nuts	20
Foods	20
Milk (aflatoxin M1)	0.5
Peanuts and Peanut products	20
Pistachio nuts	20

(FDA, 2000)

4. Trichothecenes

The trichothecene mycotoxins are mainly isolated from *Fusarium* species. They comprise a vast group of 100 fungal metabolites and are divided into two groups: macrocyclic and non-macrocyclic. Non-macrocyclic trichothenes are further sub divided into type A and type B toxins. The T-2 toxin, HT-2 toxin, and diacetoxyscirpenol are the type-A trichothecenes. The Type-B trichothecenes are fusarenone-X, deoxynivalenol and nivalenol toxins.

4.1 T-2 toxin

The T2 toxin is predominant in tropical and subtropical regions and the toxin at various doses (4 to 16 ppm) affects poultry. T-2 toxin poisoning is characterized by decreased feed intake, growth inhibition with lower weight gain, mouth lesions, depigmentation of the leg skin, changed feather quality, and neural disturbances. In laying hens, poisoning is indicated by reduced egg production (with thinner egg shell), decreased hatchability, reduced feed intake, cyanosis of the comb, leucopenia, and changed feather quality. A dose of T-2 toxin that would kill 50% of a seven day-old broiler population (LD50) is 4.97 mg/kg bw. In comparison with other mycotoxins, in seven-day old broilers, T-2 toxin is more toxic than aflatoxin (LD50=6.8 mg/kgbw) and deoxynivalenol (LD50=140 mg/kgbw), and is equally or less toxic than ochratoxin (LD50=2.1 mg/kgbw) and diacetoxyscirpenol (LD50=2.0 mg/kg to 5.9 mg/kgbw). The T-2 toxin inhibits DNA, RNA and protein synthesis in eukaryotic cells, affects the cell cycle, and induces apoptosis both *in vivo* and *in vitro.* Actively dividing cells (cells of the gastrointestinal tract, bone marrow, lymph nodes, spleen, and liver) are highly sensitive to T-2 toxin (Leeson *et al.,* 2001). The attempt by Sehata *et al.* (2005) to study the molecular mechanism of action of T-2 toxin by microarray shows increased expression of oxidative stress-related genes such as the heat shock protein 40 (HSP40), heme oxygenase and Manganese-superoxide dismutase (MnSOD) genes in the liver of pregnant rats, thioredoxin reductase, heat shock protein 70 (HSP70) and metallothionein-2 and -1 in the placenta, and metallothionein-2 and -1 in the fetal liver. Further, the expression of genes involved in apoptosis-tumor necrosis factor receptor and bax alpha; signal transduction- p38 mitogen activated protein kinase (MAPK), extracellular signal related kinase (ERK3) and MAP kinase kinase kinase1 (MEKK1); and cell growth- P21 protein , cyclin D1 and nuclear factor-kappa B are increased in liver of rats by T-2 toxin treatment. The expression of lipid metabolism-related genes such as 17-beta hydroxysteroid dehydrogenase type 2 and cholesterol 7-alpha-hydroxylase genes and drug-metabolizing enzyme genes such as P450d, P450e are down regulated by T-2 toxin. The maximal allowed concentration for T-2 toxin in poultry feed is 150 ppm and further studies are required to elucidate the mechanism of T-2 toxicity in poultry.

4.2 Deoxynivalenol

Deoxynivalenol (DON) also known as vomitoxin is one of about 150 related compounds known as the trichothecenes that are formed by a number of species of *Fusarium* and some other fungi. It is nearly always formed before harvest when crops are invaded by certain species of *Fusarium* such as *F. graminearum and F. culmorum*. These two species are important plant pathogens and cause *Fusarium* heat blight in wheat and Gibberella ear rot in maize. Deoxynivalenol (Fig. 1) is thermally stable, so once formed it is likely to persist through storage and the food chain. Because deoxynivalenol is toxic and often found in

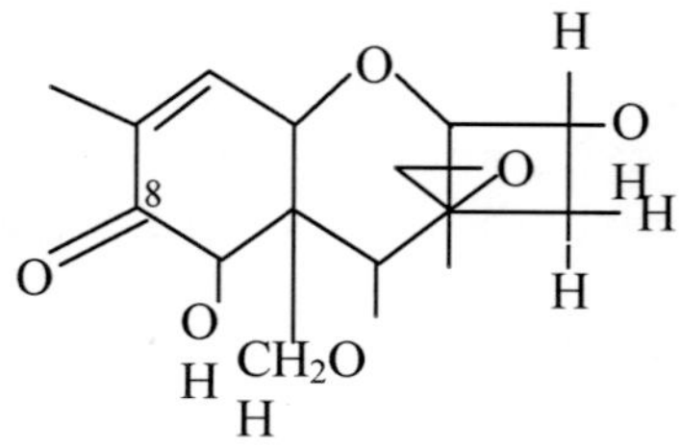

Fig. 1 : Deoxynivalenol

foodstuffs, sometimes in high concentrations, it has recently been of concern to international organizations and government food agencies.

The maximal allowed concentration for DON in poultry feed is 5 ppm (European Union, 2006) as poultry can tolerate up to 5ppm dietary DON without deleterious effects. In chickens, DON is rapidly absorbed in the upper part of the gastrointestinal tract and quickly cleared through bile, urine and feces and this makes them tolerant to DON. Feeding DON (2.5 and 5.0ppm) through naturally contaminated wheat to one day old broilers (Ross) for 23 days did not affect feed intake or body weight (Dietrich *et al.*, 2011). However, at higher levels, deoxynivalenol produces a variety of adverse health effects in poultry. Broilers fed 9.3ppm DON in the grower phase showed reduced nutrient absorption, decreased feed intake, weight gain including reduced peripheral blood monocytes (Swamy *et al.*, 2004). The fast growing broilers are more susceptible to DON than laying hens (Leeson *et al.*, 2001). Laying hens fed diets for 24 week up to 5ppm DON did not show any adverse effects on health or productivity. The DON has very low toxicity for turkeys and feeding 75 ppm dietary DON to turkey poults from 7 to 14 days of age had no effects on feed consumption or growth rate (Leeson *et al.*, 2001).

4.2.1 DON toxicity in broilers and cellular functions

Cells and tissues with high protein turnover rate, such as the liver and small intestine are most affected by DON in broilers (Awad *et al.*, 2008). The cell functions altered during DON toxicity are described below.

a) Nutrient transport

Injury to gastrointestinal tract is an important aspect of DON toxicity. The DON has an influence on intestinal morphology of chickens, especially in the duodenum and jejunum and villi of DON affected birds appear shorter and thinner (Leeson *et al.*, 2001). The solute carrier family (SLC) proteins SLC2A5, SLC7A10, SLC7A5 and SLC16A are involved in transport of nutrients, glucose and amino acids (Table 1) in liver and jejunum of broilers.

Table 2 : Transporters and their function

Transporters	Function
SLC2A5	Transports D-fructose with high affinity and glucose with very low affinity
SLC7A10	Na^+-independent transport of small neutral amino acids (glycine, alanine, serine, cystine, threonine) with high affinity and large neutral amino acids are transported with lower affinity
SLC7A5	Transports neutral amino acids with branched or aromatic side chains such as leucine
SLC16A	Transports monocarboxylates such as butyrate, lactate and pyruvate

The microarray study by Dietrich *et al.* (2011) indicates that DON (5.0ppm) decreases the expression of solute carrier family genes *viz.*, SLC2A5, SLC7A10, SLC7A5 and SLC16A and thereby decreases nutrient absorption (glucose and amino acid) in the liver and jejunum. Hence the reduction in nutrient uptake by DON is not due to cell damage but as a result of specific modulation of the membrane transporters (Lambert *et al.*, 2002; Maresca *et al.*, 2002).

b) Cell integrity

Cells are connected by intracellular complexes such as tight junctions and adherens junctions. The DON down regulates tight junction protein 1 (TJP1), essential for maintenance of transepithelial electrical resistance (TEER) and functional tight junctions. Further, *in vitro* studies indicate a decrease in transepithelial electrical resistance, disintegration of TJP1 structure and the total amount of TJP1 by DON (Diesing *et al.*, 2011). However, claudin 3 (CLDN3) that improves TEER is up regulated by DON and TJP1 is suggested to interact with CLDN3 and maintain the TEER during DON exposure (5 ppm) in broilers (Dietrich *et al.*, 2011).

c) DNA damage and repair

Under normal cellular conditions, malondialdehyde formed by peroxidation of polyunsaturated fatty acids are detoxified into non toxic alcohols by aldo-keto reductase (AKR1B1). Feeding of DON at the dose of 5.00 ppm decreases expression of AKR1B1 in liver and jejunum of broilers and this leads to accumulation of malondialdehye (Fig. 2). Malondialdehyde, thus accumulated, can react with DNA, form DNA adducts and alter gene function. Hence AKR1B1 is suggested as an *in vivo* biomarker for DON-induced alteration of gene expression (Jin and Penning, 2007; Dietrich *et al.*, 2011).

The DON increases expression of genes related to apoptosis-poly [ADP-ribose] polymerase 1 (PARP1), tumor protein 53 inducible protein 3 (TP5313) and caspase 1 in liver and jejunum of broilers, indicating an increase in the rate of apoptosis. Besides apoptotic genes, the N-methylpurine-DNA glycosylase (MPG) genes involved in recognition and excision of alkylated purine bases (Brien and Ellenberger, 2004); essential meiotic endonuclease 1 (EME1) involved in cleaving branched DNA structures (Abraham *et al.*, 2003); Chromatin assembly factor 1, subunit B (CHAF1B) responsible for nucleotide excision repair and repair of single-strand breaks (Mello *et al.*, 2002); RAP1 interacting factor homologue (RIF1) that functions as a DNA damage response factor (Silverman *et al.*,2004); xeroderma pigmentosum group A complementing gene (XPAC) involved in nucleotide excision repair are up regulated by DON. The up regulation of DNA repair proteins may be due to the mutagenic effects of DON or its decomposition products. Alternatively it may be a protective mechanism against anchorage of lipid aldehydes to the DNA due to reduced activity of AKR1B1 by DON (Dietrich *et al.,* 2011).

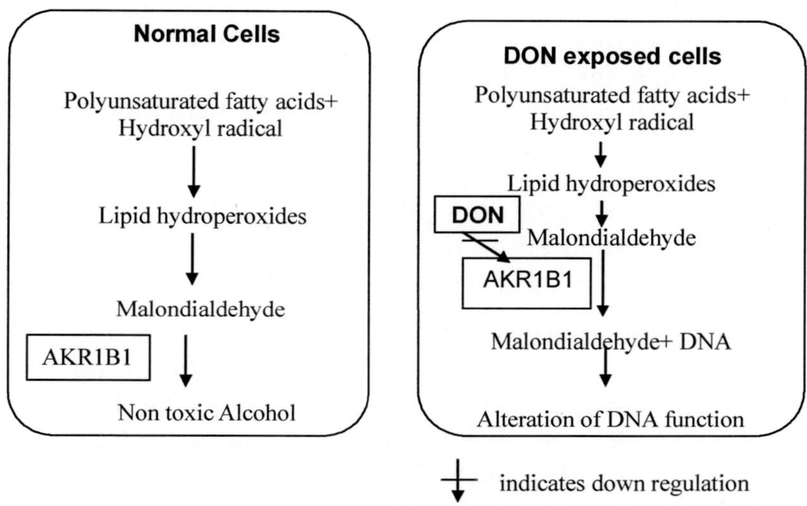

Fig. 2 : Functions of AKR1B1 in normal and DON exposed cells

d) Translation

The DON binds to 60 S ribosomal subunits and prevents initiation and elongation steps of translation process (Leeson *et al.,* 2001). The microarray study by Dietrich *et al.* (2011) indicates down regulation of translation initiation-related genes- eukaryotic translation initiation factor 2-α kinase 3 (EIF2AK3), and DnaJ homolog subfamily C member 3 (DNAJC3), and the mRNA stabilisation genes-exosome component 9 (EXOSC9) and 5′-3′ exoribonuclease (XRN1) in broilers. Down regulation of these genes is suggested to have important influence on the rate of protein synthesis and growth of broilers (Yang *et al.,* 2000; Huizen *et al.,* 2003; Schilders *et al.,* 2006; Pestka, 2010).

The main effects of DON with economic impact might be reduced expression of the nutrient transporters, translation initiation genes and mRNA stabilization genes as they have an important influence on growth rate of broilers. The increased expression of AKR1B1 might produce cytotoxic effects in tissues (Dietrich *et al.,* 2011). The DON has not generally been recognized as overtly toxic to chickens, but slight changes in cell function could affect productivity or disease susceptibility, particularly in young chickens. Hence caution should be exercised when utilizing DON contaminated feedstuffs to formulate poultry diets.

5. Ochratoxins

The fungi, *Aspergillus ochraceus, Aspergillus versicolor, Penicillium verrucosum* produce the, ochratoxins A, B, C of which ochratoxin A (OTA) is the most toxic one. The OTA is nephrotoxic in all animal species. The turkeys, chickens and ducklings are susceptible to ochratoxin. Typical signs of poultry ochratoxicosis are reduction in weight gain, poor feed conversion, reduced egg production, poor egg shell quality and nephrotoxicity. Even exposure to low levels of OTA (0.5 ppm) alters performance, including decreased feed consumption and growth rate and poor feed conversion efficiency (Wang *et al.,* 2009). Reduction in egg production and egg weight occurs in laying hens fed a diet contaminated with OTA at 2 and 3 ppm levels (Denli *et al.,* 2008; Denli and Perez, 2010). Residues of OTA are detected in the muscle of hens and chickens and even in eggs (Leeson *et al.,* 2001).

Birds fed with different doses (1–5 mg/kgbw) OTA, in varying ages, cause decreases in cholesterol, total protein, albumin, globulin, potassium, and triglyceride levels and increases in uric acid and creatine levels and in the activities of serum alkaline phosphatase and gamma glutamyl transferase (Denli and Perez, 2010). The effects depend on the level of the toxin and time of exposure. The OTA accumulates both in target and non target organs so considered as hepatotoxic, nephrotoxic, neurotoxic, immunosuppressive, cytotoxic, genotoxic, mutagenic, teratogenic, and carcinogenic agent. Its toxicity has been shown to be associated with inhibition of protein, DNA and RNA synthesis, mitochondrial dysfunction, formation of DNA adducts, disruption of calcium homeostasis, and the generation of reactive oxygen species (Farag *et al.,* 2010). Ochratoxin A possesses an L-phenylalanine moiety in its structure. The toxin inhibits specifically and competitively the activity of phenylalanine-tRNA synthetase, an enzyme involved in the initial step of translation. It also inhibits phosphoenolpyruvate carboxykinase the key enzyme in gluconeogenesis (Murray *et al.,* 2000; Leeson *et al.,* 2001).

5.1 Mechanism of OTA toxicity

Ochratoxin induced gene expression changes have not been studied in poultry so far. However, *in vitro* studies (5 µM and 12.5µM) and *in vivo* studies (1mg/kg and 10mg/kgbw) OTA) in rats show alteration in expression of genes involved in various functions (Table 3).

The OTA causes up regulation of expression of genes involved in inflammation, responses to DNA damage (like DNA repair processes, apoptosis, and cancerogenesis), oxidative stress and down regulation of genes involved in cellular metabolism and detoxification processes and thereby induce toxicity in animals (Luhe *et al.,* 2003).

Table 3 : Changes in gene expression during OTA toxicity

Name of gene	Function	Up/Down regulated	Inference
Catalase and glutathione synthetase (GlutS)	Breakdown of ROS	U	Oxidative stress
Alpha-2-macroglobulin	Protease inhibitor and positive acute phase protein	U	Inflammatory reaction
Contrapsin-like protease inhibitor	Negative acute phase protein	D	Potential for cancer development (Dobashi *et al.,* 2000)
Tissue factor (TF)	Coagulation	U	Activation of several blood clotting mechanisms
GADD 153 (growth arrest and DNA damage-inducible gene) and *GADD 45*	Blood cell development, cell cycle arrest and apoptosis	U	DNA damage (Pflumio and Dirheimer, 2000)
Nucleosome assembly protein (NAP)	unpacking of chromatin in order to replicate or repair DNA	U	Repair processes after DNA damage
Annexin V	Marking apoptotic cells for recognition by phagocytes	U	Apoptosis (Basco *et al.,* 2000)
Stem cell factor (SCF)	cell-matrix adhesion and rescue factor in mast cell apoptosis	D	Loss of cell–cell adhesion and tumor progression
Cathepsin S (Cat S)	Tumor progression	U	Loss of cell–cell adhesion
NADP-dependent isocitrate dehydrogenase, NADPH quinone oxidoreductase 1, beta-alanine synthetase, ATP-ated stimulglucocorticoid-receptor translocation promoter	Energy metabolism	D	Reduced production of energy
Alcohol dehydrogenase 1, argininosuccinate lyase, glutamine synthetase, GST's alpha, P1 and Ya, sulfotransferase K2	Biotransformation and detoxification	D	Toxic metabolites react with macromolecules and cell structures and loss of basic cell function

U-Up regulated ; D-Down regulated (Luhe *et al.*, 2003)

6. Fumonisins

Fumonisin B1 (FB1) is a mycotoxin produced by the fungus *Fusarium verticillioides.* The FB1 is neurotoxic, hepatotoxic, and nephrotoxic in animals, however, it has very low toxicity for poultry. Feeding purified (98.1% pure) fumonisin B1 (FB1) at dietary levels up to 80 ppm for three weeks to day old male broilers (Strain: *Arbor acres*) chicks did not affect body weight of chicks. But a decrease in liver lipids and increase in liver enzymes and sphinganine in serum were observed (Henry *et al.,* 2000). The study conducted by Javed *et al.* (1993) reported mortality and decreased weight in male broiler chicks fed 125 and 274 ppm purified FB1 (Strain: *Columbia :New Hampshire*), from 1 to 14 d of age. The genetic variability in susceptibility to mycotoxins is known to occur in avian species, so the difference in the results in different reports could be due to the different strain of chicken used by different groups. Decrease in the prothrombin time and an increase in the fibrinogen concentration in blood and the activity of antithrombin III, are shown in birds fed dietary FB1 at a concentration of 10 ppm for only 6 d. The hemostatic mechanism is more sensitive to FB1 than other traits, such as production parameters and tissue damage (Espada *et al.,* 1997). Feeding 15 ppm FB1 for three weeks did not influence body weight but decreased relative bursa weight, increased serum aspartate aminotransferase, and the serum levels of albumin and cholesterol. The FB1 up to 15 mg/kg does not affect growth performance, but impairs some parameters of blood biochemistry and the immuno-competence in broilers (Leeson *et al.,* 2001). Chronic effects of FB1 have been studied in turkey poults fed 75 ppm FB1 for 18 weeks and laying hens fed 100 or 200 ppm FB1 for 60weeks. However, 100 and 200 ppm FB1 did not have an effect on body weight gain (at 420 d) or relative liver weight (at 112 d) in laying hens (Leeson *et al.,* 2001). In rats long-term FB1 feeding is shown to increase expression of TGF-β1 by hepatocytes indicating prominent apoptosis and fibrosis (Lemmer *et al.,* 1999). The molecular changes induced by fumonisins in poultry needs to be elucidated.

7. Measures to protect poultry against mycotoxin toxicity

Complete prevention of mycotoxins contamination is an unattainable objective. However, following pre-harvest and post-harvest control measures helps to control the toxic effects of mycotoxins.

7.1 Pre-harvest control of mycotoxins

Mycotoxin contamination can be reduced by maintaining proper planting/ growing conditions, antifungal treatments and adequate insect and weed prevention before harvest. Using clean and dry harvesting equipment, collection/transportation equipment that are free of visible fungal growth helps to check mold growth. Breeding strategies to select *Aspergillus* resistant trait while maintaining desirable agronomic characteristics, slowed down in maize due to failure to identify expressed genes and proteins involved in resistance to *Aspergillus* microbes have been suggested to prevent mycotoxin contamination. *Trichoderma and Rhizopus species* and *Bacillus pumilus* exhibit antifungal activity against *Aspergillus. Exophiala spinefera* and *Rhizocladiella* degrade fumonisins while *Acinetobacter calcoaceticus, Phenylobacterium immobile* convert ochratoxin A into nontoxic product. Extracts of plant products, cinnamon, peppermint, basil, origanum, clove and thyme are potent inhibitors of *Aspergillus* growth in maize (Choudary and Kumari, 2010).

7.2 Postharvest control of mycotoxins

A number of approaches are available to control mycotoxins contamination after harvest. Aflatoxin contaminated grains can be physically removed, thermally inactivated and subjected to UV treatment to degrade the preformed toxins (Gowda *et al.*, 2005). Addition of individual or combinations of organic acids (propionic, benzoic and acetic acids), salts of organic acids (calcium propionate and potassium sorbate) and copper sulphate (solid or liquid forms) and ammoniation of feed reduces aflatoxin present in feed. Addition of binding agents such as mineral clay products (bentonites, zeolites and aluminosilicates) and yeast cell wall mannanoligosaccharides inhibit absorption of aflatoxin from the digestive tract of broilers. Hydrated sodium calcium alumino silicate and artichoke can effectively inhibit ochratoxin-A toxicity in broilers (Denlii and Perez, 2010). Studies indicate that plant products turmeric, silymarin from *Silybum marianum* (Chand *et al.*, 2011) and alcohol extract of *Monodora myristica* (Flora and Victor, 2004) are potential candidates to prevent aflatoxicosis in poultry (Yarru *et al.*, 2009). In addition to the above, frequent delivery of feed with shorter residence time to reduce the buildup of mycotoxins, screening of feed ingredients regularly for mycotoxin contamination and avoiding inclusion of mycotoxins contaminated feed material in mixed feeds helps to reduce the toxic effects of mycotoxins in poultry.

Conclusions

Mycotoxin contamination of food and feed is a global problem. This problem is of special significance in developing countries like India because climatic conditions and poor harvest and storage practices favor the growth of fungi and production of mycotoxins in feed. Although acute mycotoxicoses are rare in poultry production, chronic exposure to low levels of mycotoxins is responsible for reduced productivity, increased susceptibility to infectious diseases and alteration in quality of poultry products. Gene expression analysis of target organs has revealed the genes and the metabolic pathways affected by aflatoxins and deoxynivalenol in broilers; thus providing a scope for identification of novel counteractive/preventive strategies. Future research on the genomic alterations caused by different mycotoxins at different doses in laying hens, turkeys and quails may help to tackle mycotoxins in a better way. In the present scenario, contamination of feed ingredients and mixed feeds may occur at any stage of feed production. Hence it is recommended to follow integrated mycotoxin prevention and counteraction strategies to reap the health and economic benefits from poultry.

References

Abousadi M.A., Rowghani E., Honarmand E.M. (2007) The efficacy of various additives to reduce the toxicity of aflatoxin B1 in broiler chicks. *Iranian Journal of Veterinary Research* **8:** 144-150.

Abraham J., Lemmers B., Hande M.P., Moynahan M.E., Chahwan C., Ciccia A. (2003). Eme1 is involved in DNA damage processing and maintenance of genomic stability in mammalian cells. *EMBO Journal* **22:** 6137-6147.

Awad W.A., Bohm J., Razzazi-Fazeli E., Hulan H.W., Zentek J.(2004). Effects of deoxynivalenol on general performance and electrophysiological prop properties of intestinal mucosa of broiler chickens. *Poultry Science* **83:** 1964-1972.

Bedard L. L., Massey T. E. (2006). Aflatoxin B1-induced DNA damage and its repair. *Cancer Letters* **241:** 174-183.

Bintvihok A., Davitiyananda D. (2002). Aflatoxins and their metabolite residues in chicken tissues from 5 parts (10 provinces) of Thailand. *Thailand Journal of Health and Research* **16:** 37-50.

Blount W.P. (1961) Turkey "X" disease. *Journal of British Turkey Federation.* **1:** 51-62.

Brien O.P.J., Ellenberger T. (2004). Dissecting the broad substrate specificity of human 3-methyladenine-DNA glycosylase. *Journal of Biological Chemistry* **279:** 9750-9757.

Burczynski M. E., Millian M. M., Ciervo J., Li L., Parker J. B., Dunn R.T., II, Hicken S., Farr S., Johnson M. D. (2000). Toxicogenomics-based discrimination of toxic mechanism in HepG2 human hepatoma cells. *Toxicological Sciences* **58:** 399-415.

Celik I.H., Oguz O. Demet., M. Boydak., H. H. Donmez., E. Sur., F. Nizamlioglu. (2000). Embryotoxicity assay of aflatoxin produced by *Aspergullus parasiticus* NRRL 2999. *British Poultry Science* **41:** 401-409.

Celik S., Erdogan Z., Erdogan S., Bal R.(2005). Efficacy of tribasic copper chloride (TBCC) to reduce the harmful effects of aflatoxin in broilers. *Turkish Journal of Veterinary and Animal Sciences* **29:** 909-916.

Chand N., Muhammad D., Durrani F.R., Qureshi M.S., Sahibzada S.U. (2011). protective effects of Milk Thistle (*Silybum marianum*) against Aflatoxin B1 in Broiler Chicks. *Asian-Australasian Journal of Animal Science* **24:** 1011-1018.

Chang L.H., Chuang L.F., Tsai C.P., Tu C.P., Tam M.F. (1990). Characterization of glutathione S-transferases from day-old chick livers. *Biochemistry* **29:** 744-750.

Choudhary A.K., Kumari, P. (2010). Management of mycotoxins contamination in preharvest and postharvest crops: Present status and future prospects. *Journal of Phytology* **2:** 37-52.

Chukwuka O.K., Okoli I.C., Opara M.N.,. Omede A.A., Ogbuewu I. P., Iheshiulor O.O.M. (2010). The growing problems of mycotoxins in animal feed industry in West Africa: a review. *Asian Journal of Poultry Science* **4:** 122-134.

Cogburn L.A., Porter T.E., Duclos M.J., Simon J., Burgess S.C., Zhu J.J. (2007). Functional genomics of the chicken—A model organism. *Poultry Science* **86:** 2059-2094.

Denli M., Perez J.F. (2010). Ochratoxins in feed, a risk for animal and human health: Control strategies. *Toxins* **2:** 1065-1077.

Denli M., Blandon J.C., Guynot M.E., Salado S., Perez J.F. (2008). Efficacy of a new ochratoxin-binding agent (OcraTox) to counteract the deleterious effects of ochratoxin A in laying hens. *Poultry Science* **87:** 2266-2272.

Diaz G.J., Murcia H.W., Cepeda S.M. (2010). Cytochrome P450 enzymes involved in the metabolism of aflatoxin B_1 in chickens and quail. *Poultry Science*. **89:** 2461-2469.

Diaz G.J., Sugahara M. (1995). Individual and combined effects of aflatoxin and gizzerosine in broiler chickens. *British Poultry Science* **36:** 729-736.

Diesing A.K., Nossol C., Panther P., Walk N., Post A., Kluess J. (2011). Mycotoxin deoxynivalenol (DON) mediates biphasic cellular response in intestinal porcine epithelial cell lines IPEC-1 and IPEC-J2. *Toxicology Letters* **200:** 8-18.

Dietrich B., Neuenschwander S., Bucher B., Wenk C. (2011). Fusarium *mycotoxin-contaminated wheat containing deoxynivalenol alters the gene expression in the liver and the jejunum of broilers.* Animal **6:** 278-291.

Edrington T. S., Kubena L. F., Harvey R. B., Rottinghaus G. E. (1997). Influence of super activated charcoal on the toxic effects of aflatoxins or T-2 toxin in growing broilers. *Poultry Science* **76:** 1205-1211.

Espada Y., Gopegui R.R., Cuadradas C., Cabanes F. J. (1997). Fumonisin mycotoxicoses in broilers: Plasma protein and coagulation modifications. *Avian Diseases* **41:** 73-79.

European Union 2006. 2006/576/EC: Commission Recommendation of 17 August 2006 on the presence of deoxynivalenol, zearalenone, ochratoxin A, T-2 and HT-2 and fumonisins in products intended for animal feeding. *Official Journal of European Union Legislation* **49:** 7-9.

Farag I.M., Aziz, A.K.B., Nada S.A., Tawfek N.S., Farouk T., Darwish H.R. (2010). Modulation of ochratoxin-induced oxidative stress, genotoxicity and spermatotoxic alterations by *Lactobacillus rhamnosus* GG in male Albino mice. *Journal of American Science* **6:** 575-587.

Farombi E.O. (2006). Aflatoxin contamination of foods in developing countries: For hepatocellular carcinoma and chemo preventive strategies. *African Journal of Biotechnology* **5:** 1-14.

FDA compliance policy guides manual. (2000). Guidance for industry: Action levels for poisonous or deleterious substances in human food and animal feed. *http:// www.fda.gov*.

Flora O., Victor T. O. (2004). Reversal of toxigenic effects of aflatoxin B1 on cockerels by alcoholic extract of African nutmeg, *Monodora myristica*. *JSFAAE* **84:** 333-340.

Gowda N.K.S., Malathi V., Suganthi R.U., Raghavendra A. (2005). Effect of dry heat and sunlight on the aflatoxin content in compounded feed. *Indian Journal of Animal Nutrition* **22:** 132-134.

Gowda N.K.S., Malathi V., Suganthi R.U. (2002). Influence of storage condition, bag material and duration of feed storage on aflatoxin production. *Indian Journal of Animal Nutrition* **19:** 340-345.

Guengerich F.P., Gillam E.M., Shimada T. (1996). New applications of bacterial systems to problems in toxicology. *Critical Reviews in Toxicology* **26:** 551-583.

Henry M. H., Wyatt R. D., Fletcher O. J. (2000). The Toxicity of Purified Fumonisin B1 in Broiler Chicks. *Poultry Science* **79:** 1378-1384.

Hsiao C.D., Martsen E.O., Lee J.Y., Tsai S.P., Tam M.F. (1995). Amino acid sequencing, molecular cloning and modelling of the chick liver class-theta glutathione S-transferase CL1. *Biochemical Journal* **312:** 91-98.

Huff W. E., Kubena L. F., Harvey R.B., Hagler V. M., Swanson S.P., Phillips T.D., Creger C. R.(1986). Individual and combined effects of aflatoxin and deoxynivalenol (DON, vomitoxin) in broiler chickens. *Poultry Science* **65:** 1291-1298.

Huizen R., Martindale J.L., Gorospe M., Holbrook N.J. (2003). P58IPK, a novel endoplasmic reticulum stress-inducible protein and potential negative regulator of eIF2alpha signaling. *Journal of Biological Chemistry* **278:** 15558-15564.

Iheshiulor O.O.M., Esonu B.O., Chuwuka O.K., Omede A.A., Okoli I.C., Ogbuewu I.P. (2011). Effects of Mycotoxins in Animal Nutrition: A Review. *Asian Journal of Animal Science* **5:** 19-33.

Javed T., Bennett G. A., Richard J. L ., Kurtzman M. A. D., Cote L. M., Buck W. B. (1993). Mortality in broiler chicks on feed amended with *Fusarium proliferatum* culture material or with purified fumonisin B1 and moniliforme. *Mycopathology* **123:** 171-184.

Jin Y., Penning T.M. (2007). Aldo-keto reductases and bioactivation/ detoxication. *Annual Review of Pharmacology and Toxicology* **47:** 263-292.

Kamdem L.K., Meineke I., Armbrust G. U., Brockmoller J., Wojnowski L.(2006). Dominant contribution of P450 3A4 to the hepatic carcinogenic activation of aflatoxin B1. *Chemical Research in Toxicology* **19:** 577-586.

Kermanshahi H., Hazegh A.R., Afzali N. (2009). Effect of sodium bentonite in broilers fed diets contaminated with aflatoxin B1. *Journal of Animal and Veterinary Advances* **8:** 1680-5593.

Kim J.E., Bauer M.M., Mendoza K.M., Reed K.M., Coulombe Jr.R.A. (2010). Comparative genomics identifies new alpha class genes within the avian glutathione S-transferase gene cluster. *Gene* **452:** 45-53.

Klein P.J., Vleet V.T.R., Hall J.O., Coulombe Jr. R. A. (2003). Effects of dietary butylated hydroxytoluene on aflatoxin B1-relevant metabolic enzymes in turkeys. *Food and Chemical Toxicology* **41:** 671-678.

Klein P.J., Vleet V.T.R., Hall J.O., Coulombe J.R.A. (2002). Biochemical factors underlying the age-related sensitivity of turkeys to aflatoxin B1. *Comparative Biochemistry and Physiology. Toxicology and Pharmacology* **132:** 193-201.

Kubena L.F., Harvey R.B., Bailey R.H., Buckley S.A., Rottinghaus.G. E. (1998).Effects of a hydrated sodium Calcium Aluminosilicate (T-bind) on Mycotoxicosis in young broiler chickens. *Poultry Science* **77:** 1802-1509.

Lambert D.W., Wood I.S., Ellis A., Beechey S.P. (2002). Molecular changes in the expression of human colonic nutrient transporters during the transition from normality to malignancy. *British Journal of Cancer* **86:** 1262-1269.

Lee K.M., Kim J. H., Kang D. (2005). Design issues in toxicogenomics using DNA microarray experiment. *Toxicology and Applied Pharmacology* **207:** 200-208.

Lemmer E.R., Hall P., Omori N., Omori M., Shephard E.G., Gelderblom W.C. (1999) .Histopathology and gene expression changes in rat liver during feeding of fumonisin B1, a carcinogenic mycotoxin produced by *Fusarium moniliforme. Carcinogenesis* **20:** 817-824.

Leeson S., Diaz G., Summers J.D. (2001) Poultry metabolic disorders and mycotoxins. International Book Distributing Company, I[st] ed. Army Printing Press, Lucknow. pp. 251.

Lozano, M.C., Diaz G.J. (2006). Microsomal and cytosolic biotransformation of aflatoxin B1 in four poultry species. *British Poultry Science* **47:** 734-741.

Luhe A., Hildebrand H., Ute Bach DingermannT., Ahr H.J. (2003). A new approach to studying ochratoxin A (OTA) induced nephrotoxicity: expression profiling *in vivo* and *in vitro* employing cDNA microarrays. *Toxicological Sciences* **73:** 315-328.

Manafi M. (2011). Evaluation of different mycotoxins binders on aflatoxin B1 (*Aspergillus parasiticus*) produced on rice (*Oriza sativa*) on fertility, hatchability, embryonic mortality, residues in egg and semen quality. *Advances in Environmental Biology* **5:** 3818-3825.

Maresca M., Mahfoud R., Garmy N., Fantini J. (2002). The mycotoxins deoxynivalenol affects nutrient absorption in human intestinal epithelial cells. *Journal of Nutrition* **132:** 2723-2731.

Mello J.A., Sillje H.H., Roche D.M., Kirschner D.B., Nigg E.A. Almouzni G. (2002). Human Asf1 and CAF-1 interact and synergize in a repair-coupled nucleosome assembly pathway. *EMBO Reports* **3:** 329-334.

Modirsanei M., Mansoori B., Khosravi A.R., Kiaei M. M., Khazraeinia P., Farkhoy M., Masoumi Z. (2008). Effect of diatomaceous earth on the performance and blood variables of broilers chicks during experimental aflatoxicosis. *Journal of the Science of Food and Agriculture* **88:** 626-632.

Murphy P.A., Hendrich S., Landgren C., Bryant C.M. (2006). Food mycotoxins: an update. *Journal of Food Science* **71:** 51-65.

Murray R.K., Granner D.K., Mayes P.A., Rodwell.(2000). Harper's Biochemistry, (25th ed.), Appleton and Lange Publications, USA, pp 268-272.

Oguz H., Kurtoglu V., Coskun B. (2000). Preventive efficacy of clinoptilolite in broilers during chronic aflatoxin (50 and 100 ppb) exposure. *Research in Veterinary Science* **69:** 197-201.

Oguz H., Kurtoglu V. (2000). Effect of clinoptilolite on performance of broilers chickens during experimental aflatoxicosis. *British Poultry Science* **41:** 512-517.

Oguz H. (1997). The preventive efficacy of polyvinylpolypyrrolodone (PVPP) alone and its combination with the other adsorbents into broiler feeds against aflatoxicosis. PhD Thesis, University of Selcuk, Konya.

Oliveira C. A. F., E. W. Kobashigawa., T. A. Reis., L. Mestieri., R. Albuquerque., B. Correa. (2000). Aflatoxin B1 residues in eggs of laying hens fed a diet containing different levels of the mycotoxins. *Food Additives and Contaminants* **17:** 459-462.

Ortatatli M., Oguz H. (2001). Ameliorative effects of dietary clinoptilolite on pathological changes in broiler chickens during aflatoxicosis. *Research in Veterinary Science* **71:** 59-66.

Ozen H., Karaman M., Cigremis Y., Tuzcu M., Ozcan K., Erdag D. (2009). Effectiveness of melatonin on aflatoxicosis in chicks. *Research in Veterinary Science* **86:** 485-489.

Pandey I., Chauhan S. S. (2007). Studies on production performance and toxin residues in tissues and eggs of layer chickens fed on diets with various concentrations of aflatoxin AFB1. *British Poultry Science* **48:** 713-723.

Parkinson A. (2001) Biotransformation of xenobiotics, In: *Toxicology, the basic science of poisons* (C.D. Klaassen, ed), McGraw-Hill, New York, pp133-224.

Pestka J.J. (2010). Deoxynivalenol: mechanisms of action, human exposure, and toxicological relevance. *Archives of Toxicology* **84:** 663-679.

Rawal S., Kim J.E., Coulombe R.J. (2010). Aflatoxin B1 in poultry: toxicology, metabolism and prevention. *Research in Veterinary Science* **89:** 325-331.

Richard J.L., Payne G.A., Desjardin A.E., Maragos C., Norred W.P., Pestka J.J. et al. (2003). Mycotoxins: risks in plant, animal and human systems. *Council of Agricultural Science and Technology Task Force Report* **139:** 101-103.

Schilders G., Dijk V.E., Raijmakers R., Pruijn G.J. (2006). Cell and molecular biology of the exosome: how to make or break an RNA. *International Review of Cytology* **251:** 159-208.

Sehata S., Kiyosawa N., Atsumi F., Ito K., Yamoto T., Teranishi M. (2005). Microarray analysis of T-2 toxin-induced liver, placenta and fetal liver lesions in pregnant rats. *Experimental and Toxicologic Pathology* **57:** 15-28.

Shabani A., Dastar B., Khomeiri M., Shabanpour B., Hassani S. (2010). Response of broiler chickens to different levels of nanozeolite during experimental aflatoxicosis. *Journal of Biological Sciences* **10:** 362-367.

Shen H. M., Ong C., Lec B. L., Shi C. Y. (1995). Aflatoxin B1 induced 8 - hydroxy deoxy guanosine formation in rat hepatic DNA. *Carcinogenesis* **16:** 419-422.

Silverman J., Takai H., Buonomo S.B., Eisenhaber F., de Lange T. (2004). Human Rif1, ortholog of a yeast telomeric protein, is regulated by ATM and 53BP1 and functions in the S-phase checkpoint. *Genes and Development* **18:** 2108-2119.

Sun Y.J., Kuan I.C., Tam M.F., Hsiao C.D. (1998). The three-dimensional structure of an avian class-mu glutathione S-transferase, cGSTM1-1 at 1.94 A resolution. *Journal of Molecular Biology* **278:** 239-252.

Swamy H.V., Smith T.K., Karrow N.A., Boermans H.J.(2004). Effects of feeding blends of grains naturally contaminated with Fusarium mycotoxins on growth and immunological parameters of broiler chickens. *Poultry Science* **83:** 533-543.

Tiemersma E.W., Omer R. E., Bunschoten A., Veer P.V., Kok F.J., Idris M.O. (2001). Role of genetic polymorphism of glutathione-S transferase T1 and microsomal epoxide hydrolase in aflatoxin-associated hepatocellular carcinoma. *Cancer Epidemiology Biomarkers and Prevention* **10:** 785-791.

Thomson A.M., Meyer D.J., D.Hayes. (1998). Sequence, catalytic properties and expression of chicken glutathione-dependent prostaglandin D2 synthase, anovel class Sigma glutathione S-transferase. *Biochemical Journal* **333:** 317-325.

Umaya R.S., Suresh K.P., Parvatham R. (2011). Effect of aflatoxin on feed conversion ratio in broilers: A meta-analysis. *Asian Australasian Journal of Animal Science* **24:** 1757-1762.

Umaya R.S., Parvatham R. (2009). Efficacy of *Moringa oleifera* and *Aloe vera* on aflatoxin-B1 induced hepatotoxicity in rats. *Research Journal of Biotechnology* **4:** 20-24.

Umaya R.S., Bhavya S., Parvatham R. (2010). Occurrence of Aflatoxin B1 in Poultry Feed Ingredients and Mixed Feeds: A Report From South India. *Indian Journal of Animal Nutrition* **27:** 174-178.

Verma J., Johri T. S., Swain B. K., Ameena S. (2004). Effects of graded levels of aflatoxins, ochratoxin and their combinations on the performance and immune response of broilers. *British Poultry Science* **45:** 512-518.

Vleet V.T.R., Mace K., Coulombe Jr. R.A. (2002). Comparative aflatoxin B(1) activation and cytotoxicity in human bronchial cells expressing cytochromes P450 1A2 and 3A4. *Cancer Research* **62:** 105-112.

Wang H., Xue C.Y., Chen F., Ma Y. L., Zhang X.B., Bi Y.Z., Cao Y.C. (2009). Effects of combinations of ochratoxin A and T-2 toxin on immune function of yellow-feathered broiler chickens. *Poultry Science* **88:** 504-510.

Williams D.M., Phillips T.D., Jolly P.E., Stiles J.K., Curtis M.J., Aggarwal D. (2004) Human aflatoxicosis in developing countries: a review of toxicology, exposure, potential health consequences and interventions. *American Journal of Clinical Nutrition* **80:** 1106-1122.

Yang G.H., Li S., Pestka J.J. (2000). Down-regulation of the endoplasmic reticulum chaperone GRP78/BiP by vomitoxin (Deoxynivalenol). *Toxicology and Applied Pharmacology* **162:** 207-217.

Yarru L. P., Settivari R. S., Antoniou E., Ledoux D. R., Rottinghaus G.E. (2009). Toxicological and gene expression analysis of the impact of aflatoxin on hepatic function of male broiler chicks. *Poultry Science* **88:** 360-371.

❑❑❑

Chapter 33

Recent Advances in Amelioration of Anti-Nutritional Factors in Livestock Feedstuffs

S.B.N. Rao, K.S. Prasad, D. Rajendran
National Institute of Animal Nutrition and Physiology, Adugodi, Bangalore-560 030, Karnataka, India

Summary

Newer feed resources and few important feedstuffs commonly used in livestock feeding contain one or the other anti nutritional factor (ANF). In the present chapter, important ANFs present in individual or group of feedstuffs and strategies to reduce them have been discussed. The strategies can be utilized either by industry or commercial farmers who are primarily dealing with livestock. Some of ANF's have medicinal (Karanjin or Pongamol) and insecticidal uses (azadirachtin) which can reduce the cost of detoxification process.

Escalating feed costs and feed ingredient availability is limiting factors affecting successful commercial livestock production in our country. This is attributable to growing competition between humans and livestock for grains and plant proteins, particularly soybean meal (SBM) for which suitable alternatives need to be found. Many newer feed resources (NFR) are being investigated and recommended for animal feed usage after thorough nutritional evaluation. The NFR may contain certain incriminating factors which are detrimental to the health of the livestock. Compared to temperate countries, livestock under tropical conditions experience seasonal changes in quality and quantity of plant materials. Under these circumstances supplementation strategies have also to be devised by animal nutritionists to combat seasonal variations in quality of feeds depending upon the level and type of production of livestock *i.e.,* milk, meat and wool production.

1. Significance of anti-nutritional factors

Plants have co-evolved with predator populations of bacteria, insects, fungi and grazing animals, and have developed defense mechanisms for their survival. Many plants also produce chemicals which are not directly involved in the process of plant growth (secondary compounds), but act as deterrents to insects and fungal attack. These compounds also affect animals (including humans) and the nutritive value of forages. The ANFs may be defined as those substances generated in natural feed stuffs by normal metabolism of within plants and by different mechanisms like inactivation of some nutrients, diminution of the digestive process or metabolic utilization of feed which exert effects contrary to optimum nutrition. The ANFs may be regarded as a class of compounds, which are generally not lethal but reduce animal productivity and may cause toxicity during periods of scarcity or confinement when the feed rich in these substances is consumed by animals in large quantities (Cheeke and Shull, 1985). The ANFs which have been implicated in limiting the utilization of shrub and tree forages include non-protein amino acids, glycosides, phytohemagglutinins, polyphenolics, alkaloids, triterpenes and oxalic acid (Table 1).

Table 1 : Important anti nutritional factors present in commonly used alternative feed ingredients

Plant-derived nutrient	Anti-nutrients present
Soybean meal	Protease inhibitors, lectins, phytic acid, saponins, phyto-estrogens, antivitamins, allergens
Rapeseed meal	Protease inhibitors, glucosinolates, phytic acid, tannins
Lupin seed meal	Protease inhibitors, saponins, phytoestrogens, alkaloids
Sunflower oil cake	Protease inhibitors, saponins, arginase inhibitor
Cottonseed meal	Phytic acid, phytoestrogens, gossypol, antivitamins, cyclopropenoic acid
Leucaena leaf meal	Mimosine
Alfalfa leaf meal	Protease inhibitors, saponins, phytoestrogens, antivitamins
Mustard oil cake	Glucosinolates, tannins
Sesame meal	Phytic acid, protease inhibitors

Many plant components have the potential to precipitate adverse effects on the productivity of farm livestock (D'Mello, 2000). These compounds are present in the foliage and/or seeds of virtually every plant that is used in practical feeding. Typical concentrations for few important toxins are presented in Table 2. Plant toxins may be divided into a heat-labile group, comprising lectins, protease inhibitors and cyanogens, which are sensitive to standard processing temperatures and a heat-stable group which include antigenic proteins, condensed tannins, quinolizidine alkaloids, glucosinolates, gossypol, saponins, the non-protein amino acids like S-methyl cysteine sulphoxide and mimosine, and phyto-estrogens.

Table 2 : Plant toxins: sources and concentrations

Toxin	Principal sources	Typical concentrations
Lectins	Jackbean Winged bean Lima beans	73 units/mg protein 40-320 units/mg 59 units/mg protein
Trypsin inhibitors	Soybean	88 units/mg
Antigenic proteins	Soybean	-
Cyanogens	Cassava root	186 mg HCN/kg
Condensed tannins	Acacia spp. Lotus spp.	65 g/kg 30-40 g/kg
Quinolizidine alkaloids	Lupin	10-20 g/kg
Glusosinolates	Rapeseed	100 mmol/kg
Gossypol	Cottonseed	0.6-12 g/kg (free)
Saponins (steroidal)	Brachiaria decumbens; Panicum spp.	-
S-methyl cysteine sulphoxide	Kale	40-60 g/kg
Mimosine	*Leucaena leucocephala*	145 g/kg (seed) 25 g/kg (leaf)
Phyto-oestrogens	Clover; Lucerne, soybean	-

Source: Compiled from D'Mello, 1995

2. Common protein supplements, their antinutritional principles and ameliorative measures

2.1 Soybean (*Glycine max*) meal

Soybean meal is probably the best quality vegetable protein source widely used around the world for livestock rations. It is high in protein and energy and has a good amino acid profile. Raw soybeans contain protease inhibitors which inhibit proteolytic enzymes and thereby growth in non-ruminants. In soybeans, two main groups of protease inhibitors have been found namely: (1) *Kunitz* inhibitors specificity towards trypsin and (2) *Bowman-Brik* inhibitors inhibiting both trypsin and chymotrypsin. Feeding raw soybeans to pigs, chicks and rats have resulted in low growth rate, pancreatic hyperplasia and low production (Watanapa and Williamson, 1993; Herrington *et al.*, 1994). These inhibitory substances are mostly heat labile and can easily be destroyed by application of heat. The naturally occurring trypsin inhibitor is deactivated by controlled heat treatment, the biggest advantage of which is the reduced protein degradability in the rumen and increased bypass protein value. However, soybean cake presently available in the market is of solvent extracted and does not pose any danger to livestock and poultry even as sole protein supplements (Rao *et al.*, 2006).

2.2 Mustard (Rape seed) seed meal

Mustard seed meal is being used for feeding of Indian cattle and buffaloes especially in Northern and Eastern states of India. Often feeding of this cake is limited by the presence of anti-nutritional factors glucosinolates (GIs). Glucosinolates are secondary plant metabolites that occur in all *Brassica* species. The Gls contents are generally higher in rapeseed meal (RSM) varieties grown under tropical regions compared to temperate countries. The RSM from Indian sub-continent contain primarily 3-butenyl, 2-propenyl and 4-pentenyl glucosinolates. But 2-propenyl glucosinolate accounts more than 95% of their total glucosinolates present in RSM of European and other temperate countries, and did not contain 4-pentenyl glucosinolates. Depending on the pH, cofactors and Gls content and composition of RSM, the major metabolites of glucosinolates are thiocyanates (SCN), isothiocyanates (ITC), nitriles, 5-vinyl-2-oxazolidinethione (VOT) and 5-vinyl-1, 3-oxyzolodine-2-thione (5-VOT). Apart from total glucosinolate (TGls) content SCN, nitriles and VOT estimates are the chief attribute of RSM quality as these are produced upon hydrolysis of Gls following the processing of RSM (Tripathi and Mishra, 2007). Major deleterious effects of glucosinolates ingestion in animals are reduced palatability, decreased growth and production. Progoitrin and epi-progoitrin impair palatability at a level between 2.3 and 4.65mol/g diet, while higher levels decreases feed intake. Nitriles are known to affect liver and kidney functions. The thiocyanates interfere with iodine availability, whereas VOT is responsible for the morphological and physiological changes of thyroid. Rapeseed meal feeding did not impair quality traits of carcass and increased unsaturated fatty acids (C22:2 and *trans* C18:1) content in carcass and milk fat. Ruminants are less sensitive to dietary glucosinolates as they are hydrolyzed and metabolites may affect certain functions. Pigs are more severely affected by dietary glucosinolate compared to rabbit, poultry and fish. (Tripathi and Mishra, 2007).

Decomposition of glucosinolates increase with increasing moisture and period of exposure to microwave heating. It has been reported that microwave irradiation at 2450-MHz for 2.5 min of pre-conditioned (moisture 13g/kg, 24 h at 4°C) RSM inactivate myrosinase enzyme and decompose glucosinolates (Maheshwari *et al.*, 1980). The glucosinolate decomposition ranges from 70 to

254 μmol/mmol in different meals. The micronization process for 90 sec at 195°C thermal temperature of RSM was found effective in reducing glucosinolates contents. Micronization removed 370 μmol/mmol total glucosinolates, all isothiocyanates and leaving a traces of oxazolidinethione. Extrusion of RSM was more effective over microwaving in removing glucosinolates. Dry extrusion of RSM is reported to reduce total glucosinolates in range of 193–428 μmol/mmol (Smithard and Eyre, 1986; Aumaitre *et al.*, 1989; Fenwick *et al.*, 1986). Wet extrusion of high glucosinolate rapeseed meal with ammonia (150°C, 200 rpm, with 2% ammonia) resulted in more reduction (670 μmol/mmol) in total glucosinolates content (Huang *et al.*, 1995). The inclusion of extruded RSM in diet improved dry matter intake, live weight gain and biological value of protein. Heat treatment negatively affects the Gls content of RSM, wet heating/pressure cooking is more effective over dry heating. Feeding of heat treated high Gls RSM as sole protein supplement improved milk yield, protein output, and showed higher dietary nitrogen utilization in dairy cows and, improved growth performance in growing calves. Drastic heating (above 110°C, more than 30 min) of RSM impairs protein quality in non-ruminants animals (Newkirk *et al.*, 2003; Glencross *et al.*, 2004), however, this will be an advantage for ruminant feeding in providing more un-degradable ruminal protein. For non-ruminant feeding, heating of RSM should be restricted to 30 min at 100°C (Jensen *et al.*, 1995). This heating level reduced total glucosinolate by 500μmol/mmol and maintained the protein quality.

Among various RSM treatment protocols, only copper sulphate treatment was found effective, which inactivated ITC and OT of the meals. Treating RSM with copper sulphate (1 kg RSM soaked in 2:1 copper sulphate solution, 6.25 g $CuSO_4 \cdot 5H_2O$ dissolved in 2 liter H_2O and dried at 60°C) was effective in reducing TGls by 900 μmol/mmol (Das and Singhal, 2001, 2005).

Solid-state fermentation was another approach tried for detoxification of glucosinolates. The fermentation of RSM (sterilized at 121°C, 15 lb/in^2 for 15 min) using *Rhizopus oligosporus* and *Aspergillus* sp. under solid-state fermentation (meal: water ratio 1:3, at 25°C under aerobic conditions for 10 days) inactivated myrosinase, reduced total glucosinolates by 431 μmol/mmol and thiooxalidone by 340 mg/g (Vig and Walia, 2001). The complete degradation of glucosinolates occurred after 60–96 h fermentation at 30°C (Rakariyatham and Sakorn, 2002). Decomposition of glucosinolate was higher with longer fermentation period. The reduction in glucosinolates and their metabolites during fermentation may be due to utilization of glucose and sulphur moieties of these compounds by microbial enzymes.

2.3 Cotton (*Gossypium*) seed meal

Cotton belongs to genus, *Gossypium,* belonging to family Malvaceae, is distributed widely from temperate to tropical regions. Gossypol is a toxic compound found in the cotton plant. It is present in discrete bodies called 'pigment glands' (Boatner, 1948) and is distributed in leaves, stems, roots and seeds. Gossypol exists in two forms: free and bound. The free form is toxic, whereas gossypol that binds to proteins is in the 'bound' or non-toxic form. The gossypol content of Indian cottonseed varies from 0.72 to 0.92% in the seed, 1.56 to 2.35% in the kernel and 0.38 to 0.47% in the oil (Pandey and Thejappa, 1975). Whole cottonseed contains high level of free gossypol. Gossypol primarily affects heart and liver. The reproductive tract, abomasum and kidney are also affected. Ruminants can tolerate higher levels of free gossypol because gossypol binds to proteins in the rumen. Young calves and lambs are quite susceptible to gossypol toxicity. Simple stomached animals have long been known to be susceptible. Pigs and rabbits appear to be more sensitive than poultry. Gossypol leads to discolouration of egg yolk by binding with iron of the yolk to form chocolate-brown complex (Swensen *et al.*, 1942). During cold storage, 2-cycloproponoid fatty acids (CPFA) of cotton seed meal (CSM) alter the permeability of egg yolk vitelline membrane resulting in the diffusion of alkaline albumin proteins into yolk and yolk iron to albumin. It enhances brown discoloration and leads to the development of salmon or orange colored yolk and pink albumin. Minerals like iron, calcium, sodium and potassium are found to be effective in alleviating the problem. Tolerance levels of gossypol reported in literature vary widely from as much as 1000ppm (p.01%) to as little as 160 ppm (0.016%). A significant reduction in growth rate and poor feed efficiency along with depressed digestibility of DM, CP, CF and EE in growing-finishing pigs due to incorporation of CSM up to 30% in the concentrate mixtures was reported by Balogun *et al.*(1990). Ruminants become susceptible to gossypol toxicity, if the rumen detoxification is bypassed or if they receive enough CSM to tax the rumen's gossypol detoxification mechanism.

Hydraulic or expeller processing and cooking or moist heat treatment results in binding and inactivation of gossypol, which is in the free form in seed giving rise to bound and free gossypol in the final product. It was observed that CSM detoxified with 1% $Ca(OH)_2$ would be a satisfactory substitute to costly and scarce deoiled groundnut cake (DGNC) in lamb diets (Nagalakshmi *et al.*, 2003). Supplementation of vitamin E was marginally effective in overcoming the toxicity. The 1.5% $Ca(OH)_2$ treatment of CSM is capable of counteracting the deleterious effects of gossypol to a major extent with respect to nutritional, reproductive performance of rams (Author's personal observation).

2.4 Mahua (*Madhuca Indica*) seed cake

The two major species of genus Madhuca found in India are *Madhuca indica* (syn. *Bassia latifolia*) and *Madhuca longifolia* (syn. *Brassica longifolia*). Mahua is the widely accepted as local name for the fat from both these species. This plant is common in deciduous forests. *Madhuca latifolia* is a medium sized to large deciduous tree, distributed in Andhra pradesh, Gujarat, Madhya Pradesh, Orisa, Bihar and Uttar Pradesh, *Madhuca longifoia*, a large evergreen tree found in South India, and evergreen forests of the Western ghats from Konkan Southwards. The potential availability of Mahua seed cake is to the tune of 0.320 million metric tonnes (Radhakrishna, 2003). The presence of toxic and bitter saponins in mahua cake/meal prevents its utilization in poultry/animal feeds. It can be used in cattle feed when bitters and saponins are removed, since it contains 20% crude protein. It must be supplemented with essential amino acids *e.g.*, Arginine and tryptophan. A technique for removing saponins from Mahua seed cake has been developed (Varma and Singh, 1979). About 16 kg of Mahua seed cake was treated with water (1:4) for 10 min and stirred manually for 1min. A pause of 2 minutes was allowed for settling the foam which was removed by strainer. The process was repeated 10 times in a span of an hour till foam becomes oily and yellowish. The treated cake was incorporated in the rations of dairy calves could replace 50 % digestible crude protein content with no adverse effect on growth rate of cross-bred dairy calves. Various methods to detoxify mahua cake like water washing followed by foam removal, hydrochloric acid treatment, ethanol extraction did not yield any tangible success. Ensiling the cake with fertilizer grade urea @ 6-7% (w/w) for 30 d converted the cake into a palatable product and improved feed intake and nutrient utilization in crossbred bull calves (Gowda *et al.*, 1994). However, Dular *et al.* (2000) did not find any beneficial effect of incorporating processed Mahua seed cake in the rations of broiler chicken at 5, 10 and 15% levels.

2.5 Neem (*Azadirachta indica*) seed cake

The neem tree grows abundantly in the Indian subcontinent and also in parts of Africa. Mature neem berries are processed for oil that finds a ready market for a variety of purposes, whereas the residual neem kernel meal (NKM) is employed as organic manure to improve soil fertility. India has annual production potential of 0.5 million tonnes of neem seed cake (NSC) as a residue after oil extraction (Radhakrishna, 2003). The NKM is high in crude protein (36-38%) and found unsuitable for feeding due to presence of bitter and toxic triterpenoids (azadirachtin, salannin, nimbin, nimbidiol *etc.*). Azadirachtin and Salannin (%) in neem seed kernels (n=16) was found to be ranging from 0.044 to 0.135 (mean ± SD: 0.09±0.03) and 0.128 to 0.294 (mean ± SD: 0.22±0.04) (Rao *et al.*, 2009). The bitterness of neem is attributed to limonoids which are the triterpenoids. Water washing of cake converted it into a wholesome protein substitute (Agrawal *et al.*, 1987; Nath *et al.*, 1989; Sastry and Agrawal, 1992), it led to a loss of 22% DM due to washing. To avoid such loss, processing the cake in alkaline medium without water washing was tried either by soaking it in water (1:5 w/v) containing either NaOH (2% w/w) for 24 h or by ensiling with 2.5% urea (w/w) for 5-6 d (Nagalakshmi *et al.* 1996, 1999). The sundried and ground alkali treated and urea ammoniated neem seed kernel cake was found suitable in the feeding of growing lambs (Anandan *et al.*, 1999) and kids (Musalia *et al.*, 2000), broiler poultry (Nagalakshmi *et al.*, 1996, 1999) without affecting their growth, nutrient utilization, blood profile, rumen/caecal fermentation pattern, physical and chemical characteristics of carcass including organoleptic sensory score and gross and histopathology of vital organs.

2.6 Karanj (*Pongamia pinnata*) seed cake

Karanja (*Pongamia pinnata*) is a forest tree belonging to the family Leguminosae, grown in all parts of India, particularly in Tamil Nadu, Andhra Pradesh and Karnataka, for its ecological advantages. The seed contains 27-39% oil, 20–30% protein and a group of furano-flavonoids that constitutes 5-6% by weight of the oil. The oil is known for its curative effect on skin problems, such as, leucoderma, psoriasis, scabies and skin itches (Bringi, 1987). India has production potential of 0.145 million metric tonnes of Karanja seed cake (Radhakrishna, 2003). The seeds contain on average 28-30% oil. The cake is bitter and pungent in taste, is used as manure, fungicide and insecticide. Although the cake is rich in proteins, it is unpalatable and toxic due to the presence of karanjin, pongamol and an unusual amino acid, glabrin. It was found in a study (Dineshkumar *et al.* 2011) that ANF's in karanj seeds samples (n=13) collected across different locations in Karnataka were found to be ranging from 0.57 to 1.75% in case of Karanjin, 0.25 to 1.27% in case of Pongamol and 790-1278 μg/g seed meal in case of trypsin inhibitor activity.

However, raw cake is not normally used as feed for poultry and livestock since the presence of its toxic factors resulted in poor intake (Parmar *et al.*, 1976). Gupta *et al.* (1981) have reported that complete de-oiling of the cake by solvent extraction removes bitter taste and pungent odour. Such a cake has been fed to cattle calf up to 160 g/kg level in the diet without any adverse effect. However, significant reduction in the feed intake, growth, and nutrient balance is found in the animals (Mandal and Banerjee, 1974; Natanam *et al.*, 1988 and 1989) and reduced protein digestibility in growing goat kids, fed at higher levels of solvent-extracted cake, is observed (Srivastava *et al.*, 1990). Ravi *et al.* (2000) have observed significant difference in the digestibility of dry and organic matter in animals fed with expeller pressed cake, revealing that oil-soluble toxic compounds are responsible for the adverse effects in the animals. Various methods, namely, solvent extraction, water leaching, autoclaving, acid and alkali treatment, were adopted to detoxify karanja cake (Prabhu *et al.*, 2002). It is found that solvent extraction removed karanjin efficiently. Besides these, tannins, phytates and protease inhibitors, as meal constituents, are the non-nutrient components that hinder the usage of cake. Attempts have also been made to detoxify karanja seed meal by refluxing with 2% HCl (Mandal, 1985). Rats, fed on the resultant meal, at 30% level, did not suffer any toxic effects. The studies were conducted for assessment of protease inhibitors and digestibility of proteins due to detoxification by refluxing with 2% HCl. However, karanj cake, after solvent extraction followed by alkali (1% NaOH) processing, can be a wholesome protein substitute, to spare 50% nitrogen moiety of costly and scarce vegetable oil cakes for economical mutton production in short term fattening of lambs in developing countries. Panda *et al.* (2006) reported that the adverse effect of dietary incorporation of karanj cake in broiler chickens was due to synergistic effect of karanjin, tannin and trypsin inhibitor activity but not because of the furanoflavonoid, karanjin alone. Solvent extracted karanj cake could, however, be incorporated after alkali (1.5% NaOH, w/w) processing at an enhanced level of 6.43%, replacing 12.5% of soybean meal nitrogen, in the broiler diets up to 4 weeks of age, beyond which the observed growth depression on this diet could be alleviated by 0.2% methionine supplementation. Such diet, by partially sparing costly and scarce conventional oil cake, supported optimum nutritional performance and immune-competence in broiler chickens.

2.7 Jatropha (*Jatropha curcus*) seed cake

The oil plant *Jatropha curcas* (L) or purge/physic nut is a multipurpose and drought resistant large shrub or small tree. It is a native of tropical America; it now thrives throughout Africa and Asia. Being drought tolerant, it can be used to reclaim eroded areas, be grown as a boundary fence or live hedge in the arid/semi-arid areas. The seeds of Jatropha contain viscous oil, which can be used for manufacture of candles and soap, in the cosmetics industry, for cooking and lighting by itself or as a diesel/paraffin substitute or extender. Being rich in nitrogen, the seed cake is an excellent source of plant nutrients. Some constraints which could restrict the optimum utilization of seed cake from both the toxic and non-toxic variety are: very high levels of trypsin inhibitor activity (21-27 mg trypsin inhibited /g DM), lectin (51-102 when expressed as inverse of minimum concentration in mg of Jatropha meal per ml of the assay) which produces haemagglutination and phytate concentration (9-10%) (Makkar *et al.*, 1998 a,b). It was found that 3% sodium hydroxide or sodium bicarbonate was most effective in reducing the phorbol esters to 55% level but feeding trial with Deccani sheep resulted in appearance of clinical symptoms such as dullness, inappetance, diarrhea and mortality of sheep in just 4-11 days (A.V. Elangovan NIANP personal communication). The *J. curcas* seed meal (with 1-2% residual oil) contains 58-64% crude protein (90% of which is present in the form of true protein) and levels of essential amino acids except lysine are higher than for the FAO reference protein. The amino acid composition, the percentage of essential amino acids and the mineral content of the pressed cake can be compared to those of other seeds and pressed cakes used as feeds (Aderibigbe *et al.*, 1997).

There appears to be difference in variety as seed meal from the Cape Verde and Nicaragua varieties has been found to be highly toxic to fish, rats and chikens while seed meal from a Mexican variety was not (Makkar *et al.*, 1998b). In addition, experiments with rats showed that the protein efficiency ratio of the feed containing heat-treated seed meal from the non-toxic variety was about 86% of that obtained with standard protein casein. They further suggested that both toxic and non-toxic varieties must be detoxified and found to be good protein sources for livestock.

2.8 Castor (*Ricinus communis*) seed cake

Castor *(Ricinus communis)* seed cake (CSC) is a by-product of the vegetable-oil industry, contains fairly good amounts of protein (CP = 35%). CSC can be a substitute of conventional oil cakes like soybean meal (SBM) in livestock diets but for the presence of a toxic glycoprotein, ricin. In spite of its high protein content, castor cake is not used as livestock feed due to the presence of toxic factors ricin, ricinine and allergen. Of the three, ricin is the most detrimental to the animals (Ambekar and Dole, 1957). In order to detoxify the cake, a number of physical and chemical methods were employed. Soaking (3, 6 and 12h), steaming (30 and 60min), boiling (30 and 60min), autoclaving (15psi, 30min; 15psi, 60min) and heating (100°C 30min; 120°C 25min) were the physical methods employed, while the chemical methods consisted of ammonia (7.5, 12.5ml/kg of castor cake), formaldehyde (5, 10g/kg), lime (10, 20 and 40g/kg), sodium chloride (5, 10 and 20g/kg), tannic acid (5, 10g/kg) and sodium hydroxide (2.5, 5 and 10g/kg). The efficacy of the treatments was assessed, based on the qualitative and quantitative changes in ricin content. Of all the methods employed, autoclaving (15psi. for 60min) and lime treatment (40g/kg) completely destroyed the toxin (Anandan *et al.*, 2005).

3. Saponins

Saponins are widely distributed in the plant kingdom and have been identified in 500 species belonging to more than 80 different families. The important common forages which have saponins are Lucerne (*Medicago sativa*), white clover (*Trifolium repens*), red clover (*T. prateuse*) and soybean (*Glycine max*). Saponins are plant glycosides which yield on hydrolysis sugars (pentoses, hexoses and uronic acids) and aglycones derived from polycyclic ring systems and are known as sapogenins. The saponins are divided into two main groups from the point of views of chemical nature of sapogenins: Steroids (C27) or triterpenoides (C30) with the triterpenoid sapogenins further divided into three classes based on the compound ursane, oleanane or lupine. Saponins are found in a large number of plant and some animals (such as sea cucumber). In plants, they occur in different plants such as root, tuber, bark, leaves, seed and fruit. Common saponins containing plants are listed (Wina *et al.* 2005; Table 3).

Table 3 : Saponin containing forages commonly used as livestock feed.

Family and species	Plant part	Saponin or sapogenin name
Fabaceae		
Acacia auriculoformis	Fruit	acaciaside
Albezia lebbek	Pods, bark	Albiziasaponin
Ear pod tree (*Enterolobium cyclocarpum*)	Leaf, fruit	Saponin content (3.9 mg/g)
Glyricidia sepium	Root, fruit	Hederagenin
Glycine maxima (soybean)	Seed	Soyasapogenol
Lupinus spp. (lupin)	Seed	Soyasapogenol
Medicago sativa (alfalfa and lucerne)	Leaf, root, seed	Medicagenic (aglycone) Soyasapogenol
Meliotus alba (white sweet clover)	Leaf,flower, root	Melitonin
Pueraria Montana var.lobata (Kudzu)	Root	Kudzusaponins (Soyasapogenol)
Sesbania sesban	Leaf, seed	Glucuronide-oleanolic acid stigmasta galactopyranoside
Sesbania pachycarpa	Leaf	Saponin
Ladino clover (*Trifolium repens*)	Leaf	Cloversaponins (soyasapogenol)
Red Clover (*Trifolium pretense*)	Leaf	Soyasapogenin
Fenugreek (*Trigonella foenum-graecum*)	Leaf, seed	Steroid saponin
Moringa oleifera	Leaf	80g/Kg diosgenin equivalent
Oat (Avena sativa)	Leaf, root, seed	Avenacin
Signal grass (Brachiara decumbens) (signal grass)	Leaf	Dioscin, diosgenin, yamogenin

Saponins possess significant characteristics like bitter taste, foaming in aqueous solution and hemolysis of red blood cells. Saponins have characteristic properties which determine their biological activity. Structurally saponins contain a lipid soluble aglycone and a water soluble glycone part which jointly confers lower surface tension and thus form stable foam when dissolved in water. Saponins readily combine with cholesterol resulting in minimization of the activity of original saponin. Saponins tend to alter the permeability of the cell wall and thereby exert a general toxicity on many organs and tissues.

Saponins are present in all parts of the plant *i.e.*, plants, stems, roots and blossoms of the plant in varying amounts (2-3%). The levels vary due to stage of cutting (first cut Lucerne have more than second or third cuts). The levels are inversely correlated with crude fibre and hay yield. There is also an indication that leaves contain twice the amounts of saponins as that of stems and saponin contents decline as the plant gets older (Sen *et al.*, 1998).

Whenever animals consume saponin rich diets, they tend to alter the surface tension of the ruminal contents due to entrapment of countless bubbles of fermentation gases throughout ingesta. This condition is described as *frothy bloat* and gases would be difficult to expel out. Animal becomes restless and respiration rate increases. At ruminal level, saponins tend to exert antiprotozoal effects (defaunation), antimethanogenic and selective action on rumen bacteria. Rumen ammonia level may tend to reduce due to indirect result of the decreased protozoal counts caused by the added saponin. The major effects of saponins on rumen fermentation were a shift of towards increased proportion of propionate and decreased acetate to propionate ratio. The higher propionate proportion may be the result of lower acetate and butyrate, which are both major fermentation end products of protozoa. Therefore, when the number of protozoa was depressed by saponins, a significant increase in the proportion of propionate would be expected (Lu *et al.*, 1987 and Leng *et al.*, 1992).

Makkar and Becker (1996) found that the efficiency of *in vitro* microbial protein synthesis (EMPS) was linearly increased by the addition of Quilaja saponins (0.4 to 1.2 mg/mL) to a hay substrate. They concluded that saponins partition the nutrients in such a manner that a higher proportion of the digested substrate goes into the formation of microbial mass and a lower proportion to shortchain fatty acids and gas. They further reported that saponins caused a significant reduction in the apparent and true digestibility of the substrate in an *in vitro* fermentation study. At intestinal level these saponins cause inhibition of certain digestive enzymes such as α-chymotrypsin. Levels of Lucerne meal (above 7%) in poultry caused depression in weight gain in chickens and also depress egg production which can partially reversed by feeding of cholesterol and cotton seed oil in the diet for the saponins to get bound.

Removal of saponins from quinoa (*Chenopodium quinoa)* by washing and abrasion was attempted (Ridout *et al.,* 1991). The data obtained suggest differential cellular locations of the individual saponins. The processing of quinoa led to changes in sensory characteristics; removal of saponins was associated with reductions in bitterness and astringency. Microscopic analysis revealed considerable differences in washed and abraded samples, both before and after cooking; in particular the abraded samples showed a greater degree of cellular disruption. Water soaking and rinsing will remove these components in the feedstuffs. The remedial measures for bloat include feeding of dry roughage prior to feeding saponin rich fodder and spraying of oil.

4. Mimosine

Mimosine is a toxic amino acid, also called as 'leucenine' found in genus *Leucaena* which includes subabul. Concern has arisen because of the importance of *L. leucocephala,* in which the level of mimosine in the leaf is about 2-6% and varies with seasons and maturity. Mimosine cannot be degraded after absorption. The mechanism of action of mimosine in producing its effect is not clear but it may act as an amino acid antagonist or may complex with pyridoxal phosphate, leading to disruption of catalytical action of B_6-containing enzymes such as transaminases, or may complex with metals such as zinc (Hegarty, 1978). It can be extensively degraded to dihydroxy pyridone (DHP) in the rumen. Excess DHP is absorbed into the blood stream, reaches thyroid gland and inhibits biosynthesis of the hormone thyroxin. It has extensive deleterious properties in animals including disruption of reproductive processes and teratogenic effects (D'Mello, 1991). Among the various livestock, horses, sheep, pigs and even rabbits are highly sensitive to mimosine and thus subabul should not be fed to them as sole feed. The main symptoms are reduced growth and weight loss, excessive salivation, loss of hair, eroded gums, enlarged thyroid gland and poor reproductive efficiency.

The main symptoms of toxicity in ruminants are poor growth, loss of hair and wool, swollen and raw coronets above the hooves, lameness, mouth and oesophageal lesions, depressed serum thyroxine level and goitre. Some of these symptoms may be due to mimosine and others to 3, 4 dihydroxypyridine, a metabolite of mimosine in the rumen (Jones and Hegarty, 1984). Toxic signs like skin lesions also resemble Zn deficiency. Reduction in calving percentage due to leucaena feeding has also been noted (Jones *et al.,* 1989).

A solution to the mimosine problem could be the development of low mimosine cultivars. However, low mimosine types are found to be unproductive and of low vigour. The other approach is to feed Leucaena mixed with other feeds. Hiremath (1981) suggested that use of Leucaena fodder may be restricted to 30% of the green forage in the case of cattle and buffalo, and 50% for goats. The effect of Leucaena and mimosine can be reduced by heat treatment (Tangendijaja *et al.,* 1990), by supplementation with amino acids (Rosenthal and Janzen, 1979) or with metal ions such as Fe^{2+}, Al^{3+} (D'Mello and Acamovic, 1989) and Zn^{+2} (Jones *et al.,* 1978).

5. Tannins

Feedstuffs containing tannins are widely used in India especially in arid and semi-arid regions of the country, particularly during dry seasons when more nutritious feeds are in short supply. Tannins are secondary compounds of various chemical structures widely occurring in plant kingdom and are generally divided into hydrolysable and condensed tannins. Their anti-nutritional effects include interference with the digestive processes either by binding with the enzymes or by binding to feed components like proteins or minerals (Liener, 1989). Hydrolysable tannins are easily degraded in biological systems, forming smaller compounds that can enter the blood stream and over a period of time cause toxicity to the vital organs such as liver and kidney. Recommended methods for the removal of condensed tannins include de-hulling the seeds to remove the tannin rich outer layer, autoclaving or treatment with alkali (Griffiths, 1991). Polyethylene glycol (PEG) is used as a tannin blocking agent to enhance the intake of tannin rich plants (TRP) and/or to alleviate the tannin detrimental effects in ruminants (Silanikove *et al.*, 2006). In general, positive results, with regard to improved intake, were found when tannin content in the diet or plant (as a sole feed) was above 50 g/kg DM (Makkar, 2003) or when a single source of tannins was offered to small ruminants (Silanikove *et a.*, 2006). Negative effects of tannins were counteracted successfully by drenching 5 g of PEG per day in goats browsing on *Prosopis cineraria* shrub foliage for a period of 90 days. The observed beneficial effects in PEG group compared to tannin group are improved protein digestibility, blood parameters, rumen ammonia nitrogen, total volatile fatty acid concentrations and growth performance (Bhatta *et al.*, 2002). Further addition of PEG (50 g per kg DM of concentrate mixture) could substitute high protein concentrate mixture with low protein concentrate mixtures for goat kids browsing on *Prosopis cineraria* vegetation Bhatta *et al.*, 2004). Thus, nutritional strategies can be successfully devised for ruminants which had access to tannin rich forages.

6. Cyanogens (Prussic acid)

Cyanogens are glucosides of a sugar and a cyanide containing aglycone. Intact cyanogens are harmless. Cyanogens can be hydrolyzed by enzyme to release hydrocyanic acid (HCN) which is toxic. The hydrolytic reaction takes place in the rumen by microbial activity. In pig and horse, enzyme concerned in the release of HCN is destroyed by the gastric HCl. Hence, ruminants are more susceptible to cyanide than monogastric animals. The HCN is rapidly absorbed and some is eliminated through the lungs, but the greater part is rapidly detoxified in the liver by conversion to thiocyanate. Excess cyanide ion can quickly produce anoxia of the central nervous system through inactivating the cytochrome oxidase system and death can result within few seconds. Based on the intensity, animals show nervousness, abnormal breathing, trembling or jerking muscles, blue colouration of the lining of the mouth, spasms or convulsions and respiratory failure (Harris and Shearer 2003).

High levels of cyanogens can be found in certain grasses such as jowar (sorghum) and sudan grass, linseed and cassava root. In plants the glucoside is non-toxic in the intact issues and as stated earlier, when the plants are damaged or begin to decay, hydrolytic enzyme from the same plant is released and liberates HCN. This reaction can take place in the rumen by microbial activity. Forage sorghum, sorghum-Sudan hybrids, Sudan grass, and Johnson grass can accumulate cyanide under drought conditions if rain fall is scanty or irrigation is not plenty. When the plant wilts, its cells rupture and the HCN is freed from the sugar molecule. If consumed by grazing livestock, the free HCN is readily absorbed into the blood stream, where it prohibits the animal's ability to take oxygen from the blood. Even in unwilted plants, chewing and digestion in the rumen can release toxic levels of HCN.

Many other conditions adversely affecting the normal growing functions of a plant can cause accumulation of HCN, such as prolonged cloudiness, soil acidity, abnormally high or low temperature (especially sudden changes in temperature), herbicide treatments, and low soil phosphorous. Proper curing or ensiling of forages containing high levels of HCN greatly reduces or eliminates the danger because free HCN volatilizes fairly quickly after it is released. Animals which have shown much evidence of toxicity may be injected intravenously with 3 g of sodium nitrate and 15 g sodium thiosulphate in 200 ml H_2O for cattle, for sheep, 1g sodium nitrate and 2.5 g sodium thiosulphate in 50 ml H_2O (Harris and Shearer 2003).

7. Nitrates

Nitrate itself is not toxic to animals, but at elevated levels will cause a disease called nitrate poisoning. Nitrates are normally found in forages are converted by the digestion process to nitrite, and in turn the nitrite is converted to ammonia. Nitrate accumulation can occur in virtually any plant with the ability to grow rapidly and use soil nitrogen efficiently. Under normal conditions, nitrate in the soil is absorbed by plant roots, transported through the stems, and converted in leaves to proteins and other substances that are useable by the animal. Nitrate typically is used by the plant about as fast as it is absorbed from the soil. Nitrate poisoning occurs when this excessive nitrate is consumed and converted to nitrite faster than the animal can use it. Free nitrite in the rumen is readily absorbed into the blood stream, where it destroys the blood's ability to absorb and carry oxygen.

The ammonia is then converted to protein by bacteria in the rumen. If cattle rapidly ingest large quantities of plants that contain high levels of nitrate, nitrite will accumulate in the rumen. Nitrite is ten times as toxic to cattle as nitrate. It cause an acute toxicosis in cattle resulting from formation of methemoglobin (a true oxidation product of haemoglobin), which is unable to transport oxygen because the iron is in the ferric (Fe^{+++}) rather than the usual ferrous (Fe^{++}) state. Symptoms seen in acute toxicity include laboured breathing (dyspnoea), grinding of the teeth, uneasiness and excessive salivation. Drying or ensiling forages tends to have a small effect on nitrate levels. Hays and silage from high-risk plants may remain toxic. Nitrate poisoning is usually treated by intravenous injection of methylene blue. A high dose of concentrates in the daily ration and adequate feeding of Vitamin A have a protective effect (Harris and Shearer 2003).

8. Moulds and mycotoxins

Mycotoxins are the secondary metabolites of fungi that have the capacity to impair animal health and productivity (D'Mello and Macdonald, 1998). Principal mycotoxins occurring in feeds and forages are presented in Table 4. Mycotoxin contamination of forages and cereals frequently occurs in the field following infection of plants with particular pathogenic fungi or with symbiotic endophytes. Contamination may also occur during processing and storage of harvested products and feed whenever environmental conditions are appropriate for spoilage fungi. Moisture content and ambient temperature are key determinants of fungal colonization and mycotoxin production. Mycotoxigenic species may be further distinguished on the basis of geographical prevalence, reflecting specific environmental requirements for growth and secondary metabolism. Thus, *Aspergillus flavus*, *A. parasiticus* and *A. ochraceus* readily proliferate under warm, humid conditions, while *Penicillium expansum* and *P. verrucosum* are essentially temperate fungi. Consequently, the *Aspergillus* mycotoxins predominate in plant products emanating from the tropics and other warm regions, while the *Penicillium* mycotoxins occur widely in temperate foods, particularly cereal grains. *Fusarium* fungi are more ubiquitous, but even this genus contains toxigenic species that are almost exclusively associated with cereals from warm countries. A new source of neutraceuticals has some potential antifungal and cytotoxic properties have been identified (Mokhlesi *et al.*, 2012) from sea cucumber (*Holothuria leucospilota*). The common organisms are susceptible to *Aspergillus niger, Candida albicans, Pseudomonas aeruginosa, Staphylococcus aureus and Escherichia coli etc*. Methonolic extract has shown potential cytotoxic effect (LC_{50} 0.4 μg/mL). Important mycotoxin producing fungi and their principal toxin were listed in Table 4.

Table 4 : Different mycotoxin producing fungi and their principal toxin*

Fungal species	Mycotoxins
Aspergillus flavus; A. parasiticus	Aflatoxins
A. flavus	Cyclopiazonic acid
A. ochraceus; Penicillium viridicatum; P. cyclopium	Ochratoxin A
P. citrinum; P. expansum	Citrinin
P. expansum	Patulin
P. citreo-viride	Citreoviridin
Fusarium culmorum; F. graminearum	Deoxynivalenol
F. sporotrichioides; F. poae	T-2 toxin
F. sporotrichioides; F. graminearum; F. poae	Diacetoxyscirpenol
F. culmorum; F. graminearum; F. sporotrichioides	Zearalenone
F. moniliforme	
Alternaria alternata	*Neotyphodium coenophialum* *N. lolii* *Claviceps purpurea* *Phomopsis leptostromiformis* *Pithomyces chartarum*

*Adapted from D'Mello and MacDonald (1998)

9. Effect of processing on reduction of these anti-nutritive substances

Heat processing is a common procedure in feed manufacture, conferring improved properties as regards the safety and nutritive value of animal feeds. For example, heat treatment of dried poultry litter appears to be an effective method for controlling, or even eliminating, contamination with *Salmonella*, *E. coli* and *Campylobacter* (Jeffrey *et al.*, 1998). Thermal processing is also effective for denaturing proteinase inhibitors, lectins and cyanogens. However, for antigenic proteins, more complex procedures involving the uses of hot aqueous ethanol extraction are required (D'Mello, 1991).

For aflatoxin-contaminated oilseeds destined for animal feed, ammoniation appears to be the processing method of choice. The feedstuff is treated with either ammonium hydroxide or gaseous ammonia at high temperatures and pressure in commercial feed mills, or at ambient temperature and low pressure in small-scale operations in developing countries. If the ammoniation reactions are allowed to proceed to completion, the detoxification process is irreversible and aflatoxin contamination is virtually eliminated. Providing that the residual ammonia is dissipated, diets containing the decontaminated meals are readily consumed by animals without ill-effects. Sun drying of animal feeds can be viable and cheap mehod of detoxification of aflatoxins especially in tropical countries like India. Nutritionally inert adsorbents like bentonite or activated charcoal can be used in feeds at low levels to make milk free from AFM_1 or under prescribed limits. Depending on the efficacy of decontamination, residues of AFM1 in the milk of dairy cows are substantially reduced or absent altogether.

Conclusions

Most of the newer feed resources contain one or more anti-nutritional factors which can affect the animal performance. Suitable detoxification methods have to be developed for making feeding of NFR safe. Few ANF's have commercial value and have to be harvested during detoxification process for making it economically viable. In this way newer feed resources will augment the feedbase for optimum livestock production.

References

Aderibigbe A.O., Makkar H.P.S., Becker K., Foidl N. (1997). Chemical composition and effect of heat on organic matter-and nitrogen-degradability and some antinutritional components of Jatropha meal. *Animal Feed Science Technology* **67:** 223-243.

Agrawal D.K., Garg A.K., Nath K. (1987). The use of water-washed neem (*Azadirachta indica*) seed kernel cake in the feeding of buffalo calves. *Journal of Agricultural Science* **108:** 497-499.

Ambekar V.R., Dole K.K. (1957). Detoxification of castor cake. *Indian Journal of Dairy Science* **10:** 107-122.

Anandan S. Anil Kumar G.K., Ghosh J., Ramachandra K.S. (2005). Effect of different physical and chemical treatments on detoxification of ricin in castor cake. *Animal Feed Science and Technology* **120:** 159-168.

Anandan S., Sastry V.R.B., Katiyar R.C., Agrawal D.K. (1999). Growth rate and nutrient efficiency of growing goats fed urea ammoniated neem *(Azadirachta indica)* seed kernel meal as protein supplement. *Small Ruminant Research* **32:** 125-128.

Aumaitre A., Bourdon D., Peiniau J., Freire J.B. (1989). Effect of graded levels of raw and processed rapeseed on feed digestibility and nutrient utilization in young pigs. *Animal Feed Science and Technology* **24:** 275-287.

Balogun T.F., Aduku A. O., Dim N. I., Olorunju. S.A.S. (1990). Undecorticated cottonseed meal as a substitute for soyabean meal in diets for weaner and growing-finishing pigs. *Animal Feed Science Technology* **30:** 193-201.

Bhatta R., Shinde A.K., Vaithiyanathan S., Sankhyan S.K., Verma D.L. (2002). Effect of polyethylene glycol-6000 on nutrient intake, digestion and growth of kids browsing *Prosopis cineraria. Animal Feed Science and Technology* **101:** 45-54.

Bhatta R., Shinde A.K., Verma D.L., Sankhyan S.K., Vaithiyanathan S. (2004). Effect of supplementation containing polyethylene glycol (PEG)-6000 on intake, rumen fermentation pattern and growth in kids fed foliage of *Prosopis cineraria. Small Ruminant Research* **50:** 45-52.

Boatner C.H. (1948). Cottonseed and cottonseed products. Their chemistry and chemical technology (A.E. Bailey, ed.) Chapter 6, Wiley (Interscience) Publishers, New York (e.f Liener, 1980).

Bringi N.V. (1987). Non-traditional oilseeds and oils in India. Oxford and IBH Publishing Co. Pvt. Ltd, New Delhi, pp 143–166.

Cheeke P.R., Shull L.R. (1985). Natural Toxicants in Feeds and Livestock. AVI Publishing Inc., West Port, Connecticut.

Das M.M., Singhal K.K. (2001). Influence of chemical treatment of mustard oil cake on its glucosinolate content and myrosinase activity. *Indian Journal of Animal Sciences* **71:** 793-796.

Das M.M., Singhal K.K. (2005). Effect of feeding chemically treated mustard cake on growth, thyroid and liver function and carcass characteristics in kids. *Small Ruminant. Research* **56:** 31-38.

Dineshkumar, D. Rao, S. B. N. Jash, S, Elangovan, A.V., Hemalatha, S. (2011) Chemical composition and anti-nutritional factors in karanja (*Pongamia pinnata*) seed kernels and its *in vitro* evaluation. *Indian Journal of Animal Sciences* **81:** 478-483.

D'Mello J.P.F., Acamovic T. (1989). *Leucaena leucocephala* in poultry nutrition: A Review. *Animal Feed Science and Technology* **26:** 1-28.

D'Mello J.P.F. (1991). Antigenic proteins. In*: Toxic substances in crop plants.* (J.P.F. D'Mello, C.M. Duffus and J.H. Duffus, eds). Royal Society of Chemistry, Cambridge, UK, pp 107-125.

D'Mello J.P.F. (1995). Antinutritional substances in legume seeds. In*: Tropical legumes in animal nutrition.* (J.P.F. D'Mello and C. Devendra, eds). CAB International, Wallingford, UK, pp 135-172.

D'Mello J.P.F. (2000). Antinutritional factors and mycotoxins. In*: Farm animal metabolism and nutrition.* (J.P.F. D'Mello, ed), CAB International, Wallingford, UK, pp 383-403.

D'Mello J.P.F. and Macdonald A.M.C. (1998). Fungal toxins as disease elicitors. In: *Environmental toxicology: current developments.* (J. Rose, ed.) Gordon and Breach Science Publishers. Amsterdam, the Netherlands, pp 253-289.

Dular R.K. Vaishnava C.S.V., Sihag S. (2000). Effect of feeding processed Mahua cake on performance of broiler chicks. *Indian Journal of Poultry Science* **35:** 105-108.

Fenwick G.R., Spinks E.A., Wilkinson A.P., Heaney R.K., Legoy M.A. (1986). Effect of processing on the antinutrient content of rapeseed. *Journal of the Science of Food and Agriculture.* **37:** 735-741.

Glencross B, Hawkins W., Curnow J. (2004). Nutritional assessment of Australian canola meal. Part II. Evaluation of canola oil extracted methods on the protein value of canola meal fed to the red seabream (*Pagrus auratus*, Paulin). *Aquaculture Research* **35:** 25-34.

Gowda N.K.S., Katiyar R.C., Sastry V.R.B. (1994). Detoxified Mahua (Bassia latifolia) seed cake as protein source for high growth potential animals. *Indian Journal of Animal Nutrition* **11:** 1-6.

Grffiths D.W. (1991). Condensed tannins. *In: Toxic substances in crop plants (J.P.F.D'Mello, C.M. Duffus and J.H. Duffus, eds)*, Royal Society of Chemistry, Cambridge, UK, pp 180-201.

Gupta B.S., Srivastava J.P., Tripathi A.K., Verma A.K., Thakur S. (1981). Biological valuation of karanja (*P. glabra*) cake. *Indian Journal of Animal Health* **6:** 75-77.

Harris B., Shearer J.K. (2003). Nitrate, prussic acid (HCN) and grass tetany problems in cattle feeding, *Technical Document, DS6,* Animal Science Department, Florida Cooperative Extension Service, Institute of Food and Agricultural Sciences, University of Florida. *http://edis.ifas.ufl.edu*.

Hegarty M.P. (1978). Toxic amino acids of plant origin. In: *Effect of poisonous plants on livestock.* (R.F. Keeler, K.R. Van Kampen, L.F. James, eds.) Academic Press, New York, pp 575-585.

Herrington M. K. Permert J. Kazakoff R.K. Zuckerc K.A. Bilchikd A.J. Pourb M.P., Adrian, T.E. (1994) Effects of raw soya diet and cholecystokinin receptor blockade on pancreatic growth and tumor initiation in the hamster. *Cancer Letters* **82:** 7-16.

Hiremath N.B. (1981). Subabool *(Leucaena leucocephala)* - A wonder plant. *Indian Dairyman* **33:** 351-356.

Huang S., Liang M., Lardy G., Huff H.E., Kerley M.S., Hsieh F. (1995). Extrusion process of rapeseed meal for reducing glucosinolates. *Animal Feed Science and Technology* **56:** 1-9.

Jeffrey J.S., Kirk J.H., Atwill E.R., Cullor J.S. (1998). Prevalence of selected microbial pathogens in processed poultry waste used as dairy cattle feed. *Poultry Science* **77:** 808-811.

Jensen S.K., Liu Y.G., Eggum B.O. (1995). The effect of heat treatment on glucosinolates and nutritive value of rapeseed meal in rat. *Animal Feed Science and Technology* **53:** 17-28.

Jones L.A. (1985). Gossypol chemistry and plant distribution. In: *Male Fertility and its Regulation*, MTP Press, Lancaster, England, pp 93-110.

Jones R.J., Blunt C.G., Nurnberg B.I. (1978). Toxicity of *Leucaena leucocephala*. The effect of iodine and mineral supplements on penned steers fed a sole diet of Leucaena. *Australian Veterinary Journal* **54:** 387-392.

Jones R.J., Hegarty M.P. (1984). The effect of different proportion of *Leucaena leucocephala* in the diet of cattle on growth, feed intake, thyroid function and urinary excretion of 3-hydroxy-4 (IH)-pyridone. *Australian Journal of Agriculture Research* **35:** 317.

Jones R.M., McLennan M.W., Dowsett K. F. (1989). The effect of *Leucaena leucocephala* on the reproduction of beef cattle grazing leucaena/grass pastures. *Tropical Grasslands* **23:** 108-114.

Leng, R. A. Bird, S. H. Klieve, A. Choo, B. S. Ball, F. M.Asefa, G. Brumby, P. Mudgal, V. D. Chaudhry, U. B. Haryono, S. U. and Hendratno, N. (1992). The potential for tree forage supplements to manipulate rumen protozoa to enhance protein to energy ratios in ruminants fed on poor quality forages. In: *Legume trees and other fodder trees as protein sources for livestock;* FAO Animal Production and Health Review 102; Section 11 (A. Speedy, P.L. Pugliese, eds.), FAO publication, Rome. 177-191.

Liener I.E. (1989). Antinutritional factors in legume seeds: state of the art. *In: Recent advances of research in anti-nutritional factors in legume seeds. (J. Huisman, A.F.B. Van der Poel and I.E. Liener, eds)*, Pudoc, Wageningen, pp 6-14.

Lu C.D. Tsai L.S., Schaefer D.M., Jorgensen N.A. (1987) Alteration of fermentation in continuous culture of mixed rumen bacteria by isolated alfalfa saponins. *Journal of Dairy Science* **79:** 799-805.

Maheshwari P.N., Stanley D.W., Van de Van F.R. (1980). Microwave treatment of dehulled rapeseed meal to inactivate myrosinase and its effect on oil meal quality. *Journal of the American Oil Chemists' Society* **57:** 194-199.

Makkar H.P.S., Aderebigbe A.O., Becker K. (1998a). Comparative evaluation of toxic and nontoxic varieties of *Jatropha curcus* for chemical composition, digestibility, protein degradability and toxic factors. *Food Chemistry* **62:** 207-215.

Makkar H.P.S., Becker K, Schmook B. (1998b). Edible provenances of *Jatropha curcas* from Quintana Roo state of Mexico and effect of roasting on antinutrient and toxic factors in seeds. *Plant Foods and Human Nutrition* **52:** 31-36.

Makkar H.P.S., Becker K. (1996). Effect of quillaja saponins or *in vitro* rumen fermentation, In: *Saponins used in food and agriculture.* (G.R.Waller, Y.Yamasaki, eds), Plenum Press, New York, pp 387-394.

Makkar H.P.S. (2003). Effects and fate of tannins in ruminant animals, adaptation to tannins, and strategies to overcome detrimental effects of feeding tannin-rich feeds. *Small Ruminant Research* **49:** 241-256.

Mandal L., Banerjee G.C. (1974). Studies on the utilization of karanja (*Pongamia glabra*) oil cake in poultry rations. *Indian Journal of Poultry Science* **9:** 141-147.

Mokhsesi A., Saeidnia S., Gohari A.R., Shaverdi A.R., Nasrolahi A., Farahani F., Khoshnood R., Es'haghi N. (2012). Biological activities of the Sea Cucumber (*Holothuria leucospilota*). *Asian Journal of Animal and Veterinary Advances* **7:** 243-249.

Musalia L.M., Anandan S., Sastry V.R.B., Agrawal, D. K. (2000). Urea-treated neem (*Azadirachta indica A. juss*) seed kernel cake as a protein supplement for lambs, *Small Ruminant Research* **35:** 107-116.

Nagalakshmi D., Sastry V.R.B., Agrawal D.K. (2003). Relative performance of fattening lambs on raw and processed cottonseed meal incorporated diets. *Asian-Australasian Journal of Animal Sciences* **16:** 29-35.

Nagalakshmi D., Sastry V.R.B., Agrawal D.K., Katiyar R.C., Verma S.V.S. (1996) Performance of broiler chicks fed on alkali-treated neem (*Azadirachta indica*) kernel cake as a protein supplement. *British Poultry Science* **37:** 809-818.

Nagalakshmi D., Sastry V.R.B., Katiyar R.C., Agrawal D.K., Verma S.V.S. (1999). Performance of broiler chicks fed on diets containing urea ammoniated neem (*Azadirachta indica*) kernel cake. *British Poultry Science* **40:** 77-83.

Natanam R., Kedirvel R., Balagopal R. (1988). Toxic effect of pungam (Pongamia glabra Vent) kernel cake and oil in poultry. In: *Third symposium on latest trend in livestock and poultry nutrition of* Animal Nutrition Society, Banaras, India, Abstract No. 181.

Natanam R., Kedirvel R., Ravi R. (1989). Toxic effect of Karanja (*Pongamia glabra Vent*) oil and cake on growth and feed efficiency of broiler chicks. *Animal Feed Science and Technology* **27:** 95-100.

Nath K., Agrawal D.K., Hassan Q.Z, Daniel S.J., Sastry V.R.B. (1989). Water-washed neem (*Azadirachta indica*) seed kernel cake in the feeding of milch cows, *Animal Production* **48:** 497-502.

Newkirk R.W., Classen H.L., Scott T.A., Edney M.J. (2003). The digestibility and content of amino acid in toasted and non-toasted canola meal. *Canadian Journal of Animal Science* **83:** 131-139.

Panda A.K, Sastry V.R.B, Mandal A.B., Saha S.K., Kumar, A. (2006). Quantification of Karanjin, tannin and trypsin inhibitors in raw and detoxified expeller and solvent extracted Karanj (*Pongamia glabra*) cake. *Asian-Australasian Journal of Animal Sciences* **19:** 1776-1783.

Pandey S.N., Thejappa N. (1975) Study on relationship between oil, protein, and gossypol in cottonseed kernels. *Journal of the American Oil Chemists' Society* **52:** 312-315.

Parmar B.S., Sahrawat K.L., Mukherjee, S.K. (1976). Pongamia glabra: constituents and uses. *Journal of Scientific and Industrial Research* **35:** 608-611.

Prabhu, T.M., Deva Kumar C., Sastry V.R.B., Agarwal D.K. (2002). Quantification of karanjin using high performance liquid chromatography in raw and detoxified Karanj (*Pongamia glabra vent*) seed cake. *Asian-Australasian Journal of Animal Sciences* **15:** 416-240.

Radhakrishna P (2003) Tree borne oil seeds as a source of energy for decentralized planning. Government of India, Ministry of Non-Conventional Energy Sources, New Delhi, India.

Rakariyatham N., Sakorn P. (2002). Biodegradation of glucosinolates in brown mustrad meal (*Brassica juncea*) by *Aspergillus sp.* NR-4201 in liquide and solid culture. *Biodegradation* **3:** 395-409.

Rama Rao, S. V. Raju, M.V.L.N. Panda, A.K., Reddy M.R (2006) Sunflower seed meal as a replacement of soybean meal in commercial broiler chicken diets, *British Poultry Sceince* **47:** 592-598.

Rao S.B.N., Dineshkumar D., Elangovan A.V., Jash S., Anandan S., Brijpal Singh (2009) Unconventional oil seeds – potential for use as protein supplements after complete detoxification, In: *Proceedings of 13th biennial animal nutrition society conference on "Diversification of animal nutrition research in the changing scenario"*, held at NIANP, Bangalore from 17-19th December 2009), Volume II (Abstr.) p 163.

Ravi U., Singh P., Garg A.K., Agrawal D.K. (2000). Performance of lambs fed expeller pressed and solvent extracted Karanj (*Pongamia pinnata*) oil cake. *Animal Feed Science and Technology* **88:** 121-128.

Ridout C.L. Price K.R., Dupont M.S., Parker M.L., Fenwick G.R. (1991). Quinoa saponins-analysis and preliminary investigations into the effects of reduction by processing. *Journal of the Science of Food and Agriculture* **54:** 165-176.

Rosenthal G.A., Janzen D.H. (1979). Herbivores. Their interaction with secondary plant metabolites. Academic Press, New York.

Sastry V.R.B., Agrawal D. K. (1992). Utilization of water washed neem seed kernel cake as protein source for pigs. *Journal of Applied Animal Research* **1:** 103-107.

Sen S., Makkar H.P.S., Becker K. (1998) Alfalfa saponins and their implication in animal nutrition. *Journal of Agricultural and Food Chemistry* **46:** 131-140.

Silianikove N., Landau S., Or D., Kababya D., Bruckental I., Nitsan Z. (2006). Analytical approach and effects of condensed tannins in carob pods *(Ceratonia siliqua)* on feed intake, digestive and metabolic responses of kids. *Livestock Science* **99:** 29-38.

Smithard R.R., Eyre M.D. (1986). The effect of dry extrusion of rapeseed with other feedstuffs upon its nutritional value and anti-thyroid activity. *Journal of the Science of Food and Agriculture* **37:** 136-140.

Srivastava J.P., Gupta B.S., Thakur S., Verma A.K. (1990). Utilisation of deoiled karanj (*Pongamia glabra*) cake in kid grower rations. *Indian Journal of Animal Nutrition* **7:** 15-20.

Swensen A.D.Fieger E.A., Upp C.W. (1942) The Nature of egg colour discolouration produced by cottonseed meal. *Poultry Science* **21:** 374-378.

Tangendijaja B., Rahardjo Y.C., Lowry J.B. (1990). Leucaena leaf meal in the diet of growing rabbits: Evaluation and effect of a low mimosine treatment. *Animal Feed Science and Technology* **29:** 63-72.

Tripathi M.K., Mishra A.S. (2007). Glucosinolates in animal nutrition: A Review. *Animal Feed Science and Technology* **132:** 1-27.

Varma A., Singh U.B. (1979). Techniques of removing saponins from Mahua (*Bassia longifolia*) seed cake and its suitability as animal feed. *Cellular and Molecular Life Sciences* **35:** 520-521.

Vig A.P., Walia A. (2001). Beneficial effects of *Rhizopus oligosporus* fermentation on reduction of glucosinolates, fiber and phytic acid in rapeseed (*Brassica napus*) meal. *Bioresource Technology* **78:** 309-312.

Watanapa P., Williamson R.C.N. (1993) Experimental pancreatic hyperplasia and neoplasia: effects of dietary and surgical manipulation-Review, *British Journal of Cancer* **67:** 877-884.

Wina E., Muetzel S., Becker K. (2005). The impact of Saponins or Saponin-containing plant materials on ruminant production – A review. *Journal of Agricultural and Food Chemistry* **53:** 8093-8105.

❏❏❏

Chapter 34

Xenobiotics in Animal Nutrition

K.S. Prasad, S.B.N. Rao, D.T. Pal
National Institute of Animal Nutrition and Physiology, Adugodi, Bangalore-560 030, Karnataka, India

Summary

Xenobiotics are percolating into human food chain through various routes. The demand for animal origin food for human consumption is increasing and the xenobiotic compounds present in animal food products are mainly contaminating through animal feeds. Hence xenobiotics in animal feeds are in much attention and the efforts for minimizing their contamination are required. Recent trends in heavy metals (Lead, Cadmium, Arsenic and Mercury) contamination in soil, water, feeds and animal products and their maximum limits, health hazards are discussed in this chapter. The pesticide residues' persistance in environment, contamination in feeds, carryover to animal products, potential hazards, biodegradations and possible remedies are also covered.

Xenobiotics or xenobiotic compounds are manmade chemicals that are present in the environment and pollute when present in high concentrations. The word 'xeno' means 'foreign'. A compound that is normal to one organism may be xenobiotic to another. Xenobiotics are foreign to animal body, hence, expected to result in biological reactions in animal body for their elimination. Many groups of xenobiotics are present in nature/environment. The synthetic xenobiotic chemicals particularly heavy metals and pesticide residues are more relevant to animal nutrition in the country. These chemicals belong to important groups of substances such as volatile hydrocarbons, dioxins, toxic metals, pesticides, herbicides, insecticides, fungicides, chemical fertilizers, food additives, chlorine and fluoride.

The xenobiotics are increasing in environment due to more industrialization, urbanization and agricultural practices which pose threat to animal health and quality animal products. Many contaminants like pesticide residues, heavy metals *etc.* which are xenobiotic in nature, present in animal feeds are percolating into human food through animal food products. Hence, safe animal feed is important for the health of animals, the environment and for the safety of foods of animal origin. Thus there is a need to address xenobiotics problem in present scenario.

Identifying the areas of concentrations of xenobiotics is important. Latest technique like Geographical Information System (GIS) can be used to identity potentially xenobiotic contaminated areas which combines information from cartography sources (*i.e.,* maps), earthbound surveys, remote sensing (*i.e.,* aerial and satellite imagery) and creates overlapping layers that can be accessed, transformed, and manipulated interactively in one spatial structure. The GIS has also been increasingly used to monitor, analyze and model pesticide migration in the environment. GIS analysis has proved to be a valuable tool in environmental and public health studies yielding important results that may ultimately help preventing excessive or uncontrolled exposure to xenobiotics. Although GIS technology has several advantages is not commonly used in the developing countries for such studies, because of lack of knowledge and accessibility. However some studies reported the use of this technology for monitoring and analyzing pesticide pollution and its impact on public health (Kaminska *et al.,* 2004).

Environmental metabolomics is recent approach for examining metabolic finger prints, or profiles, in biological systems exposed to environmental stress. It has been used to study the biochemical impacts of xenobiotics and disease. The approach analyzes changes in the concentrations of metabolites, which are the precursors and products of enzymatic activity, and then attempts to associate these changes with biological function and/or regulation. Environmental scientists have recently applied such techniques to suggest biomarkers for the risk assessment of chemicals and for diagnosing diseases in wild animals (Lin *et al.*, 2006). Furthermore, this approach can in principle allows scientists to better understand the underlying mechanisms of toxic compound's action in the environment.

1. Impact of heavy metals on environment pollution

Metals such as arsenic, cadmium, lead and mercury are natural occurring chemical compounds present at various levels in the soil, water and atmosphere. Metals can also occur as residues in animal feedstuffs because of their presence in the environment, as a result of human activities such as farming. Livestock can be exposed to these metals from the environment or by ingesting contaminated feed or water. These accumulations in animal body can lead to harmful effects. In India, heavy mortality in cattle and buffaloes was reported due to industrial lead toxicity which leads to significant financial losses to farmers (Swarup and Dwivedi, 2002). Heavy metal contaminations are also reported from water, soil, feed and milk samples in selected sewage areas compared to non-sewage areas (Prasad and Reddy, 2005; Roy *et al.*, 2009).

1.1. Lead

Lead is a soft, dense, and ductile metal. It is a natural environmental contaminant, from anthropogenic activities including mining and smelting, soldering, battery manufacturing, ammunition, metal water pipes, and particularly used in paints and petrol. Livestock exposure to lead can occur via feed, water, soil, dust and air. Lead exists both in organic and inorganic forms. In the environment, inorganic lead predominates over organic lead. Exposure to the latter is generally limited to occupational settings. Organic and inorganic lead differs in terms of both toxicokinetics and toxicodynamics. Organo-lead compounds, such as tri-alkyl-lead and tetraalkyl-lead compounds, are more toxic than inorganic forms of lead (U.S. ATSDR, 2007; UNEP, 2008). To some extent, organic lead compounds are metabolized to inorganic lead both in humans and animals (IARC, 2006).

Table 1 : European Union legislation on permissible limits of lead in products with maximum content of 12% moisture intended for animal feed

Products intended for animal feed	mg/kg (ppm)
Feed materials in general	10
Green fodder (*)	30
Phosphates and calcareous marine algae	15
Calcium carbonate	20
Yeasts	5
Additives belonging to the functional group compounds of trace elements in general	100
Zinc oxide	400
Manganous oxide, iron carbonate, copper carbonate	200
Additives belonging to the functional groups of binders and anti-caking agents in general	30
Elinoptiolite of volcanic origin	60
Premixtures	200
Complementary feeding stuff in general	10
Mineral feeding stuffs	15
Complete feeding stuffs	5

(*) Green fodder includes products intended for animal feed such as hay, silage, fresh grass, etc.

Table 2 : Maximum permissible levels for lead as laid down in Regulation (EC) No 1881/2006

Food of Human	mg/kg wet weight
Raw milk, heat-treated milk and milk for the manufacture of milk based products	0.02
Meat (excluding offal) of cattle, buffalo,sheep, goat, pig and poultry	0.10
Fats and oils, including milk fat	0.10
Food supplements	3.0

Lead can accumulate in the body, primarily in the skeleton. From the skeleton, it is released gradually back into the blood stream, particularly during physiological or pathological periods of bone demineralization such as pregnancy, lactation and osteoporosis, even if lead exposure has already ceased. Lead can be transferred from the mother to the fetus in utero and calf through milk. Lead affects virtually every system in the body, including the blood, the cardiovascular, renal, endocrine, gastrointestinal, immune and reproductive systems. Lead is classified as a class 2A carcinogen by the (IARC, 2006).

1.2 Cadmium

Cadmium is primarily found in association with zinc ores, approximately 3 kg of cadmium being produced for each ton of zinc. As a by-product of zinc processing, cadmium production has closely followed the demand for zinc. Anthropogenic sources of cadmium include industrial emissions, non-ferrous mining and smelting, metal using industry, industrial and agricultural wastes, coal combustion, phosphate fertilizer and urban pollution (incineration of municipal solid waste, road dust, sewage water *etc.*).

Cadmium accumulation has been reported in grasses and food crops, and in earthworms, poultry, cattle, horses, and wildlife (ATSDR, 1999). In general, cadmium accumulates in the leaves of plants therefore, is more of a risk in leafy parts grown in contaminated soil than in seed or root crops (Alloway *et al.*, 1990). He and Singh (1994) reported that, for plants grown in the same soil, accumulation of cadmium decreased in the order: leafy vegetables > root vegetables > grain crops. Some studies have shown that soil pH is the major factor influencing plant uptake of cadmium from soils (Smith, 1994). Soil type also affects uptake of cadmium by plants. For soils with the same total cadmium content, cadmium has been found to be more soluble and more plant-available in sandy soil than in clay soil (He and Singh, 1994). Similarly, cadmium mobility and bioavailability are higher in non-calcareous than calcareous soils (Thornton, 1992).

Table 3 : Maximum permissible levels of cadmium in feedstuffs and products of animal origin [a]

Name of foodstuffs	mg/kg wet weight	Name of foodstuffs	mg/kg wet weight
Cereals, excluding bran, germ, wheat, and rice	0.10	Bran, germ, wheat, and rice	0.20
Soybeans	0.20	Vegetables and fruit, excluding leaf vegetables, fresh herbs, fungi, stem vegetables, root vegetables, and potatoes	0.05
Food supplements consisting exclusively or mainly of dried seaweed or of products derived from seaweed	3.0	Leaf vegetables, fresh herbs, celeriac and the following fungi: *Agaricus bisporus* (common mushroom), *Pleurotus ostreatus* (Oyster mushroom), *Lentinula edodes* (Shiitake mushroom)	0.20
Liver of cattle, buffalo, sheep, goat, pig, poultry and horse	0.50	Meat (excluding offal) of cattle, buffalo, sheep, goat, pig and poultry	0.05

[a] according to EC regulation No 1881/2006 and latest amendment EC regulation No. 629/2008.

1.3 Arsenic

Arsenic is a metalloid that occurs in different inorganic and organic forms, of which the inorganic forms are more toxic as compared to the organic arsenic occurring in food. However, so far most of the occurrence data in food collected is still reported as total arsenic without differentiating the various arsenic species. The need for speciation data is evident because especially in seafood most of the arsenic is present as organic arsenic and thus is in the less toxic form. Consequently, a risk assessment not taking into account the different species but considering the total arsenic as being present exclusively as inorganic arsenic would lead to a considerable overestimation of the health risk related to dietary arsenic exposure.

1.4 Mercury

Mercury exists in the environment as elemental mercury (metallic), inorganic mercury and organic mercury (primarily methylmercury). Elemental and inorganic mercury released into the air from mining, smelting, industrial activities, combustion of fossil fuels, is deposited to soil, water and thereby to sediments where the mercury is transformed into methylmercury which can accumulate and resulting in biomagnifications along the food chain, particularly in the aquatic food chain. Thus highest concentrations can be found in carnivorous fish and marine mammals having long life. The toxicity and toxico-kinetics of mercury in animals and humans depends on its chemical form. Elemental mercury is volatile and mainly absorbed through the respiratory tract, whereas its absorption through the gastrointestinal tract is negligible. Gastrointestinal absorption of inorganic mercury is in the 10-30% range. Following absorption, inorganic mercury distributes mainly to the kidneys and, to a lesser extent, to the liver. The critical effect of inorganic mercury is renal damage. In animals, as in humans, methylmercury and its salts are readily absorbed in the gastrointestinal tract (>80%). Absorbed methylmercury is widely distributed to all tissues, although the largest deposition occurs in the kidney. Excretion of unchanged methylmercury occurs predominantly in the faeces through biliary excretion. The enterohepatic cycle results in a long half-life for this compound compared to inorganic mercury. Methylmercury is able to cross the blood-brain and the placental barriers. As a consequence, the nervous system is the primary site of toxicity in animals and humans. Animal studies confirmed these neuro developmental effects in fetus of dams exposed to methylmercury in the diet. Goats experimentally exposed to mercuric chloride added to drinking water (average 150 mg mercury/head per day /7-7.5 kg bw) developed signs of toxicity after 43 days, such as gastrointestinal disturbances and renal dysfunction (Pathak and Bhowmik, 1998). Palmer *et al.* (1973) produced acute mercury toxicosis in yearling cattle and sheep with an ethyl-mercury fungicide, administered in capsules at 0.48 mg/kg bw (equivalent to 0.15 mg/kg elemental mercury), with deaths recorded between 7 and 27 days.

Table 4 : Maximum permissible limits of arsenic in feedstuffs having maximum moisture content of 12% (EC, 2008)

Products intended for animal feed	mg/kg or ppm
Feed materials in general	2
Meal made from grass, from dried lucerne and from dried clover, and dried sugar beet pulp and dried molasses sugar beet pulp	4
Palm kernel expeller	4
Phosphates and calcareous marine algae	10
Calcium carbonate	15
Magnesium oxide	20
Feeding stuffs obtained from the processing of fish or other marine animals	15
Sea weed meal and feed materials derived from sea weed	40
Complete feeding stuffs in general	2
Complete feeding stuffs for fish and fur animals	6
Complementary feeding stuffs in general	4
Mineral feeding stuffs	12

2. Pesticide residues

There is a growing concern over the pesticide residues entering through various routes to the livestock and thus animal products to human being. India is one of the largest manufacturer of pesticides and the second-largest producer of agrochemicals in Asia (Abhilash and Singh, 2009). It manufactures 44 types of pesticides among which DDT (dichloro-diphenyl-trichloroethylene), BHC (benzene hexa chloride), malathion, monocrotophos, chlorpyrifos, deltamethrin, cypermethrin carbofuran and endosulfan are commonly used. Though DDT and BHC are banned but still find their presence in food chain. Organo-chlorine pesticides group are highly lipophilic in nature and therefore are rapidly absorbed, stored in fatty (adipose) tissues and are not readily excreted by animals except in lipidic excreta such as milk. First calvers release a lot of lipid deposits in the milk. The pesticides not only reach milk but also deposited in tissue and hair. This renders organochlorine pesticides highly persistent and bioaccumulative. In general, the organophosphate and carbamate pesticides are more toxic to warm-blooded animals and active for shorter periods than the chlorinated hydrocarbons. Repetitive use of toxic compounds increases the incidence of pesticide poisonings among domestic animals. Carcinogenesis, poisoning, epilepsy, infertility and birth defects are some of the adverse effects of pesticide poisoning. Under *in vitro* conditions pesticides like endosulphan and chloropyriphos exhibited adverse affects on *in vitro* dry matter digestibility and reduced volatile fatty acid production (Rao *et al.,* 2010).

2.1 Reasons for more persistence of pesticides in the environment

- Presence of halogens in the place of hydrogen in the molecule; the carbon-halogen bond is highly stable and its cleavage requires considerable energy.
- Substitution of -H by other groups like nitro-, sulphonate, methoxy-, amino and carbamyl groups.
- Cyclic structures, aromatic compounds, cycloalkanes and heterocyclic compounds are more recalcitrant than linear chain or aliphatic compounds.
- Branched linear chains resist biodegradation *etc.* In general, the more complex is the structure of a xenobiotic compound, the more resistant it is to biodegradation. Many other xenobiotics resist biodegradation due to their large molecular size and insolubility in water.

2.2 Sources of contamination

The major sources of contamination of pesticides for animals are from animal feeds, fodder (Prasad and Chhabra, 2001), utensils and equipments.

Some of the pesticides used to control the ectoparasites through sprays also contribute to the intake of pesticides by the animals. Pesticides application to crops are retained in feed/fodder, when consumed by animals gets absorbed, stored in body and secreted in milk to variable extent depending upon the level of contamination, stage of lactation and parity of cow. In addition, milk/ milk products may pose danger of causing residue problem to infants. Some residues can even get recycled to crops through carcass/manure/urine (Rudra Swamy *et al.*, 2007). Hence, thorough long term monitoring of residues in the food chain will provide suitable answers to the pesticide residue problem.

2.3 Carryover of pesticides in milk

Milk contains the fat as droplets suspended in water, an emulsion separated from the blood plasma by a semi permeable membrane. Chemicals can be excreted into milk by binding to milk protein or adhering to the surface of milk fat globules, or they can be totally contained within the fat globules (Prasad and Chhabra, 2006). Together with the large amount of major and trace nutrients, a small and widely varying amount of undesired substances are also eaten by the dairy cow and partially excreted in the milk. This mechanism, called carry-over, depends on the chemical nature of the compound(s) in question and principally their ability to pass the blood-milk barrier. Molecular size, binding affinity, electrical charge and the concentration gradient between both sides of the membrane are some of the factors control the process. As the excretion competes with the metabolism, a considerable resistance to biological degradation is a further determining factor for the carry-over rate into the milk. Determination of the carry-over rate helps to identify foreign substances, which may accumulate above a certain threshold 'maximum residue limits (MRL)' in milk, when the substances are either naturally or artificially present in the feed of the dairy animal. This can lead to restrictions or abandoning of specific feeding regimes such as the exclusion of polluted areas from feed production or grazing.

3. Potential health hazards of Xenobiotics

The severity of health impact of pollution depends on kind of pollution and pollutants, presence of interacting chemicals, extent and route of exposure, and species, age, physiology and nutrition of the exposed population. Undernourished, young, old, physiologically stressed and debilitated animals are more susceptible to pollution effects. Various industrial, transport and other polluting sources release host of specific and common pollutants such as oxides of sulfur, nitrogen and carbon, halogen gases, toxic heavy metals, volatile hydrocarbons, oxidants and ozone, to name a few. Many of these pollutants persist in the environment and can build up to high levels, even if released in small quantities. Many others undergo transformation and are converted into more dangerous forms than parent compounds. For example, inorganic mercury is converted into more toxic methyl-mercury by certain bacteria in aquatic sediment. Exposure to higher concentration of toxic chemicals induces specific acute toxicities, where as long term low level exposure causes chronic toxicity.

Many xenobiotics persist in the environment and increase in concentration with time. They tend to accumulate in biological systems often by a factor of 104-106. A typical example is DDT, where it is taken up continuously by plankton from water. In a sequential manner in a food chain (plankton → small fish → large fish → sea eagles), the concentration of DDT builds up. It was found that 105 fold increases occurs in sea eagles as compared to concentration present in the aqueous environment (Tanabe *et al.*, 1994).

At low concentrations, they can cause various skin problems. They tend to accumulate in the environment and lead to bioaccumulation and biomagnification. Carbon halogenated compounds have proven to be carcinogenic in nature. One of the adverse effects of xenobiotics is endocrine disruption. Endocrine disruption from environmental contaminants has been linked to a broad spectrum of adverse outcomes. One concern about endocrine-disrupting xenobiotics is the potential for additive or synergistic (*i.e.*, greater-than-additive) effects of mixtures. Prototypic thyroid-disrupting chemicals (TDCs) such as dioxins, polychlorinated biphenyls (PCBs), and polybrominated diphenyl ethers have been shown to alter thyroid hormone homeostasis primarily by up-regulating hepatic catabolism of thyroid hormones. Dose-dependent additivity and synergism existed in TDCs that may act via different mechanisms in a complex mixture (Crofton *et al.*, 2005). It has been found that feeding xenobiotics to laboratory rats caused elevation in serum cholesterol levels and high levels of high density lipoproteins (HDL) and apolipoprotein A-I (apo A-I) and very low density lipoproteins (VLDL) rich in cholesterol and apo E (Oda *et al.*, 1994). When a foreign organism or the macromolecule enters the body, immune system may produce antibodies that interact with and destroy it. However, some xenobiotics do not trigger an antibody response. In that case, the body's numerous enzymes metabolize such foreign molecules and toxins to less reactive water-soluble metabolites that can be readily excreted (Pandit, 2007).

4. Biodegradation of xenobiotics

The compounds that resist biodegradation and thereby persist in the environment are called recalcitrant. The xenobiotic compounds may be recalcitrant due to one or more of the following reasons: They are not recognized as substrate by the existing degradative enzymes, they are highly stable, *i.e.*, chemically and biologically inert due to the presence of substitution groups like halogens, nitro-, sulphonate, amino-, methoxy- and carbamyl groups, they are insoluble in water, or are adsorbed to external matrices like soil, activated charcoal, they are highly toxic or give rise to toxic products due to microbial activity, their large molecular size prevents entry into microbial cells, inability of the compounds to induce the synthesis of degrading enzymes, and lack of the permease needed for their transport into the microbial cells.

Since xenobiotics consist of a wide variety of compounds, their degradation occurs via a large number of metabolic pathways. But these enzymes are not very specific and each enzyme oxidizes a limited range of compounds. Thus xenobiotics are degraded by a wide variety of microorganisms, each of which degrades a small range of compounds.

4.1 Microbial Bioremediation

Microorganism has the capability of degrading all naturally occurring compounds; this is known as the principle of microbial infallibility. These are also able to degrade many of the xenobiotics compounds, but they are unable to degrade many others. Bioremediation of organic contaminants is primarily based on either microorganisms naturally present at the sites, or on microbial inoculants developed in the laboratory and introduced at the site. Certain bacterial, fungal and algal species are capable of accumulating some toxic inorganic contaminants as well. However, there is no cost-effective method of removing these microorganisms from the soil after they have sequestered the inorganic ions. Therefore, bioremediation of inorganic contaminants is primarily based on suitable plant species.

The fungi were isolated from soil, which is contaminated with industrial residues containing a mixture of organochlorine compounds, mainly hexachlorobenzene in the Baixada Santista region. The fungi were grown in liquid malt extract medium with 0.02% of dye and shaken at 200 rpm for 14 days at 28 ± 2°C. Two types of behavior regarding the dye were observed: adsorption and degradation. *Eupenicillium baarnense* SSP1951 and SSP1952 and *Eupenicillium crustaceum* SSP1953 presented high RBBR decolorization and were then analyzed regarding their ability to degrade 14C-hexachlobenzene (4138.31 mg HCB per kg soil) during a 56 days culture at 28 ± 2°C. *Eupenicillium crustaceum* SSP1953 was able to reduce n-hexane soluble 14C-compounds (24.6%) and to form non-extractable 14C-residues (20.5%). The same behavior was also observed in the two *E. baarnense* strains (SSP1951 and SSP1952) but the percentages were lower than those obtained for *Eupenicillium crustaceum*. The main action of *Eupenicillium* spp on HCB is to transform it into non-extractable 14C-residues as confirmed by the gas chromatography results (Vitali *et al.,* 2006).

4.2 Phytoremediation

Phytoremediation is the use of green plants and their associated microorganisms, soil amendments, and agronomic practices to remove, contain or render harmless environmental contaminants. The first plant-based remediation system was installed over 300 years ago in Germany for the treatment of municipal sewage; since then this use of plants has become rather common.

But plants are also used to decontaminate soils polluted by organic wastes. For example, carrots are used to absorb DDT, these carrots are harvested, air-dried and incinerated to destroy the DDT. Plant roots absorb organics in nearly direct proportion to their relative lipophilicity.

Remediation may occur due to accumulation of organics in plant tissues, translocation of the organics to leaf and volatilization from the leaf surface or the organics may be metabolized in plant tissues or in the rhizosphere itself (by enzymes secreted by the plants). In addition active microbial communities associated with plants may degrade the organic contaminants. Phytoremediation has been obtained for certain pesticides, trichloroethylene and petroleum hydrocarbons, but the overall rate and quantity of degradation is relatively slow. Inherent technical limitations of phytoremediation are (1) the contaminant must be present within the root zones of actively growing plants, (2) the site must be sufficiently large for easy plant cultivation, and (3) it takes much longer than do 'dig and dump' techniques. The approach is being refined and it is hoped that genetic engineering would greatly facilitate large-scale practical application of the technology. In India, Tata Energy Research Institute, New Delhi is using phytoremediation to tackle environmental problems caused by flyash. Flyash is produced in large quantities by thermal power stations and other industries driven by coal energy.

Table 5 : Accumulation of metals by some plants (Alkorta, *et al.*, 2004)

Plant	Metal	Concentration (mg/kg shoot weight)
Thlaspi caerulenscens	Cd	1,800
Ipomoea alpina	Cu	12,300
Haumanisatrum robertii	Co	10,200
T. rotundifolium	Pb	8,200
Macadamia neurophylla	Mn	51,000
Psychotria douarrei	Ni	47,500
Sebertia acuminata	Ni	25% by weight of dried sap
T. caerulenscens	Zn	51,600

5. Possible remedial measures for xenobiotics

Current crop protection, against pests, weeds and diseases is based on the use of chemical pesticides. However, it is essential to develop pest resistant crop varities using latest biotechnology tools. The scale of pesticide use inevitably results in the occurrence of residues in food products. In case of residue problem, prevention is always better than cure. Use of bio-pesticides brings down the chemicals load in nature. Amelioration of pesticide residues in the food chain could be undertaken at various levels like, proper treatment to the soil, drinking water, feed and fodder of the animal, animal itself (Prasad and Chhabra, 2004), milk and milk products, human carefulness *etc.* Treatment of sewage water, industrial effluents, lead free fuels, judicial use of mining, use of chemical fertilizers and good manufacturing practices etc. can help in controlling heavy metals contamination in food chain. Some supplementations like vitamin E has a protective effect in arsenic contaminated diet fed to goats and zinc supplementation in the diet of Pb exposed kids had beneficial effect on oxidative stress and immunoglobulins (Ig) concentration (Kumar *et al.,* 2010).

Conclusions

Xenobiotics are more problematic for future human food chain as an outcome of increasing human activities in nature. The reason being we need more food to meet the ever growing human population which in turn requires more and more use of pesticides and insecticide for crop protection. It affects both human and animal health and the residues are available in human food. Therefore a proper monitoring and strict regulatory systems should be developed to control the availability of xenobiotics in food chain so that remedial measures can be taken to get a safe food for human consumption.

References

Abhilash P.C., Singh N. (2009). Pesticide use and application: An Indian Scenario. *Journal of Hazardous Materials* **165:** 1-12.

Alkorta J., Hernández-Allica J.M., Amezaga B.I., Albizu I., Garbisu C. (2004). Recent findings on the phytoremediation of soils contaminated with environmentally toxic heavy metals and metalloids such as Zinc, Cadmium, Lead, and Arsenic. *Reviews in Environmental Science and Biotechnology* **3:** 71-90.

Alloway B.J., Jackson A.P., Morgan H. (1990). The accumulation of cadmium by vegetables grown on soils contaminated from a variety of sources. *Science of the Total Environment* **91:** 223-236.

ATSDR (Agency for Toxic Substances and Disease Registry), (1999). Toxicological profile for Cadmium (Final Report). NTIS Acc. No. PB99-166621, p 434.

Council Regulation (EC) No. 440/2008 of 30 May 2008 Laying down test methods pursuant to Regulation (EC) No. 1907/2006 of the European parliament and of the

Council on the Registration, Evaluation, Authorization and Restriction of Chemicals (REACH).

Crofton K.M., Craft E.S., Hedge J.M., Gennings C., Simmons J.E., Carchman R.A., Carter Jr. H., DeVito M.J. (2005). Thyroid hormone–disrupting chemicals: Evidence for dose-dependent additivity or synergism. *Environmental Health Perspectives* **113:** 1549-1554.

European Commission on Arsenic as undesirable substance in feed (2008). Opinion of the Scientific Panel on Contaminants in the Food chain. *The European Food Safety Authority Journal* **654:** 1-76.

He Q.B., Singh B.R. (1994). Effect of organic matter on the distribution, extractability and uptake of cadmium in soils. *European Journal of Soil Science* **44:** 641-650.

IARC (2006) Monographs on the evaluation of the carcinogenic risk of chemicals to humans. Inorganic and organic lead compounds. *International Agency for Research on Cancer, Lyon, France,* **87:** 249-305.

Iovdijová A., Bencko V. (2010). Potential risk of exposure to selected xenobiotic residues and their fate in the food chain – Part I: Classification of Xenobiotics. *Annals of Agriculture and Environmental Medicine* **17:** 183-192.

Kaminska I.A., Anna oldak, Turski W.A. (2004). Geographical information system (GIS) as a tool for monitoring Aand analysing pesticide pollution and its impact on public health. *Annals of Agriculture and Environmental Medicine* **11:** 181-184.

Kumar M., Kaur H., Phondba B.T., Bhupender T., Mani V., Kewalramani N. (2010). Effect of Zinc supplementation to Lead exposed goat kids on immunity and blood antioxidant status. *Indian Journal of Animal Nutrition* **26:** 355-359.

Lin C.Y., Viant M.R., Tjeerdema RS. (2006). Metabolomics: Methodologies and applications in the environmental sciences. *Journal of Pesticide Science:* **31:** 245-251.

Oda H., Matsushita N., Hirabayashi A., Yoshida A. (1994). Cholesterol-rich very low density lipoprotiens and fatty liver in rats fed polychlorinated biphenyls. *Biosciences, Biotechnology & Biochemistry* **58:** 2152-2158.

Palmer J.S., Wright F.C., Haufler M. (1973).Toxicological and residual aspect of an alkyl mercury fungicide to cattle, sheep and turkeys. *Clinical Toxicology* **6:** 245-437.

Pandit N.K. (2007). Introduction to the pharmaceutical sciences. Lippincott Williams & Wilkins, Philadelphia.

Patel A.K., Kewalramani N., Mani V., Kaur H. (2009). Effect of Vitamin E supplementation in growing kids fed on arsenic containing diet. *Indian Journal of Animal Nutrition* **26:** 9-16.

Pathak S.K., Bhowmik M.K. (1998). The chronic toxicity of inorganic mercury in goats: clinical signs, toxicopathological changes and residual concentrations. *Veterinary Research and Communication* **22:** 131-138.

Prasad K.S.N., Chhbra A. (2001). Organo pesticide residues in animal feeds and fodders. *Indian Journal of Animal Science* **71:** 1178-1180.

Prasad K.S.N., Chhbra A. (2004). Effect of charcoal supplementation on organo-chlorine pesticide residues concentration in rumen liquor and excretion in crossbred cattle. *Indian Journal of Dairy and Bio Science* **15:** 9-13.

Prasad K.S.N., Chhbra A. (2006). Effect of supplementing charcoal on the Organochlorine pesticide residues in milk. *Indian Journal of Animal Nutrition.* **23:** 53-55.

Prasad K.S.N., Obi Reddy A., Garg M.R. (2006). Heavy metals in soil, feeds, fodders and milk in sewage and non sewage areas. In: *Proc.VI Biennial conference of Animal Nutrition Association held at Sher-e-Kashmir University of Agricultural Science and Technology, Jammu 15-17, Sept.*

Rao, S.B.N., Anandan, S., Giridhar, K and Sampath, K.T. (2010). Effect of pesticides on in vitro dry matter digestibility and rumen fermentation. *Indian Journal of Animal Nutrition* **27:** 217-219.

Roy D.,Bharathidasan S., Mani V., Kaur H., Kewalramani N. (2009). Heavy metals contents in cow and buffaloes milk samples from Haryana. *Indian Journal of Animal Nutrition* **26:** 29-33.

Rudraswamy M.S., Rao, S.B.N., Roy K.S. (2007). An Overview of Factors affecting pesticide contamination of milk and possible measures for their amelioration. *Indian Journal of Dairy and Biosciences* **18:** 67-70.

Smith S.R. (1994). Effect of soil pH on availability to crops of metals in sewage sludge-treated soils. II. Cadmium uptake by crops and implications for human dietary intake. *Environmental Pollutants* **86:** 5-13.

Swarup D., Dwivedi S.K. (2002). Environmental pollution and effects of lead and fluoride on animal health. Indian Council of Agricultural Research, New Delhi.

Tanabe S., Sung J.K., Choi D.Y., Baba N., Kiyota M., Yoshida K., Tatsukawa R. (1994) Persistent organochlorine residues in northern fur seal from the Pacific coast of Japan since 1971. *Environmental Pollution* **85:** 305-314.

Thornton I. (1992). Sources and pathways of cadmium in the environment. *International Agency for Research on Cancer Scientific Publication* **118:** 149-162.

United Nations Environment programme (UNEP, 2008) Geneva US Agency for toxic substances and disease registry (USATSDR, 2007).

Vitali V.M.V., Machado K.M.G., Andrea M.M. and Bononi V.L.R. (2006). Screening mitosporic fungi for organochlorides degradation. *Brazilian Journal of Microbiology.* **37:** 256-261.

❏❏❏

Chapter 35

Feed Quality, Safety and Regulation

S.B.N. Rao, K.S. Prasad, S. Jash
National Institute of Animal Nutrition and Physiology, Adugodi, Bangalore-560 030, Karnataka, India

Summary

Quality assurance for animal feeds is one of the biggest challenges which compromise the quality and safety of animal products. Adulteration of animal feeds is quite rampant in retail chains which need to be tackled by a suitable regulation. In this chapter, newer adulterants like melamine and cyanuric acid and molecular methods for detection of plant proteins commonly used as feedstuffs, status of feed quality assurance and safety aspects are discussed. Regulatory aspects on quality control of feedstuffs are also presented.

Feed quality and safety are interrelated which determine quality of animal products for safe human consumption. In the absence of suitable regulation, feed quality is at times very difficult to maintain at retail chains. However, in the organized feed industry, feed quality can be very well controlled by qualified animal nutritionists. In the era of modern agriculture, many synthetic chemicals are added to crops which leaves residues on by-products (Prasad and Chhbra, 2001; Rao *et al.*, 2011). These in turn can be excreted in to milk (Waliszewskia *et al.*, 1996; Banerjee *et al.*, 1997) causing public health problems. Adulteration is of feedstuffs also quite rampant in retails chains and mostly in unorganized sector. Newer adulterants like melamine and cyanuric acid are increasingly threatening the safety of animal products (Suchy *et al.*, 2009). A suitable regulation need to be formulated and enforced upon to maintain the quality and safety of animal feeds which in turn can result in to safe animal products. There is an urgent need to develop 'hazardanalysis and critical control points (HACCP)' concept in feed chains for the benefit of all stakeholders (Hartong, 2003).

1. Adulteration of feedstuffs

Adulteration is defined as admixture of pure substance with some cheaper and low quality substance. Costly feed ingredients like oil cakes and fishmeal are sometimes sprayed with urea to increase their protein content. Inedible protein meal or husks are mixed with oilcakes as a spurious practice. Adulteration of feedstuffs is deliberate with malicious intention of making money. Singh and Kundu (2003) collected supplies of concentrate feed ingredients from four different sources and compared with available Bureau of Indian Standard (BIS) specifications. They found that most of the feed ingredients fulfill the BIS requirements however, there are widespread adulteration in cattle feeds available in the market in which rice husk is the major adulterant. Analysis of cattle feed samples revealed that 52% samples only met the prescribed standards for calcium and urea. Rest of the samples had higher levels of calcium and urea indicating that lime stone powder and urea were being added deliberately (Punjab Dairy Development Board, Down to Earth). Nalwanga *et al.* (2009) observed serious adulteration in feed ingredients used in the fish feed such as fish meal, cottonseed cake, sunflower seed cake and maize bran which occurred along the supply chain *i.e.,* primary outlet, store or shop level in Lake Victoria region of Uganda and Kenya. The main adulterant used in the feeds is probably sand. The deterioration of the nutritional value of feed ingredients coincides with the composition of the commercial fish feeds being substantially below the values labeled; this also affects the relative costs per unit of nutrient. It is therefore suggested that a set of measures should be developed to assure feed quality. For assuring the quality of feeds, series of strategic measures need to be followed. These include, strategic sampling and regular feed analysis of purchased feed samples or feed ingredients from different locations need to be undertaken. Apart from this, retail feed ingredient dealers need to be monitored so that quality can be maintained.

Common adulterants of different feed ingredients

Feed Ingredient	Adulterant
Groundnut cake	Groundnut husk, urea
Mustard cake	*Argemona maxicana* seeds, fibrous feed ingredients, urea
Soybean meal	Urea, raw soybean
De-oiled rice bran, wheat bran	Ground rice husk, saw dust
Fish meal	Common salt, urea, sand
Mineral mixture	Common salt, marble powder, sand and limestone
Molasses	Water
Maize grain	Maize cobs
Rice Kani	Marble and grit

1.1 Melamine and cyanuric acid contamination in feeds

Recently, two important compounds like melamine and cyanuric acid have been abused during food and feed adulteration by increasing the content of nitrogen compounds in these products. Melamine (2,4,6-triamino-1,3,5-triazine) is a heterocyclic compound containing 6 nitrogen atoms and have a very high nitrogen content (66% N) and is being used as a raw material in manufacture of plastics, pesticides, cleaning agents, fertilizers and many other products, *e.g.*, melamine resin. A hydrolysis product of melamine is cyanuric acid {1,3,5-triazine-2,4,6-triol $(CNOH)_3$} – is a cyclic trimer of hydrocyanic acid (HOCN). It is a white crystalline substance produced by thermal decomposition of urea under defined conditions. It can also be obtained by hydrolysis of melamine. It is a component in various disinfectants, herbicides and bleaching agents. Melamine and cyanuric acid as individual substances do not cause any toxicity but the complex melamine-cyanurate complex, is the cause of human and animal health problems. Feeds with a high nitrogen content and low level of amino acids are to be suspected of adulteration with melamine. Protein concentrates from unknown origin are to be suspected of contamination with melamine. Modern analytical methods are to be used for detection these compounds. Samples are extracted with acetonitrile-water and purified through solid-phase-extraction (SPE) cartridge and subsequent evaporation and injecting in to liquid chromatograph coupled with mass detector (LC-MS/MS) (Vail *et al.*, 2007, Yamamoto *et al.*, 2008). A study conducted by Battaglia *et al.* (2010) revealed that more than 60% of melamine was transferred to milk within 30 h of melamine ingestion. However, melamine was not detected in milk after 7 days of treatment. However, cyanuric acid was not detected in any of the samples indicating no biological conversion of melamine in the cow. Melamine administration did not affect BUN and milk melamine was transferred mainly to the whey fraction during cheese preparation.

1.2 Urea contamination of feedstuffs

Urea is added in concentrate mixtures as a source of non-protein nitrogen for ruminant diets. Urea can be a cheap source of nitrogen but has to be added carefully by following certain nutritional procedures. Addition of urea leads to 2.87 times increase in crude protein percent of concentrate mixture (1 kg of urea yields a protein equivalent of 2.875 kg nitrogen). This is the main reason for urea adulteration in concentrate mixtures by local infamous feed manufacturers. As per BIS specification only 1% urea can be added in concentrate mixtures. Urea particles under light microscope looks like needle shaped particles which can crumble under pressure. When urea is mixed in cattle feeds it may be difficult to detect it by microscopic means as gets dissolved hence, chemical means is only the solution. The Indian standard specifies a spectrometric method for the determination of the urea content of animal feeding stuffs (IS 13399:1992).

1.3 Silica contamination of feedstuffs

Silica contamination of feedstuffs is deliberate especially in retail chains. It can be either mixed in dal chunis and brans basically to increase the weight. Fine clay (*Multani mitti)* can be added while expeller processing of oil seeds. The resultant cake contains more silica when analyzed and protein content is lower. To compensate the lower protein, urea can be even sprayed leading to multiple adulteration. Acid insoluble ash content of feedstuffs can give an indication of silica contamination in feedstuffs. No systematic reports are available on silica/sand contamination in animal feeds available in the literature.

2. Quality control and safety of feedstuffs

The objective of quality control of feeds is to ensure that consumer should obtain feeds that are unadulterated and true to their nature and produce desired results. Quality control is therefore, defined as maintenance of quality at levels and tolerances applicable to buyer while minimizing the cost of processing. In India the quality control is regulated by a statuary body Bureau of Indian Standards (BIS). It was established under BIS Act, 1986. Earlier, Indian Standard Institute (ISI) was regulating the quality control of various commodities. A sub-committee on animal feeds called 'animal feeds sectional committee' has been specifically set up to check the quality of animal feeds and feed ingredients. The members of sub-committee are taken among eminent nutritionists from Indian Council of Agricultural Research (ICAR) institutes, state agricultural universities, feed industry, Government departments having specialization in animal nutrition and feed technologist concerned with animal husbandry activities. In our country, feedstuffs used for livestock feeding are mostly homegrown especially straws and fodders. Farmers sometimes feed their livestock with individual ingredients like oil cakes (groundnut cake, GNC/ Til cake/Mustard cake), grains (maize, jowar or ragi *etc.,*) or bran like (wheat bran, rice bran). On the other hand, compound feeds produced in India contain bran, oilcakes (mostly solvent extracted) and limited amount of grains. The BIS has suggested specifications for different feedstuffs to be used in cattle feed as well as compound cattle feeds (Table 1).

The BIS also provides guidance for maximum residue limits with regard to pesticide residues that are commonly encountered in feedstuffs (Table 2).

Table 1 : Bureau of Indian Standards (BIS) specifications for few Indian feedstuffs

Name of feedstuffs	BIS specifications						Reference
	Moisture (%Max)	Crude protein (%Min)	Crude fibre (%Max)	Crude fat (%Min)	Ash (%Max)	AIA (% Max	
Decorticated groundnut oil cake - grade-1	8.0	48.0	8.0	7.0	-	2.0	IS: 1713-1986 Reaffirmed 1992
Decorticated groundnut oil cake - grade-2	8.0	43.0	12.0	6.0	-	2.5	
Solvent extracted groundnut oil cake - grade-1	8.0	51.0	7.0	-	-	2.5	IS: 3441-1982 Reaffirmed 1995
Solvent extracted groundnut oil cake - grade-2	8.0	47.0	10.0	-	-	2.5	
Solvent extracted coconut oil cake	10.0	23.0	14.0	-	-	1.5	IS: 3591-1985
Decorticated sunflower oilcake	8.0	45.0	6.0	12.0	6.0	1.0	IS: 10165-1982
Solvent extracted cottonseed oil cake	10.0	42.0	16.0	-	-	2.0	IS: 3592-1985
Guar meal	10.0	45.0	8.0	3.0	7.0	1.0	IS: 4193-1986
Rubber seed cake	7.0	30.0	7.0	5.0	7.0	1.0	IS: 9599-1980
Mango seed kernel	10.0	5.0	3.0	12.0	-	1.0	IS: 10671-1983
Mango seed kernel (solvent extracted)	8.5	6.0	1.75	-	5.0	1.0	IS: 12829-1989

contd...

table contd...

Name of feedstuffs	BIS specifications						
	Moisture (%Max)	Crude protein (%Min)	Crude fibre (%Max)	Crude fat (%Min)	Ash (%Max)	AIA (% Max	Reference
Maize gluten feed - grade I	10.0	45.0	3.0	4.0	-	0.5	IS: 2152-1972
Maize gluten feed - grade II	10.0	23.0	8.0	3.0	-	0.5	(Reaffirmed 1980)
Maize germ oil cake	8.0	18.0	10.0	8.0	3.0	0.5	IS: 2151-1985
Decorticated safflower (Kardi) oil cake	10.0	48.0	9.0	7.0	-	1.5	IS: 2503-1986
Decorticated cottonseed oilcake - grade-I	8.0	40.0	12.0	7.0	-	2.0	IS: 1712-1982
Un-decorticated cottonseed oil cake - grade-I	8.0	24.0	22.0	7.0	-	2.0	
Sesame oil cake-expeller hydraulic (high fat)	8.0	40.0	7.0	8.0	13.0	1.5	IS: 1934-1982
Maize bran - coarse	10.0	7.5	18.0	-	1.5	0.5	IS: 2153-1985
Maize bran - fine	10.0	14.0	9.5	-	1.5	0.5	
Solvent extracted rice bran - grade I	10.0	14.0	12.0	-	-	6.0	IS: 3593-1979
Gram chuni	10.0	18.0	3.5	-	4.5	0.80	IS: 3161-1965 Reaffirmed 1980

contd...

table contd...

Name of feedstuffs	BIS specifications						Reference
	Moisture (%Max)	Crude protein (%Min)	Crude fibre (%Max)	Crude fat (%Min)	Ash (%Max)	AIA (% Max	
Gram husk	10.0	3.0	50.0	-	6.0	1.0	IS: 3162-1965 Reaffirmed 1995
Rice bran - grade I	10.0	13.0	10.0	15.0	-	5.0	IS: 3648-1975 Reaffirmed 1995
Rice polish	10.0	11.0	4.0	15.0	10.0	1.5	IS: 3163-1965
Fish meal - grade-I	10.0	60.0	Chlorine as Nacl-4.0	12.0 (max)	-	3.0	IS: 4307-1983 Reaffirmed 1995
Compounded cattle feed for cattle - type I*	11.0	22.0	7.0	3.0	Urea 1% (max)	3.0	IS: 2052-1979 Reaffirmed 1995
Compounded cattle feed for cattle - type II*	11.0	20.0	12.0	2.5	Urea 1% (max)	4.0	

*Salt = 2.0 % maximum; Calcium and available Phosphorus (% max) 0.5 each; vitamin A: 5000 IU/kg

Table 2 : Suggested BIS specifications for pesticide residues in animal feedstuffs.

Residues	Max limit
Gamma BHC	20 ppb
DDT	5 ppb
Endosulfan	10 ppb
Aldrin	1 ppb

2.1 Feed quality assurance

Chemical analysis is the starting point for determining the nutritive value of feed. The methods of chemical analysis that have been described have a history of more than 100 years. Many techniques used have started in a place called in Weende, a village near the University of Goettingen in Germany. Hence, these methods are described as Weende system of analysis. The principle of analysis is to separate the feed components into groups or fractions in accordance with their feeding value. The various fractions are dry matter, total protein, ether extract or fat, crude fiber, ash and nitrogen free extract. The proximate analysis suffers from limitations as some components are in excess or missing. The basis of the scheme is that the feedstuffs contain organic and inorganic constituents. The former comprises of carbohydrates, crude fiber and nitrogen free extract, fats and oils, proteins and other nitrogenous compounds along with numerous organic compounds. The inorganic matter comprises ash composed of various minerals but the proximate analysis gives no indication about the kinds of minerals present. For example, rice straw contains 16% ash, but 85% of ash is silica which is of no value to the animal. The proximate analysis does not include many chemical factors that are important in feeding today. The ash gives no indication of the chemical elements or deficiency or excess of particular essential mineral element. The method also does not include vitamins. To overcome the limitations of proximate analysis, Dr. P.J. VanSoest in 1965 developed a method which makes the use of the concept the dry matter of plant origin consists of two principal parts: cell wall and cell contents. Total cell wall constituents composed of cellulose, hemi-cellulose, lignin and silica. The nutrient availability of this fraction depends upon the degree of lignifications of the cell walls. Cell contents represent lipids, soluble carbohydrates, most of the proteins and other water soluble substances. The procedure developed by VanSoest seems to be more meaningful and represents the advance over the older concept. The cell walls of feeds of plant origin are not uniformly nutritious, in the sense that their principal components consist of cellulose, hemicelluloses, silica and lignin *etc.*, singly or in such combinations as nitrogen-hemicellulose or lignocelluloses and differ widely in nutritional availability depending upon the kind and maturity of the plant as well as on the age and species of the animal feed (Goering and VanSoest, 1970 and VanSoest, *et al.*, 1991).

2.2 Microscopic evaluation of feedstuffs and adulterants

Feed microscopy is commonly used for confirming the adulteration and identifying the adulterants (AOAC, 2005). Feed ingredients, adulterants and contaminants must be studied under low and high magnification for distinguishing features whether coarsely or finely ground. At physical characteristics such as shape, color, and particle size, softness, hardness, and texture of the feeds are examined at low magnification. It is useful method to identify impurities/contaminants and evaluating the quality of feed ingredients. It also serves as a useful method for identifying missing ingredients in finished feed. The plant cells and structural features of the feeds will be observed at high magnification since these characters are retained after grinding or even after powdering the feed ingredients. Pretreatment of feed is sometimes required for clear histological identification. By this method, it will be possible to identify various concentrate feed materials and their possible adulteration with potential contaminants.

First hand information on the subject was collected by corresponding with feed companies. It was observed that compound cattle feed manufactured used ingredients such as maize, broken rice, rice polish, sunflower extract, soybean extract, fish meal, rapeseed extract, groundnut extract, cottonseed cake and coarse bran is powdered and mixed in feeds as a means of adulteration. In the expeller mills, common salt is being added to sunflower seeds for better facilitation of oil. In that process, salt level in cake will increase which can create problems like diarrhea especially in monogastric animals. Another adulterant commonly used in black gram bran and tapioca tippi is calcite (calcium carbonate). There is also problem of sand and silica adulteration in oilcake meals which need to be checked. Different grades of de-oiled rice bran are being mixed which increases the sand and silica content of feeds. During the process of thrashing and winnowing of wheat grain for separating it from straw and husk cleanings would be generated. This cleanings can be a source of adulteration of wheat bran.

Outer coatings of horse gram (*Macrotyloma uniflorum*) particles are red colored and have very rough surface. Broken rice (*Arachis hypogea)* particles look typically white stones under microscopes with occasional brownish bran like material. Pea *(Pisum sativum)* husk particles look somewhat smooth and having ridges. On the other hand, gram (*Cicer arietinum*) particles look somewhat similar to horsegram but having colored smooth surface (Author's unpublished data).

Expeller Indian mustard (*Brassica nigra*) cake particles are looking typically reflecting yellow coloured oil globules which are not appreciated when the same has been extracted with chloroform. Under low magnification, examined feed particles such as gram husk, Jowar (*Sorghum vulgare*) grain, cotton

(*Gossypium sp.,)* seed cake and groundnut cake are not so distinct and looks very fine. Wheat and rice bran particles under magnification look somewhat different. Fine wheat bran particles look like amoeba like structures (Fig. 1a) and can easily be distinguished from rice bran with fine longitudinal striations (Fig. 1b). Very fine particles of rice bran look like filaments under magnification. Similarly, wheat bran has irregular corrugated surface compared to rice bran which has straight edges (Author's unpublished observation).

Few potential adulterants like saw dust, paddy husk and urea and salt have been examined under microscope. Saw dust has typical serrated edges which can be easily identified under magnification (Fig. 1c). Paddy husk is also typical have straight edges as similar to rice bran (Fig. 1d). Only distinguished feature is that it has thick longitudinal edges. Urea particles are thin needle shaped particles (Fig. 1e). Salt particles look like spherical or cuboid structures (Fig. 1f). When mixed with wheat bran (in different proportions), paddy husk can be easily distinguished on the basis of characteristic structures. However at low proportions, more microscopic fields have to be observed to get a glimpse of saw dust particles.

At present, the only quantification method is described by the European Commission (EC) for protein of animal origin like fishmeal, meat and bone meal (MBM) using light microscopy (European Union 2009). Improved method suggested by Veys and Baeten (2010) is based on three elements. (1) the preparation of permanent slides with an optical adhesive preserving all morphological markers of bones necessary for accurate identification and precision counting; (2) the use of a counting grid eyepiece reticule and (3) new definitions for correction factors for the estimated portions of animal particles in the sediment. This revised quantification method was tested on feeds adulterated at different levels with bovine meat and bone meal (MBM) and fishmeal, and it proved to be effortless to apply. In this process, initially feed material is subjected with tetrachloroethylene (TCE) and the sediment (mostly bones, cartilage and minerals) is dried at in the oven. The weighed sediment is then stained with Alizarin Red solution. The sediment is gently stirred to spread it uniformly over the resin deposit and then a cover glass was immediately placed on the slide, which was directly placed for curing under an ultraviolet (UV) light source at 365nm for at least 2 min. By using this optical adhesive, it was possible to quantify the contamination of meat and bone meal and fish meal to actual added levels (Veys and Baeten 2010). The advantage over existing method is that these slides could be used as reference materials in case of disputes. With the help of feed microscopy, Haschek *et al.* (1989) detected upto 3-5% cotton seed meal in swine rations.

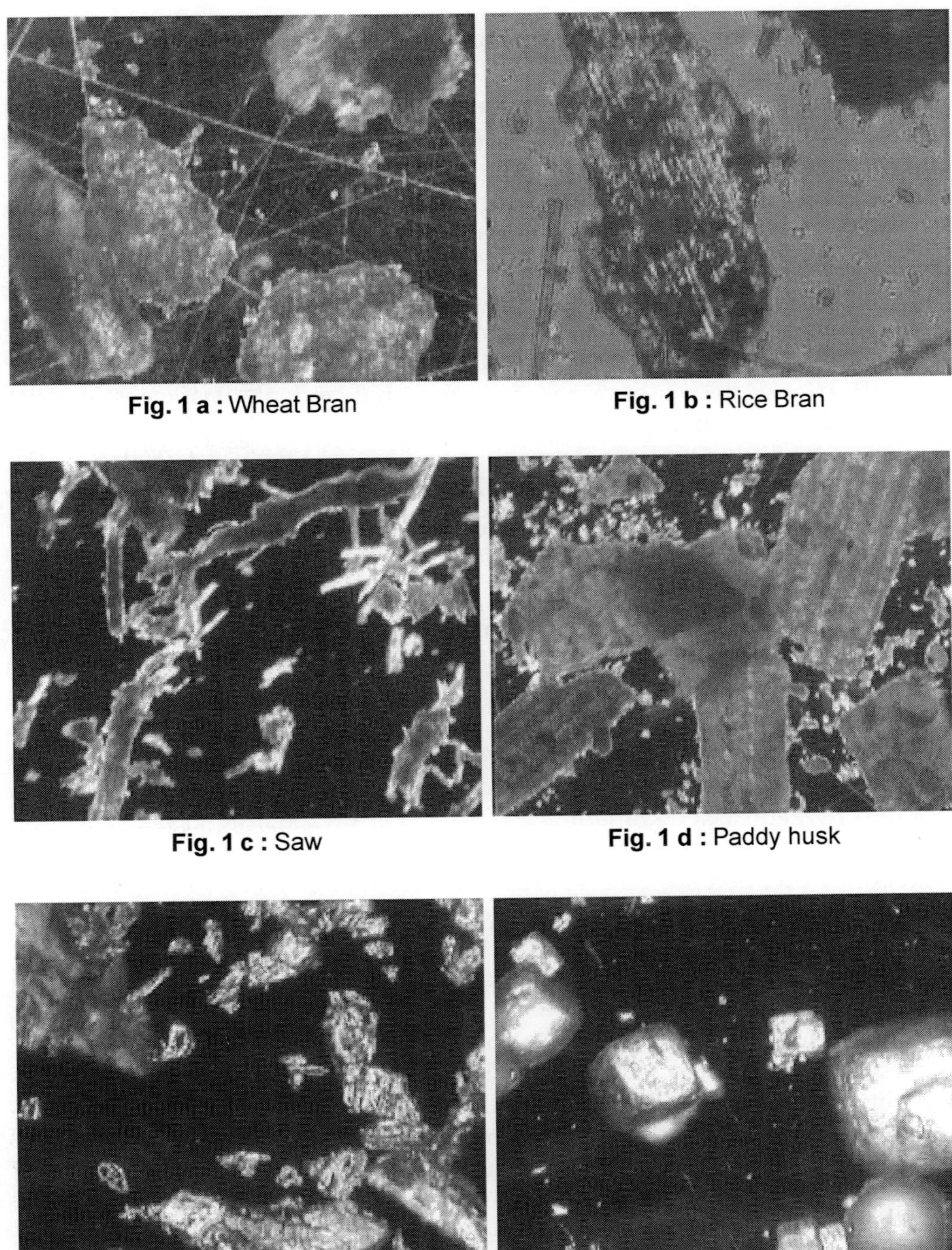

Fig. 1 a : Wheat Bran

Fig. 1 b : Rice Bran

Fig. 1 c : Saw

Fig. 1 d : Paddy husk

Fig. 1 e : Urea particles

Fig. 1 f : Salt Particles

Fig. 1 : Microphotographs of few feed stuffs and adulterants

2.3 PCR based method for identification of feed adulterants and plant proteins

A simple and rapid tubulin based polymorphism (TBP) detection by PCR method is recently used to differentiate any plant species in blends of plant origin (Cassaza *et al.,* 2011). The method relies on the presence of intron-specific DNA polymorphisms within plant β-tubulin gene family. A simple PCR reaction needs to be performed using degenerated universal primers designed on the β-tubulin exon regions flanking the intron sequences. The method involves initial processing of feed samples by reducing them to fine flour, followed by extraction of genomic DNA, quatification and quality assesment by agarose gel electrophoresis. About 15–30 ng of genomic DNA are used typically in any single PCR reaction. Based on characteristic amplification patterns obtained for each analyzed plant species, correct identification of plant is possible. Advantage of this method is that the analysis can be performed regardless of any information about the plant genome under investigation. It is easy to use, rapid in execution, reliable and reproducible (Cassaza *et al.,* 2011). All of these advantages makes the proposed method diagnostic technique with a wide range of applications in the context of feed/ food quality certification.

Bovine spongiform encephalopathy (BSE) belongs to a group of progressively degenerative neurological diseases known as transmissible spongiform encephalopathies (TSEs) associated with a variant form of Creutzfeldt-Jakob disease in humans. The TSEs are fatal diseases caused by prions (proteineous infectious particle) and are characterized by an incubation period that may range from several months to several years, depending on the host (Dragon and Arvaham, 2000). Tajima et al. (2002) suggested a method for detection of micro-contamination of feed by animal materials like meat and bone meal. Because BSE is spread through animal feed, the main strategy for preventing the establishment and spread of BSE is to prohibit the use of proteins derived from mammalian tissue in feed for ruminant animals. The PCR test for the detection of materials derived from ruminants, pigs, and chickens are developed (Tajima *et al.,* 2002) on the basis of sequences of the Art2 short interspersed repetitive element (SINE), PRE-1 SINE, and CR1 long interspersed repetitive element (LINE), respectively. The designed primers amplify the SINE or LINE from total DNA extracted of the target animals and from test feed containing commercial 'meat and bone meal (MBM)'. Detection of Art2, PRE-1, or CR1 in test feed is possible at concentrations of 0.01% MBM or less (Tajima *et al.,* 2002).

3. Importance of feed regulations

Improper procurement, manufacturing and handling of animal feed can result in the introduction of pathogens and spoilage organisms to animals and the introduction of chemical hazards such as heavy metals, pesticide residues, mycotoxins and of other contaminants which can affect the safety and suitability animal products. Therefore, proper animal feeding practices should be followed to minimize or prevent the introduction of contaminants through feed or feeding practices. There is an urgent need for development effective regulatory body to maintain quality and safety of feed. Hartog (2003) presented a quality program for Dutch animal feed Industry with a goal to produce and supply animal feeds which are safe for consumers of animal products, for the animals and for the environment. It is trustworthy for all stakeholders–the partners in the chain, the consumers and the legislators–which mean to do so demonstrably and transparently. An important part of this program is the 'good manufacturer practice (GMP)' standard animal feed, which was set up in 1992. This GMP standard contains requirements for the quality system (comparable with ISO 9002) and a number of additional generic control measures for production, trade and transport of animal feed materials focused on additives, undesirable substances and microbiological aspects. Further, it also provides provision for the integration of HACCP in the GMP standard and upstream extension of the quality assurance to all suppliers of feed ingredients. By this way the quality system of the food processing industry has been adopted in the animal feed industry. This underlines that the animal feed is part of the food chain, expressed in the slogan 'Feed for Food'. The main points of the program are food safety has a high priority worldwide, the animal feed industry, including the ingredient suppliers, is part of the food chain and responsible for the safety of its products, demonstrable and transparent quality assurance is a 'license to produce'. Further, it envisages that HACCP is a proactive approach which links the feed chain to the food chain, quality control of raw materials is a mutual concern for suppliers and the animal feed industry and trade and industry are assuming their responsibility for product safety.

3.1 Raw material sourcing

Wide ranges of raw materials are utilized by feed mills in the manufacture of animal feed. While cereals and their byproducts and oil seed cakes make up a large proportion of these raw materials. Storage times and conditions can influence quality parameters of raw materials, which, in turn, can affect feed safety. It is important, therefore, if feed quality and safety is to be assured, that only high quality raw materials must be sourced. Equally, constant monitoring and evaluation of all raw materials must be carried out to ensure that documented standards are maintained.

3.2 Transportation

Both raw materials and finished feed products of transportation, can introduce hazards that may compromise feed safety. Good, well managed stores for raw materials will not prevent the introduction of hazards if vehicles used for their transportation are not clean or have previously been used to transport hazardous materials that may contaminate the load. This applies not only to vehicular transport, but also to rail, ships, etc. Raw material importers and brokers must also carry out their own evaluation to ensure that raw materials arriving at the port are in good condition, have not been repeatedly treated with pesticides (to the extent that there are excessive pesticide residues) and have not been stored in unsatisfactory warehouses which have bird/vermin/roof leaks, *etc.*

3.3 Regulatory measures

The labeling/markings on feed bags along with existing information should also include feed does not contain unsafe additives, drugs and contaminants. There should be Hazard Analysis Critical Control Points for the production of safe animal feed as in the lines of food products. The Food Safety and Standards Authority of India (FSSAI) should also include feeds as on the lines of Food and Drug Administration, USA, for effective regulation of animal feeds.

Conclusions

Quality of feed ingredients available in retail chains is always questionable as they are subject of adulteration by unscrupulous traders. Simple microscopic techniques can be suitably applied for identification of feed materials and adulterants. A suitable regulation need to be implemented for ensuring the quality and safety of animal feeds. The concepts of 'Feed for Food' needs to be integrated with HACCP.

References

AOAC (2005). Association of analytical chemists, official methods of analysis, 17th Edition, Washington, DC, USA, pp 67-68.

Banerjee B.D., Zaidi S.S.A., Pasha S.T., Rawat D.S., Koner B. C., Hussain Q.Z. (1997) Levels of HCH Residues in Human Milk Samples from Delhi, India. *Bulletin of Environmental Contamination and Toxicology* **59:** 403-406.

Battaglia M., Cruywagen C.W., Bertuzzi T., Gallo A., Moschini M., Piva G., Masoero F. (2010). Transfer of melamine from feed to milk and from milk to cheese and whey in lactating dairy cows fed single oral doses. *Journal of Dairy Science* **93:** 5338-5347.

Casazza A.P., Gavazzi F., Mastromauro F., Gianì S., Breviario (2011). Certifying the feed to guarantee the quality of traditional food: An easy way to trace plant species in complex mixtures. *Food Chemistry* **124:** 685-691.

Down to Earth (2005). Punjab, too much limestone powder and urea: adulteration hardly a bother for feed-makers, published on June, 30.

Dragan M., Avraham R. (2000) Detection and Analysis of Animal Materials in Food and Feed. *Journal of Food Protection* **63:** 1602-1609.

European Union (2009). Regulation EC/2009/152. Commission Regulation of 27 January 2009 laying down the methods of sampling and analysis for the official control of feed. *Official Journal of European Communities* **L54:** 1-130.

Goering H.K., Van Soest P.J. (1970). Forage fiber analyses (Apparatus, reagents, procedures and some applications). ARS, *USDA Handbook* 379.

Hartog,J.D (2003)Feed for Food: HACCP in the animal feed industry. *Food Control* **14:** 95-99.

Haschek W.M, Beasley V.R, Buck W.B., Finnell J.H. (1989). Cottonseed meal (gossypol) toxicosis in a swine herd. *Journal of American Veterinary Medicine Association* **195:** 613-615.

IS 13399 (1992) *Indian Standard* : Animal feeds and feeding stuffs – determination of urea. *Bureau of Indian Standards, Manak Bhavan, 9, Bahadur Shar Zafar Marg, New Delhi – 110002,* pp 1-2.

Nalwanga R., Liti D.M., Waidbacher H., Munguti J., Zollitsch W.J. (2009). Monitoring the nutritional value of feed components for aquaculture along the supply chain – an East African case study. *Livestock Research for Rural Development* **21:** 148. http://www.lrrd.org/lrrd21/9/nalw21148.htm.

Pardíoa V.T., Waliszewskib K.N., Landína L.A., Bautista R.G. (2003). Organo-chlorine pesticide residues in cow's milk from a tropical region of Mexico. *Food Additives and Contaminants* **20:** 259-269.

Prasad K.S.N., Chhbra A. (2001). Organo pesticide residues in animal feeds and fodders. *Indian Journal of Animal Science* **71:** 1178-1180.

Rao S.B.N. Dineshkumar D., Giridhar K., Elangovan A.V., Sampath K.T. (2011) Organo-chlorine pesticide residues in feedstuffs. *Indian Veterinary Journal* **88:** 38-39.

Singh R., Kundu S.S. (2003). Quality evaluation of some animal feedstuffs available in Haryana. *Animal Nutrition and Feed Technology* **3:** 143-150.

Suchy P. Strakova E. Herzig I. Stana J. Kalusova R., Pospichalova M. (2009). Toxicological risk of melamine and cyanuric acid in food and feed. *Interdisciplinary toxicology* **2:** 55-59.

Tajima K., Enishi O., Amari M., Mitsumori M., Kajikawa H., Kurihara M.,Yanai S. Matsui H. Yasue H. Mitsuhashi T. Kawashima T., Matsumoto M. (2002). PCR Detection of DNAs of Animal Origin in Feed by Primers Based on Sequences of Short and Long Interspersed Repetitive Elements. *Bioscience Biotechnology Biochemistry* **66:** 2247-2250.

Vail T., Jones P.R., Sparkman O.D. (2008). Rapid and unambiguous identification of melamine in contaminated pet food based on mass spectrometry with four degrees of confirmation. *Journal of Analytical Toxicology* **31:** 304-312.

Van Soest P.J., Robinson J.B., Lewis B.A. (1991). Methods for dietary fiber, neutral detergent fiber, and nonstarch polysaccharides in relation to animal nutrition. *Journal of Dairy Science* **74:** 3583-3597.

Veys P., Baeten V. (2010). New approach for the quantification of processed animal proteins in feed using light microscopy. *Food additives and Contaminants* **27:** 926-934.

Waliszewskia S.M., Pardiob S.V. Waliszewskic T.,Chantiria K.K.N., Infanzona P.J.N., Ma R.R., Rivera J. (1996). Detection of some organochlorine pesticides in cow's milk. *Food Additives and Contaminants* **13:** 231-235.

Yamamoto M., Uneyama C., Toda M., Sasaki S., Morikawa K. (2008). Pet food and animal feed contaminated with melamine [Article in Japanese] *Shokuhin Eiseigaku Zasshi* **49:** 13-16. [cited by, Veys P., Baeten V. (2010). New approach for the quantification of processed animal proteins in feed using light microscopy. *Food additives and Contaminants* **27:** 926-934].

❑❑❑

Chapter 36

Fluorosis : An Endemic Toxicity, Mode of Action and Methods of Amelioration

N.K.S. Gowda, D. Rajendran, D.T. Pal, K.T. Sampath, C.S. Prasad
National Institute of Animal Nutrition and Physiology, Adugodi, Bangalore-560 030, Karnataka, India

Summary

High content of fluoride (F) in the drinking water is an endemic problem in many part of the world including India. Other source of high F includes phosphate mineral supplements and industrial emissions. Ingestion of F in excess amount and acute toxicity is rare but the continuous ingestion of small quantity both in humans and animals is common and cause chronic toxicity (Fluorosis). Almost all organs are affected but bone and teeth are the initial targets, followed by liver, kidney and thyroid. Fluoride, due to its high electronegative anionic nature complexes and displaces cations like Ca, Zn, Mn. However, this depends on the dose and extent of exposure to F. Radical property of F is the reason for its effect on lipid peroxidation and antioxidant system. Other effects in fluorosis include depressed immunity, pro-diabetic action, nervous disorders, low semen quality and mutagenesis. Defluoridation method of water using alum has been questioned due to the action of free aluminium on nervous system. Other effective methods includes use of slaked lime in water and supplementation of adequate Ca, P and Vitamin D provide some protection against F. Promising ameliorating agents include boron, antioxidants and certain plant extracts like Tamarind pulp and Moringa seeds. Conservation and preservation of surface water is the most ideal and practical method of reducing the problem of excess fluoride ingestion. Recommendation of fluoridation of water and dental care products for preventing dental caries appears to be an unsafe approach and needs a serious review.

Fluorine (F) element was first discovered in the year 1886 by Professor Henri Moissan, a Nobel Laureate (1906) from France. It is an electronegative, non-metallic halogen element with a molecular weight of 19 and atomic number of 9. It exists as a diatomic molecule with remarkably low dissociation energy and as a result it is highly reactive and has strong affinity to bind with other elements to form compounds known as fluoride. It is considered both as beneficial and harmful to man and animals. However, many studies with most sterile element environment have failed to produce F deficiency in animals. The suggested physiological functions of F are calcification of skeleton, bone cell proliferation, activation of certain enzymes like adenyl cyclase, isocitric dehydrogenase and acid/alkaline phosphatase (Swarup and Dwivedi, 1998). However, in most cases, toxicity of F is often a great concern than the deficiency as the small requirement can be easily met through water and food/feed supplements. Fluoride is widely distributed in nature as a co-constituent of metal complexes. In India, ground water in several districts of at least 22 states is reported to contain high F level (2-8ppm). Such regions are reported in states of Gujarat, Rajasthan, Bihar, Andhra Pradesh, Karnataka, Punjab, Kerala, Tamil Nadu and Jharkhand. Common source of fluoride are: high fluoride in water, industrial (cement, aluminium, brick, phosphate fertiliser factories) emission of fluoride, phosphate feed supplements and mineral mixtures, fluoride rich soils and vegetation grown on such soils (Swarup and Dwivedi, 1998). High level of F (1.5-4ppm) in drinking water in many districts of southern Rajasthan (up to 18ppm) with osteo-dental lesions have been reported (Choubisa, 2001). Aluminium smelter factories contribute fluoride to environment as evidenced by higher fluoride level in water, vegetation and prevalence of fluorosis in goats within 10 km radius (Sahoo and Ray, 2004).

In India, dental fluorosis has been reported in humans ingesting 0.5 to 1.0 ppm F in drinking water (Ray *et al.,* 1981), while at concentrations of 3.4 to 3.8 ppm, 100% dental fluorosis has been recorded (Subbareddy *et al.,* 1985). Deformities such as crippling, kyphosis, and genu varum were observed most frequently in higher age groups (>40 years) at a F concentration of 2.8 ppm in drinking water or higher at fluoride affected areas of Rajasthan. None of the fluorotic subjects showed evidence of goitre (thyroidism) or genu valgum syndrome. The occurrence of fluorosis can vary widely among different locations having almost the same F concentrations in the drinking water and can be affected by a number of other factors such as nutritional status, climate, individual susceptibility and biological response, duration of F exposure, and dissolved salts in drinking waters. Beside these factors, the difference in prevalence of fluorosis in the villages, although having almost the same F levels, appears mostly due to differences in the frequency of fluoride intake (Choubisa, 2001).

In Berhait and Sahibganj district of Jharkhand state, India where people were chromically exposed to as high as upto 29 ppm of F through drinking water, had shown lesions in teeth, deformities of bone, spine and exostocis in children and adult (Nayak *et al.,* 2009). Prevalence of dental and skeletal fluorosis in some villages of Gulbarga district in Karnataka is reported where the water F level ranged from 0.5-12.6 ppm (Shivashankara *et al.,* 2000). Recent study has indicated that about 14% of water samples in Karnataka are fluorotic in nature (>1.5ppm, range 0.4-4.0 ppm, Author's unpublished data).

1. Mode of action

Fluoride anions can easily cross cell membrane of soft tissue and alter biochemical functions. Excessive F in the diet can cause adverse health effects. Release of free radicals, lipid peroxidation and change in antioxidant defence mechanism play a great role in F toxicity. Chronic toxicity of F is called as fluorosis, which is manifested mainly by dental and skeletal lesions in humans and animals, especially in geographical locations with elevated F levels in natural resources and industrial emissions. Young animals are more susceptible to F toxicity. Poultry are the most tolerant animals. The fluoride level in plasma, urine and bone of cattle in the vicinity of aluminium and fertiliser units were higher and showed change in haemogram as compared to cattle in non-industrial areas (Senthil kumar and Aravindakshan, 2011). The organ and biochemical changes due to fluoride exposure depends on factors like duration of exposure, age and nutritional status of animals. A threefold increase in bone fluoride content does not cause a distinct change in metabolism, mineral density and mechanical resistance of bones to fluoride exposed adult male Wistar rats, more over no significant differences were found in alkaline phosphatase activity, calcium and magnesium concentration in serum, and hydroxyproline concentration in urine between control and exposed animals (Urbañska *et al.*, 2001). Liver oxidative and the antioxidant systems are altered in fluoride toxicity. Oxidative damage from oxidative stress therefore appears to be an important pathway for fluoride-induced hepatotoxicity (Guo *et al.*, 2003). Fluoride content of soft tissue and organs of rat increased in a dose and time-dependent manner. Animals receiving the higher dose of sodium fluoride (25 mg/L) show the increase about two-fold in serum, seven-fold in liver and kidney, nine-fold in brain, and twelve-fold in testes after 12 weeks of exposure. Urinary fluoride is also found increased from the beginning of exposure in a dose-dependent manner (Inkielewicz and Krechniak, 2003).

Increased serum transaminase activity with reduced serum protein was observed in rats orally treated with 10, 20 and 30 mg/kg sodium fluoride for 90 days (Qujeq *et al.*, 2002). Oral administration of F (9 mg/kg body weight) alone or in conjunction with aluminium sulfate(150 mg/kg body weight) to goats for 30 days period showed a significant decline in plasma glucose and protein levels (Kant and Shrivastava, 2009). Fluoride ingestion @ 60mg/kg diet for 90 days period caused decline in serum calcium and increase in alkaline phosphatase activity in buffaloes (Madan *et al.*, 2009). Decline in serum calcium levels in fluoride supplementation is attributed to binding of F with calcium resulting in lowered gut absorption and enhanced urinary excretion of calcium (Bhati *et al.*, 2007). This is supported by the report that urinary fluoride level is an indicator of fluoride exposure of animals in industrial areas (Garg *et al.*, 1998).

There is much evidence that superoxide free radicals and lipid peroxidation play an important role in fluorosis (Shivarajashankara *et al.*, 2001). Superoxide radicals are highly reactive and may lead to chemical modification and impairment of proteins, lipids, carbohydrates, and nucleotides in living cells (Chinoy, 2002). Increased lipid peroxidation with increase in malandialdehyde levels, increased glutathione peroxidase activity and reduced glutathione levels were observed in rats supplemented with 30 and 100 ppm of fluoride in water (Shivashankara *et al.*, 2011). Similarly, increased lipid peroxidation with free radical mediated oxidative stress and elevated antioxidant activity in blood has been recorded in children exposed to fluoride toxicity in endemic areas (Shivashankara *et al.*, 2011). The antioxidant enzyme (superoxide dismutase), ceruloplasmin and immune status were affected in rats at higher levels of fluoride ingestion (30 and 60ppm in water), beyond 6 months of period. The serum glucose level was consistently higher in all the fluoride supplemented groups compared to control. The content of fluoride in liver, bone and teeth was proportionately increased with the level of ingestion. Further, liver, spleen and kidney showed degenerative changes at 30 and 60 ppm of fluoride level after 3 months of ingestion (Gowda *et al.*, 2011). Inhibition of enzymes in glycolytic pathway (hexokinase, enolase, pyruvate kinase) by fluoride is one of the reasons for increased glucose in blood in fluorosis (Adamek *et al.*, 2005). Of late, there is a growing evidence to suggest a relationship between fluorosis and glucose intolerance due to the lower insulin secretion and mRNA expression in pancreatic beta cells with elevated glucose levels (Eliud *et al.*, 2009).

Prolonged exposure to fluoride is likely to damage male reproductive organs and semen could be another way of fluoride expulsion from the male body. Rats given 84 mg NaF/kg, had plasma fluoride concentrations as high as 12 ppm, but testicular fluoride concentration in most cases was only 10-20% of that in the plasma (Skare *et al.*, 1986). A certain concentration gradient is maintained by the blood-testis barrier, thus keeping the fluoride concentration lower in the testis than in the plasma. This permeability barrier may be crossed during prolonged exposure to fluoride, causing spermatogenic damage resulting in cessation of spermatogenesis (Susheela and Kumar, 1991). *In vitro* treatment of human spermatozoa with 250 mM sodium fluoride for 20 min showed altered lysosomal enzyme activity and glutathione levels with morphological anomalies (Chinoy and Narayana, 1994). Sodium fluoride at concentrations of 20, 100, 200 μmol/L, and 0.1 mol/L caused a significant decrease in the motility of spermatozoa and the number of intact acrosomes in ram and lower concentrations of fluoride significantly decreased the activity of acid phosphatase, lactate dehydrogenase, and gamma glutamyl transferase in comparison with the control (Zakrzewska *et al.*, 2002). Fluoride has been shown to be mutagenic, cause chromosome damage and interfere with the enzymes involved with DNA repair in a variety of cell and tissue studies. Studies have also found a correlation between fluoride exposure and chromosome damage in humans (Joseph and Gadhia, 2000). The neurotoxic changes in the brain of rabbits indicate damage to the neurones and neuroglial cells due to fluorosis and suggest direct action of fluoride upon the nervous tissue, which is responsible for paralysis, seizure, tremors, and sensory deficits and is indicative of brain dysfunction in experimental fluorosis (Shashi, 2003).

Dietary fluoride levels of 130 and 190 ppm in dairy calves for a period of 5 months declined the cell mediated immune response (Kapoor and Prasad, 1994). Similar observation of suppressed immunity in rats supplemented F at 30 and 60 ppm in water has been recorded (Gowda *et al.*, 2011). Sodium fluoride treated mice showed a 35% decrease in body weight, a 75% decrease in plasma free T4, and reduction in the cerebellar and cerebral protein concentrations by 27% and 17%, respectively causing neurotoxicity, cell damage and even cell death (Trabelsi *et al.*, 2001). Reduced thyroid activity due to fluoride could be attributed to inhibition of enzyme proteinase involved in formation of T_3 and T_4 in thyroid gland (Swarup and Dwivedi, 2002), and hence goitre is more common in populations of fluorotic areas.

2. Preventive and ameliorative measures

Regular monitoring the level of F in water, feed supplements, and vegetation surrounding metal industries is important. Defluorinated phosphate supplements are to be used in mineral mixture formulation. Slaked lime treatment of water (500-1000 mg/kg), supplementation of adequate calcium and phosphorus in diet offers some protection against excessive F ingestion. The combined use of cake alum and a polymeric anionic flocculent (PAF) in drinking water has reduced up to 99% arsenic and 77% fluoride, respectively through sedimentation (Piñón-Miramontes *et al.*, 2003). But when complexed with aluminium, fluoride interferes with G-proteins and such interactions give aluminium-fluoride complexes, the potential to interfere with many hormonal and some neurochemical signals (Li, 2003). Hence, defluoridation of drinking water with alum is often questioned and needs rethinking. The recommended safety limits of F are 1-1.5ppm in drinking water and 4-6ppm in dietary dry matter. The reported upper tolerance levels of F ranges between 30-100 ppm for cattle, 50-60 ppm for sheep, 60 ppm for horses and 70 ppm for swine (dry matter basis). Fluoride ingestion of 0.6 ppm in water is useful for bone and teeth heath and development and WHO standards permits only 1.5 ppm F in drinking water as a safety limit (WHO,

2011). However, clinical significance of low levels of F ingestion with adequate calcium and vitamin D is known to strengthen the bones. Ekambaram and Paul (2002), observed that supplementation of calcium carbonate (50m/kg) to Weister rats along with drinking water containing 500 ppm of sodium fluoride for 60 days decrease the fluoride toxicity. Their study also showed that short term fluoride exposure is reversible. Boron and aluminium sulfate alleviate F toxicity but the safety against free aluminium ions in water is still a matter of concern. Supplementation of Boron (140 ppm) to 60 ppm of F containing diet of buffaloes for 90 days showed partial amelioration against adverse effects of F (Bharti *et al.*, 2008). Use of cationic silicated binders appears to covalently bind anionic F and need to be tested for efficacy.

Ascorbic acid, calcium and vitamin E administration alone or in combination is found to reverse sodium fluoride toxicity in mice and ascorbic acid being the most beneficial in bringing about pronounced recovery (Chinoy and Memom, 2001). Extract of polyphenolic flavinoid rich *Primula heterochroma* plant, native to some regions in Iran has shown moderate protective action against fluorosis (Alinezhad *et al.*, 2011). Tamarind intake led to significant increase ($P<0.001$) in the excretion of fluoride in 24 h urine (4.8 ± 0.22 mg/day) as compared to excretion on control (3.5 ± 0.22 mg/day) diet (Khandare *et al.*, 2002). This is supported by the report that supplementation of aqueous extracts of either *Tamarindus indica* fruit pulp (100 mg/kg body weight) or *Moringa oleifera* seeds (50mg/kg body weight) to rabbits along with drinking water containing 90 ppm of F showed some protective effect (Ranjan *et al.*, 2009), which could be due to high calcium content in tamarind pulp or presence of cationic polyelectrolyte and/or presence of tartaric acid resulting in alkaline urine that promote excretion of F. These findings indicate the possibility of using such traditional food items in the diet for their supportive role in ameliorating fluorosis.

Conclusions

On perusal of many studies, it can be recommended that less than 1.5 ppm F in drinking water or 4-6 ppm F in dietary dry matter appears to be safe for different categories of livestock. Much variation in biological effects of F, particularly on biochemical parameters could be attributed to difference in level of F used in studies, duration of exposure and age/category of animals used. It can be conclusively ascertained that more often F is a cumulative toxin with a specific affinity to bone, teeth and biochemical functions of glucose and thyroid metabolism. Other consequential effects on antioxidant, immune and nervous systems appear to be the secondary actions. Fluoride being a strong anion, while depositing in organs, there is a possibility of it replacing the cations (Ca, Cu, Zn), however, this depends on the dose of F ingested and duration of exposure. Defluoridation of water through aluminium sulphate (alum) suggested and employed elsewhere needs to be reviewed as presence of aluminium could pose much greater hazard than the F alone. Similarly, the fluoridation of drinking water and dental care products recommended many years back as a measure to prevent dental caries need to be reviewed. The biochemical essentiality of F is a known fact, but the need of dietary supplementation is a question. Looking into the natural level of F in water and food/feed supplements, there is unlikely need to supplement F to humans and animals. On the other hand, efforts must focus on reducing the F level in water and mineral supplements to safer limits. Future research and application attempts lies in the use of water purification techniques with ion-exchange principles, competitive absorption inhibitors or alleviators like boron, lime, silicated binders and ameliorating agents like antioxidants, adequate mineral supplements particularly calcium and phosphorus. The prospects and consequences of these technical interventions need to be cautiously followed and proved for their efficacy, economics, biosafety and social acceptability. The most simple and natural approach is to conserve the surface water (lakes, river, rain water) and preserve the layers of earth crust (avoid deep bore wells, deep mining). Technocrats, policy makers and administrators should make a serious thinking on these issues to adopt a scientific and practical approach; otherwise, the present endemic problem will become epidemic and later pandemic.

References

Adamek E., Pawlowska-Goral K., Bober K. (2005). *In vitro* and *in vivo* effects of fluoride ions on enzyme activity. *Annales Academiae Medicae Stetinensis* **51:** 69-85.

Alinezhad H., Mahboobehzare Z., Nabavi S.F., Naqinezhad A., Nabavi S.M. (2011). Assessing the protective effect of *Primula heterochroma* stapf extracts against sodium fluoride-induced hemolysis in rat erythrocytes. *Fluoride* **44:** 238-242.

Bharti V.K., Gupta M., Lall D. (2008). Ameliorative effects of boron on serum profile in buffalo (*Bubalis bubalis*) fed high fluoride ration. *Tropical Animal Health and Production* **40:** 111-116.

Bhati V.K., Gupta M., Lall D., Balamurugan T.C., Imam S. (2007). Effect of boron on urinary and fecal excretions of minerals in buffalo calves fed high fluoride ration. *Animal Nutrition and Feed Technology* **7:** 125-130.

Chinoy N. J. Memon M. R. (2001). Bene?cial effects of some vitamins and calcium on ?uoride and aluminium toxicity on gastrocnemius muscle and liver of male mice. *Fluoride* **34:** 21-33.

Chinoy N.C., Narayana M.V. (1994). *In vitro* fluoride toxicity in human spermatozoa. *Reproductive Toxicology* **8:** 155-159.

Chinoy N.J. (2002). Studies on fluoride, aluminium and arsenic toxicity in mammals and amelioration by some antidotes In: *Modern Trends in Environmental Biology* (G. Tripathi, ed.). New Delhi: CBS Publishers and Distributors, pp 164-193.

Choubisa S.L. (2001). Endemic fluorosis in southern Rajasthan, India. *Fluoride* **34:** 61-70.

Ekambaram P., Paul V. (2002). Modulation of fluoride toxicity in rats by calcium carbonate and by withdrawl of fluoride exposure. *Pharmacology and Toxicology* **90:** 53-58.

Eliud A., Garcia-Montalvo., Reyes-Perez. H., Luz M. Del Razo. (2009). Fluoride exposure impairs glucose tolerance via decreased insulin expression and oxidative stress. *Toxicology* **263:** 75-83.

Garg M.R., Bhanderi B.M., Sherasia P.L. (1998). Interrelationships between dietary fluorine, blood serum and urinary fluorine in adult ruminants. *Indian Journal of Animal Nutrition* **15:** 78-82.

Guo X., Sun G., Sun Y. (2003). Oxidative stress from fluoride-induced hepatotoxicity in rats. *Fluoride* **36:** 25-29.

Inkielewicz I., Krechniak J. (2003). Fluoride content in soft tissues and urine of rats exposed to sodium fluoride in drinking water. *Fluoride* **36:** 263-266.

Joseph S., Gadhia P.K. (2000). Sister chromatid exchange frequency and chromosome aberrations in residents of fluoride endemic regions of South Gujarat. *Fluoride* **33:** 154-158.

Kant V., Shrivastava A.K. (2009). Alterations in biochemical parameters during subacute toxicity of fluoride alone and in conjunction with aluminium sulfate in goats. *Biological Trace Element Research* **130:** 20-30.

Kapoor T., Prasad T. (1994). Effect of fluorine ingestion on cell-mediated immune response in calves. *Fluoride* **27:** 3-6.

Khandare A.L., Rao G.S., Lakshmaiah N. (2002). Effects of tamarind ingestion on fluoride excretion in humans. *European Journal of Clinical Nutrition* **56:** 82-85.

Li L. (2003). The biochemistry and physiology of metallic fluoride: action, mechanism, and implications. *Critical Reviews of Oral Biology and Medicine* **14:** 100-114.

Madan J., Puri J.P., Singh J.K. (2009). Growth, feed efficiency and blood profile of buffalo calves consuming high levels of fluoride. *Tropical Animal Health and Production* **41:** 295-298.

Nayak B., Roy M.M., Das B., Pal A., Sengupta M.K., De S.P., Chakraborti D. (2009). Health effects of ground water fluoride contamination. *Clinical Toxicology* **47:** 292-295.

Piñón-Miramontes M., Bautista-Margulis R.G., Pérez-Hernández A. (2003). Removal of arsenic and fluoride from drinking water with cake alum and a polymeric anionic flocculent. *Fluoride,* **36:** 122-128.

Qujeq D., Laghaie B., Gholipour A., Solimani N., Hassenzadeh S. (2002). Effects of sodium fluoride on total serum protein levels and transaminase activity in rats. *Biomedicine and Pharmacotheraphy* **56:** 169-172.

Ranjan R., Swarup D., Patra R.C., Chandra V. (2009). *Tamarindus indica* L. and *Moringa olifera* M. extract administration ameliorates fluoride toxicity in rabbits. *Indian Journal of Experimental Biology* **47:** 900-905.

Ray S.K., Ghosh S., Nagchauduri J, Tiwari I.C., Kaur P. (1981). Prevalence of fluorosis in rural community near Varanasi. *Fluoride* **14:** 86-90.

Sahoo N., Ray S.K. (2004). Fluorosis in goats near an aluminium smelter plant in Orissa. *Indian Journal of Animal Sciences* **74:** 48-50.

Senthil Kumar P., Aravindakshan C.M. (2011). Effects of industrial fluoride pollution on haemogram of cattle. *Indian Veterinary Journal* **88:** 47-49.

Shashi A. (2003). Histopathological investigation of fluoride- induced neurotoxicity in rabbits. *Fluoride* **36:** 95-105.

Shivarajashankara Y.M., Shivashankara A.R., Gopalakrishna P.B., Rao S.H. (2001). Effect of fluoride intoxication on lipid peroxidation and antioxidant systems in rats. *Fluoride* **34:** 108-113.

Shivashankara A.R., Shivashankara Y.M., Rao H.S., Bhat G.P. (2000). Clinical and biochemical study of chronic fluoride toxicity in children of kheru thanda of Gulbarga district, Karnataka, India. *Fluoride* **33:** 66-73.

Shivashankara Y.M., Shivashankara A.R., Rao H.S., Bhat G.P. 2011. Oxidative stress in children with endemic skeletal fluorosis. *Fluoride* **34:** 103-107.

Skare J.K., Schrotel K.R., Nixon G.A. (1986). Lack of DNA-Strand breaks in rat testicular cells after *in vivo* treatment with sodium fluoride. *Mutation Research* **170:** 85-92.

Subbareddy V.V., Tiwari A. (1985). Enamal mottling at different levels of fluoride in drinking water: In endemic area. *Journal of Indian Dental Association* **57:** 205-212.

Susheela A.K., Kumar A. (1991). A study of the effect of high concentrations of fluoride on the reproductive organs of male rabbits, using light and scanning electron microscopy. *Journal of Reproduction Fertility* **92:** 353-360.

Swarup D., Dwivedi S.K. (1998). Research effects of pollution on livestock. *Indian Journal of Animal Sciences* **68:** 814-824.

Swarup D., Dwivedi S.K. (2002). Fluorine pollution and fluorosis. In: Environmental pollution and effects of lead and fluoride on animal heatlh (D. Swarup and S.K. Dwivedi, eds). Indian Council of Agricultural Research, New Delhi, India, pp 68-106.

Trabelsi M., Guermazi F., Zeghal N. (2001). Effect of fluoride on thyroid function and cerebellar development in mice. *Fluoride* **34:** 165-173.

Urbañska B., Czarnowski W., Krechniak J., Inkielewicz I., Stolarska K. (2001). Skeletal metabolism and bone mineral density in fluoride-exposed rats. *Fluoride* **34:** 95-102.

World Health Organisation. (2011). Guidelines for drinking water. 4th edition.

Zakrzewska H., Uda³a J., Blaszczyk B. (2002). *In vitro* influence of sodium fluoride on ram semen quality and enzyme activities. *Fluoride* **35:** 153-160.

❑❑❑

Index

A

B

C

D

E

H

I

K

L

M

N

O

P

Q

R

S

T

U

□□□

About the Editors

Dr K.T. Sampath, Ph.D (Animal Nutrition) is former Director of National Institute of Animal Nutrition and Physiology (NIANP), Bangalore. He has served as research Scientist under Indian Council of Agricultural Research (ICAR) in various capacities at ICAR Research for NEH region, Barapani, National Dairy Research Institute and at NIANP, Bangalore. His research works are mainly in the areas of feed and fodder resources, improvement of nutritive value of poor quality roughages, bypass nutrients, feed quality and safety and manipulation of rumen microbes for improving the digestibility of fiber. He is recipient of ICAR Team Research award, Hari Om Trust Award, Fakhruddin Ali Ahmed award and CLFMA Award. He is fellows of Indian Dairy Association and National Academy of Veterinary Sciences and is associated with many policy making bodies. He has served as President of Animal Nutrition Society of India for two terms.

Dr Jyotirmoy Ghosh, Senior Scientist, National Institute of Animal Nutrition and Physiology a graduate (BVSc & AH) of College of Veterinary and Animal Sciences, Bidhan Chandra Krishi Viswa Vidhyalaya, Nadia, West Bengal, Master of Veterinary Sciences and PhD in Veterinary Gynaecology and Reproduction from Indian Veterinary Research Institute, Bareilly, UP. He was a national merit scholarship holder during graduation, recipient of Junior and Senior Research Fellows during post graduation and doctoral studies. During his 12 years long service he has many publications in peer reviewed international and national journals. He has conducted and associated with many training courses on various aspects of reproduction for the middle level scientists, university teaching faculties and veterinary officers. He has guided many students reviewed research and review articles for Indian and foreign journals. He has been awarded for outstanding team research by Indian Council of Agricultural Research and has been involved in technology transfer and contract research. His research interest is centered on ovarian and uterine biology especifically identification of pregnancy marker in large ruminants, uterine antioxidant mechanism and development of marker for mineral deficiency in animals. He has been the recipient of overseas fellowship from Department of Biotechnology, Government of India, under Niche areas of Biotechnology for one year during which he visited Center for Regenerative Biology, University of Connecticut, USA for learning stem cell research.

Dr. Raghavendra Bhatta, Senior Scientist, National Institute of Animal Nutrition and Physiology, Bangalore obtained graduation (BVSc & AH), Master of Veterinary Science and PhD in Animal Nutrition from University of Agricultural Sciences, Bangalore. He was recipient of ICAR Junior Research Fellowship during MVSc and CSIR, Senior Research Fellowship during PhD and awarded University Gold Medal both in master and doctorate degree. He has been awarded the prestigious Japan Society for the Promotion of Science (JSPS) fellowship for post doctoral studies at the National Institute of Livestock and Grassland Science, Japan where he worked on estimation and regulation of methane emission from ruminants for two years. He obtained 3 months training on mitigation strategies for methane production from livestock at United States Department of Agriculture Laboratory, Texas, USA, under National Agricultural Innovative Project. He has worked at the Central Sheep and Wool Research Institute, Avikanagar for 10 years before moving to NIANP, Bangalore. He has more than 18 years of research experience in the field of ruminant nutrition with specialization in manipulation of rumen fermentation using natural tannins, methane estimation and mitigation strategies. He is a member of the editorial board of the Asian Australasian Journal of Animal Science since 2003 and sectional editor of Research Journal of Dairy Science and Research Journal of Animal science. He has more than 60 research articles in journals of national and international repute, presented invited papers in various national and international conferences and chaired a technical sessions at Busan, South Korea in 2006.